THE COMPLETE & UP-TO-DATE

CARB
BOOK

THE COMPLETE & UP-TO-DATE

CARB

BOOK

*A Guide to Carb, Calorie,
Fiber, and Sugar Content*

Karen J. Bellerson

AVERY
a member of Penguin Group (USA) Inc.
NEW YORK

AVERY
Published by the Penguin Group
Penguin Group (USA) Inc., 375 Hudson Street, New York, New York 10014, USA ❖ Penguin Group (Canada),
90 Eglinton Avenue East, Suite 700, Toronto, Ontario M4P 2Y3, Canada (a division of Pearson Penguin Canada Inc.) ❖
Penguin Books Ltd, 80 Strand, London WC2R 0RL, England ❖ Penguin Ireland, 25 St Stephen's Green, Dublin 2,
Ireland (a division of Penguin Books Ltd) ❖ Penguin Group (Australia), 250 Camberwell Road, Camberwell,
Victoria 3124, Australia (a division of Pearson Australia Group Pty Ltd) ❖ Penguin Books India Pvt Ltd, 11 Community
Centre, Panchsheel Park, New Delhi–110 017, India ❖ Penguin Group (NZ), Cnr Airborne and Rosedale Roads, Albany,
Auckland 1310, New Zealand (a division of Pearson New Zealand Ltd) ❖ Penguin Books (South Africa) (Pty) Ltd,
24 Sturdee Avenue, Rosebank, Johannesburg 2196, South Africa

Penguin Books Ltd, Registered Offices: 80 Strand, London WC2R 0RL, England

Most Avery books are available at special quantity discounts for bulk purchase for sales promotions, premiums,
fund-raising, and educational needs. Special books or book excerpts also can be created to fit specific needs.
For details, write Penguin Group (USA) Inc. Special Markets, 375 Hudson Street, New York, NY 10014.

ISBN 1-58333-243-X

Printed in the United States of America
1   3   5   7   9   10   8   6   4   2

While the author has made every effort to provide accurate telephone numbers and Internet addresses at the time of
publication, neither the publisher nor the author assumes any responsibility for errors, or for changes that occur after
publication. Further, the publisher does not have any control over and does not assume any responsibility for author or
third-party websites or their content.

Neither the publisher nor the author is engaged in rendering professional advice or services to the individual reader.
The ideas, procedures, and suggestions contained in this book are not intended as a substitute for consulting with your
physician. All matters regarding your health require medical supervision. Neither the author nor the publisher shall be
liable or responsible for any loss or damage allegedly arising from any information or suggestion in this book.

For Brandon Clark and Kaitlyn Grace.
You bring priceless joy to my life
and you are loved and adored by your Grams.

Contents

Acknowledgments

As always, my appreciation goes to those food manufacturers who make nutritional information about their products available and who have listened to consumers' requests for tastier healthful food choices.

For all of you who take the time to write me (whether to ask questions, make comments, or offer suggestions), I want you to know that your letters are of great help to me. Thank you very much for allowing me to play a small part in your endeavors to pursue a healthier, nutritionally sound lifestyle.

Preface

Low-carbohydrate diets are not new phenomena. And, contrary to what many may believe, they were not the brainchild of Dr. Atkins. The low-carbohydrate diet has been around for many years, with such names as the Mayo Clinic Diet (popular in the 1960s) and many more. What is new, however, is the wider acceptance of watching one's carbohydrate intake as a viable way of losing and controlling one's weight.

Now, with The Complete & Up-to-Date Carb Book, *the countless people on low-carb and healthy-carb diets have a tool to use in their quest for a healthy lifestyle. With this book, I bring to you the most comprehensive and timely nutritional data available with the hope that I can educate not only you but myself as well. By this I mean that the constantly changing food industry keeps me on my toes with its ingenuity in manufacturing new food products. It is an endless challenge, which I gladly accept, to keep up with the extraordinary abundance of food products making their debut on our grocery shelves.*

Many food manufacturers, along with nutritional watchdogs such as the Center for Science in the Public Interest, the National Cancer Institute, the American Heart Association, and the publishers of numerous nutrition and health newsletters, take our nutritional habits very seriously. They persevere in keeping the public aware of what we eat and how it affects all aspects of our lives. As much as I agree with so many of the recommendations from these sources, there is one that is, sadly, missing from most of the health literature published in this country. I am referring to the proven fact that healthful eating habits have benefits beyond just sustained physical well-being and involve more than just what we eat. I thought you might like to see the following recommendations, found in published dietary guidelines from some other countries, that reinforce this fact.

- *Britain's number-one dietary guideline is: Enjoy your food.*
- *Japanese dietary advice includes: Avoid too much salt and, furthermore, happy eating makes for happy family life. Sit down and eat together and talk. Treasure family taste and home cooking.*
- *The Norwegian government tells its people: Food and joy equal health.*
- *Vietnam advocates preparing a healthy family meal that is delicious and serving it "with affection."*

As charming as the above advice is, it also makes perfect sense. Why? As you will find, following it often leads to a welcome bonus of more harmony within the family circle. And those of you who have teenagers may very well enjoy a double bonus by following any of these guidelines. Research strongly indicates that teenagers who eat with adult family members an average of five times a week tend to be more mentally alert, more motivated to do well in school, and less likely to use drugs or experience depression than those who eat with their parent/parents only three times a week or less.

As you read this book and plan your meals, keep in mind that it is your total diet that counts, not the nutrient content of a single food. Educating yourself in what nutrients are in the foods you eat will enable you to make wise choices and keep your eating habits balanced and in moderation to make room for all your favorite foods. Remember, too, that small, gradual changes can add up to lifelong eating habits. Choose foods that fit in with your personal tastes and preferences, balancing good nutrition, variety, and great taste! Also, keep in mind that it is important for you to know that any calories eaten beyond what your body burns will be stored as fat.

Bottom line? What is most important is that you do both what is healthy and what works for you. Once again, I wish you wellness, I wish you happiness, and I wish all of us peace.

Until next time,

Introduction

All carbohydrates are not created equal. There are the complex/natural carbohydrates, and then there are the simple/refined carbohydrates. Your best and healthiest choices for carbohydrates should be from foods that are complex/natural. These are carbohydrates in which hundreds and/or thousands of sugar units are linked together in one single molecule. Complex carbohydrates fall into two separate groups: low fiber and high fiber. High-fiber vegetables, beans, and legumes are the best choices for our nutritional needs. Lower-fiber food examples are tomato, squash, rice, bread, potatoes, cereals, and grains.

Simple/refined carbohydrates are one, two, or three units of sugar linked together in single molecules. These carbohydrates break down easily in the stomach and intestines to enter the bloodstream quickly. This causes a rise in glucose levels, and the process slows down weight loss. So, simple/refined carbohydrates should be chosen less often than the more complex carbohydrate foods. Simple carbohydrates are almost always detected by their sweet taste (e.g., syrup, processed foods, fruit juice, candy, dried fruit, cookies, pastry, honey, ice cream, jam, and fresh fruits).

As you look at nutritional labels and try to determine the health value of the foods you are eating, it will be helpful to know that whether the carbohydrate is complex or simple, each gram of carbohydrate equals 4 calories. Each fat gram equals 9 calories, each gram of protein equals 4 calories, and a gram of sugar alcohols equals 2 calories.

THE GLYCEMIC INDEX

The Glycemic Index is a rating system that ranks foods according to their effect on the level of glucose in the blood. It can help you choose which foods fall into the desirable category of complex/unrefined sources of carbohydrates and help you avoid simple/refined carbohydrate sources. It was originally developed to help diabetics with their food choices and is also a great tool for those who are watching their carbohydrate consumption or trying to lose weight.

The foods you will find listed in the Glycemic Index were tested and ranked according to their effect on the blood glucose levels two to three hours after they were consumed. Those foods that caused a rapid and marked rise in blood sugar levels were given higher index numbers. Those foods that had less effect on blood sugar were given lower index numbers. The index is based on a scale of 0 to 150. A low score is within the range of 0 to 35, a medium score is within the range of 36 to 70, a high score is from 71 to 100, and a very high score is any number over 100. You can find a complete listing of foods ranked by the Glycemic Index at **www.glycemicindex.com**.

NET CARBOHYDRATES

When you count up the number of carbs in your food, you get a reward for those carbs that contain fiber. Fiber—at least most fiber—and sugar alcohols do not affect blood sugars. Therefore, you can subtract the total amount of fiber (and in some cases sugar alcohols) from the amount of carbohydrates in any food to get a new "net carb," or low-impact carb, content. The concept of net carbs is somewhat controversial. So far, listings for net carbs appear only on the labels of "diet" food products. However, that may very well change in the near future! In the meantime: When you see fiber listed on the nutritional label of your chosen food product, deduct it from the total amount of carbohydrates shown. This gives you a "net carb" content.

SUGAR ALCOHOLS

Sugar alcohols are sweeteners, and they are a type of carbohydrate found in some sweetened foods. On food labels, sugar alcohols are sometimes called sorbitol, xylitol, maltitol, mannitol, erythritol, hydrogenated starch hydrolysates, and isomalt. Since it appears that they have no effect on blood sugars, they, like fiber, can be subtracted from the total amount of carbohydrates shown to be in foods. This, as noted above, will give you a net carb total. You will not find a column for sugar alcohols in this book. Since it is a nutrient not mandatory to list on the nutritional food label, very few manufacturers spend the money it takes to analyze its content in their products. Furthermore, grams of sugar alcohols are required on the label only when a claim is made about sugar alcohols or sugars on the packaging. On some diet-food packaging, you may find a sugar alcohol content listed when it is present. If there are a number of carbohydrates listed on a food label but the sugar is either not listed or listed as 0, you can, more often than not, rest assured that the sweetener used in the product is a sugar alcohol.

Your copy of *The Complete & Up-to-Date Carb Book* will be a valuable companion as you take control of your eating habits. You will discover that by adjusting the foods you choose to eat, you will reap many rewards—rewards such as more energy, better sleep, more control over your weight, and perhaps most important, vibrant health and a more satisfying quality of life as a whole!

How to Use This Book

This is a well-researched, in-depth, and comprehensive nutritional guide. As you shop for and prepare your new food choices, it will be a valuable source of information for your healthy eating lifestyle. Although extreme care has been taken in recording the data in this book, you may come across occasional discrepancies between the information here and the nutritional data on product labels or other sources of nutritional information. There are a number of possible reasons for this.

First, manufacturers are given a little flexibility, so they may round off their data and still be in accordance with governmental regulations on product labeling. If a certain product contains 2.3 grams of carbohydrates, for example, the manufacturer may list the carbohydrate content as 2 grams, dropping the .3. The same is done with data on calories and the rest of the nutrient contents of each food product. For example, if a product serving has 134 calories, the manufacturer may list the calorie content as either 130 or 135.

Second, when I gathered data from product labels and compared this with data I received directly from manufacturers, there was, at times, a difference between the two because the labels listed the nutritional data of old product formulas while the manufacturer provided up-to-date information reflecting a change in the formulas. In these cases, the book gives the more recent data obtained directly from the manufacturer. Also, product serving sizes may change and, in turn, alter the nutritional data.

When comparing products, be sure that you are comparing them in the same serving size—that is, a quarter-cup of one product against a quarter-cup of another. Other discrepancies may be due to differences in the analytical methods and sampling techniques used by various food manufacturers.

As you can see, data in this book are listed in six columns. The first column contains each food product. "Amount" means the serving size of food served or used in a recipe. Remember that any deviation in serving size will mean a change in the data in all the other columns. The remaining columns are Total Calories, Total Carbohydrates, Fiber, and Sugars. The content of each food is listed under each appropriate column heading, expressed as the number of grams (the measurement used for weighing the nutrient content of food) per serving.

You will find both generic and brand-name products in these tables. The listing of a product by brand name is not an endorsement. If certain brand-name products are not listed, it means that there was no nutritional data available at the time the list was compiled, and they were not included for that reason only. Data are given for food products available in wholesale clubs and through wholesale distributors; these are identified as "food service products."

Food Description, Amount, Total Calories, Total Carbs, Fiber and Sugars are provided for most products listed. There are, however, a few entries marked "na." This means that the nutritional information for that particular nutrient was unavailable at the time of my researching the book. In most cases, the entries are listed alphabetically for easy reference. Where appropriate, some types of foods are presented in groups, such as "Frozen Entrée/Dinner," "Mexican Food," and "Asian Food." After the A-to-Z list, you will find a separate section on fast foods, organized alphabetically by individual franchise name.

The book features main headings for foods in uppercase boldface letters. In some instances, subheadings (smaller and bold) with solid boxes before them have been added for clarity. Descriptions of foods are in upper/lowercase, with brand names in parentheses.

If you are unable to find a particular food, look for the entry of a similar food. The nutritional data should be similar, if not exactly the same. When comparing foods, make sure you are comparing the same serving size, weight measure, and/or volume. The Table of Equivalent Measures (page 6) should help you not only in comparing serving sizes but in making exchanges as well. Finally, note that all servings of cooked vegetables are drained of liquid unless otherwise specified.

Abbreviations and Symbols

~	=	approximately
<	=	less than
"	=	inch
–	=	trace amount or less
dia	=	diameter
fl oz	=	fluid ounce
lb	=	pound
na	=	not available
oz	=	ounce
pkg	=	package
pkt	=	packet
sdw	=	sandwich
sec	=	second
Tbs	=	tablespoon
tsp	=	teaspoon
w/	=	with
w/o	=	without

Table of Equivalent Measures

VOLUME

1 tablespoon	=	½ fluid ounce
		3 teaspoons
1 fluid ounce	=	2 tablespoons
¼ cup	=	2 fluid ounces
		4 tablespoons
⅓ cup	=	5⅓ tablespoons
½ cup	=	4 fluid ounces
		8 tablespoons
⅔ cup	=	10⅔ tablespoons
¾ cup	=	6 fluid ounces
		12 tablespoons
1 cup	=	½ pint
		8 fluid ounces
		16 tablespoons
1 pint	=	2 cups
		16 fluid ounces
1 quart	=	2 pints
		4 cups
		32 fluid ounces
1 gallon	=	4 quarts
		8 pints

WEIGHT

1 ounce	=	28.35 grams
100 grams	=	3.5 ounces
4 ounces	=	¼ pound
8 ounces	=	½ pound
12 ounces	=	¾ pound
1 pound	=	16 ounces
		454 grams

Sources of Nutritional Information

United States Department of Agriculture Handbook No. 8 (revised), "Composition of Foods Raw, Processed, Prepared," sections 8-1 through 8-22; Handbook No. 456, "Nutritive Value of American Foods in Common Units"; Home and Garden Bulletin No. 232, "Nutrition and Your Health: Dietary Guidelines for Americans"

Food manufacturers and processors, as well as their product labels

Individual fast-food chains

A–Z Listing of Basic Foods

A

Food and Description	Amount	Total Calories	Total Carbs	Fiber	Sugars
ABALONE					
fried	3 oz	161	9	–	0
raw	3 oz	90	5	0	0
ACEROLA/raw	1 medium	2	0	0	0
ACEROLA JUICE	8 fl oz	51	12	1	0
ACORN					
dried	1 oz	145	15	na	na
raw	1 oz	105	12	na	na
ADUKI/ADZUKI BEAN					
(Arrowhead Mills) raw	¼ cup	160	29	6	0
(Eden)	½ cup	110	19	5	0
AGAR (*See* SEAWEED)					
ALE (*See* BEER, ALE & MALT LIQUOR)					
ALFALFA SPROUTS/raw	1 cup	10	0	0	0
ALLIGATOR/raw	3.5 oz	145	1	0	0
ALLSPICE	1 tsp	6	0	0	0
ALMOND					
(Azar)	1 oz	170	6	3	0
(Blue Diamond)					
barbecue	1.1 oz	170	5	3	1
blanched/whole	1 oz	190	6	4	0
chopped/natural	1 oz	180	6	4	1
dry-roasted	1 oz	170	6	3	1
honey-roasted	1 oz	170	8	3	4
roasted/salted	1 oz	190	5	3	1
slivered	1 oz	200	6	4	1
smokehouse	1 oz	170	5	3	1
barbecue	1 oz	180	5	4	1
honey-roasted	1 oz	180	8	4	4
(Fisher)					
ground/fine	1 oz	170	6	3	1
sliced natural	1 oz	170	6	3	1
slivered	1 oz	170	6	3	1
Salad Buddies	1 oz	160	10	3	1
whole/natural	1 oz	170	6	3	1
(Frito-Lay) smoke-flavored	1 oz	190	6	3.5	<1
(Planters)					
Gold Measure/slivered	2 oz	340	12	3	2

Food and Description	Amount	Total Calories	Total Carbs	Fiber	Sugars
honey-roasted	1 oz	160	7	4	0
regular	1 oz	170	5	3	1
salted	1 oz	160	5	3	0
sliced	2.25 oz	200	6	4	1
slivered	2-oz pkg	340	11	6	2
smoked	1 oz	170	6	3	0
ALMOND BUTTER					
(Arrowhead Mills)	2 Tbs	210	7	2	0
(Erewhon)	1 Tbs	90	3	0	0
(Hain)					
natural/raw	2 Tbs	190	3	0	0
toasted-blanched	2 Tbs	220	3	0	0
(Kettle) Roaster Fresh all styles	1 oz	184	6	0	0
(Westbrae Natural) all styles	2 tbs	190	7	0	0
ALMOND MEAL/partially defatted	1 oz	116	8	2	0
ALMOND PASTE	1 Tbs	127	14	1	na
AMARANTH					
(Arrowhead Mills) seeds	¼ cup	170	29	3	0
ANASAZI BEAN					
(Arrowhead Mills) dry	¼ cup	150	27	9	0
ANCHOVY, EUROPEAN					
canned/in oil..drained	5 fish	42	0	0	0
fresh/raw	3 oz	110	0	0	0
ANCHOVY PASTE	1Tbs	42	0	0	0
ANISE	1 tsp	7	1	0	0
APPLE					
CANNED, JAR, or BAG					
(Lucky Leaf)					
Dutch-baked	5 oz	170	41	3	40
fried	4.6 oz	170	43	2	39
rings..red spiced	1.5 oz	35	9	0	8
sliced	4 oz	50	12	2	9
spiced crab	2 oz	35	8	1	5
(Musselman's)					
100% natural apples					
by the slice	2.8 oz	45	12	2	10
crab/spiced	2 oz	35	8	1	5
diced	4 oz	50	12	1	8
sliced..sweetened in syrup	4 oz	50	12	1	8
spiced	2 oz	35	8	1	5
(Whitehouse)					
cinnamon/escalloped	5 oz	160	35	0	25
sliced	5 oz	100	22	2	16
spiced rings	1 ring	30	9	0	8
DRIED					
(Mariani)	¼ cup	110	26	3	18
(Seneca) apple chips					
1-oz bags..all flavors	1 bag	140	20	2	11
1.5-oz ounce bags..all flavors	1 bag	210	30	3	17

Food and Description	Amount	Total Calories	Total Carbs	Fiber	Sugars
(Sun-Maid) Washington	1.25 oz	110	26	3	18
(Tree Top) fat-free..all flavors	1 oz	110	26	3	22
FRESH					
cooked..w/o skin..sliced	1 cup	95	24	5	na
microwaved/sliced..peeled	½ cup	65	12	2.5	na
raw					
(Dole) w/skin	1 medium	80	22	5	16
sliced	1 cup	64	16	2	11
APPLE BUTTER					
(Dutch Girl)	1 Tbs	35	9	0	7
(Eden) organic	1 Tbs	20	4	1	4
(Lucky Leaf) old-fashioned spiced	1 Tbs	30	8	0	6
(Mary Ellen)	1 Tbs	35	9	0	7
(Musselman's)	1 Tbs	30	8	0	6
(Smuckers) all types	1 Tbs	45	11	0	10
(Welch's) Bama..original recipe	1 Tbs	40	9	0	6
APPLE FRITTERS/frozen					
(Mrs. Paul's) home-style	4 oz	240	33	1	14
APPLE JUICE/NECTAR					
BOTTLED, BOXED, or CANNED					
(Apple & Eve)	8 fl oz	110	26	0	22
(Hood)	8 fl oz	120	31	0	26
(Knouse) Apple Time					
100% from concentrate	8 fl oz	120	31	0	26
premium	8 fl oz	120	31	0	26
(Knudsen)					
apple	8 fl oz	110	26	0	22
Thirst Quencher..nectar	8 fl oz	120	31	0	26
(Libby's)					
Juicy Juice	4.23 fl oz	60	15	0	13
46-oz bottle..100% juice	8 fl oz	110	28	0	26
(Lincoln) premium	8 fl oz	120	31	0	26
	6.75 fl oz	100	23	0	22
(Lucky Leaf)	5.5 fl oz	80	20	0	17
	6.75 fl oz	100	23	0	22
(Martinelli's) 100% pure					
natural/unfiltered	8 fl oz	140	35	0	31
organic	8 fl oz	140	35	0	31
sparkling	10 fl oz	180	43	0	39
apple cranberry	8 fl oz	110	27	0	22
apple grape	8 fl oz	120	31	0	28
from fresh apples	8 fl oz	150	37	0	33
(Minute Maid)					
100% pure	11.5 oz	160	39	0	36
apple pure	12 fl oz	170	41	0	38
(Mott's) natural	8 fl oz	120	29	0	23
	9.5 fl oz	140	34	0	32
	10 fl oz	150	37	0	33

Food and Description	Amount	Total Calories	Total Carbs	Fiber	Sugars
(Odwalla) Essentials					
organic	8 fl oz	110	34	0	32
pressed	8 fl oz	140	34	0	32
(Seneca) country apple	8 fl oz	110	30	0	26
(TreeTop)					
Grower's Best	8 fl oz	120	29	0	26
single-serve	5.5 fl oz	80	20	0	18
	6.75 fl oz	100	25	0	22
	10 fl oz	140	36	0	33
	11.5 fl oz	170	42	0	38
(Tropicana) chilled	6 fl oz	80	21	0	19
	8 fl oz	110	28	0	26
	10 fl oz	140	34	0	32
(Welch's) single-serve..100% juice	5.5 fl oz	80	30	0	19
	10 fl oz	140	36	0	35
	11.5 fl oz	160	41	0	39
FROZEN..PREPARED..UNLESS OTHERWISE NOTED					
(Minute Maid)	8 fl oz	110	28	0	26
(Seneca)					
100% apple juice concentrate	2 oz	110	28	0	28
country-style	8 fl oz	120	30	0	26
(TreeTop)..all styles	8 fl oz	120	29	0	26

APPLE JUICE BLEND/DRINK

(NOTE: Unless stated otherwise, data are for prepared serving amounts.)

BOTTLED, BOXED, or CANNED

Food and Description	Amount	Total Calories	Total Carbs	Fiber	Sugars
(Dole)					
apple cherry cocktail	8 fl oz	120	29	0	27
apple cranberry	10 fl oz	180	45	0	44
(Full Circle) cranberry apple	8 fl oz	130	30	0	29
(Hi-C) Jammin' Apple	8.45 fl oz	120	31	0	31
(Knudsen) all styles	8 fl oz	120	30	0	26
(Libby's) Juicy Juice..apple grape	8 fl oz	100	24	0	21
(Mott's)					
apple juice drink	9.5 fl oz	150	36	0	35
	10 fl oz	160	41	0	39
apple cranberry juice	8 fl oz	120	29	0	27
apple grape juice	8 fl oz	120	31	0	29
apple raspberry juice	6 fl oz	85	20	0	18
	10 fl oz	140	36	0	35
(Old Orchard) frozen concentrate..prepared					
apple cherry	8 fl oz	130	31	0	29
apple cranberry	8 fl oz	120	29	0	27
apple kiwi strawberry	8 fl oz	130	31	0	29
apple passion mango	8 fl oz	130	31	0	29
apple peach mango	8 fl oz	120	29	0	27
(TreeTop)					
apple berry juice	8 fl oz	130	31	0	26
apple cranberry juice	10 fl oz	180	45	0	44
apple grape juice	8 fl oz	130	32	0	26
apple raspberry juice	5.5 fl oz	80	20	0	18

Food and Description	Amount	Total Calories	Total Carbs	Fiber	Sugars
(Tropicana)					
blends..cranberry apple	8 fl oz	130	33	0	32
Twister..apple berry blast	8 fl oz	130	31	0	28
(Welch's)					
juice cocktail..juice drink					
apple cranberry					
low-cal	10 fl oz	15	3	0	2
regular	8 fl oz	150	36	0	35
	10 fl oz	180	45	0	44
	11.5 fl oz	210	52	0	51
APPLESAUCE					
(Del Monte)					
light	½ cup	50	13	2	8
sweetened	½ cup	90	21	1	17
(Lucky Leaf)					
cherry	4-oz cup	90	21	1	17
chunky	4.8 oz	100	25	2	21
cinnamon	4-oz cup	80	21	2	19
light	4.6 oz	50	13	2	8
old-fashioned natural	4.6 oz	50	13	2	8
orange mango	4-oz cup	100	26	2	19
raspberry	4-oz cup	80	20	2	18
(Mott's)					
chunky	5 oz	110	26	2	22
cinnamon	5 oz	120	29	1	24
fruit snacks					
cinnamon	4 oz	90	23	1	19
Dutch apple spice	4 oz	70	18	1	16
strawberry	4 oz	80	22	1	18
sweetened	4 oz	90	22	1	18
(Musselman's)					
chunky home-style	4.8 oz	100	25	2	21
cinnamon					
deluxe	4.8 oz	100	25	2	21
light	4.3 oz	50	13	2	8
regular	6-oz cup	130	31	3	28
fruit & sauce/light					
cherry	4-oz cup	60	15	1	10
natural	6-oz cup	70	18	3	12
orange mango	4-oz cup	60	14	1	9
peach	4-oz cup	60	14	2	9
raspberry	4-oz cup	60	14	1	9
strawberry	4-oz cup	60	14	1	9
unsweetened..natural	4.6 oz	50	13	2	8
(Santa Cruz) Organic					
apple cinnamon	4-oz cup	80	19	2	16
other flavors..all types	4-oz cup	50	13	2	11
(Seneca)					
100% natural	4.5 oz	60	15	3	13
cinnamon	4.5 oz	100	24	3	18

Food and Description	Amount	Total Calories	Total Carbs	Fiber	Sugars
Golden Delicious	4.5 oz	100	24	3	18
McIntosh	4.5 oz	100	24	3	18
regular	4.5 oz	100	24	2	18
wild berry	4-oz cup	80	20	1	18
(Walnut Acres) Fruit Squeezies					
berry wild	2 oz	40	10	1	8
wild apple	2 oz	35	9	0	8
(Whitehouse)					
cinnamon	4 oz	100	25	1	18
Fruitastics peach	4 oz	70	13	1	13
regular	4.5 oz	90	23	2	18
APRICOT					
CANNED					
(Del Monte) halves/unpeeled					
almond-flavored	½ cup	90	22	1	20
in heavy syrup	½ cup	100	26	1	25
light	½ cup	60	16	1	15
individual pull-top can	1 can	60	16	1	15
Orchard Select	½ cup	80	21	1	20
(Libby's)					
halves..in juice	½ cup	80	21	1	19
unpeeled halves in heavy syrup	½ cup	60	13	1	11
(S&W)					
almond in light syrup	½ cup	90	22	1	19
whole/peeled..in heavy syrup	½ cup	120	28	1	24
DRIED					
(Ann's House of Nuts) Turkish	5 pieces	90	22	3	19
(Del Monte) sun-dried	⅓ cup	80	25	6	19
(Dole) Sun Giant Turkish	6 pieces	90	22	3	19
(Mariani)					
California	1.5 oz	110	25	2	17
Mediterranean	1.4 oz	100	24	3	21
(Sonoma)	10 pieces	130	31	3	20
(Sun Maid)					
bag					
California	1.5 oz	110	25	2	17
Mediterranean	1.42 oz	100	24	3	21
cannister					
Mediterranean	1.4 oz	100	24	2	21
FRESH					
(Dole)	3 medium	60	11	1	1
halves	1 cup	74	17	4	na
APRICOT JUICE/NECTAR					
BOTTLED, BOXED, or CANNED					
(Del Monte)	6 fl oz	100	24	0	22
(Goya)	6 fl oz	120	29	0	26
	8 fl oz	130	31	0	29
(Kern's)	5.5 oz	100	24	0	22
	6.59 fl oz	120	29	0	26
	7.6 fl oz	140	35	0	32

Food and Description	Amount	Total Calories	Total Carbs	Fiber	Sugars
	11.5 fl oz	210	52	0	44
(Libby's)	5.5 oz	100	24	0	22
	11.5 fl oz	210	52	0	44
(S&W)	12 fl oz	200	50	0	45
(Walnut Acres)	8 oz	130	32	0	29
ARROWHEAD..plant					
COOKED	medium corm	9	2	<1	na
RAW	medium corm	12	2.5	<1	na
ARTICHOKE (*See also* JERUSALEM ARTICHOKE)					
CANNED or JARRED					
(Cara Mia)					
in water	1 oz	15	3	1	0
marinated					
crowns	1 oz	12	3	1	0
hearts	1 oz	25	3	1	0
(Native Forest)					
artichoke hearts					
marinated	1 oz	35	2	<1	9
quartered	4 oz	35	6	4	1
whole	4 oz	35	6	4	1
hearts of palm..organic	1 oz	15	2	1	0
(Progresso) hearts in brine	3 oz	30	6	1	1
(Reese)					
bottoms	2 pieces	35	7	1	1
hearts	4.5 oz	50	9	2	1
(S&W)					
bottoms..in water	3 pieces	25	4	2	<1
hearts					
in water	3 pieces	30	6	1	<1
marinated	2 pieces	20	2	1	<1
FRESH					
(Dole) 1 medium	2 oz	25	6	3	1
FROZEN					
(Birds Eye) hearts..deluxe	14 pieces	40	7	5	0
ARTICHOKE HEART (*See* ARTICHOKE)					
ARUGULA..fresh..chopped	½ cup	2	0	0	0
ASIAN FOOD (*See also* FROZEN ENTRÉE/DINNER; PASTA ENTRÉE/DINNER; RICE DISH; VEGETARIAN FOODS; individual listings)					
■ **BEEF DISHES** (*See also* Chow Mein; Fried Rice; Sweet & Sour in this section)					
(Chun King) canned..beef pepper					
divider pack entrée..prepared	1 cup	100	12	2	<1
(La Choy) canned..prepared					
beef pepper..bi-pack	¾ cup	80	10	2	0
beef pepper Oriental entrée	¾ cup	100	12	2	<1
■ **CHICKEN DISHES** (*See also* Chow Mein; Fried Rice; Sweet & Sour in this section)					
(Chun King) frozen entrée					
imperial chicken	13 oz	460	59	5	17
walnut chicken	13 oz	460	56	5	15

Food and Description	Amount	Total Calories	Total Carbs	Fiber	Sugars
(La Choy) canned/prepared					
chicken teriyaki..bi-pack	¾ cup	85	8	1	na
sweet & sour					
bi-pack	¾ cup	120	13	2	na
entrée	¾ cup	240	47	1	na
■ **CHOW MEIN** (*See* Vegetables/Vegetable Dishes in this section)					
■ **EGG ROLL**					
(Chun King) frozen..mini					
pork & shrimp	6 pieces	210	27	2	4
shrimp	6 pieces	190	28	2	3
(La Choy) frozen					
bite-size..pork & shrimp	6 pieces	210	27	2	4
mini					
chicken	6 pieces	210	25	2	3
pork & shrimp	6 pieces	210	27	2	4
shrimp	6 pieces	190	28	2	6
vegetable w/lobster	6 pieces	190	27	2	3
restaurant-style/6 oz					
chicken	1 piece	210	25	2	4
shrimp	1 piece	180	25	2	6
(Minh) frozen					
chicken white meat	3 oz	150	20	2	3
pork	3 oz	170	18	2	2
pork & shrimp	3 oz	140	19	2	3
vegetable	3 oz	140	21	2	3
(Pagoda Cafe) frozen					
chicken					
sweet & sour	¼ box	160	23	2	4
white meat	¼ box	160	20	2	2
white meat/mini	½ box	180	24	2	3
pork/savory					
& vegetable	⅓ box	170	18	2	2
mini	½ box	200	22	2	2
pork & shrimp	¼ box	170	19	2	2
vegetable	¼ box	150	20	2	2
(Schwan's) frozen					
chicken	2 pieces	220	22	2	2
mini	4 pieces	200	22	2	2
pork	2 pieces	240	25	2	3
Southwest chicken	2 pieces	260	35	2	4
wonton pizza-flavored	5 pieces	410	45	3	3
(Yu Sing) frozen					
chicken	6 rolls	180	23	1	2
pork & shrimp	6 rolls	200	23	1	3
shrimp	6 rolls	180	24	2	5
sweet & sour chicken	6 rolls	190	26	1	4
sweet & sour pork	6 rolls	210	25	1	4
■ **EGG ROLL WRAPPER**					
(Azumaya Pasta)	1 large	160	31	1	1

Food and Description	Amount	Total Calories	Total Carbs	Fiber	Sugars
(Nasoya)	3 wrappers	170	35	1	1
■ ETHNIC GOURMET					
(Heinz) frozen entrées					
Chinese-style					
kung pao chicken	12 oz	420	61	3	9
kung pao tofu wrap	8 oz	410	48	4	5
shrimp fried rice	11 oz	460	63	4	5
Szechuan vegetarian					
chicken	12 oz	380	69	6	10
Japanese-style					
teriyaki chicken	11 oz	340	63	2	9
vegetarian teriyaki	12 oz	330	71	4	12
Korean-style	10 oz	350	36	2	10
Singaporean-style	10 oz	290	44	8	4
Thai-style					
chicken massaman	11 oz	330	44	4	13
chicken pad Thai	10 oz	430	71	3	20
lemongrass & basil chicken	11 oz	400	53	4	11
pad Thai..w/shrimp	10 oz	350	64	3	13
Vietnamese-style	10 oz	330	43	1	14
■ FORTUNE COOKIE					
(La Choy)	4 cookies	120	23	1	na
■ FRIED RICE (*See also* Yu Sing in this section)					
(Chun King)					
w/chicken	8 oz	270	44	4	9
w/pork	8 oz	290	48	5	11
(La Choy) fried rice..prepared	1 cup	235	53	2	2
(Lugiano's)					
chicken	1 pkg	250	38	2	2
pork	1 pkg	250	37	2	2
shrimp	1 pkg	220	38	2	2
shrimp & pork	1 pkg	250	39	2	2
(Tyson) Meal Kit					
chicken fried rice..w/sauce	½ kit	440	69	5	15
■ NOODLE (*See also* PASTA; PASTA ENTRÉE/DINNER)					
(Annie Chun's)					
basil	1 cup	210	50	0	<1
chow mein	1 cup	200	39	3	<1
original	1 cup	210	50	0	<1
pad Thai	1 cup	210	50	0	<1
(China Bowl)					
cellophane..cooked	½ cup	70	17	0	<1
Chinese..cooked	½ cup	150	34	6	<1
rice sticks	½ cup	150	33	1	<1
(China Boy) dry					
chow mein					
classic	~1 oz	125	16	1	0
wide	~1 oz	130	16	1	0
rice..thin	~1 oz	130	16	1	1

Food and Description	Amount	Total Calories	Total Carbs	Fiber	Sugars
(Eden) organic					
Japanese traditional noodles..pasta					
bifun	2 oz	200	44	0	0
kuzu	2 oz	200	48	2	0
lotus root soba	2 oz	190	37	4	2
mugwort soba	2 oz	190	37	2	2
mung bean	2 oz	190	47	0	0
wild yam sobam soba	2 oz	190	37	4	2
(Ka-Me)					
Chinese egg	2 oz	210	40	2	0
Chinese..lo mein wide	2 oz	200	45	1	0
Chinese plain	2 oz	200	45	1	0
Chuka soba curly	2 oz	200	42	1	0
Py Mai fun rice sticks	2 oz	195	48	0	0
Soba Shin Shu Japanese buckwheat	2 oz	200	40	2	2
Tomoshiraga Somen	2 oz	190	41	1	0
(La Choy)					
chow mein	½ cup	140	16	<1	0
crispy wide	½ cup	150	16	<1	0
rice	½ cup	120	21	<1	0
(Pagoda Cafe) frozen					
noodle pot					
golden Thai-style chicken	11 oz	410	54	4	9
golden Thai-style vegetable	11 oz	410	63	5	9
■ POTSTICKERS					
(Ling Ling) frozen chicken & vegetable					
dumplings, dumplings only	5 pieces	280	49	2	na
(Pagoda Cafe) frozen..savory pork	3.25 oz	240	21	1	3
■ SAUCES & SEASONINGS (*See also* SAUCE; SEASONINGS)					
(China Bowl)					
chili paste w/garlic	2 Tbs	15	3	<1	<1
hoisin	1 tsp	10	4	0	3
oyster	½ tsp	5	1	0	1
soy	½ tsp	<5	0	0	0
(Chun King)					
hot teriyaki sauce	2 Tbs	30	6	0	4
soy sauce	1 Tbs	10	4	0	3
(Dynasty) oyster sauce	1 Tbs	30	6	<1	4
(House of Tsang)					
oil					
hot chili sesame	1 tsp	45	0	0	0
Mongolian Fire Oil	1 tsp	45	0	0	0
pure sesame	1 tsp	45	0	0	0
Singapore curry	1 tsp	45	0	0	0
wok	1 Tbs	130	0	0	0
sauce					
Bangkok padang	1 Tbs	45	4	0	3
classic stir-fry	1 Tbs	25	4	0	3
hibachi grill sauce					

Food and Description	Amount	Total Calories	Total Carbs	Fiber	Sugars
Hunan smokehut	1 Tbs	40	8	0	7
Kobe steak	1 Tbs	50	2	0	2
sweet ginger sesame	1 Tbs	40	8	0	7
teriyaki	1 Tbs	40	10	0	8
Thai peanut	1 Tbs	50	4	0	4
hoisin sauce	1 tsp	15	4	0	3
imperial citrus stir-fry	1 Tbs	25	5	0	5
Korean teriyaki	1 Tbs	30	6	0	4
Mandarin marinade	1 Tbs	25	6	0	5
oyster-flavored stir-fry	1 Tbs	30	7	0	6
Saigon sizzle	1 Tbs	40	8	0	6
soy sauce					
ginger-flavored					
low-sodium	1 Tbs	10	4	0	2
regular	1 Tbs	20	4	0	3
low-sodium	1 Tbs	5	0	0	0
spicy brown bean	1 tsp	15	3	0	2
sweet & sour stir-fry	1 Tbs	35	4	0	3
sweet ginger sesame hibachi	1 Tbs	40	9	0	7
Szechuan spicy stir-fry	1 Tbs	20	4	0	3
(Ka-Me) sauce					
black bean	1 Tbs	10	2	1	1
chili..hot garlic	1 Tbs	15	4	1	2
duck	2 Tbs	80	20	0	16
fish	1 Tbs	20	1	0	1
goisin	2 Tbs	45	10	1	8
hot	1 tsp	0	0.5	0	0
lemon	1 Tbs	45	11	0	5
mandarin orange	2 Tbs	80	21	0	3
oyster	1 Tbs	10	3	0	2
plum	2 Tbs	80	19	0	17
stir-fry	1 Tbs	10	1	0	1
sweet & sour	2 Tbs	50	13	0	11
Szechuan	1 Tbs	20	2	2	1
tamari	1 Tbs	10	1	0	1
tempura	2 Tbs	15	3	0	3
teriyaki	1 Tbs	10	2	0	1
(Kikkoman)					
soy sauce					
light	1 Tbs	10	0	0	0
regular	1 Tbs	10	0	0	0
sushi & sashimi	1 Tbs	15	2	0	2
stir-fry	1 Tbs	20	4	0	3
sukiyaki	1 Tbs	20	4	0	4
sweet & sour	2 Tbs	35	9	0	7
dipping sauce	1 Tbs	35	9	0	7
tempura	1 tsp	5	1	0	1
teriyaki					
baste & glaze					

Food and Description	Amount	Total Calories	Total Carbs	Fiber	Sugars
original	2 Tbs	50	11	0	9
w/honey & pineapple	2 Tbs	80	18	0	14
light	1 Tbs	15	3	0	3
original	1 Tbs	15	2	0	2
roasted garlic	1 Tbs	25	5	0	3
(Lighthouse) Sagawa's sauce					
Polynesian BBQ	2 Tbs	60	13	0	11
stir-fry	1 Tbs	25	5	0	4
sweet & sassy	2 Tbs	60	14	0	12
sweet & sour	2 Tbs	50	11	0	10
teriyaki	1 Tbs	30	7	0	6
(Premier Japan)					
ginger tamari	1 Tbs	5	1	0	1
sesame garlic tamari	1 Tbs	10	1	0	1
wasabi tamari	1 Tbs	5	1	0	1
wheat-free..hoisin or teriyaki	1 Tbs	15	3	0	2
(A Taste of Thai)					
fish seasoning/sauce	1 Tbs	15	1	0	0
garlic chili pepper sauce	1 tsp	10	2	0	2
peanut satay sauce	2 Tbs	80	9	1	5
■ SEA VEGETABLES					
(Eden)					
hiziki sea vegetable	¼ cup	30	6	6	0
kombu	½ sheet	10	2	1	0
sushi nori sea vegetable	1 sheet	10	1	1	0
wakame	½ cup	25	4	4	0
wakame flakes	½ cup	25	4	4	0
■ SEASONINGS (See Sauces & Seasonings in this section)					
■ STIR-FRY (See also VEGETABLES, MIXED)					
(Birds Eye) frozen..as packaged					
stir-fry					
asparagus	2 cups	80	15	2	0
crisp green bean	1¾ cups	100	19	2	0
pepper	1 cup	25	5	1	0
7-vegetable	1 cup	30	5	2	0
sugar snap	1 cup	40	7	2	0
(C&W) frozen					
potsticker stir-fry feast					
w/o sauce	2 cups	160	23	4	3
w/sauce	2 cups	200	30	4	8
ultimate stir-fry					
w/o sauce	1½ cups	160	20	2	5
w/sauce	1½ cups	190	25	3	9
(Green Giant) frozen..as packaged					
Create A Meal!					
garlic herb chicken	2⅓ cups	230	30	3	3
stir-fry					
garlic & ginger	1⅔ cups	130	25	4	14
lo mein	2⅓ cups	170	33	3	9
sweet & sour	1½ cups	180	43	3	31

Food and Description	Amount	Total Calories	Total Carbs	Fiber	Sugars
Szechuan	1¾ cups	150	20	4	12

■ **VEGETABLES/VEGETABLE DISHES** (*See also* Chow Mein; Fried Rice; Sea Vegetables; in this section)

Food and Description	Amount	Total Calories	Total Carbs	Fiber	Sugars
(Empress)					
bamboo shoots/sliced	2 oz	13	2	<1	<1
water chestnuts..all styles	2 oz	14	3	0	0
(Geisha)					
bamboo shoots	4 oz	25	3	2	1
bean sprouts	~2 oz	25	3	2	1
water chestnuts					
sliced	5.3 oz	50	12	4	3
whole	5.3 oz	45	11	3	0
(La Choy)					
bamboo shoots	3 oz	10	2	<1	0
	¼ cup	6	1	<1	0
bean sprouts	6 oz	15	3	<1	0
water chestnuts					
sliced	2 Tbs	10	3	1	0
	¼ cup	18	4	<1	0
whole	2 medium	10	3	<1	0

■ **WON TON SOUP** (*See* SOUP)

■ **WRAPPER..PASTA**

Food and Description	Amount	Total Calories	Total Carbs	Fiber	Sugars
egg roll & won ton wrappers					
(Asumaya) large square	1 wrapper	170	35	1	1
(Nasoya) egg roll..16-oz bag	1 wrapper	170	35	1	1

■ **(YU SING)**

Food and Description	Amount	Total Calories	Total Carbs	Fiber	Sugars
frozen bowls					
beef					
spicy beef & broccoli	1 bowl	380	78	2	11
teriyaki steak	1 bowl	370	64	3	16
chicken					
honey ginger	1 bowl	350	60	3	15
sesame	1 bowl	390	67	2	10
sweet & sour w/rice	1 bowl	420	82	2	26
teriyaki	1 bowl	400	77	2	13
vegetables & white chicken	1 bowl	360	59	3	2
shrimp fried rice	1 bowl	430	76	3	5
frozen entrées					
beef					
Oriental beef & peppers w/rice	1 meal	290	44	2	4
pepper steak w/green peppers	1 meal	280	46	1	5
teriyaki w/rice	1 meal	260	57	2	7
chicken					
fried rice	1 meal	360	58	2	3
garlic w/rice	1 meal	240	43	2	4
lo mein	1 meal	230	33	2	3
sweet & sour w/rice	1 meal	360	70	1	23
pork					
fried rice	1 meal	440	69	2	4
pork & shrimp fried rice	1 meal	440	69	2	4

Food and Description	Amount	Total Calories	Total Carbs	Fiber	Sugars
shrimp lo mein	1 meal	210	37	3	5
ASPARAGUS					
CANNED					
(Del Monte) tender green..all cuts	½ cup	20	3	1	0
(Green Giant) all cuts	½ cup	20	3	1	1
(LeSueur) extra-large spears	4.5 oz	20	3	1	1
(Libby's) cut spears	4.5 oz	20	3	2	1
(Native Forest) all cuts & tips	4.5 oz	20	3	1	1
(Reese) white spears	⅓ can	20	3	1	1
(S&W)					
all green cut spears	½ cup	25	3	1	1
blended	6 pieces	15	2	1	1
(Stokely)					
cut green spears	½ cup	25	3	1	1
no salt or sugar added	½ cup	20	3	1	1
(Thank You) whole spears	½ cup	25	3	1	1
FRESH					
(Chiquita) Walla Walla					
cuts & tips	½ cup	25	3	3	0
whole	½ cup	15	2	1	1
(Dole) raw spears..trimmed	5 spears	25	4	2	1
FROZEN					
(Birds Eye)					
cuts	3.3 oz	25	4	2	2
spears..whole	½ cup	25	4	1	2
(C&W) spears	7 spears	20	3	2	2
AVOCADO					
FRESH/RAW					
California					
mashed	1 cup	407	16	11	<1
whole/medium	1 fruit	324	12	8	<1
(Calavo) medium avocado					
all types	⅕ fruit	55	3	3	0
Florida/medium	1 fruit	340	27	16	0

B

Food and Description	Amount	Total Calories	Total Carbs	Fiber	Sugars
BACON (*See also* BACON, CANADIAN-STYLE; BACON BITS, CHIPS & PIECES; BACON SUBSTITUTE)					
(Armour) ready					
crisp/fully cooked	2 slices	70	0	0	0
hickory-smoked..original	2 slices	90	0	0	0
regular	2 slices	60	0	0	0
(Boar's Head) fried					
domestic	2 slices	70	0	0	0
imported	2 slices	60	0	0	0
(Bob Evans) thick-sliced					
hickory-smoked	2 slices	80	0	0	0
(Bryan)					
precooked..pan-fried..extra thick	2 slices	90	0	0	0
single pan-fried slices..all types	2 slices	90	0	0	0
thin slices	4 slices	90	0	0	0
(Butterball) turkey bacon..original	1 slice	35	0	0	0
smoke-cured dark & white	2 slices	70	0	0	0
(Farmer John)					
regular-sliced..all types	2 slices	80	0	0	0
thick-sliced	1 slices	60	0	0	0
(Gwaltney) cooked..all types	2 slices	60	0	0	0
(Hormel) cooked					
applewood-smoked	2 slices	110	1	0	1
Black Label					
center cut	3 slices	70	0	0	0
low-salt	2 slices	80	0	0	0
regular	2 slices	80	0	0	0
Canadian-style	2 oz	70	0	0	0
fully cooked	2.5 slices	70	0	0	0
mesquite..sliced	2 slices	80	0	0	0
microwave	4 slices	70	0	0	0
lower-sodium	2 slices	80	0	0	0
PillowPack..Canadian					
bacon	2 slices	80	2	0	1
Range Brand..cooked	2 slices	110	0	0	0
Red Label	2 slices	80	0	0	0
(Jimmy Dean)					
diced	1 Tbs	90	0	0	0
precooked center piece					
regular-sliced	3 slices	80	0	0	0

Food and Description	Amount	Total Calories	Total Carbs	Fiber	Sugars
thick-sliced	2 slices	80	0	0	0
single-sliced/cooked	1 slice	60	0	0	0
single-sliced					
applewood	1 slice	50	0	0	0
heavy smoke..pan-fried	2 slices	80	0	0	0
(Louis Rich) cured..dark & light	1 slice	35	0	0	0
(Oscar Mayer) cooked					
¼"-thick cut	1 slice	60	0	0	0
lower-sodium	2 slices	70	1	0	0
original	2 slices	70	0	0	0
Ready Crisp..shelf	3 slices	70	0	0	0
(Tyson) ready-to-cook..hickory	2 slices	90	0	0	0
BACON, CANADIAN-STYLE					
(Boar's Head) extra lean	2 oz	70	1	0	1
(Dak) 98% fat-free	2 oz	60	1	0	1
(Hormel) cooked..1-oz slices	2 slices	70	0	0	0
(Jones) uncooked	3 slices	70	1	0	1
(Oscar Mayer)..cooked	2 slices	50	0	0	1
BACON, VEGETARIAN (*See* VEGETARIAN FOODS)					
BACON BITS, CHIPS & PIECES					
IMITATION					
(Betty Crocker) BacOs..all styles	1½ Tbs	30	2	0	0
(Durkee) all styles	1 Tbs	25	1	0	0
(McCormick/Schilling) all styles	1 Tbs	25	1	0	0
REAL					
(Hormel)					
bits	1 Tbs	30	0	0	0
bits..less fat	1 Tbs	35	0	0	0
crispy real bacon chips	1 Tbs	45	0	0	0
pieces	1 Tbs	25	0	0	0
(Jimmy Dean)					
applewood ends & pieces	0.5 oz	80	<1	0	1
bits	1 Tbs	90	0	0	0
diced	1 Tbs	90	0	0	0
kettle-cooked	1 tsp	20	0.5	0	0
(Oscar Mayer)..all styles	1 Tbs	25	0	0	0
BACON SUBSTITUTE (*See* BACON BITS, CHIPS & PIECES; VEGETARIAN FOODS)					
BAGEL					
(CarbXtract)					
blueberry	½ bagel	67	10	2.35	0
chocolate chip	½ bagel	67	10	2.35	0
cinnamon raisin	½ bagel	95	11	2.35	0
garlic onion	½ bagel	67	10	2.35	0
onion	½ bagel	67	10	2.35	0
plain	½ bagel	86	9	2	0
poppy seed	½ bagel	67	10	2.35	0
sesame	½ bagel	67	10	2.35	0
(Dunkin' Donuts) (*See* FAST FOOD)					

Food and Description	Amount	Total Calories	Total Carbs	Fiber	Sugars
(Lender's)					
Bagel Shop..fresh					
apple cranberry	1 bagel	310	64	3	15
blueberry	1 bagel	270	55	2	9
cinnamon raisin	1 bagel	280	54	2	12
egg	1 bagel	280	54	2	4
honey wheat	1 bagel	270	55	3	9
onion	1 bagel	270	55	2	5
plain	1 bagel	280	56	2	7
standard tomato	1 bagel	300	58	3	6
Bagel Shop..refrigerated					
blueberry	1 bagel	200	42	2	8
cinnamon raisin	1 bagel	230	44	2	11
egg	1 bagel	220	41	2	6
honey wheat	1 bagel	190	39	1	5
onion	1 bagel	220	42	2	6
plain	1 bagel	220	42	2	7
Big 'n' Crusty..frozen					
blueberry	1 bagel	250	51	2	11
cinnamon raisin	1 bagel	260	52	2	11
egg	1 bagel	260	52	1	9
honey wheat	1 bagel	230	49	2	7
onion	1 bagel	250	52	2	9
plain	1 bagel	250	52	1	3
New York--style					
blueberry	1 bagel	250	51	2	11
cinnamon raisin	1 bagel	260	52	2	11
onion	1 bagel	250	52	2	3
plain	1 bagel	230	47	3	3
original..frozen					
blueberry swirl	1 bagel	160	32	1	6
chocolate chip swirl	1 bagel	160	33	2	8
cinnamon raisin	1 bagel	160	32	1	7
cinnamon swirl	1 bagel	150	32	1	8
egg	1 bagel	160	30	1	3
garlic	1 bagel	150	29	2	4
onion	1 bagel	150	30	1	3
plain	1 bagel	150	30	1	2
plain bagelette	2 bagels	140	27	1	2
poppy	1 bagel	150	30	2	3
pumpernickel	1 bagel	150	31	1	3
rye	1 bagel	150	30	2	3
sesame seed	1 bagel	150	29	1	3
soft original 2.5 oz	1 bagel	210	37	2	6
strawberry swirl	1 bagel	160	33	2	6
(Pepperidge Farm) food service/Bountiful Bagels					
cinnamon raisin	1 bagel	280	58	3	11
brown sugar cinnamon..mini	1 bagel	120	24	2	6
everything	1 bagel	310	60	3	9

Food and Description	Amount	Total Calories	Total Carbs	Fiber	Sugars
onion	1 bagel	290	60	2	6
plain					
mini	1 bagel	120	24	<1	2
regular	1 bagel	290	60	2	6
(Sara Lee)					
16-oz bag					
apple cinnamon	1 bagel	310	64	3	16
banana walnut	1 bagel	350	61	4	10
cranberry orange	1 bagel	310	64	3	16
sun-dried tomato basil	1 bagel	300	61	2	6
20-oz bag					
blueberry	1 bagel	260	53	2	7
cinnamon raisin	1 bagel	260	55	4	9
honey wheat	1 bagel	250	50	4	7
onion	1 bagel	250	51	2	5
plain	1 bagel	250	52	2	5
mini					
blueberry	1 bagel	70	15	1	2
cinnamon raisin swirl	1 bagel	70	15	1	2
plain	1 bagel	70	15	1	2
(Thomas')					
Carb Counting					
plain	1 bagel	140	23	5	0
whole wheat	1 bagel	140	22	6	1
New York–style					
blueberry	1 bagel	300	59	3	13
cinnamon swirl	1 bagel	290	57	4	9
plain	1 bagel	280	56	2	7
plain..mini..presliced	1 bagel	130	26	1	3
(Wonder)					
blueberry	1 bagel	220	45	2	7
cinnamon raisin	1 bagel	210	45	2	7
onion	1 bagel	210	44	2	5
plain	1 bagel	210	43	1	4
BAGEL CHIPS					
(New York–style)					
chip mix..baked					
fat-free	1 oz	100	21	1	1
garlic	~1 oz	130	18	1	2
chips..garlic pita	7 chips	130	18	1	2
crisps..all flavors	7 pieces	130	18	1	2
(Old London)..bagel snacks					
cinnamon	5 pieces	60	12	1	na
garlic	5 pieces	60	9	2	na
original	5 pieces	60	9	2	na
poppy seed	5 pieces	60	8	2	ba
BAKE & FRY MIX (*See also* SEASONINGS)					
(Arrowhead) all-purpose baking mix/dry					
regular	¼ cup	140	30	2	2

Food and Description	Amount	Total Calories	Total Carbs	Fiber	Sugars
wheat-free	¼ cup	120	27	1	2
(Bisquick) dry mix only					
original	⅓ cup	160	21	0	2
reduced-fat	⅓ cup	140	27	<1	3
(Carb Sense)..baking mix..dry mix only	½ cup	125	4	4	2
(Golden Dipt) dry mix only					
Breaders & Batters					
Fry Easy/Mix					
all-purpose batter	¼ cup	100	20	0	0
beer batter	¼ cup	100	20	0	0
Cajun-style	1⅓ Tbs	35	6	0	0
cracker meal fry	¼ cup	130	23	0	0
extra-crispy chicken fry	1½ Tbs	60	9	0	0
fish & chips batter	¼ cup	100	20	0	0
fish fry	1½ Tbs	35	6	0	0
funnel cake batter	¼ cup	120	23	9	6
herbs & spices chicken fry	2 Tbs	70	13	0	<1
hot 'n' spicy chicken fry	2 Tbs	50	9	0	0
hush puppy w/onion	¼ cup	130	25	0	0
onion ring batter	¼ cup	100	20	0	1
original home-style chicken fry	2 Tbs	50	9	0	0
seafood fry	1⅔ Tbs	50	9	0	<1
tempura batter	¼ cup	100	20	0	0
Oven Easy/coating					
Cajun-style	¼ cup	90	11	0	0
garlic & herb	3 Tbs	100	13	na	2
lemon & pepper	¼ cup	90	12	0	2
shrimp & seafood	2 Tbs	70	8	0	1
Pre-Dip Egg & Milk Replacement	¼ cup	140	30	1	0.5
(Jiffy) Dry mix only	¼ cup	130	22	1	<1
(Krusteaz) dry mix only					
bake & fry mix	¼ cup	100	20	1	4
baking mix	⅓ cup	180	27	<1	2
tempura mix	¼ cup	110	23	0	0
BAKING BARS, BITS, CHIPS, CHUNKS & PIECES					
(Baker's) baking chocolate					
bars					
bittersweet	½ oz	70	7	1	5
German sweet	½ oz	60	8	<1	8
semisweet	½ oz	40	8	1	7
unsweetened	½ oz	70	4	2	0
white	½ oz	80	9	0	9
chips					
chocolate-flavored..semisweet	½ oz	70	10	0	9
real					
milk chocolate	½ oz	70	9	0	8
semisweet	½ oz	60	8	1	8

Food and Description	Amount	Total Calories	Total Carbs	Fiber	Sugars
chunks					
milk chocolate	½ oz	70	9	0	8
real semisweet	½ oz	60	9	1	8
white chocolate	½ oz	80	9	0	9
dipping chocolate					
real dark semisweet	½ oz	70	9	1	8
real milk	½ oz	80	9	0	8
real semisweet	1 Tbs	70	10	1	8
(Ghirardelli) baking chocolate					
bars					
bittersweet	1.5 oz	210	24	3	18
classic white	1.5 oz	210	25	2	21
dark w/mint	5 squares	190			
milk	½ oz	70	9	1	8
	1.5 oz	130	25	2	21
blocks..all types	3 sections	210	25	2	21
chips..premium					
classic white	2 Tbs	70	9	0	9
milk chocolate	2 Tbs	70	9	1	8
semisweet	2 Tbs	70	9	0	9
(Hershey's)					
bars					
semisweet	½ bar	70	9	1	8
unsweetened	½ bar	90	4	2	0
chips					
butterscotch	1 Tbs	80	10	0	9
chocolate					
milk	1 Tbs	80	9	0	8
mint	1 Tbs	80	10	0	8
semisweet					
mini	1 Tbs	80	9	0	8
regular	1 Tbs	80	10	1	8
cinnamon	1 Tbs	80	9	0	9
Heath bits..toffee..all types	1 Tbs	80	9	0	9
premier white milk	1 Tbs	80	9	0	9
raspberry	1 Tbs	80	10	0	8
Reese's peanut butter	1 Tbs	80	8	1	6
special dark	1 Tbs	80	9	1	8
Kisses..milk chocolate..mini	1 Tbs	80	9	0	8
(M&M * Mars) M&M Baking Bits					
milk chocolate	0.5 oz	70	10	0	9
semisweet chocolate	0.5 oz	70	9	1	8
(Mrs. Fields) premium baking chips					
milk chocolate	1 tsp	70	9	0	8
semisweet	1 tsp	70	9	<1	8
white	1 tsp	70	9	0	9
(Nestlé)					
chunks/real semisweet	½ oz	70	9	0	9
morsels..baking					
butterscotch	1 Tbs	80	10	0	10

Food and Description	Amount	Total Calories	Total Carbs	Fiber	Sugars
chocolate					
milk	1 Tbs	80	9	0	8
mint	1 Tbs	70	9	2	7
peanut butter & milk chocolate	1 Tbs	80	8	0	7
Nestlé Crunch baking pieces					
premier white	1 Tbs	80	9	0	9
semisweet..all styles	1 Tbs	70	9	1	7
(Reese's)					
peanut butter chips	1 Tbs	80	8	1	6
peanut butter cup sprinkles	1 Tbs	80	8	0	7
BAKING CHOCOLATE (*See* BAKING BARS, BITS, CHIPS, CHUNKS & PIECES)					
BAKING POWDER					
(Calumet)	1 tsp	4	0	0	0
(Davis)	1 Tbs	15	0	0	0
BAKING SODA	1 tsp	5	0	0	0
BALSAM PEAR					
pods					
cooked	½ cup	12	3	1	0
raw	½ cup	8	2	1	0
BAMBOO SHOOT (*See also* ASIAN FOOD)					
canned	1 cup	25	4	0	0
fresh					
cooked	½ cup	15	2	<1	0
raw	½ cup	21	4	1	0
BANANA					
dried	¼ cup	90	22	2	20
fresh					
red					
sliced	½ cup	70	18	2	na
whole	1 medium	120	30	3	15
yellow					
mashed	½ cup	105	27	3	15
whole	1 medium	105	27	3	15
(Chiquita)	1 medium	110	29	4	21
(Dole)	1 medium	110	29	4	21
BANANA, COOKING OR BAKING (*See* PLANTAIN/BAKING BANANA/COOKING BANANA)					
BANANA NECTAR/NECTAR BLEND					
(After The Fall) Banana Casablanca	8 fl oz	100	19	0	19
(Kern's/Libby's) nectar	11.5 oz	190	47	0	44
strawberry banana	8 fl oz	150	36	0	33
(R. W. Knudsen) strawberry banana	8 fl oz	120	30	0	27
BARBECUE SAUCE (*See also* SAUCE; SEASONINGS)					
(Annie's Naturals) smoky maple	2 Tbs	45	9	0	5
(Bull's Eye)					
grilled onion w/garlic	2 Tbs	60	14	1	12
honey garlic	2 Tbs	60	14	1	12
original..easy squeeze	~1 oz	60	13	0	12
regular	2 Tbs	60	13	0	11
smokehouse hickory	2 Tbs	60	13	0	12

Food and Description	Amount	Total Calories	Total Carbs	Fiber	Sugars
spicy					
honey	2 Tbs	50	12	0	11
hot	2 Tbs	60	13	0	11
sweet hickory smoke	2 Tbs	60	15	0	13
Texas-style mesquite	2 Tbs	60	13	0	12
(Carb Option) by Lawry's					
hickory	1 Tbs	5	1	0	0
original	2 Tbs	10	3	0	0
(Chicken 'n' Ribs)					
hickory smoke	1 Tbs	45	45	0	11
honey	1 Tbs	50	13	0	12
hot-style	1 Tbs	45	11	0	9
original	1 Tbs	50	11	0	9
(Heinz)					
chicken & rib	2 Tbs	30	9	1	7
garlic	2 Tbs	40	9	0	5
honey garlic	2 Tbs	45	11	0	9
regular	2 Tbs	40	9	1	7
(Hunt's)					
hickory..regular	2 Tbs	45	11	<1	9
hickory & brown sugar	2 Tbs	70	16	1	15
honey					
hickory	2 Tbs	50	12	<1	11
mustard	2 Tbs	50	12	1	10
hot & spicy	2 Tbs	45	11	<1	8
mesquite	2 Tbs	40	9	<1	6
original					
bold	2 Tbs	45	11	<1	9
regular	2 Tbs	50	13	<1	10
(K. C. Masterpiece)					
hickory	2 Tbs	60	13	0	12
honey					
mesquite	2 Tbs	60	13	0	12
original					
regular	2 Tbs	60	15	0	13
spicy original	2 Tbs	60	14	0	10
steakhouse	2 Tbs	60	14	0	10
teriyaki	2 Tbs	60	14	0	10
(Kraft)					
regular					
Char-Grill	2 Tbs	60	13	0	11
hickory smoke					
regular	2 Tbs	40	9	0	7
w/onion bits	2 Tbs	45	11	0	9
honey					
hickory smoke	2 Tbs	60	14	0	12
mustard	2 Tbs	60	13	0	11
roasted garlic	2 Tbs	50	12	0	10
hot					
hickory smoke	2 Tbs	40	9	0	7

Food and Description	Amount	Total Calories	Total Carbs	Fiber	Sugars
regular	2 Tbs	40	9	0	7
Kansas City–style	2 Tbs	50	11	0	9
mesquite smoke	2 Tbs	40	9	0	7
onion bits	2 Tbs	45	11	0	9
original	2 Tbs	40	9	0	7
roasted garlic	2 Tbs	50	12	0	10
spicy					
Cajun	2 Tbs	50	12	0	11
honey	2 Tbs	60	14	0	13
steakhouse-style	2 Tbs	60	14	0	12
Sweet Recipes					
brown sugar	2 Tbs	60	15	0	13
hickory smoke	2 Tbs	60	14	0	13
teriyaki	2 Tbs	60	12	0	10
Thick 'N Spicy					
brown sugar	2 Tbs	60	15	0	13
hickory					
bacon	2 Tbs	60	13	0	11
smoke	2 Tbs	60	12	0	10
honey	2 Tbs	60	13	0	11
Kansas City–style	2 Tbs	50	11	0	9
mesquite smoke	2 Tbs	50	12	0	10
original	2 Tbs	50	12	0	10
(Open Pit)					
Thick & Tangy					
brown sugar & spice	2 Tbs	50	13	0	11
chile lime	2 Tbs	60	14	0	12
original..regular	2 Tbs	50	12	0	9
sweet	2 Tbs	50	13	0	11
(Sweet Baby Ray's)					
hickory	2 Tbs	50	11	0	8
honey	2 Tbs	70	16	0	15
hot	2 Tbs	50	11	0	9
onion	2 Tbs	50	11	0	10
original	2 Tbs	50	11	0	9
sweet	2 Tbs	50	11	0	10
w/pure honey	2 Tbs	40	10	0	9
(Texas Best)					
hickory	2 Tbs	70	16	0	16
original rib style	2 Tbs	50	11	0	10
BARLEY (*See also* CEREAL)					
(Arrowhead Mills)					
flakes/rolled	¼ cup	110	28	5	<1
flour	¼ cup	93	19	3	0
hull-less	¼ cup	140	35	6	0
pearled	¼ cup	170	37	6	<1
(Quaker/Scotch)					
pearled/quick	⅓ cup	170	37	5	0
regular/medium	¼ cup	170	37	5	0

Food and Description	Amount	Total Calories	Total Carbs	Fiber	Sugars
BARLEY MALT..syrup					
(Eden)	1 Tbs	60	14	0	8
BASIL					
DRIED					
crumbled	1 tsp	3	0	0	0
ground	1 tsp	5	1	0	0
(McCormick/Schilling)	¼ tsp	1	<1	0	0
FRESH	2 Tbs	1	<1	0	0
BASS					
freshwater..raw	3 oz	97	0	0	0
mixed species..raw	3 oz	97	0	0	0
striped..cooked—dry heat	3 oz	82	0	0	0
BAY LEAF/crumbled	1 tsp	5	0	0	0
BEAN (*See* individual bean listings)					
BEAN DISH (*See also* BEANS, BAKED & VARIETY; FROZEN ENTRÉE/DINNER; MEXICAN FOOD; individual bean listings)					
CAN, JAR, or MICROWAVE CONTAINER					
(Aunt Nellie's) 3-bean salad	2.3 oz	160	13	2	8
(Green Giant) 3-bean salad	½ cup	90	20	4	10
(Hanover) 3-bean salad	½ cup	100	22	3	10
(S&W) bean salads					
deli-style	½ cup	90	17	6	8
marinated dill garden	½ cup	50	14	3	6
BEAN SPROUTS (*See also* individual bean listings)					
FRESH					
kidney..raw	1 cup	53	8	1	0
mung..mature seeds					
boiled	½ cup	105	19	8	0
raw	1 cup	31	6	2	0
stir-fried	½ cup	31	6	2	0
navy..raw	1 cup	70	14	1	0
pinto					
boiled	4 oz	25	4	0	0
raw	4 oz	70	12	0	0
soy					
boiled	½ cup	38	3	<1	0
raw	10 sprouts	12	1	0	0
	½ cup	3	0	0	0
steamed	1 cup	75	6	1	0
BEANS, BAKED & VARIETY (*See also* BEAN DISH; MEXICAN FOOD)					
(The Allens) baked beans					
barbecue	½ cup	150	29	8	6
home-style	½ cup	130	29	8	6
maple-cured bacon	½ cup	150	29	8	10
onion	½ cup	150	29	8	6
original	½ cup	150	29	8	10
vegetarian	½ cup	130	29	8	6
(Amy's) organic vegetarian baked					
in hearty tomato sauce	½ cup	120	24	6	9

Food and Description	Amount	Total Calories	Total Carbs	Fiber	Sugars
(B&M) baked beans					
bacon & onion w/brown sugar	½ cup	190	36	8	14
barbecue	½ cup	210	42	9	19
maple	½ cup	150	28	6	12
original	½ cup	170	30	6	10
vegetarian	½ cup	150	28	4	12
(Bush's Best) baked beans					
barbecue	½ cup	160	32	6	13
bold & spicy	½ cup	120	24	5	9
Boston recipe	½ cup	170	32	6	6
country-style	½ cup	170	33	7	16
home-style	½ cup	150	28	8	8
maple-cured bacon	½ cup	150	28	7	11
onion	½ cup	150	26	6	6
original	½ cup	150	29	7	5
vegetarian	½ cup	130	24	6	4
(Campbell's) baked beans					
brown sugar & bacon	½ cup	160	28	6	13
pork & beans	½ cup	140	27	7	9
(Hunt's) Big John's Beans & Fixins	½ cup	150	29	8	10
(S&W) baked beans					
barbecue					
country	½ cup	140	28	6	11
honey mustard	½ cup	140	28	6	11
maple syrup	½ cup	150	29	6	13
ranch recipe	½ cup	140	25	8	9
sweet bacon	½ cup	140	29	6	12
(Van Camp's) baked beans					
honey-smoked ham	½ cup	140	29	6	11
pork & beans	½ cup	110	24	6	7
sweet hickory & bacon	½ cup	150	29	8	10
sweet onion w/brown sugar	½ cup	140	29	6	11
BEAR..simmered	4 oz	355	0	0	0
BEAVER..roasted	4 oz	220	0	0	0
BEECHNUT..dried	1 oz	164	9	0	0
BEEF					

(NOTE: All serving sizes are for cooked portions, unless otherwise stated. "Lean" means beef trimmed of separable fat before cooking. "Lean & fat" means untrimmed and cooked or eaten as purchased. In most cases, 4 ounces of raw beef yields approximately 3 ounces cooked. Prime cuts have the most fat; choice cuts less; and select cuts the least amount of fat of all.

■ **BEEF CUTS/FRESH**

brisket/all grades/braised					
flat half					
lean					
0" fat	3 oz	160	0	0	0
¼" fat	3 oz	190	0	0	0
lean & fat					
¼" fat	3 oz	310	0	0	0

Food and Description	Amount	Total Calories	Total Carbs	Fiber	Sugars
whole					
lean					
0" fat	3 oz	185	0	0	0
¼" fat	3 oz	210	0	0	0
lean & fat					
¼" fat	3 oz	330	0	0	0
chuck					
arm pot roast/braised					
lean					
0" fat					
choice	3 oz	187	0	0	0
select	3 oz	170	0	0	0
¼" fat					
choice	3 oz	190	0	0	0
select	3 oz	175	0	0	0
lean & fat					
¼" fat					
choice	3 oz	295	0	0	0
select	3 oz	270	0	0	0
blade roast/braised					
lean					
0" fat					
choice	3 oz	225	0.	0	0
select	3 oz	205	0	0	0
¼" fat					
choice	3 oz	225	0	0	0
select	3 oz	200	0	0	0
lean & fat					
¼" fat					
choice	3 oz	310	0	0	0
select	3 oz	280	0	0	0
corned beef..brisket					
boneless/roasted	3 oz	215	0	0	0
flank/braised					
lean/0" fat/choice	3 oz	175	0	0	0
lean & fat/0" fat/choice	3 oz	195	0	0	0
ground					
extra-lean (17% fat)					
baked					
medium	3 oz	215	0	0	0
well-done	3 oz	235	0	0	0
broiled					
medium	3 oz	215	0	0	0
well-done	3 oz	225	0	0	0
pan-fried					
medium	3 oz	220	0	0	0
well-done	3 oz	225	0	0	0
lean (20% fat)					
baked					
medium	3 oz	230	0	0	0

Food and Description	Amount	Total Calories	Total Carbs	Fiber	Sugars
well-done	3 oz	250	0	0	0
broiled					
medium	3 oz	230	0	0	0
well-done	3 oz	240	0	0	0
pan-fried					
medium	3 oz	235	0	0	0
well-done	3 oz	235	0	0	0
regular (27% fat)					
baked					
medium	3 oz	245	0	0	0
well-done	3 oz	270	0	0	0
broiled					
medium	3 oz	245	0	0	0
well-done	3 oz	250	0	0	0
pan-fried					
medium	3 oz	260	0	0	0
well-done	3 oz	245	0	0	0
loin/top/broiled					
lean					
0" fat					
choice	3 oz	180	0	0	0
¼" fat					
choice	3 oz	185	0	0	0
select	3 oz	165	0	0	0
lean & fat					
¼" fat					
choice	3 oz	255	0	0	0
select	3 oz	225	0	0	0
London broil/100% lean					
choice/broiled	3 oz	167	0	0	0
porterhouse/broiled					
lean					
0" fat					
choice	3 oz	190	0	0	0
select	3 oz	165	0	0	0
lean					
¼" fat					
choice	3 oz	185	0	0	0
select	3 oz	175	0	0	0
lean & fat					
¼" fat					
choice	3 oz	280	0	0	0
select	3 oz	265	0	0	0
rib					
large end/roasted					
lean					
0" fat					
choice	3 oz	215	0	0	0
select	3 oz	190	0	0	0

Food and Description	Amount	Total Calories	Total Carbs	Fiber	Sugars
lean					
¼" fat					
choice	3 oz	205	0	0	0
prime	3 oz	240	0	0	0
select	3 oz	185	0	0	0
lean & fat					
¼" fat					
choice	3 oz	326	0	0	0
select	3 oz	290	0	0	0
small end/broiled					
lean					
0" fat					
choice	3 oz	190	0	0	0
select	3 oz	170	0	0	0
¼" fat					
choice	3 oz	200	0	0	0
select	3 oz	180	0	0	0
lean & fat/					
¼" fat					
choice	3 oz	300	0	0	0
select	3 oz	275	0	0	0
whole/roasted					
lean					
¼" fat					
choice	3 oz	210	0	0	0
select	3 oz	180	0	0	0
lean & fat					
¼" fat					
choice	3 oz	320	0	0	0
select	3 oz	290	0	0	0
rib eye					
small end/broiled	3 oz	190	0	0	0
lean..0" fat					
choice	3 oz	190	0	0	0
lean & fat..0"					
choice	3 oz	260	0	0	0
round					
bottom/roasted					
lean					
0" fat					
choice	3 oz	165	0	0	0
select	3 oz	145	0	0	0
¼" fat					
choice	3 oz	170	0	0	0
select	3 oz	155	0	0	0
lean & fat					
0" fat					
choice	3 oz	175	0	0	0
select	3 oz	150	0	0	0

Food and Description	Amount	Total Calories	Total Carbs	Fiber	Sugars
¼" fat					
choice	3 oz	220	0	0	0
select	3 oz	200	0	0	0
eye of/roasted					
lean					
¼" fat					
choice	3 oz	150	0	0	0
select	3 oz	135	0	0	0
lean & fat					
¼" fat					
choice	3 oz	205	0	0	0
select	3 oz	185	0	0	0
full cut/broiled					
lean					
¼" fat					
choice	3 oz	165	0	0	0
select	3 oz	145	0	0	0
lean & fat					
¼" fat					
choice	3 oz	205	0	0	0
select	3 oz	190	0	0	0
shank crosscuts/simmered					
lean/choice	3 oz	175	0	0	0
lean & fat/¼" fat/choice	3 oz	225	0	0	0
sirloin					
top/broiled					
lean					
0" fat					
choice	3 oz	170	0	0	0
select	3 oz	155	0	0	0
¼" fat					
choice	3 oz	175	0	0	0
select	3 oz	160	0	0	0
lean & fat					
0" fat					
choice	3 oz	195	0	0	0
select	3 oz	165	0	0	0
¼" fat					
choice	3 oz	230	0	0	0
select	3 oz	210	0	0	0
steaks/broiled					
porterhouse/broiled					
lean					
0" fat					
choice	3 oz	190	0	0	0
select	3 oz	165	0	0	0
lean					
¼" fat					
choice	3 oz	185	0	0	0
select	3 oz	175	0	0	0

Food and Description	Amount	Total Calories	Total Carbs	Fiber	Sugars
lean & fat					
⅛" fat					
choice	3 oz	255	0	0	0
select	3 oz	250	0	0	0
¼" fat					
choice	3 oz	275	0	0	0
select	3 oz	265	0	0	0
T-bone/choice					
lean					
choice	3 oz	175	0	0	0
select	3 oz	170	0	0	0
lean & fat/¼" fat	3 oz	265	0	0	0
choice	3 oz	265	0	0	0
select	3 oz	240	0	0	0
tenderloin/roasted..unless noted					
lean					
0" fat...broiled					
choice	3 oz	180	0	0	0
select	3 oz	170	0	0	0
¼" fat					
choice	3 oz	200	0	0	0
select	3 oz	180	0	0	0
½" fat					
prime..short loin	3 oz	220	0	0	0
lean & fat					
¼" fat					
choice	3 oz	290	0	0	0
select	3 oz	275	0	0	0
tip/roasted					
lean					
0" fat					
choice	3 oz	155	0	0	0
select	3 oz	145	0	0	0
¼" fat					
choice	3 oz	160	0	0	0
select	3 oz	155	0	0	0
lean & fat					
¼" fat					
choice	3 oz	210	0	0	0
select	3 oz	190	0	0	0
top/broiled					
lean					
¼" fat					
choice	3 oz	160	0	0	0
select	3 oz	145	0	0	0
½" fat					
select	3 oz	155	0	0	0
lean & fat					
¼" fat					
choice	3 oz	190	0	0	0

Food and Description	Amount	Total Calories	Total Carbs	Fiber	Sugars
select	3 oz	175	0	0	0
■ **BEEF CUTS, LEAN/BRAND NAME**					
(Boar's Head)					
beef/Italian-style/choice	2 oz	80	0	0	0
corned beef brisket/first cut					
cooked..choice	2 oz	80	0	0	0
top round/choice cap-off	2 oz	80	1	0	0
eye of round roasted beef					
Cajun-style seasoned	2 oz	80	0	0	0
pepper-seasoned	2 oz	90	0	0	0
oven-roasted no salt added	2 oz	90	0	0	0
pastrami/choice brisket	2 oz	90	2	0	0
red	2 oz	80	1	0	0
round	2 oz	70	1	0	0
top round/cap off	2 oz	70	0	0	0
top round/deluxe cap off	2 oz	80	<1	0	0
(Coleman Natural Meats) fresh/uncooked					
bottom round steak	4 oz	250	0	0	0
brisket/flat cut	4 oz	330	0	0	0
chuck					
arm roast	4 oz	290	0	0	0
blade roast	4 oz	310	0	0	0
roast					
rib roast (large end)	4 oz	390	0	0	0
tip roast	4 oz	240	0	0	0
steak					
eye of round	4 oz	250	0	0	0
rib steak (small end)	4 oz	360	0	0	0
sirloin	4 oz	260	0	0	0
tenderloin	4 oz	330	0	0	0
top loin	4 oz	300	0	0	0
top round	4 oz	210	0	0	0
(Heinman & Stern)					
corned beef brisket					
bottom round/deli-faced	2 oz	90	0	0	0
choice/whole	4 oz	240	1	0	0
round/whole					
eye of round	2 oz	80	0	0	0
top round	2 oz	80	0	0	0
(Hillshire Farm)					
corned beef brisket (cooked unless otherwise noted)					
choice/whole					
dry	2 oz	130	0	0	0
raw	4 oz	240	4	0	4
mesquite/whole..smoked..choice	3 oz	260	1	0	1
select					
bottom round	2 oz	90	1	0	0
whole/raw	4 oz	230	2	0	2
pastrami/choice..eye of round	2 oz	100	1	<1	0

Food and Description	Amount	Total Calories	Total Carbs	Fiber	Sugars
rib eye					
choice/rare	3 oz	240	1	0	0
select/rare	3 oz	220	1	0	1
round/bottom..select					
medium	2 oz	90	1	0	1
pot roast	3 oz	130	1	0	0
round/top..choice					
medium/split	3 oz	140	1	0	1
medium-well/seasoned	3 oz	100	1	0	0
medium/whole	3 oz	100	1	0	0
(Laura's Lean) (uncooked unless otherwise noted)					
ground beef					
92% lean	4 oz	160	0	0	0
96% lean	4 oz	140	0	0	0
roasts					
eye of round	4 oz	135	0	0	0
pot roast au jus—fully cooked	3 oz	100	1	0	na
top round	4 oz	135	0	0	0
steaks					
flank	4 oz	140	0	0	0
rib eye	4 oz	175	0	0	0
rib eye w/separable					
fat	4 oz	175	0	0	0
sirloin	4 oz	145	0	0	0
strip	4 oz	150	0	0	0
tenderloin fillet	4 oz	145	0	0	0
(Lean & Free) raw					
burger	4 oz	175	0	0	0
rib eye	4 oz	120	0	0	0
round steak	4 oz	110	0	0	0
sirloin steak	4 oz	110	0	0	0
strip steak/loin	4 oz	115	0	0	0
T-bone	4 oz	125	0	0	0
tenderloin steak/fillet	4 oz	120	0	0	0
top round	4 oz	135	0	0	0
■ BEEF CUTS, ORGAN/OTHER					
brain					
fried	3 oz	167	0	0	0
simmered	3 oz	136	0	0	0
heart/braised	3 oz	148	0	0	0
kidney/simmered	3 oz	122	0	0	0
liver					
braised	3 oz	137	0	0	0
fried	3 oz	184	0	0	0
lung/braised	3 oz	102	0	0	0
pancreas/braised	3 oz	232	0	0	0
spleen/braised	3 oz	123	0	0	0
sweetbreads/braised	3 oz	230	0	0	0
thymus/braised	3 oz	273	0	0	0
tongue/simmered	3 oz	241	0	0	0

Food and Description	Amount	Total Calories	Total Carbs	Fiber	Sugars
tripe (Armour Star)/canned	3 oz	90	1	0	0

BEEF, DRIED (*See* MEAT SNACK; individual meat listings)
BEEF BROTH (*See* SOUP)
BEEF DISH/ENTRÉE (*See also* ASIAN FOOD; FROZEN ENTRÉE/DINNER; HAMBURGER; MEXICAN FOOD; PASTA ENTRÉE/DINNER; RICE DISH; individual listings)

CANNED/POUCH/SHELF STAPLE

Food and Description	Amount	Total Calories	Total Carbs	Fiber	Sugars
(Armour Star)					
beef stew	1 cup	210	20	2	0
corned beef hash	1 cup	440	23	2	2
(Castleberry's)					
beef stew	8 oz	340	16	3	2
corned beef hash	7.5 oz	430	25	3	1
(Dinty Moore)					
beef stew	1 cup	180	19	2	3
meatball stew	1 cup	240	17	2	3
(Kid's Kitchen) shelf-staple entrées					
beefy macaroni	1 cup	180	24	2	4
mini beef ravioli	1 cup	240	35	1	6
pizza wedges cheeseburger	1 cup	250	41	3	12
(Mountain House) canned					
beef teriyaki	1 cup	260	44	3	11
chili mac w/beef	1 cup	250	30	5	3
diced beef/cooked	⅔ cup	130	0	0	0
lasagna w/meat sauce	1 cup	220	20	2	8
spaghetti w/meat sauce	1 cup	230	32	2	7
stew					
beef	1 cup	210	24	3	3
vegetable w/beef	1 cup	230	26	4	5
stroganoff w/beef & noodles	1 cup	260	31	2	2
FROZEN					
(Schwan's)					
burgers					
cheeseburger	1 burger	360	29	1	4
chopped beef steak	1 burger	260	0	0	0
ground chuck	1 burger	320	0	0	0
quarter pound	1 burger	200	0	0	0
chopped BBQ beef w/sauce	1 cup	220	17	1	13
creamed chipped beef	1 cup	310	21	7	4
diced beef tips w/gravy	1 cup	240	9	3	1
goulash..home-style	1 cup	280	31	3	5
lasagna/single-serve	1 tray	500	50	4	10
meatballs					
Italian-style	6 pieces	260	6	3	1
Swedish	6 pieces	260	9	3	1
steaks					
battered cubed	1 steak	320	12	0	0
New York strip	1 steak	470	1	0	1
(Tyson)					
beef strips/seasoned	3 oz	140	1	0	1

Food and Description	Amount	Total Calories	Total Carbs	Fiber	Sugars
meatballs					
home-style	6 pieces	240	5	2	0
Italian-style	6 pieces	240	5	1	0
Swedish-style	6 pieces	240	4	1	0
meat loaf/seasoned	5 oz	270	12	1	3
MICROWAVEABLE CONTAINER					
(Dinty Moore)					
American Classics bowls					
beef ravioli	1 bowl	300	34	3	8
beef stew	1 bowl	250	22	2	3
pot roast	1 bowl	200	19	2	3
roast beef w/mashed potatoes	1 bowl	240	24	2	3
Salisbury steak	1 bowl	320	28	3	2
spaghetti w/meatballs	1 bowl	290	44	3	17
MICROWAVEABLE CUPS					
beef stew	1 cup	160	16	2	2
burger stew/hearty	1 cup	240	19	3	5
corned beef hash	1 cup	350	19	2	1
noodles & beef Stroganoff	1 cup	240	16	0	2
(Hormel) micro cup meal..beef stew	1 cup	150	14	2	2
MIX					
(Betty Crocker) Hamburger Helper					
bacon cheeseburger	1 cup	380	23	2	7
beef pasta	1 cup	290	25	2	4
beef Romanoff	1 cup	290	27	0	5
beef stew	1 cup	270	26	2	6
beef taco	1 cup	310	28	1	4
cheddar and broccoli	1 cup	350	27	1	4
cheddar cheese melt	1 cup	310	28	1	7
cheeseburger macaroni	1 cup	350	31	1	7
cheesy hash browns	1 cup	410	38	2	5
cheesy shells	1 cup	330	28	1	5
chili macaroni	1 cup	290	26	1	4
double-cheese pizza	1 cup	330	33	1	7
fettuccini Alfredo	1 cup	320	24	1	5
4-cheese lasagne	1 cup	330	27	1	5
Italian Parmesan Bake/Oven Favorites	1 cup	460	54	2	11
Italian Parmesan w/rigatoni	1 cup	310	29	1	5
lasagna	1 cup	280	26	1	5
lasagna/Oven Favorites	1 cup	290	29	1	7
meat loaf & mashed potatoes/ Oven Favorites	⅙ loaf	360	30	2	5
Philly cheese steak	1 cup	330	24	<1	3
potatoes Stroganoff	1 cup	290	23	2	4
ravioli & cheese	1 cup	320	33	1	7
rice Oriental	1 cup	300	31	0	2
Salisbury	1 cup	280	24	1	3
soft taco bake/Oven Favorites	⅙ cup	420	32	0	2
spaghetti	1 cup	290	24	1	3

Food and Description	Amount	Total Calories	Total Carbs	Fiber	Sugars
Stroganoff	1 cup	330	29	1	7
three cheeses	1 cup	350	30	1	6
zesty Italian	1 cup	300	30	1	7
REFRIGERATED					
(Hormel)					
Always Tender entrées					
peppercorn beef fillet	4 oz	130	2	0	2
tequila lime beef fillet	4 oz	120	3	0	1
teriyaki beef fillet	4 oz	130	4	0	2
beef roast	5 oz	200	3	0	3
beef tips	5 oz	160	5	1	3
beef tips & gravy..family pack	5 oz	160	5	1	3
meat loaf	5 oz	250	13	2	7
sliced beef steak & gravy	5 oz	160	3	0	2
Southwestern shredded beef	2 oz	50	3	0	1
BEEF JERKY STICKS & STRIPS (*See* MEAT SNACKS)					
BEEF SAUSAGE (*See* LUNCHEON MEAT; SAUSAGE)					
BEEF TALLOW	1 Tbs	115	0	0	0
	1 cup	1,849	0	0	0
BEER, ALE & MALT LIQUOR					
(Amstel) light	12 fl oz	95	3	0	0
(Anheuser-Busch)					
Bacardi Silver	12 fl oz	220	35	0	0
Bud					
dry	12 fl oz	130	6.5	0	0
ice	12 fl oz	148	9	0	0
ice light	12 fl oz	110	6.5	0	0
light	12 fl oz	110	9	0	0
Budweiser	12 fl oz	145	10.5	0	0
Busch	12 fl oz	133	10	0	0
ice	12 fl oz	169	12.5	0	0
light	12 fl oz	110	7	0	0
nonalcoholic	12 fl oz	60	11	0	5
Doc's Hard Lemon	12 fl oz	165	16.5	0	0
Hurricane	12 fl oz	158	9.5	0	0
Michelob	12 fl oz	155	13	0	0
amber bock	12 fl oz	166	15	0	0
black and tan	22 oz	168	16	0	0
golden draft	12 fl oz	152	14	0	0
golden draft light	12 fl oz	110	7	0	0
Hefeweizen	12 fl oz	176	17	0	0
honey lager	12 fl oz	175	18	0	na
light	12 fl oz	134	11.5	0	0
ultra	12 fl oz	95	2.5	0	0
Natural					
ice	12 fl oz	157	9	0	0
light	12 fl oz	110	6.5	0	0
O'Doul's					
amber	12 fl oz	90	18	0	0
original	12 fl oz	70	13	0	0

Food and Description	Amount	Total Calories	Total Carbs	Fiber	Sugars
Tequiza	12 fl oz	127	9	0	0
(Blatz)					
LA	12 fl oz	75	6	0	0
light	12 fl oz	110	8	0	<1
regular	12 fl oz	145	13	0	<1
(Blue Moon)					
Belgian white ale	12 fl oz	171	14	0	<1
pumpkin ale	12 fl oz	185	18	0	<1
(Budweiser) (See (Anheuser-Busch) in this section)					
(Busch) (See (Anheuser-Busch) in this section)					
(Carlsberg)					
light	12 fl oz	110	7	0	0
regular	12 fl oz	149	12	0	0
(Colt 45)	12 fl oz	150	14	0	0
(Coors)					
Extra Gold lager	12 fl oz	145	11	0	<1
light	12 fl oz	102	5	0	<1
nonalcoholic	12 fl oz	65	14	0	7
original	12 fl oz	142	11	0	<1
Winterfest	12 fl oz	190	17	0	<1
(Foster's) lager	12 fl oz	140	9	0	0
(George Killian's)..Irish Red	12 fl oz	163	14	0	1
(Guinness)					
extra stout	12 fl oz	192	14	0	na
regular	12 fl oz	160	10	0	0
(Löwenbrau)	12 fl oz	160	14	0	0
(Meister Brau)					
light	12 fl oz	100	4	0	0
regular	12 fl oz	140	13	0	0
(Miller)					
Genuine Draft	12 fl oz	145	13	0	0
High Life	12 fl oz	145	13	0	0
Lite	12 fl oz	95	4	0	0
Magnum	12 fl oz	165	10	0	0
(Old Milwaukee)					
ice	12 fl oz	180	15	0	0
lager	12 fl oz	145	13	9	0
light	12 fl oz	110	8	0	0
(Pabst)					
Blue Ribbon	12 fl oz	135	12	0	0
extra light	12 fl oz	70	6	0	0
light	12 fl oz	110	8	0	0
(Red Stripe) Jamaican ale	12 fl oz	155	14	0	0
(St. Pauli Girl) light	12 fl oz	135	9	0	0
(Stroh's)					
American lager	12 fl oz	145	12	0	0
light	12 fl oz	120	10	0	0
(Zima)					
cherry	12 fl oz	234	30	0	28.5
lemon lime	12 fl oz	231	30	0	27.0

Food and Description	Amount	Total Calories	Total Carbs	Fiber	Sugars
orange	12 fl oz	231	30	0	28.5
BEERWURST (*See* SAUSAGE)					
BEET					
CANNED or JARRED					
(Aunt Nellie's) pickled					
Harvard	⅓ cup	60	14	2	10
ruby red					
sliced	~1 oz	15	4	0	4
whole	~1 oz	20	5	1	4
(Blue Boy)					
Harvard	½ cup	100	27	1	19
pickled					
sliced	½ cup	100	24	1	20
whole	~1 oz	25	6	0	5
(Greenwood)					
Harvard..sweet & tangy					
original recipe	½ cup	100	27	1	19
pickled..sweet & tangy					
original recipe	1 oz	25	6	0	5
(LeSueur) baby/whole	½ cup	35	8	2	5
(Libby's)..with or w/o onion..pickled					
sliced	½ cup	20	8	2	5
whole	½ cup	35	5	<1	5
(S&W)					
pickled..all types	1 oz	15	4	1	3
regular..julienne..all styles	½ cup	30	7	1	6
(Stokely)					
Harvard	~1 oz	25	8	0	4
marinated/sliced	~1 oz	25	6	0	5
pickled	~1 oz	25	6	0	5
regular..all styles	½ cup	40	9	2	7
FRESH					
cooked					
sliced	½ cup	35	8	2	5
whole	2 medium	45	10	2	7
raw					
sliced	½ cup	30	13	4	5
whole	1 medium	35	8	2	5
BERLINER SAUSAGE (*See* SAUSAGE)					
BERRY DRINK/BLEND (*See also* FRUIT PUNCH; SOFT DRINK; SOFT DRINK MIX; individual drink listings)					
BOTTLED, BOXED, or CANNED					
(Fruitopia) all berry flavors	8 fl oz	110	29	0	29
(Hawaiian Punch)					
Berry Blue Typhoon	8 fl oz	120	29	0	29
Bodacious Berry	8 fl oz	110	29	0	28
Green Berry Rush	8 fl oz	120	30	0	29
(Hi-C) Boppin' Berry..drink box	8.45 fl oz	140	33	0	33
(Minute Maid) berry punch drink box	8.45 fl oz	130	31	0	30
(Tropicana) berry punch	8 fl oz	120	29	0	28

Food and Description	Amount	Total Calories	Total Carbs	Fiber	Sugars
FROZEN/PREPARED					
(After The Fall) Oregon berry	8 fl oz	100	19	0	19
(Minute Maid)					
berry punch	8 fl oz	110	31	0	30
mixed berry	6.75 fl oz	100	25	0	23
(Sesame Street) Bert & Ernie's..berry	8 fl oz	120	29	0	25
(Tropicana) smoothie..mixed berry	11 fl oz	250	59	5	46
(V8 Splash) berry blend					
diet	8 fl oz	10	3	0	2
original	8 fl oz	110	27	0	27
BIRCH BEER (*See* SOFT DRINK)					
BISCOTTI (*See* COOKIE)					
BISCUIT (*See also* BAKE & FRY MIX; BREAKFAST SANDWICH)					
FROZEN					
(Bob Evans)					
buttermilk/restaurant recipe	1 biscuit	190	30	0	3
cinnamon..w/icing	1 biscuit	290	42	1	18
(Mary B's) fresh-bake					
buttermilk	1 biscuit	190	20	1	2
jumbo buttermilk	1 biscuit	300	36	2	3
Mexican-style	1 biscuit	280	30	1	4
Southern-made	1 biscuit	190	25	1	2
tea/bite-size	1 biscuit	173	18	1	2
(Rhodes) buttermilk	1 biscuit	200	25	<1	3
(Sister Schubert's)					
angel biscuits..10-count bag	1 biscuit	170	20	<1	2
buttermilk..prebaked	1 biscuit	150	20	<1	1
(White Lily)					
buttermilk or taste of butter	1 biscuit	190	24	1	3
Southern-style	1 biscuit	190	24	1	2
MIX					
(Arrowhead Mills) biscuit mix only	¼ cup	120	23	3	4
(Bisquick) mix only..complete					
buttermilk	⅓ cup	150	21	0	1
cheese garlic	⅓ cup	160	22	0	2
cinnamon swirl	⅓ cup	150	26	0	7
3-cheese	⅓ cup	160	21	0	2
original	⅓ cup	160	25	0	1
pouch mix	½ cup	160	25	0	1
reduced-fat	⅓ cup	150	27	<1	3
(Health Valley) buttermilk..mix only	1 oz	100	20	3	<1
(Jiffy) buttermilk..prepared	1 biscuit	170	29	<1	2
(Krusteaz) all-purpose..prepared.. 2" biscuit	2 biscuits	180	27	<1	2
(Martha White) Quick & Easy					
mix only...all styles	⅓ cup	190	20	1	3
(White Lily) buttermilk	¼ pkt	160	28	1	1
PACKAGED/READY-TO-SERVE					
(Arnold) old-fashioned buttermilk	3 biscuits	190	27	<1	5

Food and Description	Amount	Total Calories	Total Carbs	Fiber	Sugars
(Awrey's) buttermilk..round					
1 oz	2 biscuits	190	29	1	<1
2 oz	1 biscuit	180	29	<1	<1
REFRIGERATED					
(Pillsbury)					
1869/buttermilk	1 biscuit	100	12	0	1
Big Country					
butter tastin'	1 biscuit	100	13	0	2
buttermilk	1 biscuit	100	13	0	2
Southern-style	1 biscuit	100	13	0	2
biscuits					
buttermilk	3 biscuits	150	12	0	1
country	3 biscuits	150	29	1	3
tender layer	3 biscuits	160	27	1	3
Grands!					
butter tastin'	1 biscuit	190	25	1	5
buttermilk					
original	1 biscuit	190	24	1	4
reduced-fat	1 biscuit	170	26	1	4
corn	1 biscuit	190	28	1	8
crescent	1 biscuit	270	22	<1	5
extra-rich	1 biscuit	220	25	1	6
flaky	1 biscuit	200	25	1	3
home-style	1 biscuit	180	24	<1	5
Southern-style	1 biscuit	190	23	<1	5
wheat/reduced-fat	1 biscuit	190	27	2	6
BLACK BEAN					
(Bush's Best)	½ cup	100	20	7	<1
(Eden)					
black soy	½ cup	120	8	7	1
original	½ cup	100	18	6	0
(Fantastic Foods) big cup spicy					
Jamaican w/black beans	½ pkg	190	39	6	8
(Goya) frijoles negros	½ cup	90	16	4	0
(Knorr)					
refried	7.5 oz	140	17	0	0
regular	7.5 oz	190	30	11	2
(Progresso)	½ cup	110	17	7	0
(S&W)..all styles	½ cup	70	17	6	1
(Westbrae)..Heirloom..black beluga	½ cup	100	16	4	0
BLACK CHERRY JUICE/JUICE DRINK					
BOTTLED, BOXED, or CANNED					
(After The Fall) black cherry spritzer	12 fl oz	180	45	0	36
(Knudsen) ..100% juice	8 fl oz	180	43	0	32
BLACK TURTLE BEAN (Hain)	½ cup	100	17	7	0
BLACKBERRY					
CANNED					
(Allens) in light syrup	½ cup	60	13	9	3
(Oregon) in light syrup	½ cup	130	30	6	na

Food and Description	Amount	Total Calories	Total Carbs	Fiber	Sugars
FRESH					
(Allens)	½ cup	40	4	9	na
FROZEN					
(Big Valley)	⅔ cup	70	15	4	8
(Cascadian Farm)	1 cup	80	20	3	10
BLACKBERRY JUICE/JUICE DRINK					
(Smucker's) Mountain Berry blackberry	8 fl oz	140	35	0	33
BLACK-EYED PEA					
CAN..BAG					
(Allens) all styles	½ cup	120	21	6	1
(Allens Sunshine) w/pork	½ cup	120	20	5	0
(Bush's Best)					
jalapeño	½ cup	110	18	5	0
regular	½ cup	100	19	4	0
seasoned w/bacon	½ cup	110	18	5	0
w/snaps	½ cup	110	17	5	0
(Eden) organic	½ cup	90	16	4	1
(Glory) Southern-style	½ cup	60	10	3	<1
(Luck's) seasoned w/pork	½ cup	130	18	3	0
(Trappey's)					
w/bacon	½ cup	120	19	5	3
w/bacon & jalapeño	½ cup	110	19	5	2
FROZEN					
(Birds Eye) McKenzie's field peas all styles	2.66 oz	110	21	4	1
(Veg-All)	3.3 oz	130	40	14	1
BLOOD SAUSAGE (*See* SAUSAGE)					
BLUEBERRY					
CANNED					
(S&W) wild Maine in heavy syrup	⅓ cup	70	16	0	na
DRIED					
(Frieda's)	? cup	140	33	4	17
(Sonoma)	? cup	140	33	4	17
FRESH	1 pint	225	55	11	na
FROZEN					
(Big Valley)	⅔ cup	70	12	4	8
(C&W)	¾ cup	70	17	4	12
(Cascadian Farm)	1 cup	90	22	2	11
BLUEBERRY JUICE/NECTAR					
(After The Fall) Maine Coast	8 fl oz	90	25	0	19
(Knudsen) nectar	8 fl oz	130	30	0	29
(Walnut Acres) organic	8 fl oz	130	31	<1	28
BOLOGNA (*See* LUNCHEON MEAT)					
BORAGE					
FRESH					
cooked	½ cup	25	4	0	0
raw	½ cup	9	1.5	<1	0
BORSCHT (*See* SOUP)					

Food and Description	Amount	Total Calories	Total Carbs	Fiber	Sugars
BOYSENBERRY					
CANNED					
in heavy syrup	½ cup	115	28	3.5	na
in light syrup	½ cup	120	27	3	na
FROZEN..no sugar added	1 cup	66	16	5	na
BOYSENBERRY JUICE/NECTAR					
(Knudsen) nectar	8 fl oz	110	33	0	30
(Smucker's) juice	8 fl oz	120	30	0	30
BRAN (*See* CEREAL)					
BRANDY (*See* LIQUEUR)					
BRATWURST (*See* SAUSAGE)					
BRAZIL NUT					
(Best Yet)	1.5 oz	260	4	2	1
(Diamond)	1 oz	190	4	2	1
BREAD (*See also* BAGEL; BISCUIT; BREADSTICK; CROISSANT; MUFFIN; ROLL)					
■ **BROWN & SERVE**					
(Arnold) San Francisco sourdough	1 oz	70	15	1	0
(Colombo) French					
extra-sour	2 oz	150	27	0	0
sweet	2 oz	70	13	1	1
(Earth Grains) Bake & Serve International French Bread					
premium roasted garlic	1 piece	130	28	1	1
(Fisherman's Wharf) sour French	½ slice	120	25	0	0
(San Francisco) sourdough					
baguette	¼ roll	140	29	0	0
French bread	⅛ loaf	290	29	1	1
■ **CANNED**					
(B&M) all styles	½" slice	130	29	2	15
■ **FROZEN**					
(Bridgeford)					
white	1 oz	75	14	0	2
white..enriched	2 oz	150	28	0	2
w/honey	2 oz	150	27	0	3
(Mama Bella)					
garlic bread..home-style.. 5 servings	1" slice	150	16	1	0
home-style Parmesan	1" slice	160	17	1	0
garlic toast					
cheese/9-count	1 piece	190	17	1	0
5-cheese/8-count	1 piece	200	18	0	0
traditional/9-count	1 piece	140	16	1	0
(Marie Callender's)					
garlic..original	1 piece	190	23	2	1
Parmesan Romano	1 piece	200	23	2	1
(Marzetti)					
garlic breadstick	1 stick	180	29	1	3
original	2 1" slices	190	29	1	1
reduced-fat	2 1" slices	160	29	1	1

Food and Description	Amount	Total Calories	Total Carbs	Fiber	Sugars
Texas garlic toast					
6-carb	1-oz slice	120	7	1	0
Parmesan	1" slice	190	19	1	1
w/cheese	1" slice	180	17	1	1
w/5 cheeses	1" slice	200	18	0	0
w/o cheese	1" slice	170	16	1	1
(New York)					
garlic breadstick	1 stick	180	29	1	3
original	2 1" slices	190	29	1	1
reduced-fat	2 1" slices	160	29	1	1
Texas garlic toast					
6-carb	1-oz slice	120	7	1	0
Parmesan	1" slice	190	19	1	1
w/cheese	1" slice	180	17	1	1
w/5 cheeses	1" slice	200	18	0	0
w/o cheese	1" slice	170	16	1	1
(Pepperidge Farm)					
garlic	⅛ loaf	160	14	1	0
garlic & olive oil					
garlic Parmesan	⅛ loaf	160	20	2	1
loaves/reduced-fat..½" slice	2 slices	170	15	1	1
(Rhodes) dough/baked					
sweet	1 slice	145	24	1	3
wheat	1 slice	130	24	2	2
white	1 slice	140	24	2	2
(Schwan's)					
cheese-stuffed bread..w/sauce	3" wedge	160	20	1	6
French bread..5-cheese garlic	1 piece	330	26	1	1
ready-to-heat French baguette	¼ loaf	120	25	1	1
■ MIX					
(Arrowhead Mills) mix only					
corn bread	¼ cup	120	24	4	3
multigrain	⅓ cup	160	31	3	0
rye	⅓ cup	160	33	3	0
spelt	⅓ cup	150	31	5	0
white	⅓ cup	150	31	2	0
whole wheat	⅓ cup	150	31	5	0
(Betty Crocker) prepared					
golden corn muffin mix..pouch	1 muffin	190	27	1	19
Quick Bread mixes..pouch					
banana	1 slice	170	25	0	13
cinnamon streusel	1 slice	180	28	0	15
cranberry	1 slice	160	29	0	26
lemon poppy seed	1 slice	170	25	0	12
(Calhoun Bend Mill) mix only					
corn bread & muffin	3 Tbs	100	24	2	2
honey butter..corn bread	3 Tbs	108	21	2	8
Mexican/mix only	3 Tbs	110	23	2	2

Food and Description	Amount	Total Calories	Total Carbs	Fiber	Sugars
(Eagle Mills) bread machine mixes..mix only					
breakfast					
apple walnut	1/12 pkg	150	24	1	6
cinnamon sunrise	1/12 pkg	150	26	2	8
harvest fruit	1/12 pkg	140	26	1	8
classic Italian	1/9 pkg	160	29	1	2
country French	1/9 pkg	160	29	1	2
dessert					
chocolate nugget	1/12 pkg	150	26	1	7
lemon poppy seed	1/12 pkg	140	25	1	6
harvest wheat	1/11 pkg	140	28	3	4
hearty multigrain	1/11 pkg	150	28	2	4
home-style white	1/9 pkg	160	39	1	5
honey oat	1/11 pkg	150	28	1	5
Old World rye	1/11 pkg	150	26	2	2
San Francisco sourdough	1/9 pkg	160	29	1	2
(Krusteaz) bread machine mixes..prepared					
CarbSimple/prepared					
classic wheat	1/12 loaf	140	16	7	0
cornbread/home-style	1 piece	160	21	4	1
country white	1/12 loaf	140	16	7	0
cornbread/honey	1 piece	120	27	1	8
cornbread & muffin/fat-free honey	1 slice	120	20	1	6
cinnamon raisin	1 slice	180	35	2	10
honey wheat berry	1 slice	150	28	1	5
Italian herb	1 slice	150	28	1	5
oat bran	1 slice	150	26	3	4
savory rye	1 slice	150	29	2	5
sourdough	1 slice	150	28	1	5
12-grain	1 slice	170	31	2	6
wheat/cracked	1 slice	150	28	1	5
white/country	1 slice	150	28	1	5
(Marie Callender's) corn bread..mix only	1/4 cup	150	26	1	6
(Martha White) corn bread..prepared					
buttermilk	1 piece	130	23	1	3
cheddar cheese	1 piece	130	28	1	4
Cotton Pickin' buttermilk	1 piece	130	23	1	3
enriched					
white self-rising	1 piece	110	22	2	0
yellow self-rising	1 piece	110	23	2	1
gladiola yellow	1 piece	110	19	0	2
Mexican	1 piece	110	19	1	1
plain enriched yellow	1 piece	120	25	2	1
sweet yellow	1 piece	140	24	0	8
(Pillsbury) mix only					
quick bread & muffin mix					
apple cinnamon	1/12 pkg	130	27	1	16
banana	1/12 pkg	130	26	1	14
blueberry	1/14 pkg	110	24	1	13
cinnamon swirl	1/12 pkg	180	32	0	20

Food and Description	Amount	Total Calories	Total Carbs	Fiber	Sugars
cranberry	⅟₁₂ pkg	140	30	1	16
lemon poppy seed	⅟₁₂ pkg	150	28	1	14
pecan swirl	⅟₁₂ pkg	180	30	0	17
pumpkin	⅟₁₂ pkg	130	27	1	14
(Shawnee Mills) mix only					
Mexican	⅕ pkg	130	23	3	1
traditional	⅕ pkg	120	21	1	1
yellow buttermilk	⅕ pkg	130	25	2	1
■ PACKAGED/READY-TO-SERVE					
(Alvarado Street)					
bakery sprouted barley	1 slice	70	15	2	3
California-style	1 slice	60	10	2	1
French	1 slice	80	15	2	2
multigrain	1 slice	60	11	2	2
oat berry	1 slice	70	13	2	2
raisin	1 slice	80	15	2	6
rye seed	1 slice	60	11	2	1
sourdough	1 slice	80	15	2	2
soy crunch	1 slice	70	11	2	1
whole wheat	1 slice	90	18	3	3
(Arnold)					
Arnold Brand Brick Oven					
100% whole wheat	1 slice	130	25	1	4
cinnamon French toast	1 slice	100	15	1	4
country					
buttermilk	1 slice	110	21	1	4
potato	1 slice	110	21	1	3
wheat	1 slice	110	20	2	4
white enriched	1 slice	110	21	1	4
Health Nut	1 slice	110	20	2	3
healthy multigrain	1 slice	120	24	3	4
honey wheat berry	1 slice	110	21	2	4
marble rye & pumpernickel	1 slice	90	16	1	1
Master's Best					
3-seed	1 slice	100	14	2	3
winter wheat	1 slice	100	14	3	3
natural					
oat	1 slice	90	17	3	3
100% whole wheat					
low-fat	1 slice	80	19	5	3
9-grain	1 slice	100	18	3	3
oat nut	1 slice	110	19	1	4
oatmeal..low-fat	1.5 oz	80	21	4	3
100% whole wheat stone-ground	1 slice	70	12	2	2
potato/soft	1 slice	110	22	1	3
pumpernickel	1 slice	80	15	1	1
raisin cinnamon	1 slice	90	15	1	7
rye..Jewish caraway..seeded	1 slice	80	15	1	1
melba thin/real	2 slices	110	21	1	2
rye..Jewish..w/o seeds	2 slices	80	15	1	1

Food and Description	Amount	Total Calories	Total Carbs	Fiber	Sugars
sandwich sesame	1 slice	130	22	1	3
7-grain	1 slice	100	20	2	4
12-grain	1 slice	110	21	2	4
Bran'nola					
country oat	1 slice	100	19	3	3
honey wheat berry	1 slice	80	13	2	0
nutty grains	1 slice	90	14	3	0
original	1 slice	90	18	3	3
7-grain white	1 slice	90	20	3	<1
12-grain wheat	1 slice	110	19	3	3
dark	1 slice	90	15	3	0
hearty	1 slice	100	15	3	0
Francisco International					
French bread/sliced	1 slice	120	22	1	1
French stick	1 oz	70	12	2	2
Italian bread/sliced	2 slices	100	20	1	4
sheepherders	1 slice	110	21	1	2
sourdough/24-oz loaf	1 slice	90	19	1	0
Levy's					
melba thin-sliced rye	2 slices	90	16	<1	0
pumpernickel	1 slice	80	15	1	0
Real Jewish Rye					
w/caraway seeds	1 slice	90	16	1	1
w/o seeds	1 slice	90	16	1	1
(Awrey's) fruit breads					
blueberry	1 slice	250	31	<1	15
lemon poppy seed	1 slice	270	32	<1	16
orange walnut	1 slice	270	32	<1	16
(Brownberry)					
Brick Oven					
100% whole wheat	1 slice	130	25	1	4
cinnamon French toast	1 slice	100	15	1	4
country					
buttermilk	1 slice	110	21	1	4
potato	1 slice	110	21	1	3
wheat	1 slice	110	20	2	4
white enriched	1 slice	110	21	1	4
Health Nut	1 slice	110	20	2	3
healthy multigrain	1 slice	120	24	3	4
honey wheat berry	1 slice	110	21	2	4
marble rye & pumpernickel	1 slice	90	16	1	1
Master's Best					
3-seed	1 slice	100	14	2	3
winter wheat	1 slice	100	14	3	3
natural					
oat	1 slice	90	17	3	3
100% whole wheat					
low-fat	1 slice	80	19	5	3
9-grain	1 slice	100	18	3	3
100% whole wheat stone-ground	1 slice	70	12	2	2

Food and Description	Amount	Total Calories	Total Carbs	Fiber	Sugars
oatmeal..low-fat	1.5 oz	80	21	4	3
oat nut	1 slice	110	19	1	4
potato/soft	1 slice	110	22	1	3
premium/white					
enriched	1 slice	130	22	1	4
low-fat	1.5 oz	80	21	4	3
pumpernickel	1 slice	80	15	1	1
raisin cinnamon	1 slice	90	15	1	7
rye..Jewish caraway..seeded	1 slice	80	15	1	1
melba thin/real	2 slices	110	21	1	2
rye..w/o seeds	2 slices	80	15	1	1
sandwich sesame	1 slice	130	22	1	3
7-grain	1 slice	100	20	2	4
12-grain	1 slice	110	21	2	4
Bran'nola					
country oat	1 slice	100	19	3	3
honey wheat berry	1 slice	80	13	2	0
nutty grains	1 slice	90	14	3	0
original	1 slice	90	18	3	3
7-grain white	1 slice	90	20	3	<1
12-grain	1 slice	110	19	3	3
wheat					
dark	1 slice	90	15	3	0
hearty	1 slice	100	15	3	0
Francisco International					
French bread/sliced	1 slice	120	22	1	1
French stick	1 oz	70	12	2	2
Italian bread/sliced	2 slices	100	20	1	4
sheepherders	1 slice	110	21	1	2
sourdough/24-oz loaf	1 slice	90	19	1	0
Levy's					
melba thin-sliced rye	2 slices	90	16	<1	0
pumpernickel	1 slice	80	15	1	0
Real Jewish Rye					
w/caraway seeds	1 slice	90	16	1	1
w/o seeds	1 slice	90	16	1	1
wheat					
dark	1 slice	90	15	3	0
hearty	1 slice	100	15	3	0
(CarbXtract)					
cinnamon raisin	1 slice	76	6	1.5	0
cinnamon raisin swirl	1 slice	51	6	1.5	0
cornmeal-crusted	1 slice	42	6	1.5	0
French	1 slice	42	6	1.5	0
marble rye & pumpernickel	1 slice	42	6	1.5	0
multigrain	1 slice	42	6	1.5	0
pumpernickel	1 slice	42	6	1.5	0
rye	1 slice	76	6	1.5	0
sourdough	1 slice	42	6	1.5	0
wheat	1 slice	42	6	1.5	0

Food and Description	Amount	Total Calories	Total Carbs	Fiber	Sugars
Xbread	1 slice	69	7	1.5	0
(D'Italiano) enriched real Italian					
light	1.6 oz	40	9	2	5
original	1.6 oz	70	12	0	1
(Earth Grains)					
100% stone-ground whole wheat	1 slice	100	20	2	4
buttermilk..premium	1 slice	120	20	1	4
French bread..premium	2 oz	130	28	1	1
gold'n bran	1 slice	70	12	0	na
honey oat & nut	1 slice	80	14	0	na
honey wheat berry..premium	1 slice	100	19	2	2
honey whole grain	1 slice	120	20	1	4
oat & nut..premium	1 slice	120	20	1	4
rye..light..very thin slices	1 oz	70	14	0	<1
(Father Sam's)..pocket bread					
onion	1 pita	130	27	1	5
wheat					
medium	½ pita	120	25	2	3
mini	1 pita	100	22	2	3
white					
medium	½ pita	110	27	<1	3
mini	1 pita	110	24	<1	3
wraps (10")..all flavors	1 wrap	160	26	1	1
white	1 wrap	160	25	<1	<1
(Francisco International)					
French..sliced	1 slice	120	22	1	1
Italian..sliced	1 slice	100	20	1	4
sheepherders	1 slice	110	21	1	2
(Freihofer's)					
100% whole wheat stone-ground	1 slice	90	17	3	3
12-grain	1 slice	120	23	2	4
Canadian white	1 slice	110	21	1	3
country					
potato	1 slice	100	19	1	3
white	1 slice	100	19	1	2
hearty nut	1 slice	120	22	2	3
Italian					
rye..no seeds	1 slice	70	14	1	1
soft sourdough	1 slice	90	16	1	1
(Garden of Eatin')					
Bible bread/pita					
original	1 pita	160	31	2	1
very low salt	1 pita	160	30	1	1
Chapati Indian					
flatbread	1 piece	120	29	2	<1
(Home Pride)					
buttermilk & biscuit white	1 slice	100	18	<1	2
golden grain	1 slice	70	13	2	2
hearty					
deli rye	1 slice	140	26	3	1

Food and Description	Amount	Total Calories	Total Carbs	Fiber	Sugars
golden honey wheat	1 slice	90	18	2	2
oats & cracked wheat	1 slice	100	19	2	2
stone-ground..100% whole wheat	1 slice	90	18	3	2
(Iron Kids) all styles	1 slice	60	13	2	2
(J. J. Nissen)					
butter top	1 slice	100	19	1	4
oatmeal	1 slice	70	13	1	2
Canadian					
brown	1 slice	100	19	1	4
multigrain	1 slice	110	20	2	3
white	1 slice	100	19	1	4
original recipe..giant loaf	1 slice	70	13	0	1
potato	1 slice	90	18	0	2
sourdough	1 slice	160	17	0	1
split top					
wheat	1 slice	70	14	0	2
white	1 slice	80	14	0	1
wheat	1 slice	70	13	1	2
(Kangaroo) pocket/pita bread					
bread wraps/white	1 wrap	190	35	3	0
breakfast pita					
4" mini/whole wheat	1 pita	70	12	4	1
Greek pita flatbread					
white	1 pita	145	30	3	1
whole wheat	1 pita	145	30	3	1
pita pocket					
onion	1 pocket	90	18	1	1
wheat 'n' honey	1 pocket	90	16	4	1
white	1 pocket	90	18	1	1
salad pocket					
wheat 'n' honey	1 pocket	80	18	1	1
white	1 pocket	90	18	1	1
(King of Pita)					
gyros	1 pita	250	45	5	6
thyme	1 slice	180	34	3	<1
(King's Hawaiian) center slice	½" slice	180	29	2	7
(Labrea Bakery)					
French					
baguette	2 oz	130	27	<1	<1
loaf	4" slice	130	27	<1	<1
Italian boule	⅛ loaf	130	27	<1	<1
organic wheat	1/12 loaf	150	35	2	<1
pain rustique	⅛ loaf	160	30	2	<1
pecan raisin	⅛ loaf	180	21	2	6
roasted garlic	⅛ loaf	130	25	<1	<1
rosemary olive oil	2 oz	140	23	0	<1
seeded rye	1/12 loaf	120	25	3	2
sourdough baguette	⅛ loaf	150	31	1	1
Tuscan Italian	⅛ loaf	170	32	2	1
whole grain	1/12 loaf	130	25	2	3

Food and Description	Amount	Total Calories	Total Carbs	Fiber	Sugars
Levy's (*See* (Arnold); (Brownberry) in this section)					
(Monk's Bread)					
cinnamon	1 slice	70	10	0	na
golden rice bran	1 slice	70	14	2	na
raisin	1 slice	70	10	0	na
sunflower & bran	1 slice	60	11	2	0
white	1 slice	60	12	2	2
whole wheat..100% stone-ground	1 slice	70	13	0	1
(Natural Ovens)					
100% whole grain	1 slice	80	15	4	1
7-grain herb	1 slice	90	13	2	1
Better White	1 slice	80	19	2	1
cracked wheat	1 slice	80	19	2	1
English muffin bread	1 slice	80	16	1	2
Glorious Cinnamon Raisin	1 slice	70	16	2	4
Golden Crunch Carb Conscious	1 slice	80	7	4	2
Golden Crunch..low-carb	1 slice	70	7	4	2
Happiness Raisin Pecan	1 slice	80	15	2	4
Health Max	1 slice	80	15	2	2
Hunger Filler	1 slice	60	13	4	1
mild rye	1 slice	70	13	4	0
multigrain	1 slice	60	13	4	1
Nutty Natural	1 slice	70	13	3	1
oatmeal	1 slice	80	16	2.5	2
original..low-carb	1 slice	60	8	5	2
Right Wheat	1 slice	60	13	4	1
Soft Wheat Carb Conscious	1 slice	70	9	4	1
Sunny Millet	1 slice	70	13	4	1
(Nature's Path) manna bread					
carrot raisin	1 slice	130	27	5	10
cinnamon date	1 slice	150	29	5	10
fruit & nut	1 slice	140	27	6	16
millet rice	1 slice	130	28	6	9
multigrain	1 slice	130	26	4	9
sun seed	1 slice	160	29	7	11
whole rye	1 slice	150	32	5	7
whole wheat	1 slice	150	32	5	7
(Oroweat)					
Oroweat					
carb counting					
100% whole wheat	1 slice	60	9	3	1
multigrain	1 slice	60	9	3	1
whole wheat & oat	1 slice	60	18	3	3
natural					
100% whole wheat	1 slice	100	18	3	3
100% whole wheat & oat	1 slice	100	18	3	3
raisin cinnamon swirl	1 slice	120	22	2	9
Schwarzwalder dark rye	1 slice	70	13	<1	<1
(Panera) breads					
artisan breads					

Food and Description	Amount	Total Calories	Total Carbs	Fiber	Sugars
3-cheese	2 oz	120	21	<2	1
3-seed	2 oz	130	23	1	1
country	2 oz	120	25	1	1
French	2 oz	110	23	<1	1
Kalamata olive	2 oz	140	26	1	1
multigrain	2 oz	120	24	1	1
raisin pecan	1 oz	140	25	1	5
sesame semolina	2 oz	120	24	1	1
Asiago cheese					
demi loaf	2 oz	140	21	<1	1
ciabatta	6 oz	430	70	3	2
cinnamon raisin	2 oz	160	31	1	12
focaccia					
Asiago cheese	2 oz	150	19	1	1
rosemary & onion	2 oz	140	19	1	1
holiday bread	2 oz	150	33	<1	23
honey wheat berry	2 oz	140	25	1	3
Lower Carb					
golden original	1.2 oz	80	10	4	0
Italian herb	1.1 oz	80	10	4	0
breadstick	1.2 oz	120	13	7	0
pumpkin	1.1 oz	90	9	4	0
rosemary walnut	1.1 oz	80	9	5	0
rye	2 oz	140	25	1	3
sourdough					
2-oz slice	1 slice	120	28	1	1
baguette	2 oz	120	28	1	1
soup bowl	8 oz	500	102	4	2
sunflower	2 oz	160	24	1	4
tomato basil	2 oz	130	27	1	1
(Panne) Provincio					
black bean & salsa	⅛ loaf	130	27	2	1
country Italian	⅛ loaf	130	28	1	<1
rye..organic peasant	⅛ loaf	130	29	2	<1
sesame semolina..organic	⅛ loaf	140	29	1	<1
(Pepperidge Farm)					
banana swirl	1 slice	90	15	<1	5
cinnamon					
raisin	1 slice	80	14	1	6
swirl	1 slice	90	14	2	4
deli swirl	1 slice	80	15	1	<1
family pumpernickel	1 slice	80	15	2	<1
Farmhouse Hearty Slices					
buttermilk wheat	1 slice	120	21	1	4
butter-topped wheat	1 slice	110	21	2	3
country wheat	1 slice	110	21	2	3
crunchy oat	1 slice	110	19	2	2
sesame wheat	1 slice	110	19	2	2
7-grain	1 slice	110	20	2	3
white	1 slice	110	22	1	3

Food and Description	Amount	Total Calories	Total Carbs	Fiber	Sugars
French toast swirl					
brown sugar & cinnamon	1 slice	140	25	1	8
French vanilla	1 slice	140	23	<1	7
maple syrup & cinnamon	1 slice	130	25	2	7
hot & crusty bread					
garlic	2" slice	170	21	1	2
italian	2" slice	150	28	1	1
thin-sliced French	2 slices	150	29	1	<1
twin French	4" slice	15-	20	1	2
Italian bread	1 slice	90	15	<1	1
Jewish rye party bread	5 slices	120	25	3	2
large sandwich white	2 slices	150	27	0	3
Lifeworks					
wheat bread	2 slices	170	27	3	1
white bread	2 slices	170	28	2	3
light-style					
oatmeal	3 slices	140	27	2	2
7-grain	3 slices	140	27	2	3
wheat	3 slices	130	27	3	3
white	3 slices	140	27	3	3
natural whole grain					
multigrain	1 slice	90	15	3	2
oatmeal raisin	1 slice	60	11	1	1
original white/thin	1 slice	70	13	0	2
party pumpernickel	5 slices	130	24	3	2
rye					
seeded	1 slice	80	15	2	<1
seedless	1 slice	80	15	1	<1
very thin sliced					
white	3 slices	120	24	1	2
whole wheat	3 slices	120	21	3	2
white sandwich bread	2 slices	130	23	<1	3
whole wheat	1 slice	70	11	2	1
(Rubschlager)					
bagel bread	1 slice	90	16	2	2
cocktail breads					
honey whole grain	3 slices	80	14	2	2
pumpernickel	3 slices	80	14	2	2
rye	3 slices	80	14	2	2
regular					
pumpernickel Danish	1 slice	70	14	2	1
Westphalian	1 slice	70	14	2	1
rye sandwich	1 slice	90	17	2	2
Rye-ola sunflower bread	1 slice	100	19	3	2
sandwich					
pumpernickel	1 slice	90	17	2	2
stone-ground honey-wheat	1 slice	90	17	2	2
whole grain..European-style	1 slice	70	14	3	1

(Sahara) (*See* (Thomas') in this section)
(San Francisco) French Bread

Food and Description	Amount	Total Calories	Total Carbs	Fiber	Sugars
breadsticks					
garlic	1 stick	110	21	0	1
regular	1 stick	110	21	0	1
breadsticks/sourdough	1 stick	140	28	1	1
cheddar cheese	⅕ loaf	170	22	1	0
ciabatta	⅐ loaf	140	29	1	1
Fisherman's Wharf French bread					
extra sour	1 slice	110	22	0	0
sour	1 slice	110	21	1	0
focaccia	⅛ loaf	150	27	0	1
French, sweet loaf..stick	⅒ loaf	120	23	0	1
Le Bout/sourdough	⅜ slice	140	30	1	1
Old Italy					
bread stick	1/16 stick	140	28	1	2
sliced	1 slice	70	15	0	1
pesto garlic	⅕ loaf	190	23	1	1
Pugliese	⅕ loaf	140	29	1	1
rye/light	2 slices	120	23	1	1
sheepherders sourdough	1 slice	110	21	0	1
cracked wheat	1 slice	100	21	0	0
cracked wheat bâtard	1 slice	120	25	0	0
squaw bread	1 slice	120	22	1	3
wheat bread					
cracked	1 slice	70	13	1	2
regular	1 slice	70	14	0	2
wheat berry	2 slices	130	24	0	4
white bread	1 slice	80	14	0	2
(Sara Lee)					
Delightful..white or whole wheat	1 slice	45	9	2	<1
Heart Healthy 100% whole wheat					
classic	1 slice	70	13	2	2
home-style	1 slice	100	20	2	3
multigrain	1 slice	100	19	2	4
Heart Healthy Plus 100% whole wheat					
regular	1 slice	80	14	4	3
w/honey	1 slice	110	19	5	4
(Spring Mill)					
cinnamon	1.5 oz	100	22	1	4
honey & oats	1.5 oz	100	21	3	4
honey whole wheat	1.5 oz	90	21	3	4
Italian tomato	1.5 oz	90	20	2	2
onion dill	1.5 oz	100	22	3	4
peasant white	1.5 oz	100	21	1	2
7-grain..pan-shaped	1.5 oz	100	20	3	<1
spinach feta	1.5 oz	90	18	2	2
(Sun Maid) raisin cinnamon swirl	1 slice	90	17	1	8
(Thomas')					
cinnamon loaves..swirl/toasting	1 slice	130	20	1	6
cinnamon loaves..swirl/toasting raisin	1 slice	120	22	1	10

Food and Description	Amount	Total Calories	Total Carbs	Fiber	Sugars
Sahara pita bread					
Carb Counting					
original	1 pita	90	20	10	0
wheat	1 pita	90	20	10	1
whole wheat	1 pita	140	27	5	2
white					
mini..8 per pkg	1 pita	80	16	1	1
regular..6 per pkg	1 pita	160	32	1	2
whole wheat					
mini..8 per pkg	1 pita	60	13	2	1
regular..6 per pkg	1 pita	130	27	5	2
Sahara wraps					
Carb Counting					
original..6 per pkg	1 wrap	110	18	8	<1
wheat..6 per pkg	1 wrap	110	18	8	<1
white..6 per pkg	1 wrap	170	29	1	1
whole wheat..6 per pkg	1 wrap	170	27	4	1
(Toufayan)					
breadsticks/Grissini-style					
cheese	3 sticks	50	9	1	1
garlic	3 sticks	50	10	1	1
plain	3 sticks	50	10	1	1
flatbread					
corn & jalapeño	1 flat	210	40	2	1
Mediterranean	1 flat	270	37	1	1
pita pockets					
mini petites..regular or whole wheat	4 pieces	70	16	1	1
regular	½ pocket	110	23	1	1
(Wenner)					
corn rye	2 sices	120	27	2	1
focaccia	2 slices	140	24	<1	<1
onion pita pockets	1 pocket	150	25	1	4
scala..large	2 slices	130	26	<1	<1
(Wolferman's)					
English muffin breads					
cinnamon & raisin	1 slice	130	26	1	7
cranberry citrus	1 slice	130	27	1	5
1910 original	2 slices	120	24	4	1
San Francisco sourdough	1 slice	120	25	<1	<1
tea breads					
apple strudel	1 slice	160	28	<1	17
banana nut	⅛ loaf	190	26	1	14
gingerbread	⅛ loaf	230	31	0	20
tangy lemon	⅛ loaf	150	21	0	2
(Wonder)					
Beefsteak					
cinnamon raisin	1 slice	70	12	0	5

Food and Description	Amount	Total Calories	Total Carbs	Fiber	Sugars
French					
granola	1 slice	100	19	2	2
light-style	2 slices	80	18	5	<1
regular	1 slice	80	15	<1	1
pumpernickel	1 slice	70	13	1	0
rye					
hearty	1 slice	70	13	1	<1
light/soft	2 slices	70	17	5	2
mild	2 slices	90	18	2	1
soft	1 slice	70	13	1	0
wheat					
hearty	1 slice	70	13	1	<1
soft	1 slice	70	13	1	<1
white robust	1 slice	70	13	<1	<1
Home Pride					
7-grain	1 slice	60	12	1	<1
7-grain multigrain	1 slice	100	17	2	1
golden honey wheat	1 slice	90	18	2	2
honey oats & cracked wheat	1 slice	100	19	2	2
honey wheat	1 slice	70	14	1	1
potato	1 slice	70	13	0	2
wheat	1 slice	80	14	1	2
white	1 slice	70	13	<1	2
whole wheat..stone-ground	1 slice	90	18	3	2
Italian					
family	1 slice	70	13	0	1
light	2 slices	80	19	5	2
regular	1 slice	80	15	<1	1
seeded	1 slice	70	13	0	1
oatmeal..light	2 slices	90	19	4	2
rye					
light	2 slices	70	17	5	2
regular	1 slice	70	13	1	<1
sourdough					
light	2 slices	80	18	5	<1
regular	1 slice	90	17	<1	1
Texas toast	1 slice	100	19	1	1
■ REFRIGERATED					
(Bread du Jour)					
Austrian wheat	3" slice	130	26	2	2
breadstick	1 stick	130	25	1	3
twin French loaves	3" slice	130	26	1	2
(Pillsbury)					
breadsticks					
cornbread twists	1 twist	130	17	0	4
crusty French loaf	⅓ pkg	150	27	<1	3
garlic w/herbs	2 pieces	160	25	<1	3
original	2 pieces	140	25	1	3
Parmesan w/garlic	2 pieces	180	24	<1	3
French loaf	⅙ loaf	150	27	<1	3

Food and Description	Amount	Total Calories	Total Carbs	Fiber	Sugars
BREAD COATING (*See* BAKE & FRY MIX; SEASONINGS)					
BREAD CRUMBS (*See also* BAKE & FRY MIX; SEASONINGS)					
(4-C)					
plain	1 oz	110	22	2	2
plain kosher	1 oz	120	24	0	2
seasoned	1 oz	110	20	2	2
seasoned kosher	1 oz	110	23	0	2
seasoned salt-free	1 oz	110	23	2	2
(Contadina)					
seasoned Italian-style	¼ cup	100	19	1	2
all other styles	¼ cup	110	19	1	1
(Devonsheer) all styles	⅛ cup	110	20	1	1
(Golden Dipt)					
All-purpose breading..seasoned	¼ cup	137	29	1	<1
Modern Maid..light 'n' crunchy					
American-style/fine	¼ cup	140	29	1	1.4
Japanese-style	¼ cup	45	9	<1	0.5
Redi-Breader	¼ cup	141	29	1	1.4
Oriental/fine	¼ cup	45	9	<1	0.5
Panko..plain	¼ cup	45	9	<1	0.5
(Kellogg's) cornflake crumbs	2 Tbs	40	9	0	1
(Old Bay) seasoned..Dip & Crisp	⅓ can	110	15	0	0
(Old London)					
lemon pepper	⅛ cup	120	23	2	0
plain	⅛ cup	110	19	1	0
roasted garlic	⅛ cup	110	21	2	0
seasoned	⅛ cup	110	19	1	0
(Progresso)					
garlic herb	¼ cup	100	18	1	1
Italian	¼ cup	110	20	1	1
Parmesan	¼ cup	110	19	1	2
plain	¼ cup	110	19	1	1
BREAD CUBES (*See* CROUTONS; STUFFING/DRESSING)					
BREAD STUFFING (*See* STUFFING/DRESSING)					
BREADFRUIT/raw	¼ small	99	26	5	na
	1 cup	227	60	11	na
BREADSTICK (*See also* BREAD)					
(Angonoa)					
mini					
cheese	1 oz	120	20	1	<1
pizza	1 oz	120	21	1	<1
sesame	1 oz	130	18	2	<1
whole wheat	1 oz	130	19	3	<1
regular					
cheese	1 oz	120	20	1	<1
garlic	1 oz	120	20	1	<1
Italian	1 oz	120	20	1	<1
onion	1 oz	120	21	1	<1
sesame royal	1 oz	130	18	2	<1

Food and Description	Amount	Total Calories	Total Carbs	Fiber	Sugars
(Bread du Jour) brown & serve					
original	1 piece	130	25	1	3
sourdough	1 piece	130	25	1	3
(Fattorie & Pandea)					
sesame	3 pieces	65	10	0	<1
all other styles	3 pieces	60	10	0	<1
(New York) frozen..garlic Parmesan	1 piece	180	29	1	2
(Pepperidge Farm) brown & serve					
5-cheese	1 piece	200	22	<1	0
crusty garlic	1 piece	170	15	1	2
garlic	1 piece	160	25	1	2
mozzarella	1 piece	200	24	1	2
Parmesan garlic	1 piece	170	20	2	3
(Pillsbury)..soft..refrigerated					
cornbread twists	1 twist	130	17	0	4
crusty French loaf	⅛ pkg	150	27	<1	3
garlic and herb	2 pieces	180	25	<1	3
Parmesan	2 pieces	180	24	<1	3
plain	2 pieces	140	25	2	3
(Stella D'Oro)					
cracked pepper..mini	4 pieces	70	11	0	1
garlic					
roasted	1 piece	45	8	0	1
traditional/fat-free	2 pieces	70	12	1	1
original					
mini	4 pieces	70	12	1	1
sodium-free	1 piece	45	7	0	1
traditional/fat-free	2 pieces	70	12	1	1
sesame					
low-fat	2 pieces	70	14	1	1
mini	4 pieces	80	11	1	1
(Toufayan) Grissini-style					
cheese	3 sticks	50	9	1	1
garlic	3 sticks	50	10	1	1
plain	3 sticks	50	10	1	1
BREAKFAST/CEREAL BAR (*See also* GRANOLA/GRANOLA-TYPE BAR)					
(Atkins) Breakfast Bars..Morning Start					
apple crisp	1 bar	170	13	6	1
(Barbara's Bakery)					
Multigrain Cereal Bars..all flavors	1 bar	120	25	2	13
Puffins Cereal & Milk Bars					
blueberry yogurt	1 bar	120	24	3	8
strawberry yogurt	1 bar	130	24	3	8
(Carbolight)..all flavors	1 bar	110	22	2	0
(General Mills)					
MILK 'N' CEREAL BARS					
Chex	1 bar	160	26	0	13
Cinnamon Toast Crunch	1 bar	180	31	1	19
Cocoa Puffs	1 bar	160	26	1	16

Food and Description	Amount	Total Calories	Total Carbs	Fiber	Sugars
Honey Nut Cheerios	1 bar	160	26	1	16
OATMEAL CRISP FRUIT 'N' CEREAL BARS					
apple cinnamon	1 bar	150	45	4	19
blueberry	1 bar	150	31	1	14
strawberry	1 bar	140	30	1	14
(Health Valley)					
BAKES/FAT-FREE..all flavors	1 bar	70	19	3	11
CAFÉ CREATIONS..all flavors	1 bar	130	27	2	17
COBBLER CEREAL BARS					
low-fat..all flavors	1 bar	130	27	1	13
regular..all flavors	1 bar	130	27	1	13
FRUIT BARS/FAT-FREE..all flavors	1 bar	140	35	3	14
TARTS/LOW-FAT..all flavors	1 tart	130	28	1	14
(Kellogg's) Breakfast Bars					
CEREAL & MILK BARS					
Cocoa Rice Krispies	1 bar	95	17	<1	12
Frosted Flakes	1 bar	110	19	<1	11
Froot Loops	1 bar	100	16	<1	10
NUTRI-GRAIN CEREAL BARS					
all flavors	1 bar	140	27	1	13
NUTRI-GRAIN/MUFFIN BARS					
banana	1 bar	160	30	1	16
cinnamon raisin	1 bar	170	32	1	18
NUTRI-GRAIN TWISTS					
apple cobbler	1 twist	140	27	1	12
cappuccino & cream	1 twist	140	26	1	15
strawberry cheesecake	1 twist	140	26	<1	13
NUTRI-GRAIN YOGURT BARS					
mini yogurt icing..all flavors	1 pouch	160	32	1	18
regular-size..all flavors	1 bar	140	27	1	14
(Special K) cereal bars					
apple	1 bar	90	17	<1	9
blueberry	1 bar	90	18	<1	8
cranberry apple	1 bar	90	17	<1	9
peaches & berries	1 bar	90	17	<1	9
strawberry	1 bar	90	18	<1	8
(Rice Krispies Treats) square bars					
chocolate drizzle	1 bar	100	16	0	9
double chocolate chunk	1 bar	100	15	<1	9
original	1 bar	90	18	0	8
rainbow	1 bar	100	17	0	9
(Post) cereal bar					
Carb Well					
cinnamon					
crunch	1 bar	110	14	5	5
raisin	1 bar	140	15	3	7
cranberry almond	1 bar	140	15	3	7
golden crunch	1 bar	110	14	5	5
peanut butter	1 bar	140	15	3	5

Food and Description	Amount	Total Calories	Total Carbs	Fiber	Sugars
(Quaker) breakfast squares					
NUTRITION FOR WOMEN					
banana bread	1 bar	220	41	2	19
oatmeal raisin	1 bar	220	41	2	19
REGULAR					
baked apple	1 bar	220	44	3	18
brown sugar cinnamon	1 bar	220	43	2	20
oatmeal raisin	1 bar	220	43	3	21
(SunBelt) cereal bars..fruit & grain	1 bar	140	28	1	18
BREAKFAST DRINK (*See also* NUTRITIONAL LIQUID SUPPLEMENT)					
(NOTE: Unless otherwise noted, mixes are prepared according to package directions)					
(Carnation) Instant Breakfast					
liquid/ready-to-drink					
Carb Conscious..All flavors	10 fl oz	150	15	2	12
original					
chocolate milk	10 fl oz	250	40	1	38
French vanilla	10 fl oz	240	34	0	30
strawberry cream	10 fl oz	250	37	0	36
powdered					
Carb Conscious..all flavors	1 pkt	70	12	<1	7
regular					
cappuccino	1 pkt	130	26	0	20
classic					
chocolate malt	1 pkt	130	27	<1	19
French vanilla	1 pkt	130	27	0	18
Strawberry Sensation	1 pkt	130	27	0	19
BREAKFAST SANDWICH (*See also* FROZEN ENTRÉE/DINNER; VEGETARIAN FOODS;					
individual FAST FOOD listings)					
(Bob Evans) Snackwich					
bacon, egg & cheese burrito	1 burrito	330	26	1	1
sausage biscuits					
6-count	2 biscuits	380	24	1	0
12-count	2 biscuits	380	24	1	0
16-count	2 biscuits	330	23	0	0
sausage, egg &					
cheese biscuits					
4-count	2 biscuits	430	25	<1	1
4-count..large	2 biscuits	370	25	0	0
(Nestlé USA)					
Hot Pockets					
bacon, egg & cheese	1 sdw	170	20	1	4
ham, egg & cheese	1 sdw	150	17	1	4
sausage, egg & cheese	1 sdw	170	19	1	4
Lean Pockets					
bacon, egg & cheese..low-fat	1 sdw	150	21	2	2
(Owens)					
Border Breakfasts/tacos					
bacon/egg/cheese	2 tacos	330	26	1	1
chorizo/egg/cheese	2 tacos	350	28	1	2

Food and Description	Amount	Total Calories	Total Carbs	Fiber	Sugars
sausage/egg/cheese					
2 count	1 taco	350	28	1	1
6 count	2 tacos	350	28	1	2
12 count	2 tacos	350	28	1	2
sandwiches..biscuits					
bacon/egg/cheese..large..					
5 ct	1 biscuit	340	25	0	0
egg/bacon/cheese..large	1 biscuit	350	24	1	2
sausage	2 biscuits	380	24	1	0
sausage/egg/cheese..					
4 count	2 biscuits	430	25	1	1
(Papetti) Chef's Omelet					
ham & cheese	1 omelet	180	5	0	0
sausage & cheese	1 omelet	240	4	0	0
3-cheese	1 omelet	230	5	0	0
Western-style	1 omelet	150	6	0	0
(Schwan's) frozen					
country sausage biscuit	2 biscuits	340	22	1	2
personal pouches/sausage					
breakfast bagel	1 bagel	300	37	2	5
pigs in a blanket	4 pieces	310	21	<1	6
(Swanson) Great Starts/frozen					
croissant w/sausage, egg & cheese	1 croissant	470	27	1	5
muffin w/egg, Canadian-style					
bacon & cheese	1 muffin	270	26	0	2
(Weight Watchers) Smart Ones					
English muffin sandwich	1 muffin	210	28	2	1
BREATH MINT (See CANDY)					
BREWER'S YEAST (See YEAST)					
BROAD BEAN					
CANNED					
(Progresso) fava beans	½ cup	110	20	5	0
FRESH					
boiled	½ cup	93	16	4.5	0
raw..mature..boiled	½ cup	95	50	5	0
BROCCOLI (See also BROCCOLI DISH; VEGETABLES, MIXED)					
FRESH					
(Dole)					
florets..chopped	1 cup	25	5	3	0
stalk...7" long	1 medium	45	8	5	0
FROZEN					
(Big Valley)..all cuts	¾ cup	25	3	2	1
(Birds Eye)					
baby broccoli					
chopped	½ cup	25	4	2	1
florets	1 cup	30	4	2	0
spears	4 spears	30	4	2	0
(C&W)					
florets	5 florets	25	4	2	1
microwave Brocclettes	1 cup	30	5	1	1

Food and Description	Amount	Total Calories	Total Carbs	Fiber	Sugars
(Cascadian Farm)	⅔ cup	20	4	2	<1
(Green Giant)					
chopped/cooked	½ cup	25	4	2	1
cuts/cooked	⅔ cup	25	4	2	1
florets/select	1½ cups	25	4	2	1

BROCCOLI DISH (*See also* BROCCOLI; FROZEN ENTRÉE/DINNER; VEGETABLES, MIXED; VEGETARIAN FOODS)

FROZEN

Food and Description	Amount	Total Calories	Total Carbs	Fiber	Sugars
(Birds Eye) in cheese sauce	⅔ cup	90	8	1	0
(Green Giant) boil-in-bag					
broccoli cuts..no sauce	⅔ cup	25	4	2	1
broccoli spears..no sauce	3 spears	25	4	2	1
broccoli in cheese-flavored sauce	⅔ cup	80	9	2	5
spears in butter sauce	4 oz	50	6	2	3

BROWNIE/BROWNIE-LIKE BARS (*See also* CAKE; CAKE, SNACK; COOKIE)

FROZEN..REFRIGERATED

Food and Description	Amount	Total Calories	Total Carbs	Fiber	Sugars
(Atkins) Endulge..iced chocolate	1 brownie	180	16	4	<1
(Nestlé Toll House)					
ready-to-bake					
fudgy..12-count	1 brownie	180	26	2	18
walnut..12-count	1 brownie	170	23	1	17
(Sara Lee) Brownie Bites					
triple chocolate fudge	1 serving	90	12	1	8
(Weight Watchers) Smart Ones					
brownie à la mode	1 brownie	190	33	2	15
double fudge brownie parfait	1 brownie	260	43	1	23

MIX

Food and Description	Amount	Total Calories	Total Carbs	Fiber	Sugars
(Arrowhead Mills) prepared					
fat-free	1 brownie	120	28	2	19
regular	1 brownie	110	27	2	19
(Betty Crocker) prepared					
dark chocolate fudge	1 brownie	170	24	0	17
fudge brownie...pouch	1 brownie	190	27	1	19
Supreme					
chocolate chunk	1 brownie	180	25	1	18
dark chocolate fudge	1 brownie	170	25	0	18
frosted	1 brownie	210	30	1	22
fudge	1 brownie	170	23	0	17
German chocolate	1 brownie	190	29	1	21
original	1 brownie	160	26	1	19
peanut butter chunk w/Reese's Pieces	1 brownie	180	23	0	17
pecan	1 brownie	170	22	<1	15
triple chunk	1 brownie	180	24	1	17
turtle	1 brownie	170	23	1	16
walnut chocolate chunk	1 brownie	140	24	1	17
(Duncan Hines)					
Candy Shop					
peanut butter cup	1/16 pkg	130	23	<1	16

Food and Description	Amount	Total Calories	Total Carbs	Fiber	Sugars
w/real M&M's	⅟₁₆ pkg	120	22	<1	15
Chocolate Lover's					
double fudge	⅟₁₆ pkg	130	26	2	18
milk chocolate chunk	⅟₁₆ pkg	130	25	1	18
turtle	⅟₁₆ pkg	130	23	<1	15
walnut	⅟₁₆ pkg	130	24	2	16
chocolate marble swirl	⅟₁₆ pkg	110	22	<1	16
(Eagle Brand) premium dessert kits					
Decadent Fudge Bar	1 bar	190	23	2	20
Magic Cookie Bars	1 bar	130	16	1	9
Peanut Butter Passion	1 bar	170	20	1	15
(Estee) prepared	2 pieces	100	23	1	1
(Ghirardelli) mix..double chocolate	⅟₂₀ pkg	150	27	1	21
(Jiffy) mix only	⅕ pkg	150	28	<1	18
(Krusteaz) prepared fudge brownie					
fat-free	1 brownie	120	28	<1	19
original	1 brownie	190	30	1	23
(Pillsbury)					
Brownie Classics..mix only					
fudge toffee	⅟₂₀ pkg	120	23	1	15
traditional fudge	⅟₂₀ pkg	120	23	1	15
Fudge Supreme..mix only					
chocolate					
chunk	⅟₁₆ pkg	120	22	1	15
double	⅟₁₆ pkg	110	23	1	16
extreme	⅟₁₆ pkg	120	22	1	16
frosted	⅟₁₆ pkg	140	27	1	19
fudge toffee					
vanilla-frosted	⅟₁₆ pkg	140	27	1	20
walnut	⅟₁₂ pkg	140	24	1	16
white fudge chunk	⅟₁₆ pkg	120	21	1	15
Snack Batch fudge..mix only	⅑ pkg	130	26	1	18
Thick 'n' Fudge					
cheesecake swirl	⅟₁₈ pkg	110	19	1	15
chocolate chunk	⅟₁₆ pkg	120	22	1	15
double chocolate	⅙ pkg	120	23	1	16
walnut	⅟₁₂ pkg	150	24	1	15
white fudge chunk	⅟₁₆ pkg	120	21	1	15
READY-TO-SERVE					
(Awrey's)					
chocolate decadent..individual	1 brownie	210	32	<1	24
chocolate peanut sensation	1 brownie	240	29	<1	22
home-style fudge nut	1 brownie	210	29	<1	22
no nut brownie	1 brownie	420	61	1	47
(Better Low Carb) brownies					
all styles and flavors	1 brownie	47	2	0	0
(Entenmann's) Little Bites Brownies					
fudge	⅕ pouch	280	34	2	24
golden...w/chocolate chips	⅕ pouch	250	37	<1	25

Food and Description	Amount	Total Calories	Total Carbs	Fiber	Sugars
(Gourmet Baker) Food Service					
Bengal	1 brownie	230	31	1	16
Blondie Obsession	1 brownie	260	30	0	20
Caramel Rage	1 brownie	290	36	1	27
Caramel Silk	1 bar	240	37	0	23
Chocolate Macaroon	1 bar	280	35	2	22
Chocolate Silk	1 bar	240	37	0	23
Double Fudge	1 brownie	260	37	1	24
Obsession	1 brownie	250	29	1	7
(Hostess)					
brownie bites..all styles	3 brownies	170	21	1	17
fudge brownies	1 brownie	330	54	1	11
low-fat	1 brownie	140	28	1	19
(Little Debbie)					
Be My Valentine	1 brownie	200	29	0	18
Christmas Tree	1 brownie	200	23	<1	13
Cosmic	2.5 oz	320	46	1	25
Fall	1 pkg	270	39	1	25
fudge	2 oz	260	37	1	20
	2.5 oz	320	46	1	25
reduced-fat	1 brownie	190	38	1	27
loaves	1 loaf	270	39	1	22
Stars & Stripes	1 pkg	290	40	1	25
(Mrs. Fields) (*See* FAST FOOD)					
(Otis Spunkmeyer)					
Café Collection..bars					
double chocolate caramel bar w/Snickers	2 oz	240	35	<1	26
lemon bar	2.8 oz	260	37	0	26
pecan pie	3.25-oz bar	390	53	2	37
raspberry	3.25-oz bar	330	50	2	32
Café Collection.. brownies					
café au lait	3.25 oz	390	53	2	42
double chocolate	2 oz	260	37	1	26
turtle	33.25 oz	420	49	3	33
(Sara Lee) food service					
Bistro Collection					
blondie	1 brownie	180	24	0	20
Bourbon Street chocolate	2.5-oz bar	290	40	3	22
	1.4-oz bar	170	23	2	12
chocolate pecan	2.5-oz bar	290	40	3	22
	1.4-oz bar	170	23	2	12
chocolate raspberry cordial	1 brownie	180	25	<1	18
marbled chocolate caramel	3-oz bar	390	47	2	33
	2.7-oz bar	360	48	1	31
peanut butter & chocolate	1 brownie	170	24	<1	13
Seven Layers of Heaven	2.78-oz bar	360	44	2	36
	1.5-oz bar	190	24	1	20

Food and Description	Amount	Total Calories	Total Carbs	Fiber	Sugars
Ultimate Brownie Bar	2.78-oz bar	360	48	1	31
	1.5-oz bar	190	26	1	17
fruit bars					
Classic Caramel Apple	1 bar	110	23	<1	18
Lemon Lover's	2.78-oz bar	320	43	1	33
	1.5-oz bar	170	23	<1	18
raspberry shortbread	1 bar	160	27	<1	15
BRUSSELS SPROUTS					
FRESH					
cooked..drained	½ cup	30	7	2	0
raw	½ cup	20	4	2	0
(Dole)	½ cup	20	4	2	0
FROZEN					
(Birds Eye) all styles	3 oz	35	7	3	2
(C&W) petite	3.2 oz	30	5	3	2
BRUSSELS SPROUTS DISH					
(Birds Eye) frozen in butter sauce	4 oz	70	9	3	4
(Green Giant) baby in butter sauce	⅔ cup	45	6	3	4
BUCKWHEAT GROATS/KASHA					
(Arrowhead Mills) brown	¼ cup	100	31	3	0
(Wolff's) roasted kernels..cooked	½ cup	170	35	2	0
BUFFALO/BISON					
COOKED					
(Denver Buffalo Co.)					
buffalo burgers	4 oz	130	0	0	0
ground	4 oz	250	0	0	0
RAW	4 oz	112	0	0	0
(New West)					
buffalo & beef hot Polish sausage	1 link	210	1	0	1
buffalo steak	4 oz	130	0	0	0
ROASTED	3 oz	148	0	0	0
BULGUR/HARD RED WINTER WHEAT					
COOKED (Arrowhead Mills)	¼ cup	150	33	4	0
UNCOOKED	1 cup	480	105	25	0
BURBOT..cooked—dry heat	3 oz	100	0	0	0
BURDOCK ROOT					
COOKED..DRAINED	1 cup	110	26	2	0
RAW	1 cup	85	20	4	0

BURGER (*See* BEEF; BUFFALO/BISON; HAMBURGER; TURKEY; VEGETARIAN FOODS)
BURGER MIX (*See* BEEF DISH/ENTRÉE; VEGETARIAN FOODS)
BURRITO (*See* BREAKFAST SANDWICH; MEXICAN FOOD; VEGETARIAN FOODS)
BUTTER (*See also* BUTTER BLEND/SPREAD; BUTTER-FLAVORED SEASONING;
  MARGARINE, MARGARINE SPREAD & SPRAY)

(Breakstone) salted or unsalted					
stick	1 Tbs	100	0	0	0
whipped	1 Tbs	60	0	0	0
(Challenge) salted or unsalted					
light	1 Tbs	50	0	0	0
sweet	1 Tbs	100	0	0	0
whipped	1 Tbs	70	0	0	0

Food and Description	Amount	Total Calories	Total Carbs	Fiber	Sugars
(Horizon) organic..salted or unsalted	1 Tbs	100	0	0	0
(Hotel Bar)	1 tsp	35	0	0	0
(Keller's)	1 tsp	35	0	0	0
(Land O' Lakes) salted or unsalted					
honey butter	1 Tbs	90	4	0	3
light					
stick	1 Tbs	50	<1	0	0
whipped	1 Tbs	35	<1	0	0
regular					
stick	1 Tbs	100	0	0	0
whipped	1 Tbs	70	0	0	0
roasted garlic	1 Tbs	100	0	0	0
soft baking w/canola oil	1 Tbs	100	0	0	0
spreadable w/canola oil	1 Tbs	110	0	0	0
sweet cream	1 Tbs	100	0	0	0
ultra creamy	1 Tbs	110	0	0	0
BUTTER BEAN (*See also* LIMA BEAN)					
CANNED					
(Aunt Nellie's) Reber	½ cup	140	25	6	4
(Bush Bros.)					
baby	½ cup	120	19	5	0
green	½ cup	110	19	6	0
large	½ cup	100	18	5	0
small	½ cup	100	16	5	0
speckled	½ cup	110	18	5	9
(Eden)..baby lima	½ cup	100	17	4	0
(Glory)..seasoned					
butter beans	½ cup	120	20	5	0
lima beans	½ cup	140	24	7	0
(Trappey's)					
baby green..w/bacon	½ cup	120	22	6	2
w/sausage..large white	½ cup	110	21	6	0
DRIED					
(Hurst) ham beans..all styles	½ cup	120	22	9	1
FROZEN					
(Birds Eye)					
baby	½ cup	130	24	6	2
fordhook	½ cup	100	19	5	3
(Green Giant) baby lima & butter	⅔ cup	110	20	4	1
BUTTER BLEND/SPREAD (*See also* MARGARINE, MARGARINE SPREAD & SPRAY)					
(Blue Bonnet) stick w/tub	1 Tbs	90	0	0	0
	4 oz	360	0	0	0
(Buttery Blend) liquid	1 Tbs	120	0	0	0
(Downey's) honey butter..all styles	1 Tbs	60	11	0	11
(Kraft) Touch of Butter					
bowl	1 Tbs	50	0	0	0
squeeze bottle	1 Tbs	80	0	0	0
stick/50% fat	1 Tbs	90	0	0	0

Food and Description	Amount	Total Calories	Total Carbs	Fiber	Sugars
(Land O' Lakes)					
Country Morning Blend					
stick..light	1 Tbs	50	0	0	0
stick..regular..salt or no salt	1 Tbs	100	0	0	0
tub..light	1 Tbs	50	0	0	0
tub..regular..salt or no salt	1 Tbs	100	0	0	0
BUTTERBUR					
canned..chopped	½ cup	2	<1	0	0
raw	1 cup	13	3	na	0
BUTTERFISH..cooked—dry heat	3 oz	160	0	0	0
BUTTER-FLAVORED SEASONING (*See also* SEASONINGS)					
(Best O' Butter)					
cheddar cheese flavor	½ tsp	6	2	0	0
other flavors..all	½ tsp	4	1	0	0
(Butter Buds) butter-flavored					
granules or mix	1 tsp	5	2	0	0
salt	any amount	0	0	0	0
(Molly McButter) sprinkles					
all styles	1 tsp	5	1	0	0
BUTTERNUT/dried	1 oz	175	3.5	1.5	1

C

Food and Description	Amount	Total Calories	Total Carbs	Fiber	Sugars
CABBAGE					
CANNED or JARRED					
(Aunt Nellie's) red..sweet & sour	2 Tbs	20	5	0	2
(Libby's) red..sweet & sour	2 Tbs	20	5	0	4
(S&W) red..sweet & sour	2 Tbs	15	3	0	2
FRESH					
Chinese/bok choy/napa					
cooked	½ cup	10	1.5	1.5	0
raw/shredded	½ cup	5	1	<1	0
(Dole)					
bok choy	½ cup	5	1	<1	0
Danish					
shredded	½ cup	10	2	<1	0
whole/2-lb head	1 head	220	50	20	0
red/raw/shredded	1 cup	20	4	1	0

Food and Description	Amount	Total Calories	Total Carbs	Fiber	Sugars
savoy/raw	1 cup	20	4	2	0
skunk..swamp..cooked..drained	1 cup	20	4	2	0
CACTUS					
(Embassa)	⅔ cup	5	1	0	0
(La Costena)					
Napolitos tender cactus	1 cup	20	4	0	0
CAKE (*See also* BROWNIE/BROWNIE-LIKE BARS; CAKE, SNACK; DONUT; MUFFIN; PASTRY; POPCORN CAKES; RICE CAKES)					
■ **FROZEN OR REFRIGERATED**					
(Atkins) Endulge Cheesecake					
chocolate swirl	3-oz slice	250	3	0	1
pumpkin	3-oz slice	210	3	0	1
vanilla pound	3-oz slice	250	3	0	1
(Edward's)					
cheesecake					
caramel dulce de leche..2-count	1 cake	290	26	0	16
chocolate marble..2-count	1 cake	290	26	0	16
harvest pumpkin..limited edition	⅙ cake	520	51	2	35
original..2-count	1 cake	290	23	0	14
strawberry marble..2-count	1 cake	280	25	0	16
gourmet cheesecake					
pecan	⅛ cake	530	59	1	32
(Kraft) Philadelphia..cheesecake bars	1 bar	180	19	0	13
(Mrs. Smith's)					
carrot	1 piece	240	29	1	21
Flip-It cakes					
apple caramel	1 cake	480	90	2	58
strawberry delight	1 cake	380	73	1	47
(Pepperidge Farm) 3-layer cakes					
chocolate fudge	1 piece	250	31	1	20
coconut classic	1 piece	250	35	1	24
(Sara Lee)					
retail					
cheesecake					
chocolate swirl	⅙ cake	470	45	1	23
French chocolate swirl	⅕ cake	430	52	2	31
classic	⅕ cake	410	27	6	17
strawberry French	⅙ cake	320	43	1	26
New York–style classic	⅙ cake	350	35	1	25
original					
cream cherry	¼ cake	350	55	2	35
cream classic	¼ cake	340	38	1	29
cream strawberry	¼ cake	330	49	2	36
cheesecake bites					
chocolate-dipped..original	1 piece	100	8	0	6
	5 pieces	500	40	0	30
chocolate praline pecan	1 piece	100	8	1	6
	5 pieces	480	40	5	30
coffee cake					
butter streusel	⅙ cake	190	25	1	10

Food and Description	Amount	Total Calories	Total Carbs	Fiber	Sugars
crumb	⅛ cake	190	30	1	18
pecan	⅙ cake	140	23	1	9
pound cake..all butter					
family-size	⅙ cake	220	34	1	19
regular	¼ cake	240	34	1	19
free & light	¼ cake	200	39	1	21
strawberry swirl	¼ cake	290	44	1	25
shortcake/strawberry/filled w/real strawberries	⅛ cake	180	27	1	15
Food Service					
breakfast cakes					
blueberry	1 slice	180	30	<1	19
French crumb cake	1 slice	180	33	0	20
home-style blueberry yogurt	1 slice	300	47	1	32
lemon poppy seed	1 slice	300	45	2	28
cheesecake					
French cream					
home-style	1/14 cake	280	31	<1	18
round	1/16 cake	360	35	<1	20
New York–style					
creamy	1/16 cake	420	29	1	27
high-profile	1/14 cake	530	38	2	34
plain	1/16 cake	410	32	1	18
Gourmet Desserts/Bistro Collection					
cheesecakes					
caramel pecan	1 slice	520	40	2	21
chocolate mousse	1 slice	520	62	3	50
Chocolate Raspberry Rumble	1 slice	450	48	3	36
Key Lime Breeze	1 slice	510	40	0	31
mint chocolate chip	1 slice	560	51	2	42
mocha swirl	1 slice	500	39	3	19
New York–style vanilla bean	1 slice	530	42	<1	35
White Chocolate Tuxedo	1 slice	420	37	2	22
chocolate/chocolate dessert torte	1 slice	370	36	2	13
chocolate truffle mousse	1 slice	440	46	3	42
tarts/individual					
pecan	1 tart	860	120	11	62
rustic apple	1 tart	540	71	7	23
tiramisu desserts					
pan	4.5 oz	430	38	<1	24
Viva	5.5 oz	500	48	1	38
(Weight Watchers) Smart Ones					
carrot cake	1 serving	220	33	2	21
cheesecake					
French-style	1 serving	170	28	2	19
New York–style	1 serving	150	21	1	18
double fudge cake	1 serving	150	20	2	1
■ MIX					
(Banquet) Dessert Bakes					
Chocolate Cherry Decadence	⅙ pkg	310	62	0	43

Food and Description	Amount	Total Calories	Total Carbs	Fiber	Sugars
Chocolate Lava Cake	1 slice	370	73	0	53
(Betty Crocker) prepared					
Classic Dessert					
gingerbread cake & cookie	1/12 cake	230	39	1	18
pineapple upside-down cake	1/6 cake	400	64	4	3
pound cake	1/8 cake	260	45	0	26
Snackin' Cake					
banana walnut	1/9 cake	180	31	0	17
chocolate chunk	1/9 cake	80	32	1	19
cinnamon swirl	1/9 cake	190	34	0	20
German chocolate	1/9 cake	180	32	1	20
SuperMoist					
angel food					
confetti	1/12 cake	150	34	0	25
one-step white	1/12 cake	140	32	0	24
butter chocolate	1/12 cake	250	35	2	22
butter pecan	1/12 cake	240	35	0	20
butter yellow	1/12 cake	250	36	0	20
carrot cake	1/10 cake	320	42	0	25
cherry chip	1/10 cake	300	41	0	23
chocolate chip	1/12 cake	250	35	0	20
chocolate fudge	1/12 cake	270	35	1	21
devil's food	1/12 cake	270	35	2	21
double chocolate swirl	1/12 cake	270	35	1	21
French vanilla	1/12 cake	240	35	1	21
fudge marble	1/10 cake	290	42	0	25
German chocolate	1/12 cake	270	36	0	21
golden vanilla	1/12 cake	240	35	0	20
lemon	1/12 cake	240	35	0	20
milk chocolate	1/12 cake	240	34	1	21
party rainbow white	1/10 cake	300	41	0	24
party swirl	1/12 cake	240	35	0	20
pineapple	1/12 cake	250	35	0	20
sour cream white	1/10 cake	280	41	0	23
spice	1/12 cake	250	35	0	20
strawberry	1/12 cake	250	35	0	21
white	1/12 cake	230	34	0	19
yellow	1/12 cake	250	335	0	20
(Dromedary) prepared					
carrot	1/12 cake	232	23	0	na
pound cake	1 slice	150	21	0	na
(Duncan Hines)					
Moist Deluxe					
angel food..prepared	1/12 cake	140	31	0	23
banana supreme..mix only	1/12 pkg	180	36	0	20
devil's food..mix only	1/12 pkg	180	35	1	20
red velvet..prepared	1/12 cake	180	35	1	20
tres leches (three milk)..prepared	1/12 cake	140	28	<1	18
yellow classic..mix only	1/12 pkg	180	36	0	20

Food and Description	Amount	Total Calories	Total Carbs	Fiber	Sugars
Signature Desserts..mix only					
Boston cream	1/6 pkg	270	53	1	32
Chocolate Silk Torte	1/10 pkg	190	29	<1	22
Orange Dreamsicle	1/12 pkg	220	42	<1	25
Strawberry Swirl	1/12 pkg	270	50	0	4
(Jell-O) No-Bake Desserts..mix only					
Chips Ahoy	1/6 pkg	260	46	1	28
Oreo	1/6 pkg	270	48	2	30
peanut butter cup	1/8 pkg	290	38	2	26
no-bake cheesecake..mix only					
cherry	1/9 pkg	200	41	1	24
real	1/6 pkg	220	40	1	25
strawberry	1/9 pkg	200	42	1	28
strawberry swirl/reduced-fat	1/8 pkg	180	39	1	28
(McCormick) funnel cake..mix only	1/4 cup	120	23	<1	6
(Pillsbury) mix only, unless noted otherwise (*See also* Ready-to-Serve, this section)					
Funfetti	1/12 pkg	180	35	1	22
Easter	1/12 pkg	190	35	1	19
Halloween..yellow					
cake	1/12 pkg	190	35	1	19
cupcake kit	1/12 pkg	200	36	1	26
holiday	1/12 pkg	190	35	1	20
spring	1/12 pkg	190	35	1	19
Stars & Stripes	1/12 pkg	190	35	1	20
Valentine's	1/12 pkg	190	35	1	20
Moist Supreme					
angel food/prepared	1/12 cake	140	31	0	23
banana	1/12 pkg	180	35	1	21
butter recipe chocolate	1/12 pkg	180	35	1	21
chocolate chip	1/12 pkg	190	35	1	20
devil's food	1/12 pkg	170	34	1	20
German chocolate	1/12 pkg	170	34	1	18
lemon	1/12 pkg	170	34	1	20
strawberry	1/12 pkg	180	35	1	21
white	1/12 pkg	180	35	1	22
Ultimate Dessert Kits					
chocolate caramel cake	1/9 kit	180	36	1	23
stawberry 'n' cream cake	1/9 kit	170	35	1	26
triple chocolate cake	1/9 kit	200	35	1	23
■ READY-TO-SERVE					
(Awrey's) food service					
International Marquise cakes					
Cajeta caramel	1 slice	340	44	0	35
French mint	1 slice	300	43	<1	32
pistachio lime	1 slice	270	35	<1	25
strawberry guava snow puff	1 slice	270	34	0	27
Marquise cakes					
banana chocolate chip	1 slice	320	45	1	34
Cherries Cordial	1 slice	280	36	<1	26
Chocolate Peanut Fantasy	1 slice	360	42	1	31

Food and Description	Amount	Total Calories	Total Carbs	Fiber	Sugars
French espresso	1 slice	330	33	<1	23
Georgia peach	1 slice	280	37	0	26
Killer Chocolate	1 slice	320	47	2	36
Lemon Whisper	1 slice	280	38	0	28
raspberries 'n' cream	1 slice	270	36	<1	25
raspberry extraordinaire	1 slice	370	53	<1	42
red velvet layer	1 slice	340	38	0	30
tropical chocolate	1 slice	270	40	<1	26
torte cakes					
black forest	1 slice	430	39	0	26
double chocolate	1 slice	390	59	1	41
strawberry supreme	1 slice	310	47	<1	32
(Entenmann's)					
all-butter loaf	⅙ loaf	210	30	1	18
Carb-Counting butter loaf	⅛ loaf	170	21	1	0
cheesecake..deluxe French	⅕ cake	460	46	1	30
chocolate fudge	⅛ cake	260	39	2	30
coffee/crumb cakes					
crumb	⅒ cake	250	33	1	13
crumb delight..light	⅑ cake	210	37	1	20
little bites	1 cake	280	36	1	19
ultimate for crumb lovers	⅒ cake	250	33	1	17
walnut Danish ring	⅙ cake	240	25	1	12
cupcakes..holiday	1 cupcake	280	40	1	33
Danish ring					
pecan	⅙ cake	250	26	1	12
walnut	⅙ cake	240	25	1	12
Louisiana crunch..original	⅑ cake	330	48	1	35
(Mrs. Fields) bundt cakes					
banana walnut	1 slice	350	35	3	18
banana walnut w/chocolate chips	1 slice	370	39	3	25
blueberry	1 slice	270	36	1	19
raspberry	1 slice	270	36	1	19
white cake w/chocolate chips	1 slice	350	45	1	27
(Pepperidge Farm)					
chocolate fudge	⅛ cake	250	31	1	20
coconut	⅛ cake	250	35	<1	24
devil's food	⅛ cake	250	34	<1	24
German chocolate	⅛ cake	250	31	<1	20
golden	⅛ cake	250	33	<1	21
guava	⅛ cake	190	36	<1	25
mango	⅛ cake	190	35	0	22
strawberry stripe	⅛ cake	250	32	<1	21
vanilla	⅛ cake	250	35	<1	25
CAKE, SNACK					
■ READY-TO-SERVE					
(Drake's)					
all-butter pound cake	1 piece	280	43	2	30

Food and Description	Amount	Total Calories	Total Carbs	Fiber	Sugars
Boston cream	1 cake	180	25	1	17
coffee cakes					
large	1 cake	270	39	1	23
mini	4 pieces	210	32	1	17
original	1 cake	140	20	0	11
Devil Dogs					
original	1 piece	180	26	1	15
reduced-fat	1 cake	160	29	1	18
Funny Bones					
mini	5 pieces	270	45	2	30
regular	2 cakes	300	41	4	25
Ring Dings					
mini	5 pieces	310	45	4	31
original	2 cakes	340	43	2	30
Sunny Doodles	2 cakes	220	33	1	28
Yankee Doodles..mini	4 pieces	190	30	1	22
Yodels	2 cakes	290	34	1	24
(Hostess)					
angel food cake	⅛ cake	160	33	1	28
Brownie Bites	3 pieces	170	21	1	17
brownie					
fudge	1 brownie	330	54	1	11
low-fat	1 brownie	140	28	1	19
Chocodiles	1 cake	240	33	1	22
coconut cakes	1 cake	260	32	1	23
crumb coffee cake					
light	1 cake	90	19	0	16
regular	1 cake	130	19	0	10
cupcakes					
chocolate					
light	1 cupcake	140	18	1	19
regular	1 cupcake	180	30	1	17
golden	1 cupcake	200	33	0	25
orange	1 cupcake	160	27	0	20
Ding Dongs	2 cakes	360	44	2	32
Ho Ho's	2 cakes	250	34	1	23
Leopards	1 cake	210	31	0	22
Shortcake Dessert Cups	1 cake	100	17	0	10
Snoballs	1 cake	180	31	1	19
Suzy Q's	1 cake	230	35	1	22
Twinkies					
light	1 cake	130	27	0	16
original	1 cake	150	25	0	14
(Lance) fig cake..low-fat	½ cake	110	21	1	14
(Little Debbie)					
angel cake/low-fat raspberry	1 pkg	130	29	0	23
apple flips	1.25 oz	150	24	<1	13
banana nut loaves	2 oz	220	31	<1	13
banana twins	2.2 oz	250	39	0	26

Food and Description	Amount	Total Calories	Total Carbs	Fiber	Sugars
Be My Valentine cake/boxed					
chocolate	1 cake	280	38	<1	25
vanilla	1 cake	290	38	0	26
blueberry loaves	2 oz	220	29	<1	16
Boston cream rolls	2.2 oz	270	40	0	25
cherry cordial	1 pkg	170	23	<1	15
chocolate chip cake	1 pkg	310	41	<1	29
cupcakes..cream-filled					
chocolate	1 cake	200	26	<1	18
	3.1 oz	380	51	2	35
lemon	1 cake	210	29	0	22
orange ginger spice	1 cake	210	29	0	22
strawberry	1 cake	210	29	<1	22
devil cream cake	3.25-oz pkg	190	29	0	20
devil squares	1 pkg	280	38	<1	26
fall party cakes					
chocolate	2.4 oz	300	41	<1	29
vanilla	2.5 oz	320	43	0	31
fancy cakes	2.4 oz	310	42	0	33
fig bars/low-fat	1 pkg	150	31	1	20
frosted fudge cake	1 cake	250	25	<1	18
fudge rounds	1.2 oz	150	23	<1	14
	2.5 oz	310	48	1	30
holiday cake roll..cherry cream	1 pkg	270	38	<1	21
holiday snack cake					
chocolate	1 pkg	300	41	<1	29
vanilla	1 pkg	320	43	0	31
marshmallow crispy bars	1.25 oz	140	26	9	13
	1.67 oz	190	35	1	18
marshmallow supremes	1.1 oz	140	22	<1	15
Nutty Bar	2 oz	310	32	1	20
	2.14 oz	330	32	1	31
oatmeal cream pie	1 pkg	170	26	<1	14
oatmeal lights..reduced-fat	1 pkg	130	29	<1	16
PB&J oatmeal	1 pkg	140	22	<1	12
peanut butter crunch bar	1 pkg	280	32	1	19
peanut cluster	1 pkg	200	23	<1	16
pound cake	1 pkg	220	31	0	18
raisin cream pie	1 pkg	140	23	0	16
Star Crunch Cosmic Snacks	1 pkg	150	22	0	12
Stars & Stripes cakes	1 pkg	310	42	0	33
strawberry shortcake roll..boxed	1 pkg	240	41	2	29
Swiss cake roll					
boxed	1 pkg	270	38	1	25
double chocolate	1 pkg	280	41	1	26
	3.3 oz	430	60	1	36
Zebra Cake	1 pkg	340	46	<1	30
	2.1 oz	270	38	1	25
	3.67 oz	460	63	1	46

Food and Description	Amount	Total Calories	Total Carbs	Fiber	Sugars
(Otis Spunkmeyer)					
Café Collection					
cakes					
chocolate truffle	2.65 oz	320	33	2	25
orange ginger spice	4-oz slice	420	57	<1	29
vanilla pound	4-oz slice	460	54	<1	31
yogurt lemon poppy	4-oz slice	440	54	<1	31
coffee cakes					
apple cinnamon	3.25 oz	370	50	2	30
cheese	3.25 oz	340	46	2	24
crumb cakes					
apple	4-oz cake	410	61	2	33
blueberry	4-oz cake	400	61	2	31
cheese	4-oz cake	450	61	2	31
mini loaves					
apple spice	3.75 oz	370	58	4	31
banana walnut	3.75 oz	450	51	2	27
chocolate fudge pecan	3.75 oz	420	53	3	30
pound cake	3.5 oz	390	47	<1	26
(TastyKake)					
Creamies					
banana	1 cake	180	23	0	16
Bunny Trail Treats	2 cakes	220	29	0	21
chocolate	2 cakes	190	24	0	1
Cupid	2 cakes	220	29	0	21
Kringle Kake	2 cakes	220	29	0	21
Sparkle Kake	2 cakes	220	29	0	21
St. Patty	2 cakes	220	29	0	21
Witchy Treats	1 cake	150	24	0	16
cupcakes					
butter cream iced..cream-filled	2.28 oz	260	40	<1	26
	3.4 oz	380	59	1	39
chocolate..iced/cream-filled	2 cakes	240	38	<1	24
	3 cakes	370	58	1	38
low-fat cream-filled					
chocolate	2 cakes	190	42	0	28
vanilla	2 cakes	200	42	1	30
Juniors					
chocolate	2 cakes	340	54	<1	35
coconut	2 cakes	400	46	0	37
Koffee Kake	2 cakes	270	42	<1	21
lemon	2 cakes	310	53	9	36
orange	2 cakes	340	58	9	37
Pound Kake	2 cakes	350	50	1	31
Kandy Kakes					
Boston cream	1 cake	180	24	0	17
chocolate	1 cake	180	24	1	15
coconut	1 cake	170	21	1	15
mint	1 cake	180	24	1	16
peanut butter	2 cakes	180	31	<1	20

Food and Description	Amount	Total Calories	Total Carbs	Fiber	Sugars
peppermint	1 cake	180	23	<1	17
raspberry	1 cake	180	23	0	19
strawberry	1 cake	180	24	1	16
Koffee Kake	2.1 oz	270	35	0	22
Kreepy Kakes	2 cakes	240	37	0	26
Krimpets					
butterscotch-iced	2 cakes	210	37	0	24
jelly-filled	2 cakes	180	34	0	21
Kreme Krimpies	2 cakes	250	31	0	19
strawberry-iced	2 cakes	220	36	0	22
Tasty Tweets	2 cakes	240	37	0	26
Tropical Delights					
coconut	2 cakes	230	29	0	19
guava	2 cakes	190	30	0	20
papaya	2 cakes	190	30	0	20
pineapple	2 cakes	200	32	0	22
Snowballs	1 cake	220	36	0	22
CAKE FROSTING/ICING					
(Betty Crocker)					
MIX..prepared..fluffy frosting..white	6 Tbs	100	24	1	23
READY-TO-SPREAD					
Rich & Creamy					
butter cream	2 Tbs	150	20	0	18
cherry	2 Tbs	150	20	0	18
chocolate	2 Tbs	150	18	0	15
chocolate almond	2 Tbs	150	18	0	15
coconut pecan	2 Tbs	140	17	0	16
cream cheese	2 Tbs	150	20	0	18
dark chocolate	2 Tbs	150	17	1	16
dulce de leche	2 Tbs	150	20	0	18
French vanilla	2 Tbs	140	23	0	20
lemon	2 Tbs	150	20	0	18
milk chocolate	2 Tbs	150	18	0	16
mint chocolate chip	2 Tbs	130	22	0	19
original	2 Tbs	150	20	0	18
rainbow chip	2 Tbs	140	23	0	20
sour cream chocolate	2 Tbs	150	18	0	15
sour cream white	2 Tbs	150	20	0	18
strawberry cream cheese	2 Tbs	150	20	0	18
triple chocolate fudge	2 Tbs	140	22	1	20
vanilla chocolate chip	2 Tbs	140	23	0	20
white chocolate	2 Tbs	140	23	0	20
READY-TO-SPREAD					
Whipped Deluxe					
butter cream	2 Tbs	110	14	0	13
chocolate	2 Tbs	100	13	1	12
cream cheese	2 Tbs	110	14	0	13
fluffy white	2 Tbs	110	14	0	13
lemon	2 Tbs	110	14	0	13
milk chocolate	2 Tbs	100	14	0	12

Food and Description	Amount	Total Calories	Total Carbs	Fiber	Sugars
strawberry	2 Tbs	110	14	0	13
vanilla	2 Tbs	110	14	0	13
(Duncan Hines) creamy home-style/ready-to-spread					
classic vanilla	2 Tbs	140	22	0	21
cream cheese	2 Tbs	140	22	0	21
milk chocolate	2 Tbs	130	20	0	19
(Pillsbury) ready-to-spread					
Creamy Supreme					
banana cream	2 Tbs	150	23	0	21
chocolate	2 Tbs	140	21	0	18
chocolate fudge	2 Tbs	140	21	0	18
chocolate mocha	2 Tbs	140	21	0	18
classic white	2 Tbs	140	22	0	20
coconut pecan	2 Tbs	160	17	1	14
cookies & cream	2 Tbs	150	23	0	21
cream cheese	2 Tbs	150	24	0	21
French vanilla	2 Tbs	160	26	0	23
Funfetti/Confetti w/candy bits..					
all flavors	2 Tbs	150	25	0	23
hot fudge	2 Tbs	140	21	0	18
milk chocolate	2 Tbs	140	21	<1	18
milk chocolate swirl w/fudge glaze	2 Tbs	140	22	0	29
strawberry cream	2 Tbs	150	23	0	21
vanilla	2 Tbs	150	23	0	21
white	2 Tbs	140	22	0	20
CALAMARI (*See* SQUID)					
CALZONE (*See* PIZZA)					
CANADIAN BACON (*See* BACON, CANADIAN-STYLE)					
CANDY (*See also* FRUIT SNACK)					
■ **ABRA CA BUBBLE** (*See* (Brach's) in this section)					
■ **(Allen Wertz)**					
coconut haystacks	2 pieces	180	13	0	0
rocky road sticks	1 piece	140	16	<1	0
■ **ALMOND JOY** (*See* (Hershey) in this section)					
■ **ALMOND ROCA** (*See* (Brown & Haley) in this section)					
■ **ALPINE WHITE** (*See* (Nestlé USA) in this section)					
■ **(Andes)**					
CDM Changemaker	3 pieces	190	20	<1	18
cherry jubilee thins	8 pieces	200	22	<1	20
crème de menthe wafers	8 pieces	200	22	1	19
mint parfait	8 pieces	210	22	0	20
mint patties	3 pieces	180	38	0	36
parfait thins	8 pieces	200	21	0	20
toffee crunch thins	8 pieces	190	23	0	22
Zotz strings	1 piece	15	5	0	3
■ **(Atkins)**					
Endulge					
caramel nut chew	1.23 oz	140	17	1	1
crisp wafers					
chocolate cream	2 bars	120	15	3	0

Food and Description	Amount	Total Calories	Total Carbs	Fiber	Sugars
mint	1 oz	120	15	3	0
peanut butter	2 bars	120	14	3	0
peanut butter cups	3 cups	160	17	0	0

■ **BABY RUTH** (*See* (Nestlé USA) in this section)
■ **BIT-O-HONEY** (*See* (Nestlé USA) in this section)
■ **(Brach's)**
Chocolate Candy

almond supremes	11 pieces	220	22	2	19
bridge mix	16 pieces	190	26	<1	22
California raisins	35 pieces	170	28	1	26
caramel clusters	3 pieces	210	23	1	19
double dippers	15 pieces	210	23	2	19
malts	15 pieces	190	30	1	21
Milk Maid..chocolate caramels	18 pieces	160	28	0	26
mint patties	3 pieces	140	29	0	26
mint pearls	24 pieces	160	35	0	31
peanut butter meltaways	3 pieces	200	19	1	17
peanut clusters	3 pieces	210	21	2	16
rich & dreamy assorted creams	3 pieces	170	36	<1	31
Sprinkles	17 pieces	200	29	1	26
Stars/chocolate	10 pieces	200	24	0	23

Other Candies

A&W root beer barrels	3 pieces	70	17	0	11
Abra Ca Bubble	1 piece	45	10	0	7
butterscotch hard candy	3 pieces	70	17	0	11
candy corn	26 pieces	140	35	0	28
cinnamon hard candy	3 pieces	70	17	0	10
cinnamon imperials	52 pieces	60	15	0	11
circus peanuts	6 pieces	160	39	0	34
dessert mints	14 pieces	60	15	0	15
French burnt peanuts	31 pieces	170	29	1	25
fruit slices	3 pieces	150	38	0	29
gummy fruits	13 pieces	110	25	0	18
ice blue mint coolers	3 pieces	70	17	0	10
jelly beans	14 pieces	150	37	0	27
jelly nougats	5 pieces	160	34	0	23
Jube Jels	12 pieces	140	34	0	17
Kentucky mints	7 pieces	60	16	0	15
maple nut goodies	7 pieces	200	30	1	23
Milk Maid					
caramels	4 pieces	160	30	0	18
Christmas..caramel chews	5 pieces	140	28	0	17
flavored caramel roll	5 pieces	140	28	0	17
orange slices	2 pieces	130	32	0	23
Party Mix	3 pieces	70	17	0	11
root beer barrels	3 pieces	70	17	0	11
Smucker's jelly beans	3 pieces	70	17	0	11
Spearmint Leaves	5 pieces	130	34	0	23
Special Treasures/toffees					
coffee-flavored	3 pieces	70	14	0	10

Food and Description	Amount	Total Calories	Total Carbs	Fiber	Sugars
fruit & cream	3 pieces	60	13	0	9
golden butter	3 pieces	80	15	0	10
spice drops	12 pieces	130	33	0	23
Star Brites disks					
butterscotch	3 disks	60	16	0	10
cinnamon	3 disks	60	16	0	10
peppermint	3 disks	60	15	0	8
spearmint	3 disks	60	15	0	8
Sundaes Neapolitan Coconuts	3 pieces	160	28	1	19
sugar-free candy					
butterscotch hard candy	3 pieces	30	17	0	0
cinnamon hard candy	3 pieces	35	17	0	0
Star Brites peppermint	3 pieces	30	17	0	0
■ **(Breath Savers)**					
breath mints/sugar-free..all flavors	1 piece	10	2	0	2
■ **(Brown & Haley)**					
Carbs In-Line Chocolatey Indulgence					
w/mint	1 bar	110	14	7	<1
w/soy crunches	1 bar	110	16	8	<1
w/toffee	1 bar	110	14	6	<1
original almond roca	3 pieces	210	18	<1	17
sugar-free almond roca	3 pieces	160	16	1	13
■ **BUNCHA CRUNCH** (*See* (Nestlé USA) in this section)					
■ **BUTTERFINGER** (*See* (Nestlé USA) in this section)					
■ **(Cadbury)**					
Bassett's/licorice..all sorts	1.46 oz	120	27	1	21
Caramello chocolate	6 blocks	200	27	<1	25
chocolate wafer	6 blocks	200	27	<1	25
dairy milk chocolate bar	9 blocks	220	21	1	18
fruit & nut bar/chocolate bar	10 blocks	200	25	1	22
roasted almond bar..chocolate	10 blocks	220	21	1	18
■ **CARAMELLO** (*See* (Cadbury) in this section)					
■ **(Carb Solutions)** chocolate					
caramel	1 oz	130	18	1	0
crisp	1 oz	140	16	1	0
raspberry	1 oz	120	17	1	0
w/almonds	1 oz	140	15	1	0
■ **(Carborite)**					
At Last! 1g Net Carb					
chocolate bars					
almond	1 oz	120	13	6	0
crisp	1 oz	110	16	<1	0
mint	1 oz	110	15	<1	0
truffle	1 oz	100	17	1	0
chocolate-covered peanuts	1.25 oz	150	18	5	0
other chocolate bars					
caramel nougat	1 oz	100	20	1	0
chocolate almond	1.75 oz	230	25	1	0
chocolate crisp	1.75 oz	250	27	1	0
chocolate peanut butter	1.75 oz	250	27	2	0

Food and Description	Amount	Total Calories	Total Carbs	Fiber	Sugars
chocolate truffle	1.75 oz	190	30	2	0
dark chocolate	1.75 oz	230	25	1	0
milk chocolate	1.75 oz	240	27	3	0
sugar-free chocolate candy bars					
chocolate almond	1 oz	130	15	1	0
chocolate crisp	1 oz	120	16	<1	0
chocolate mint	1 oz	140	15	<1	0
chocolate peanut butter	1 oz	140	15	<1	0
chocolate truffle	1 oz	122	17	1	0
coconut & almonds	1.1 oz	120	17	2	0
dark chocolate	1 oz	130	15	2	0
milk chocolate	1 oz	140	15	<1	0
peanut butter cups bar	1.2 oz	170	17	1	0
■ (Cella) (*See* (Tootsie Roll) in this section)					
■ (Certs)					
Breath Mints	1 mint	5	2	0	2
Cool Mints	1 mint	5	1	0	1
Powerful Mints	1 mint	<1	0	0	0
■ (Charms)					
Blow Pop					
junior	1 pop	50	17	0	14
regular	1 pop	60	18	0	17
super	1 pop	130	36	0	34
Charm's Way w/Sour Blow Pop	junior	50	17	0	17
	regular	60	18	0	17
	super	140	36	0	34
Charm's Zip-A-Dee-Doo-Da Pop	3 pops	50	14	0	10
Sour Pop/flat					
junior	1 pop	50	14	0	10
regular	1 pop	70	17	0	13
Sweet Pop/flat					
junior	1 pop	50	14	0	10
regular	1 pop	70	17	0	13
■ CHUNKY BAR (*See* (Nestlé USA) in this section)					
■ (Clark) Clark Bar	1.75 oz	220	37	2	29
■ CRUNCH (*See* (Nestlé USA) in this section)					
■ DOVE (*See* (M&M * Mars) in this section)					
■ (Edward & Sons) Let's Do Organics					
black licorice bears	1 bag	80	22	0	18
gummy bears/all flavors					
classic	1 bag	80	22	0	18
fruit juicy	16 pieces	130	34	0	29
jelly	1 bag	80	22	0	18
super sour gummy	1 bag	80	22	0	18
gummy worms..sour	7 pieces	130	34	0	29
Hard Organic candies					
butterscotch..old-fashioned	3 pieces	50	13	0	10
cool peppermints	6 pieces	50	13	0	10
exotic jelly fruits	15 pieces	130	35	0	30
fruit flavors/all	6 pieces	50	13	0	10

Food and Description	Amount	Total Calories	Total Carbs	Fiber	Sugars
intense breath mints	1 piece	5	2	0	1
■ (Estee)					
caramel/chocolate or vanilla	5 pieces	150	26	0	3
chocolate bar					
dark chocolate	7 squares	200	23	0	15
milk chocolate					
crisp rice	1 bar	370	29	0	24
plain	7 squares	230	16	0	15
w/almonds	7 squares	230	16	0	14
w/fruit & nuts	7 squares	220	18	0	15
mint	7 squares	200	23	0	15
peanut brittle	⅓ box	210	28	1	<1
peanut butter cups	5 candies	200	19	1	13
sugar-free gumdrops..all flavors	23 pieces	140	36	0	0
■ (Fifty/50)					
no-sugar-added candy					
candy bars..chocolate					
almond	7 pieces	210	20	1	5
chocolate-covered peanut	2 bars	200	16	2	2
crunch	7 pieces	160	17	<1	4
fruit & nut	7 pieces	200	21	1	7
minis	8 bars	140	16	0	2
■ (Ghirardelli)					
chocolate drops					
chocolate nonpareils	10 pieces	190	30	2	25
milk chocolate	11 pieces	210	26	<1	24
filled bars					
dark chocolate w/orange filling	5 squares	200	24	<1	21
milk chocolate					
w/caramel center filling	6 squares	200	24	<1	21
w/double chocolate filling	5 squares	200	24	<1	18
Legend Boxes..nonpareils	10 pieces	190	30	2	25
Premier chocolate bars					
Premier/2.5 oz..milk w/crisp	1 bar	360	44	1	35
Premier/3 oz					
dark chocolate					
plain	6 sections	210	26	2	21
w/raspberries	6 sections	210	26	3	21
milk chocolate					
w/almonds	6 sections	230	23	1	20
w/crisp	1 bar	360	44	1	35
mint chocolate	6 sections	220	26	1	23
squares..milk chocolate					
plain	4 squares	230	25	<1	23
w/caramel filling..natural flavor	3 squares	220	26	<1	23
w/caramelized almonds	4 squares	230	23	1	20
w/double chocolate filling	3 squares	220	26	<1	20
w/white mint filling	3 squares	210	30	2	25
■ (Godiva)					
bouchée					

Food and Description	Amount	Total Calories	Total Carbs	Fiber	Sugars
chocolate hazelnut	1 piece	140	13	1	11
dark chocolate	2 pieces	200	22	3	17
raspberry	2 pieces	190	25	2	20
raspberry cashew	1 piece	150	16	1	13
vanilla nut caramel or pecan	1 piece	150	13	1	12
white chocolate cream	4 pieces	200	22	1	20
cordials					
cherry	3 pieces	160	25	2	22
raspberry	3 pieces	190	32	5	22
demitasse					
dark chocolate	8 pieces	220	25	4	20
milk chocolate	8 pieces	220	23	1	23
truffles					
dark chocolate	8 pieces	220	25	4	20
milk chocolate	8 pieces	220	23	1	23

■ **GOOBERS** (*See* (Nestlé USA) in this section)
■ **GOOD & PLENTY** (*See* (Hershey) in this section)
■ **GUMMY BEARS** (*See* (Brach's and other brands) in this section)
■ **(Hershey)**

Food and Description	Amount	Total Calories	Total Carbs	Fiber	Sugars
Almond Joy	0.69-oz bar	90	11	0	9
Carmello	0.66-oz bar	90	12	0	21
Cookies 'n' Creme..bites	18 pieces	210	23	0	21
crispy rice snacks..peanut butter	3 bars	180	27	<1	14
5th Avenue	0.58-oz bar	80	10	0	8
Good & Plenty	1 box	170	43	0	27
Heath Bar	1.32 oz	200	23	<1	22
snack bar	1 piece	50	6	0	22
Hershey's					
Bites					
Almond Joy	18 pieces	230	23	2	21
milk chocolate w/almond	17 pieces	220	20	1	18
Reese's Peanut Butter	16 pieces	220	23	1	20
Cookies 'n' Creme	18 pieces	210	23	0	21
York Peppermint Patty	15 pieces	160	33	<1	29
Miniatures/chocolate bars					
milk chocolate	5 pieces	230	26	1	22
special dark	5 pieces	230	26	1	22
Nuggets					
Cookies 'n' Creme	4 pieces	190	21	0	18
dark chocolate..w/almonds	4 pieces	220	20	3	16
milk chocolate					
w/almonds	4 pieces	210	20	1	16
w/almonds & toffee	4 pieces	220	21	1	19
w/raisins & almonds	4 pieces	200	23	1	21
w/o almonds	4 pieces	230	24	1	21
1 gram sugar carb					
chocolate candy	1.1 oz	130	18	7	1
w/almonds	1.1 oz	140	16	7	1
w/soy crisps	1.1 oz	120	16	6	1
sugar-free chocolate candy					

Food and Description	Amount	Total Calories	Total Carbs	Fiber	Sugars
chocolate candy	5 pieces	170	24	2	0
dark chocolate	5 pieces	170	24	3	0
peanut butter cup					
miniatures..Reese's	5 pieces	170	23	1	0
w/almonds	5 pieces	180	23	3	0
Hugs/chocolate	9 pieces	210	23	0	21
Jolly Ranchers					
hard assorted candies	3 pieces	70	17	0	11
lollipops	1 piece	60	16	0	12
Kisses					
plain	9 pieces	230	24	1	21
w/almonds	9 pieces	230	21	1	19
Kit-Kat wafer bar	king-size	410	51	2	41
	1.45 oz	210	28	<1	24
Krackel	1 bar	90	12	0	10
	1.45 oz	210	28	<1	24
milk chocolate bar					
plain	0.3 oz	90	10	0	9
w/almonds	0.6 oz	90	9	1	14
Milk Duds	13 pieces	170	28	0	19
Mr. Goodbar	0.6 oz	100	9	0	8
	1.75 oz	270	27	2	23
Mounds	0.68 oz bar	90	11	0	19
	1.75 oz	240	29	2	23
Nibs					
cherry	2.25-oz pkg	220	51	0	33
licorice	2.25-oz pkg	210	48	0	31
Pay Day	1.85 oz	260	28	2	22
	snack bar	90	10	<1	8
Reese's					
Nutrageous	1.8 oz	280	27	2	20
	0.6 oz	190	18	1	14
peanut butter					
cup/miniatures	5 pieces	210	22	1	19
eggs	1 piece	90	9	0	8
regular	1.75 oz	270	27	2	23
pieces	1 pouch	190	22	1	20
Rolo chocolate caramels					
in milk chocolate	7 pieces	210	29	0	27
	1.7 oz	230	33	0	31
Skor	1.4 oz	220	24	0	23
Symphony/milk chocolate	1.5 oz	230	24	<1	23
Swoops					
Almond Joy	1 cup	200	20	1	18
Hershey's milk chocolate	1 cup	190	20	1	18
Reese's	1 cup	180	17	2	14
York Peppermint Patty	1 cup	190	21	2	18
Twizzlers					
cherry	3 pieces	130	30	0	18
chocolate	5 pieces	160	34	0	18

Food and Description	Amount	Total Calories	Total Carbs	Fiber	Sugars
licorice	4 pieces	150	34	0	18
strawberry	4 pieces	160	36	0	18
Whatchamacallit	0.57-oz bar	80	10	0	8
	1.6-oz bar	230	28	<1	22
Whoppers malted milk balls	18 pieces	190	31	<1	25
York Peppermint Patty					
bites	15 pieces	160	33	<1	29
patties	1.4 oz	160	33	<1	26
Zagnut	0.5 oz	70	9	0	6
Zero	1.85 oz	230	36	0	31
snack-size	0.6 oz	70	12	0	10
■ (Jelly Belly)					
Bertie Botts..all flavors	35 pieces	160	42	0	32
Gourmet Jelly Beans					
coconut	35 pieces	150	37	0	28
other flavors..all	35 pieces	140	37	0	28
sugar-free jelly beans..all flavors	35 pieces	80	37	8	0
■ JOLLY RANCHERS (*See* (Hershey) in this section)					
■ JUNIOR MINTS (*See* (Tootsie Roll) in this section)					
■ KRACKEL (*See* (Hershey) in this section)					
■ (Kraft)					
Altoid mints/curiously strong					
cinnamon w/character	1 mint	10	2	0	2
cinnamon/peppermint/spearmint	1 mint	10	2	0	2
fruit sours	1 mint	20	5	0	5
caramels..all flavors	1.4 oz	160	30	0	28
Creme savers					
chocolate & caramel..soft	1.375 oz	170	33	0	22
orange & cream	½ oz	70	13	0	11
raspberries & cream	½ oz	60	13	0	13
strawberries & cream	½ oz	60	13	0	13
Creme Savers/sugar-free..all flavors	½ oz	45	13	0	0
LifeSaver's					
assorted flavors	2 pieces	20	5	0	4
Easter jelly beans..all flavors	1.4 oz	150	37	0	32
Terry's chocolate orange					
dark	1.5 oz	240	28	3	24
milk	1.5 oz	230	27	1	25
pure milk	1.5 oz	230	27	0	24
Toblerone candy					
Swiss bittersweet w/honey & almond nougat	1.16 oz	170	21	1	18
Swiss milk chocolate w/honey & almond nougat	1.4 oz	170	21	1	18
	1.8 oz	260	32	1	27
w/honey & almond nougat bow	1.4 oz	210	26	1	22
Swiss white confection w/honey & almond nougat	1.16 oz	180	20	0	20
Trolli/Gummi					

Food and Description	Amount	Total Calories	Total Carbs	Fiber	Sugars
Classic Bears	1.4 oz	130	31	0	27
Hot Sting'n Red Ants	1.4 oz	130	30	0	27
Peachie-O's	1.4 oz	120	28	0	20
truffle peaks	1.4 oz	240	23	1	21
■ KUDOS (*See* (M&M * Mars) in this section)					
■ (La Nouba) Belgian chocolate bars					
coconut	1 bar	204	3.7	3.7	0
dark/dairy-free	1 bar	190	1.1	4.2	0
milk	1 bar	204	3.7	3.7	0
mint	1 bar	204	3.7	3.7	0
white/caffeine-free	1 bar	205	3.5	0	0
■ LAFFY TAFFY (*See* (Nestlé USA) in this section)					
■ (Lance)					
chews..all flavors	11 pieces	120	28	0	26
peanut bar	1 bar	340	29	3	19
■ LIFESAVERS (*See* (Planters) in this section)					
■ (Lindt)					
bittersweet hazelnut	14 blocks	220	18	0	16
Fairy Tales	14 blocks	210	22	0	17
mocha bar	14 blocks	210	21	0	18
pistachio	5 blocks	230	19	<1	18
Surfin' Bittersweet	14 blocks	210	21	0	19
Swiss milk chocolate	14 blocks	210	22	0	17
w/almonds	12 blocks	220	18	1	13
w/cherry	5 blocks	190	25	<2	24
w/hazelnuts	15 blocks	220	18	0	13
w/orange	5 blocks	200	24	<1	23
w/raspberry	5 blocks	190	24	<1	24
■ (M&M * Mars)					
Celebrations/mixed					
3 Musketeers	1 piece	30	5	0	4
Dove					
dark chocolate	1 piece	40	5	0	4
milk chocolate	1 piece	45	5	0	5
milk chocolate caramel	1 piece	40	5	0	5
Milky Way	1 piece	35	6	0	5
Milky Way/midnight	1 piece	30	5	0	4
Snickers	1 piece	40	5	0	4
Twix	1 piece	50	7	0	5
Celebrations..pkg..boxed..tin					
all types	5 pieces	190	26	1	22
Cookie Bars					
M&M's	1 bar	170	20	1	13
Milky Way	1 bar	180	21	1	13
Snickers	1 bar	180	20	1	12
Twix	1 bar	180	21	0	14
Dove					
dark chocolate					
Promises	5 pieces	210	24	2	20

Food and Description	Amount	Total Calories	Total Carbs	Fiber	Sugars
single	1.3 oz	200	22	2	19
6-oz bar	¼ bar	230	25	1	24
milk chocolate					
Promises	5 pieces	220	24	1	22
single	1.3 oz	200	22	1	20
6-oz bar	¼ bar	230	26	3	26
Kudos					
apple nut crunch	1 bar	90	15	1	8
chocolate chip	1 bar	130	20	1	13
milk chocolate	1 bar	130	20	1	13
Snickers bar	1 bar	100	16	0	10
M&M's					
almond..singles	1 bag	200	21	2	18
baking bits	0.5 oz	70	10	0	9
crispy	singles bag	200	31	1	25
minis	singles bag	150	21	1	19
peanut	singles bag	250	30	2	25
peanut butter	singles bag	240	26	2	22
plain	singles bag	240	34	1	31
Milky Way candy bars					
chocolate-covered caramels	2 oz	200	30	0	26
Midnight	1.76 oz	220	36	1	30
milk chocolate	2.05 oz	270	41	1	35
Musketeers (See (3 Musketeers) this section)					
Skittles					
Fresh Mint/bite-size	1.5 oz	170	37	0	31
singles (1.6-oz tube)	1 tube	180	40	0	33
original	1.5 oz	170	37	0	31
singles (2.17-oz bag)	1 bag	240	54	0	45
sour	1.5 oz	160	36	0	31
singles (1.8-oz bag)	1 bag	200	44	0	37
tropical..singles (2.17-oz bag)	1 bag	240	54	0	45
Snickers/singles					
almond	1.76 oz	240	32	1	27
Cruncher	1.66 oz	230	25	1	17
Marathon					
multigrain-crunch	1.56 oz	230	25	1	17
original	1.94 oz	229	26	2	18
	2.07 oz	280	35	1	30
Starburst					
California fruits	1 pack	240	48	0	3
chew pops..all flavors	1 pop	50	13	0	10
fruit & cream..all flavors	1 pack	240	48	0	34
jelly beans..all flavors	1.5 oz	150	38	0	30
3 Musketeers	2.13 oz bar	260	46	1	40
Chewlicious/chocolate-flavor chews	1 bar	100	18	0	15
fun-size	2 bars	140	25	1	22
miniatures	7 pieces	180	31	1	27

Food and Description	Amount	Total Calories	Total Carbs	Fiber	Sugars
Twix/cookie bars					
caramel	2 bars	280	37	1	27
peanut butter	2 bars	280	28	2	19
■ **MILK DUDS** (*See* (Hershey) in this section)					
■ **MILKY WAY** (*See* (M&M * Mars) in this section)					
■ **MR. GOODBAR** (*See* (Hershey) in this section)					
■ **MOUNDS** (*See* (Hershey) in this section)					
■ **(Nestlé USA)**					
Baby Ruth					
beast (5 oz)	1.25 oz	160	22	1	18
full-size	2.1 oz	280	37	2	31
fun-size	1 oz	130	17	<1	13
king-size	1.25 oz	160	22	1	18
Bit O'Honey	1.7 oz	190	40	0	23
Buncha Crunch	1.4 oz	200	26	1	20
crunchy movie pack	1.28 oz	190	24	1	19
Butterfinger					
BB's	1.7 oz	220	34	1	28
king-size	1.85 oz	190	30	1	22
snack pack	1.57 oz	190	30	1	22
candy bars					
beast (5 oz.)	1.25 oz	160	25	1	18
full-size (6 oz)	1 oz	270	44	1	30
fun-size (.75 oz)	1 bar	100	15	0	1
king-size	1.85 oz	190	30	1	22
minis/4 pieces	1.37 oz	180	29	1	20
single (2.14 oz)	1 bar	270	44	1	30
snack pack (5.5 oz)	1.57 oz	190	30	1	22
Chunky Bar	1.4 oz	200	24	1	21
milk chocolate	1.6 oz	230	29	1	24
beast (3.5 oz)	1.16 oz	160	22	1	18
king (2.8 oz)	2.8 oz	400	50	2	41
milk chocolate/extra crunchy..king	2.8 oz bar	400	50	2	41
white chocolate	1.4 oz	220	23	0	20
Crunch					
assorted minis	4 pieces	210	28	1	23
milk chocolate	1.85 oz	230	29	1	24
fun-size bag	1.4 oz	200	26	1	21
milk chocolate..w/caramel	1.52 oz	210	28	1	23
white chocolate/fun-size	1 bar	50	6	0	5
Flipz/2-oz pkg..all flavors	.5 oz	70	10	0	5
Goobers/milk chocolate-covered	1.38 oz bag	210	20	1	17
fun-size	2.5 oz	53	6	1	5
milk chocolate bar	1.45 oz	220	21	2	18
On-the-Go box	1.4 oz	220	21	2	18
	1.5 oz	210	23	2	21
Nips..all flavors	2 pieces	60	10	0	7
O'Henry!	1.8 oz	230	32	2	30
Raisinets	1.58 oz	200	31	1	28
fun-size	2 oz	280	38	2	25

Food and Description	Amount	Total Calories	Total Carbs	Fiber	Sugars
On-the-Go	1.75 oz	200	31	1	28
Signatures Treasures					
chocolate crème	1.33 oz	170	21	1	19
creamy caramel	3 pieces	160	22	1	19
peanut butter	1.33 oz	190	19	1	17
Sno-Caps/box	2.3 oz	300	48	3	38
semisweet chocolate	1.40 oz	190	29	2	23
On-the-Go	1.55 oz	180	30	2	24
1000 Grand Bar					
fun-size	1 bar	200	29	1	20
super-size	2.8 oz	370	57	1	51
Toll House Candy Bars/chocolate					
brownie	1 oz	120	17	1	11
cookie	1 oz	120	18	1	12
Turtles					
original	1.16 oz	160	20	1	15
original/bite-size	1.4 oz	210	25	1	19
peanut	1.76 oz	240	30	1	22
peanut/sugar-free	1.3 oz	150	150	18	0
Wonder Ball/milk chocolate..all types	1 oz	140	21	0	20
Wonka					
Bottle Caps	10 pieces	60	15	0	15
Gobstoppers..all types	9 pieces	50	14	0	14
Gumball	1 ball	45	11	0	11
Nerds	1 Tbs	60	14	0	14
Nerds Rope	1 rope	100	24	0	22
Shocktarts	9 pieces	60	13	0	11
Wonka/Laffy Taffy..all flavors	1.4 oz	170	38	0	26
■ (Newman's Own Organics)					
Organics chocolate bars					
espresso chocolate	½ bar	200	20	2	17
milk chocolate	½ bar	240	22	1	20
butter toffee	½ bar	210	22	1	20
crispy rice	½ bar	200	23	1	20
orange chocolate	½ bar	200	24	2	20
sweet dark chocolate	½ bar	200	24	2	20
Organics cups					
peanut butter cups					
dark chocolate	1 pkg	280	18	1	14
milk chocolate	1 pkg	180	17	<1	14
peppermint cups					
dark chocolate	1 pkg	170	20	1	18
■ (Nutcracker)					
chocolate					
caramel cups	⅕ oz	180	22	2	17
covered almonds	1.4 oz	220	18	2	16
covered cashews	1.4 oz	220	20	1	14
dark..w/peppermint center	1.25 oz	200	24	1	20
peanut caramel clusters	1.60 oz	220	24	2	13
ultimate tropical	1 oz	160	20	2	16

Food and Description	Amount	Total Calories	Total Carbs	Fiber	Sugars
■ **NUTRAGEOUS** (*See* (Hershey) in this section)					
■ **(OH HENRY!)** (*See* (Nestlé USA) in this section)					
■ **(Old Dominion)**					
cashew brittle	1.5 oz	190	32	1	15
peanut brittle	1.5 oz	190	32	5	12
peanut candy	1.5 oz	200	31	3	15
■ **PAY DAY** (*See* (Hershey) in this section)					
■ **(Pearson's)**					
Bun Bars..all sorts	1.75 oz	240	33	1	27
Mint Patties	5 pieces	150	33	1	27
Nut Goodie	1.75 oz	240	32	1	28
Salted Nut Roll	1.8 oz	240	27	2	20
	2.5 oz	340	40	2	29
	3.5 oz	470	31	<1	27
■ **(Planters)**					
LifeSavers					
candy cane, big tablet	4 pieces	60	16	0	13
Gummy Savers					
5-flavor	1.5-oz pkg	140	33	0	25
mixed berry	1.5-oz pkg	140	33	0	25
Tangy Fruit	1.5-oz pkg	130	33	0	25
Wacky Frootz	1.5-oz pkg	130	33	0	25
Holes..all flavors	20 pieces	20	20	0	20
LifeSavers/regular roll					
butter rum	3 pieces	60	15	0	13
Egg-Sortment	1 roll	40	10	0	10
5-flavor	2 pieces	20	5	0	4
Fruits on Fire	2 pieces	20	5	0	4
Pep-O-Mint	3 pieces	20	5	0	4
Spear-O-Mint	3 pieces	20	5	0	4
Sunshine Fruits	2 pieces	20	5	0	4
Tangy Fruit Swirls	4 pieces	40	5	0	4
Tangy Fruits	2 pieces	20	5	0	4
tropical fruits	2 pieces	20	5	0	4
watermelon	2 pieces	20	5	0	4
Wint-O-Green	2 pieces	20	5	0	4
lollipops/assorted	1 pop	40	10	0	10
Sack'it/assorted	4 pieces	60	15	0	13
■ **RAISINETS** (*See* (Nestlé USA) in this section)					
■ **(Rapunzel)**					
organic chocolate					
Swiss bittersweet..70% cocoa	½ bar	224	12	4	11
Swiss espresso..chocolate	½ bar	218	18	4	17
Swiss milk chocolate					
w/nut truffle..cream bar	½ bar	230	18	1	17
w/rum raisin bar	½ bar	217	18.5	1	18
Swiss semisweet					
w/almonds	½ bar	222	16	4	15
w/hazelnuts	½ bar	216	16	4	15

Food and Description	Amount	Total Calories	Total Carbs	Fiber	Sugars
■ REESE'S (*See* (Hershey) in this section)					
■ REGAL DYNASTY					
imported chocolate..assorted	4 pieces	200	21	1	18
Vivani Premium Organic					
dark chocolate..72% cocoa	1.5 oz	228	13	3	18
milk chocolate	1.5 oz	235	18	<1	18
w/hazelnuts	1.5 oz	239	17	<1	18
w/praline filling	1.5 oz	240	19	1	18
white chocolate..w/crispy rice	1.5 oz	236	22	0	18
■ RIESEN (*See* (Storck) in this section)					
■ (Ross)					
low-carb/sugar-free chocolate bars					
Almond Delight	1.2 oz	180	3.9	0	0
Belgian	1.2 oz	167	3	0	0
milk	1.2 oz	170	2.7	0	0
White Delight	1.2 oz	170	2.9	0	0
coconut	1.2 oz	180	3.7	0	0
Coconut Delight	1.2 oz	180	3.9	0	0
Crunchy Delight	1.2 oz	152	3.2	0	0
Dark Delight..only 1 gram bar	1.2 oz	161	1	0	0
Mint Delight	1.2 oz	167	3	0	0
Orange Delight	1.2 oz	167	3	1	0
■ (Russell Stover)					
almond delights	2 pieces	210	22	1	na
caramels	3 pieces	170	26	1	na
assorted	3 pieces	190	30	0	26
cherry cordials	3 pieces	170	25	2	na
chocolate assortments					
gift box..regular	3 pieces	180	26	0	na
milk chocolate	3 pieces	190	27	0	na
low-carb/sugar-free candies					
butter nut toffee sticks	4 pieces	160	22	1	0
chocolate-covered					
almonds	15 pieces	210	15	3	1
peanuts	25 pieces	210	17	2	1
mint patties	2 pieces	130	19	1	0
mousse medallions	2 pieces	120	28	1	0
peanut butter					
crunch	4 pieces	180	29	1	0
cups	4 pieces	180	18	2	6
medallions	2 pieces	130	14	1	0
Pecan Delights	4 pieces	180	24	2	0
	2 pieces	130	16	2	0
toffee squares	2 pieces	110	16	0	0
truffle cups	4 pieces	170	23	1	0
wafers	2 pieces	130	16	1	0
mints..French chocolate..boxed	4 pieces	220	20	2	na
Mint Dream	1 bar	160	28	1	na
Pecan Delights..boxed	2 pieces	220	19	1	na
pecan roll	1 roll	300	26	3	21

Food and Description	Amount	Total Calories	Total Carbs	Fiber	Sugars
sugar-free					
almond clusters	3 pieces	200	17	1	9
coconut miniatures	5 pieces	190	20	3	0
crispy miniatures	6 pieces	180	23	1	0
dark chocolate/solid	5 pieces	220	21	2	0
French mint miniatures	5 pieces	190	22	1	0
Liberty Orchards fruit softies	3 pieces	140	27	0	0
milk chocolate & almonds	5 pieces	200	21	1	0
milk chocolate miniatures	5 pieces	190	22	2	0
mint patties	3 pieces	190	27	1	0
orange cream miniatures	5 pieces	170	23	1	0
peanut clusters	4 pieces	170	18	2	0
Peanut Delights	2 pieces	140	17	1	0
Pecan Delights	2 pieces	170	17	0	0
strawberry cream	5 pieces	170	23	1	0
■ **SKITTLES** (*See* (Hershey) in this section)					
■ **SNO-CAPS** (*See* (Nestlé USA) in this section)					
■ **STARBURST** (*See* (Hershey) in this section)					
■ **(Storck)**					
Mamba/fruit chews..all sorts	6 pieces	110	23	0	12
Riesen/chocolate caramel					
in rich chocolate	1.25 oz	180	29	2	16
Toffifay hazelnut in caramel	1.43 oz	210	26	2	20
w/chocolate	1.16 oz	170	21	2	16
Werther's					
caramels chewy	1.8 oz	210	39	0	19
hard	½ oz	60	13	0	11
original	3 pieces	60	13	1	11
sugar-free	½ oz	40	14	0	0
toffee & milk chocolate	1.25 oz	220	21	2	18
■ **SUGAR BABIES** (*See* (Tootsie Roll) in this section)					
■ **SUGAR DADDY** (*See* (Tootsie Roll) in this section)					
■ **(Sweet 'N Low)**					
hard candies					
butter toffee	5 pieces	28	14	0	0
cinnamon	5 pieces	30	15	0	0
coffee...all flavors	5 pieces	30	14	0	0
fruit flavors	5 pieces	30	15	0	0
international coffee flavors	5 pieces	30	14	0	0
peppermint	5 pieces	30	15	0	0
Spectations wafer bars..peanut butter	3 bars	160	21	1	0
■ **SYMPHONY** (*See* (Hershey) in this section)					
■ **TAFFY TARTS** (*See* (Concorde) in this section)					
■ **3 MUSKETEERS** (*See* (M&M * Mars) in this section)					
■ **(Tootsie Roll)**					
Cella chocolate-covered cherries	2 pieces	110	18	2	17
Charleston Chew bar..all flavors	1.9 oz	230	43	0	30
Fluffy Stuff/small bag	1 oz	120	30	0	30
Hot Dots	12 dots	140	35	0	21
Junior Mints	16 pieces	170	35	<1	1

Food and Description	Amount	Total Calories	Total Carbs	Fiber	Sugars
Mason Dots	12 dots	140	35	0	21
Pops					
candy cane	1 pop	60	15	0	11
caramel apple	1 pop	60	15	0	10
fruit smoothie	1 pop	60	15	0	11
hot chocolate	1 pop	70	17	0	14
orange cream	1 pop	70	17	0	14
Sugar Babies	30 pieces	180	41	0	32
Sugar Daddy					
junior pop	3 pops	160	34	0	23
large pop	1 pop	200	43	0	29
Sugar Daddy Junior	3 pops	160	34	0	23
Tootsie Flavor Rolls	6 pieces	160	34	0	24
Tootsie Frooties	12 pieces	140	29	0	21
Tootsie Pop					
miniature	3 pops	50	13	0	9
regular	1 pop	60	15	0	10
small	1 pop	45	12	0	8
Tootsie Roll bars	1.1-oz pkg	110	23	<1	16
	1.5-oz pkg	150	30	0	21
■ **WERTHER'S** (*See* (Storck) in this section)					
■ **(WHATCHAMACALLIT** (*See* (Hershey) in this section)					
■ **(Whitman's)**					
assorted	3 pieces	190	27	0	22
dark chocolate	3 pieces	200	25	1	19
Little Ambassadors	7 pieces	190	26	1	22
Pecan Delight Bar	1 bar	310	27	2	17
Pecan Roll	1 bar	300	26	1	21
■ **WHOPPERS** (*See* (Hershey) in this section)					
■ **WONKA** (*See* (Nestlé USA) in this section)					
■ **YORK** (*See* (Hershey) in this section)					
CANNELLINI BEAN (*See* KIDNEY BEAN)					
CANTALOUPE/MUSKMELON					
FRESH					
cubed	1 cup	57	15	1	2
whole/~ 9.5 oz	½ melon	94	22	2	2
CAPERS					
(Crosse & Blackwell)	1 Tbs	5	1	0	0
(Peloponnese) wild	½ oz	0	0	0	0
CAPON					
giblets/simmered	5 oz	238	1	0	0
meat & skin/roasted	4 oz	260	0	0	0
CARAMBOLA (*See* STAR FRUIT)					
CARAWAY SEED	1 tsp	8	1	0	0
CARDAMOM SEED					
ground	1 Tbs	20	4	2	0
whole	1 tsp	6	1	<1	0
CARDOON					
cooked	3 oz	19	4	1	0
raw/shredded	1 cup	35	9	3	0

Food and Description	Amount	Total Calories	Total Carbs	Fiber	Sugars
CARISSA/NATAL PLUM..raw	1 medium	12	3	na	na
CAROB CHIPS					
regular	1 oz	140	15	0	na
mini	1 oz	140	15	0	na
CARP/cooked—dry heat	3 oz	138	0	0	0
CARP ROE/raw	3 oz	111	1	0	0
CARROT (*See also* VEGETABLES, MIXED)					
CANNED					
(Del Monte)					
honey-glazed	½ cup	70	18	1	12
julienne French-style	½ cup	30	5	2	4
sliced	½ cup	35	8	3	5
(Libby's) all styles	½ cup	25	6	2	3
(S&W) all styles	½ cup	30	5	2	4
(Stokely) all styles	½ cup	30	6	2	4
FRESH					
(Dole)					
shredded	½ cup	24	5.5	2	0
whole/1¼" dia	7" long	35	8	1	0
FROZEN					
(Birds Eye)					
sliced	½ cup	35	8	1	6
whole baby	½ cup	40	9	2	6
(C&W)					
Parisienne	⅔ cup	40	10	3	2
whole baby	⅔ cup	35	6	2	3
(Cascadian Farm) honey-glazed	1 cup	60	14	3	10
(Green Giant) boil-in-bag					
glazed family-size	¾ cup	70	47	2	4
honey-glazed	1 cup	90	13	2	10
(Schwan) maple-glazed	4.5 oz	140	11	2	7
CARROT JUICE					
CANNED					
(Hain)	1 cup	80	17	0	14
(Hollywood)	12 fl oz	120	27	1	25
(Odwalla)					
carrot blend..carrot/orange/apple	8 fl oz	100	23	1	21
Essentials	8 fl oz	70	15	1	13
CASABA MELON					
FRESH					
cubed	1 cup	45	11	1	<1
whole/8" melon	2" slice	45	11	1	<1
CASHEW					
(Beer Nuts) sweet & salty	1 oz	170	8	1	2.5
(Fisher)					
halves & pieces	1 oz	160	8	1	2
honey-roasted..whole	1 oz	150	11	1	4
oil-roasted	1 oz	170	8	1	0
Snack 'n' Serve Nut Bowl					
jumbo whole	1 oz	170	8	1	0

Food and Description	Amount	Total Calories	Total Carbs	Fiber	Sugars
whole/premium	1 oz	160	8	1	2
(Kettle) roasted..salt or unsalted	1 oz	160	8	1	2
(Lance)	1.125 oz	200	8	3	3
(Nutcracker)					
halves & pieces	1 oz	190	9	1	2
pieces..salted	1.18 oz	190	8	1	2
whole..salted	1 oz	190	9	1	2
(Planters)					
fancy	1 oz	170	8	1	2
halves & pieces	1 oz	170	7	1	0
honey-roasted..whole	1 oz	150	11	1	4
whole	1 oz	170	8	1	0
whole honey-roasted	1 oz	150	11	1	4
CASHEW BUTTER					
(Arrowhead Mills) all styles	2 Tbs	160	8	1	2
(Hain)					
raw	2 Tbs	190	8	0	0
toasted	2 Tbs	210	7	0	0
unsalted	2 Tbs	210	8	0	0
(Kettle) Roaster..fresh..unsalted	1 oz	165	9	0	0
CASSAVA					
raw/trimmed..chopped or sliced pieces	1 cup	330	78	4	0
CATFISH (*See also* SEAFOOD ENTRÉE/DINNER)					
channel/fresh/meat only..farmed					
baked or broiled	3 oz	130	0	0	0
breaded & fried	3 oz	195	7	1	0
CATSUP/KETCHUP					
(Atkins) Ketch-A-Tomato	1 Tbs	10	2	1	0
(Del Monte) all styles	1 Tbs	15	4	0	4
(Hain) natural..all styles	1 Tbs	16	4	0	4
(Heinz)					
light	1 Tbs	10	3	0	3
regular	1 Tbs	15	4	0	4
w/onions	1 Tbs	20	4	0	4
(Hunt's)					
no salt added	1 Tbs	20	4	0	4
regular or squeeze	1 Tbs	15	4	0	4
(Westbrae)					
fruit-sweetened					
regular	1 Tbs	10	3	0	1
squeeze	1 Tbs	20	4	0	4
unsweetened	1 Tbs	5	1	0	0
CAULIFLOWER					
FRESH..white					
cooked	½ cup	17	3	2	0
raw					
chopped	½ cup	12	3	2	0
(Dole)	3.5 oz	20	5	5	0
whole/medium head	⅙ head	25	5	2	2
FROZEN					

Food and Description	Amount	Total Calories	Total Carbs	Fiber	Sugars
(Birds Eye)	½ cup	25	5	2	1
(Green Giant) florets/cooked	⅔ cup	20	3	2	1
JARRED					
(Arnold's) pickled	1 oz	10	1	0	0
(Mrs. Klein's) hot	1 oz	4	1	0	0
(Vlasic)					
hot & spicy	1 oz	4	1	0	<1
sweet	1 oz	35	9	0	4
CAULIFLOWER DISH (*See also* FROZEN ENTRÉE/DINNER; VEGETABLES, MIXED)					
(Birds Eye) frozen..w/garlic sauce	1¼ cup	60	6	2	0
(Green Giant) frozen in cheese sauce	½ cup	60	7	1	4
CAVIAR					
(Romanoff)					
beluga	2 Tbs	74	1	0	0
black lumpfish	1 Tbs	15	0	0	0
black whitefish	1 Tbs	25	1	0	0
red lumpfish	1 Tbs	15	0	0	0
salmon	1 Tbs	35	0	0	0
(T. Marzetti)					
black					
lumpfish	1 Tbs	15	0	0	0
whitefish	1 Tbs	25	1	0	0
golden					
lumpfish	1 Tbs	15	0	0	0
whitefish	1 Tbs	25	1	0	0
red lumpfish	1 Tbs	15	0	0	0
salmon..all types	1 Tbs	35	0	0	0
CELERIAC/CELERY ROOT/WILD CELERY					
raw	½ cup	31	7	1.5	0
	4–5 medium	40	10	2	0
CELERY					
Chinese/diced	1 cup	15	3	1	0
fresh/medium stalks					
cooked	½ cup	13	6	2	0
raw	1 stalk	6	1	1	0
diced	½ cup	9	1	0	0
(Dole)	2 stalks	20	4	2	
CELERY ROOT (*See* CELERIAC)					
CELERY SEED/whole	1 tsp	8	1	0	0
CELERY SOUP (*See* SOUP)					
CEREAL (*See also* BARLEY; BULGUR; CORN GRITS)					
■ **COLD/READY-TO-EAT**					
Alpha-Bits (*See* (Post) in this section)					
(Arrowhead Mills)					
amaranth flakes	1 cup	140	26	3	4
bran flakes	1 cup	110	22	5	3
cornflakes	1 cup	120	27	2	2
kamut flakes	1 cup	120	25	2	2
maple buckwheat flakes	1 cup	170	35	1	5
multigrain flakes	1 cup	170	33	3	3

Food and Description	Amount	Total Calories	Total Carbs	Fiber	Sugars
Nature O's	1 cup	130	25	2	1
oat bran flakes	1 cup	140	24	4	3
Perfect Harvest	1 cup	140	25	5	2
puffed corn	1 cup	60	12	2	0
puffed kamut	1 cup	50	11	2	0
puffed millet	1 cup	60	11	1	0
puffed rice	1 cup	60	14	<1	0
puffed wheat	1 cup	60	12	2	0
raisin bran	1 cup	190	41	10	17
rice flakes	1 cup	180	40	1	8
shredded wheat					
sweetened	1 cup	200	42	5	12
unsweetened	1 cup	190	38	6	2
spelt flakes	1 cup	120	24	3	3
wheat bran	¼ cup	35	10	6	0
wheat germ/raw	3 Tbs	50	10	2	0
(Atkins) Morning Start Breakfast Cereal					
Banana Nut Harvest	~¾ cup	100	11	6	1
Crunchy Almond Crisp	~¾ cup	100	8	5	1
(Barbara's)					
2 Good	1 cup	120	24	<1	1
Alpen/Swiss-style					
no sugar or salt added	⅓cup	200	40	4	7
original	⅔ cup	200	41	4	11
Apple Cinnamon Toasted O's	¾ cup	110	24	2	11
Breakfast O's	1¼ cups	110	22	3	2
Brown Rice Crisps	1 cup	120	25	1	2
Cornflakes	1 cup	110	26	2	3
Fruity Punch	¾ cup	120	26	0	9
GrainShop	⅔ cup	90	24	9	1
Honey Crunch'n Oats	¾ cup	120	24	2	6
Honey Nut Toasted O's	¾ cup	120	23	2	11
Organic					
Crispy Wheats	¾ cup	110	25	3	6
Weetabix Biscuits	2 biscuits	120	28	4	2
Wild puffs	1 cup	100	23	<1	12
Puffins					
cinnamon	¾ cup	100	26	6	6
honey rice	¾ cup	120	25	2	6
original	¾ cup	90	23	5	5
peanut butter	¾ cup	110	23	2	6
shredded					
oats/bite-size	1¼ cups	220	46	5	12
Spoonfuls/multigrain	¾ cup	120	24	4	5
vanilla almond	1 cup	220	42	4	15
wheat biscuits	2 biscuits	140	31	5	0
SoyEssence	¾ cup	110	25	5	5
(Breadshop) granola					
blueberries 'n' cream	½ cup	220	32	4	7
cinnamon raisin	½ cup	220	37	4	15

Food and Description	Amount	Total Calories	Total Carbs	Fiber	Sugars
crunchy oat bran	½ cup	210	31	5	9
Honey Gone Nuts	¾ cup	240	33	4	6
mocha almond crunch	¾ cup	210	34	4	4
pralines 'n' cream	¾ cup	210	34	4	8
raspberries 'n' cream	½ cup	220	32	4	7
strawberries 'n' cream	½ cup	220	32	4	7
Super Natural w/almonds	½ cup	220	31	3	11
Tripleberry Crunch	⅔ cup	220	36	4	9
Vermont maple	¾ cup	210	33	4	11
Cap'n Crunch (*See* (Quaker) in this section)					
Cheerios (*See* (General Mills) in this section)					
(Erewhon)					
amaranth/Aztec Corn	1 cup	110	26	1	1
Apple Stroodles	¾ cup	110	25	1	4
cornflakes	1¼ cups	210	45	3	<1
crispy brown rice					
gluten-free	¾ cup	110	25	0	<1
no salt added	¾ cup	110	25	1	1
original	¾ cup	110	25	1	1
w/mixed berries	¾ cup	120	27	1	6
Fruit 'n' Wheat	¾ cup	170	39	5	12
kamut flakes	⅔ cup	110	25	4	1
oat bran..w/toasted wheat germ	⅓ cup	170	31	5	1
raisin bran	1 cup	170	40	6	10
rice twice	¾ cup	120	26	0	8
whole wheat flakes	1 cup	180	42	6	<1
Fruit & Fiber (*See* (Post) in this section)					
(General Mills) Big G Cereals					
Basic 4	1 cup	200	42	3	14
Boo Berry	1 cup	120	27	0	14
Cheerios					
apple cinnamon	¾ cup	120	25	1	13
Berry Burst..all flavors	1 cup	110	24	2	11
frosted	1 cup	120	25	1	13
Honey Nut	1 cup	120	24	2	11
multigrain plus	1 cup	110	24	3	6
original	1 cup	110	22	3	1
Team	1 cup	110	25	2	11
Chex					
corn	1 cup	110	25	0	3
frosted mini	¾ cup	110	27	0	10
honey nut	¾ cup	120	26	0	9
morning mix..all styles & flavors	1 pouch	130	24	1	9
multibran	1 cup	200	49	8	12
rice	1¼ cups	120	27	0	2
wheat	1 cup	180	40	5	5
Cinnamon Grahams	¾ cup	120	26	1	11
Cinnamon Toast Crunch	¾ cup	130	24	1	10
Cocoa Puffs	1 cup	120	26	0	14
Cookie Crisp	1 cup	120	26	0	13

Food and Description	Amount	Total Calories	Total Carbs	Fiber	Sugars
Count Chocula	1 cup	120	26	0	14
Country Corn Flakes	1 cup	110	26	0	2
Fiber One	½ cup	60	24	14	0
Frankenberry	1 cup	120	27	0	14
French Toast Crunch	¾ cup	120	20	0	12
Gold Medal Raisin Bran	1⅓ cups	170	41	6	12
Golden Grahams	¾ cup	120	25	1	10
Harmony	1½ cups	200	43	2	11
Honey Nut Clusters	1 cup	210	46	3	17
Kaboom	1¼ cups	120	26	0	6
Kix					
Berry Berry	¾ cup	120	25	0	9
original	1⅓ cups	120	25	1	3
Lucky Charms	1 cup	120	25	1	13
Multi-bran Chex	1 cup	200	49	8	12
Nature Valley low-fat fruit granola	⅔ cup	210	44	3	19
Nesquik chocolate	¾ cup	120	25	0	12
Oatmeal Crisp					
almond	1 cup	220	42	4	16
apple cinnamon	1 cup	210	45	4	19
raisin	1 cup	210	44	4	18
Peanut Butter					
Toast Crunch	¾ cup	130	23	1	10
Raisin Nut Bran	¾ cup	200	41	4	16
Reese's Peanut Butter Puffs	¾ cup	130	23	0	13
Rice Chex	1¼ cups	120	27	0	2
Total					
brown sugar & oats	¾ cup	110	23	1	9
cornflakes	1½ cups	110	24	0	4
raisin bran	1 cup	170	41	5	20
whole wheat	¾ cup	110	23	3	5
Trix	1 cup	120	27	1	13
Wheaties					
Energy Crunch	1 cup	210	42	4	13
honey-frosted	¾ cup	110	27	0	12
original	1 cup	110	24	3	4
raisin bran	1 cup	180	44	5	18
(Golden Temple) part organic					
granola					
cinnamon apple raisin	½ cup	220	33	4	12
fruit & nut	½ cup	220	33	4	12
ginger snap	½ cup	220	36	3	15
super nutty	½ cup	220	33	4	12
wild blueberry	½ cup	230	33	4	8
low-fat					
apple cinnamon raisin	½ cup	190	38	4	14
strawberry/ raspberry	½ cup	200	39	4	14
(Health Valley)					
low-fat granola					
date almond flavor	⅔ cup	180	43	6	10

Food and Description	Amount	Total Calories	Total Carbs	Fiber	Sugars
raisin cinnamon	⅔ cup	180	43	6	10
tropical fruit	⅔ cup	180	43	6	10
non-organic cereal					
Banana Gone Nuts	¾ cup	200	41	4	11
Corn Crunch-Ems!	1 cup	110	26	2	2
Cranberry Crunch	¾ cup	200	41	4	11
Empower	1 cup	200	42	6	12
HeartWise	1 cup	200	36	5	12
Honey Crunches & Flakes	¾ cup	130	31	4	6
Raspberry Rhapsody	¾ cup	200	41	4	11
Real Oat Bran Almond Crunch	¾ cup	200	34	5	9
Rice Crunch-Ems!	1 cup	110	26	2	2
soy flakes					
original	1¼ cups	190	35	5	7
raisin	1 cup	190	39	4	15
Soy O's					
apple cinnamon	1 cup	180	31	3	7
honey nut	1 cup	180	31	3	7
original	1 cup	180	31	4	2
organic cereal					
amaranth flakes	¾ cup	100	24	4	4
blue corn flakes	¾ cup	100	24	3	5
Fiber 7/multigrain flakes	¾ cup	100	24	4	4
Golden Flax	¾ cup	190	38	6	9
Healthy Fiber/multigrain flakes	¾ cup	100	23	4	3
Honey Fiber 7 Flakes	¾ cup	110	27	4	7
Just Flakes..1-lb. box					
multigrain	¾ cup	100	24	4	4
oats	¾ cup	100	19	3	2
oat bran flakes	¾ cup	100	24	4	5
w/raisins	¾ cup	110	25	4	7
Oat Bran O's	¾ cup	100	23	3	14
raisin bran flakes	1¼ cups	190	46	6	13
raisin crunch bran	¾ cup	160	40	6	10
(Kashi)					
Go-lean					
crunchy	¾ cup	120	28	10	7
regular	1 cup	190	36	8	13
Good Friends					
Cinna-raisin	1 cup	120	39	10	11
regular	¾ cup	90	24	8	6
Heart to Heart	¾ cup	110	25	5	5
Kashi					
Baby & Me/dry	4 Tbs	50	11	2	0
Medley	½ cup	120	15	1	0
Pilaf	½ cup	170	30	6	0
Puffed	1 cup	70	25	2	7
Promise/organic					
Autumn Wheat	1 cup	190	45	6	7
Cranberry Sunshine	1 cup	110	26	2	9

Food and Description	Amount	Total Calories	Total Carbs	Fiber	Sugars
Strawberry Fields	1 cup	120	28	1	9
Seven in the Morning	½ cup	210	47	7	3
(Kellogg's)					
All Bran					
Bran Buds	⅓ cup	70	24	13	8
original	½ cup	80	23	10	6
w/extra fiber	½ cup	50	20	13	0
Apple Jacks	1 cup	130	30	<1	17
Cinnamon Crunch Crispix	½ cup	120	26	<1	9
Marshmallow Scooby-Doo	1 cup	140	25	1	13
Cocoa Rice Krispies	½ cup	120	27	1	14
Complete					
oat bran flakes	¾ cup	110	23	4	6
wheat bran flakes	¾ cup	90	23	5	5
Corn Pops	1 cup	120	28	1	14
Cracklin' Oat Bran	¾ cup	200	35	5	15
Crispix	1 cup	110	26	1	3
Froot Loops					
marshmallow-blasted	1 cup	120	26	0	16
original	1 cup	120	28	1	15
Frosted Flakes	¾ cup	120	28	1	12
Fruit Harvest					
apple cinnamon	1 cup	190	42	3	19
peach strawberry	¾ cup	110	26	1	9
strawberry blueberry	¾ cup	110	25	1	10
granola..low-fat w/raisins	⅔ cup	220	48	3	17
Honey Crunch cornflakes	¾ cup	120	26	1	10
Just Right..w/fruit & nuts	1 cup	200	43	3	13
Kellogg's					
Corn Flakes	1 cup	100	24	1	2
Frosted Flakes	1 cup	120	28	1	12
S'morz	1 cup	120	25	<1	13
Mini-Wheats..frosted					
bite-size	~24 biscuits	200	48	6	12
maple & brown sugar	24 biscuits	190	44	5	13
original	~5 biscuits	180	41	5	10
raisin	¾ cup	180	42	5	11
strawberry	¾ cup	170	40	5	9
Mueslix w/raisins, dates & almonds	⅔ cup	200	40	4	17
Product 19	1 cup	100	25	1	4
Raisin Bran	1 cup	190	45	7	19
Raisin Bran Crunch	1 cup	190	45	4	20
Rice Krispies					
original	1¼ cups	120	29	0	3
Treats	¾ cup	120	26	0	9
Smacks	¾ cup	100	24	1	15
Smart Start					
original	1 cup	190	43	3	14
soy protein	1 cup	200	40	4	14

Food and Description	Amount	Total Calories	Total Carbs	Fiber	Sugars
Special K					
original	1 cup	110	22	<1	4
red berries	1 cup	110	25	1	10
Tony's Cinnamon Krunchers	1 cup	110	23	<1	10
(Kretschmer)					
wheat bran	¼ cup	30	10	7	0
wheat germ					
honey crunch	1⅔ Tbs	50	8	1	3
regular	2 Tbs	50	6	2	1
Life (See (Quaker) in this section)					
(Malt-O-Meal)					
Apple Zings	1 cup	130	30	1	16
Balance w/berries	1 cup	110	25	5	10
Berry Colossal Crunch	¾ cup	120	26	1	13
Cinnamon Toasters	¾ cup	130	24	1	10
Cocoa Dyno-Bites	¾ cup	120	26	0	13
Cocoa Roos	¾ cup	190	45	5	11
Corn Bursts	1 cup	120	29	0	14
crispy rice	1¼ cups	130	29	0	3
frosted					
flakes	¾ cup	120	28	1	14
mini spooners	1 cup	190	45	6	11
Fruity Dyno-Bites	¾ cup	100	24	0	12
Golden Puffs	¾ cup	100	25	1	15
Honey Buzzers	1⅓ cups	110	26	1	11
Graham Squares	¾ cup	120	25	1	14
Nut Toasty O's	1 cup	110	24	2	11
puffed rice	1 cup	60	13	0	0
puffed wheat	1 cup	50	11	1	0
raisin bran	1 cup	190	45	8	17
toasted cinnamon twists	¾ cup	130	25	1	10
Tootie Fruities	1 cup	120	28	1	15
(Mother's)					
Bumpers					
cocoa	1 cup	120	29	1	14
peanut butter	1 cup	130	26	1	10
Cinnamon Oat crunch	1 cup	230	48	5	15
Honey					
Grahams	¾ cup	100	24	1	13
Roundups	¾ cup	110	25	1	14
Toasted Oat Bran	¾ cup	120	24	3	5
Nature Valley (See (General Mills) in this section)					
(Nature's Path)					
EnviroKid					
Amazon Frosted Flakes	⅔ cup	120	26	2	6
Cheetah Chomps	¾ cup	130	24	2	6
Gorilla Munch	¾ cup	115	26	2	9
Koala Crisp	⅔ cup	120	26	1	10
Orangutan-O's	¾ cup	120	26	2	9
Peanut Butter Panda Puffs	¾ cup	130	24	2	7

Food and Description	Amount	Total Calories	Total Carbs	Fiber	Sugars
Organic Flakes					
8-Grain synergy multigrain corn	⅔ cup	100	23	6	5
honey'd	⅔ cup	120	26	2	4
original	¾ cup	120	25	2	3
Flax Plus					
original	¾ cup	100	22	7	6
raisin bran	¾ cup	180	41	11	16
Heritage	¾ cup	100	22	4	6
Kamut Krisp	¾ cup	100	24	3	5
Mesa Sunrise	¾ cup	120	24	3	4
Millet rice oat bran	⅔ cup	100	23	6	5
multigrain oat bran					
flakes	⅔ cup	100	24	5	5
& raisins	⅔ cup	100	23	4	9
raisin bran/honey'd	¾ cup	100	24	6	9
spelt	¾ cup	120	23	3	3
Organic Muesli					
blueberry almond	½ cup	210	42	7	10
Heritage	½ cup	220	41	6	9
Organic Eco Pacs					
cornflakes	¾ cup	120	25	2	3
Heritage	¾ cup	100	23	6	4
bites	¾ cup	100	22	4	6
honey'd cornflakes	¾ cup	120	26	2	4
honey'd raisin bran	¾ cup	100	24	6	9
Kamut Krisp	¾ cup	100	24	3	5
Mesa Sunrise	¾ cup	120	24	3	4
Millet rice oat bran flakes	⅔ cup	110	21	3	3
Multigrain oat bran					
flakes	⅔ cup	100	24	5	5
flakes & raisins	⅔ cup	100	23	4	9
Oaty Bites	¾ cup	120	24	3	7
Organic Granola					
Ginger Zing	½ cup	150	20	2	7
Hemp Plus	½ cup	140	20	3	6
Pumpkin Flax Plus	½ cup	140	19	4	8
Raspberry Heritage	½ cup	130	22	3	5
Soy Plus	½ cup	130	22	2	7
Organic Optimum					
Power breakfast	1 cup	190	40	10	16
Slim cereal	1 cup	180	38	11	10
Zen	¾ cup	200	43	10	14
(New Morning)					
cocoa crispy rice	¾ cup	120	26	1	10
Cocomotion	¾ cup	100	22	<1	9
cornflakes					
frosted	1 cup	120	27	2	6
plain	1 cup	120	26	2	3
w/strawberries	1 cup	120	27	2	7
Cornfetti	¾ cup	110	24	<1	6

Food and Description	Amount	Total Calories	Total Carbs	Fiber	Sugars
Kamutios	1 cup	120	25	5	3
Fruit-e-O's	1 cup	120	25	2	7
Oatios					
apple cinnamon	1 cup	120	18	2	9
cocoa	¾ cup	110	17	2	9
honey almond	1 cup	120	17	2	9
Ultimate Oat Bran	⅔ cup	110	22	3	3
Wafflers	⅔ cup	110	26	2	9
(Post)					
Alpha-Bits					
original	1 cup	130	27	1	13
w/marshmallows	1 cup	120	26	1	13
bran flakes	¾ cup	100	24	5	5
Cocoa Pebbles	¾ cup	120	26	0	13
Fruit & Fiber					
dates/raisins/walnuts	1 cup	200	42	6	15
peaches/raisins/almonds	1 cup	190	42	6	14
Fruity Pebbles	¾ cup	110	24	0	12
Golden Crisp	¾ cup	110	25	1	14
Grape-Nuts					
flakes	¾ cup	110	24	3	4
original	½ cup	200	47	6	5
O's	¾ cup	120	28	2	11
Honey Bunches of Oats					
honey-roasted	¾ cup	120	25	1	6
w/almonds	¾ cup	130	24	1	7
w/real strawberries	¾ cup	120	26	2	7
Honeycomb	1 cup	110	26	1	11
strawberry-blasted	1 cup	120	26	1	12
Hulk w/marshmallow bits	1 cup	110	27	0	13
Post Toasties	1 cup	100	24	1	2
raisin bran	1 cup	190	46	8	20
Selects Cereal					
Banana Nut Crunch	1 cup	240	44	5	11
Blueberry Morning	1¼ cups	230	48	2	15
Cranberry Almond Crunch	1 cup	210	43	3	14
Great Grains					
crunchy pecan	⅔ cup	220	38	4	8
raisins, dates & pecans	⅔ cup	200	39	4	13
shredded wheat					
Frosted spoon-size	1 cup	180	43	5	12
Honey nut spoon-size	1 cup	200	43	4	12
original					
regular	2 biscuits	160	36	6	0
spoon size	1 cup	170	40	6	0
Waffle Crisp	1 cup	130	25	0	13
(Quaker)					
Apple Zaps	1 cup	120	27	1	14
bran/unprocessed	⅓ cup	35	11	8	1
Cinnamon Crunch	1 cup	120	25	1	12

Food and Description	Amount	Total Calories	Total Carbs	Fiber	Sugars
Cap'n Crunch					
Crunchberries	¾ cup	100	22	1	12
Oops! Choco Donut	¾ cup	100	23	1	11
peanut butter	¾ cup	110	22	1	9
regular	¾ cup	110	23	1	12
Cocoa					
Blasts	1 cup	130	29	1	16
Bronto Blasts	¾ cup	110	26	1	13
Cranberry Macadamia Nut	1 cup	240	46	4	17
Crispy Corn Puffs	1 cup	110	25	1	6
Crunchy Corn Bran	¾ cup	90	23	5	6
Frosted					
Flakes	¾ cup	120	28	0	13
Oats	1 cup	110	23	1	12
Fruitangy O's	1 cup	120	27	1	13
Honey Crisp Corn Flakes	¾ cup	110	27	1	12
Honey Dipps	1¼ cups	130	28	1	12
Honey Graham O's	¾ cup	110	23	1	11
Honey Nut Oats	¾ cup	110	24	1	11
King Vitaman	1½ cups	120	26	1	6
Life..cinnamon	¾ cup	120	26	2	9
Marshmallow Safari	¾ cup	140	29	1	15
Oat Bran High Fiber	1¼ cups	210	43	6	9
Oat Squares					
cinnamon	1 cup	230	48	5	14
original	1 cup	210	44	4	9
100% natural granola					
low-fat w/raisins	½ cup	210	44	3	18
regular					
oats & honey	½ cup	220	31	3	13
w/raisins	½ cup	230	34	3	16
Quaker Oatmeal cereals..all flavors	1 cup	190	39	3	12
Quaker Squares					
cinnamon	1 cup	230	48	5	14
regular	1 cup	210	44	4	9
Quisp	1 cup	110	23	1	12
Rice Crisps	1 cup	110	26	0	3
Shredded Wheat					
frosted	1 cup	190	45	5	11
original	3 pieces	220	50	7	1
Sweet Crunch	1 cup	110	23	1	12
Sweet Puffs	1 cup	130	30	2	16
Toasted Oats	1 cup	110	23	2	2
(Ralston)					
bran flakes/enriched	¾ cup	90	23	5	5
Confruity Crisp	¾ cup	110	25	0	12
Cocoa Crisp Rice	¾ cup	120	27	0	14
Cocoa Crunchies	1 cup	120	26	0	14
Corn Biscuits	1 cup	110	27	2	2
Corn Flakes	1 cup	100	24	<1	2

Food and Description	Amount	Total Calories	Total Carbs	Fiber	Sugars
Crisp Crunch Berry	¾ cup	120	27	<1	13
Crisp Crunch Treets	1 cup	120	27	<1	14
Crisp Rice	1¼ cups	120	29	0	3
Crispy Hexagons	1 cup	110	25	0	3
Freaky Fruits	1 cup	120	27	0	13
Frosted Flakes/Sugar	¾ cup	120	28	<1	12
Fruit Rings	1 cup	120	28	0	15
Magic Stars	¾ cup	120	27	1	13
Oats & More..w/almonds	¾ cup	130	27	1	6
Raisin Bran	1 cup	200	47	8	18
Rice Biscuits/natural	1¼ cups	110	26	2	2
Shredded wheat..frosted..spoon-size	1¼ cups	200	47	5	11
Silly Spheres	1½ cups	110	25	0	3
Tasteeos..apple cinnamon	¾ cup	120	26	1	13
(Skinner) raisin bran	1 cup	170	41	7	13
(Sunbelt)..granola					
banana nut	½ cup	250	37	4	13
berry basic	½ cup	240	41	5	12
fruit & nut	½ cup	240	40	3	19
low-fat cinnamon					
raisin	½ cup	220	44	3	20
raisin almond crunch	½ cup	220	43	3	15
Total (See (General Mills) in this section)					
(U.S. Mills) Uncle Sam					
original	1 cup	190	38	10	<1
w/mixed berries	1 cup	220	39	10	5
Weetabix (See (Barbara's Bakery) in this section)					

■ HOT/COOKED

NOTE: All cereals are either dry or prepared with water per directions on packaging. If milk is used, calorie and fat content increase accordingly. For additional information on milk, see MILK.)

Food and Description	Amount	Total Calories	Total Carbs	Fiber	Sugars
(Arrowhead Mills) dry					
Bear Mush	¼ cup	150	32	2	0
Bits of Barley	¼ cup	160	34	6	1
corn grits					
white	¼ cup	150	33	1	0
yellow	¼ cup	130	30	1	0
4-grain plus flax	¼ cup	150	28	9	0
old-fashioned oatmeal	⅓ cup	130	23	4	<1
oat					
bran	⅓ cup	130	21	4	0
flakes	⅓ cup	130	23	4	<1
oats/oatmeal					
instant					
cinnamon raisin almond	1 pkg	140	24	3	3
maple apple spice	1 pkg	140	26	3	5
regular	1 pkg	110	19	2	0
regular/steel-cut	¼ cup	160	27	8	0
Rice & Shine	¼ cup	150	32	2	0
7-grain cereal					

Food and Description	Amount	Total Calories	Total Carbs	Fiber	Sugars
regular	⅓ cup	140	28	6	0
wheat-free	¼ cup	150	30	3	0
wheat bran	¼ cup	35	10	6	0
wheat germ/raw	3 Tbs	50	10	2	0
Cream of Rice (*See* (Post) in this section)					
Cream of Wheat (*See* (Post) in this section)					
(Erewhon)					
Barley Plus/dry	¼ cup	170	37	4	0
cream of brown rice/dry	¼ cup	170	36	1	0
oat bran w/toasted wheat germ	1 pkg	170	31	5	1
oatmeal/instant dry					
apple cinnamon	1 pkg	130	24	3	4
apple raisin	1 pkg	140	26	3	6
dates & walnuts	1 pkg	130	24	3	6
maple spice	1 pkg	130	26	3	6
oatmeal w/added bran	1 pkg	130	25	4	1
raisins, dates & nuts	1 pkg	130	24	3	6
w/added oat bran	1 pkg	130	25	4	1
farina..prepared	1 cup	120	22	<1	0
(Highspire)					
Maltex	¼ cup	135	29	2	0
Wheatena	¼ cup	125	26	5	0
(Gram's Gourmet)..cream of flax	½ cup	140	11	8	1
(H-O)					
farina/quick/dry	3 Tbs	120	26	3	0
oatmeal/instant/dry					
apple cinnamon	1 pkg	130	22	3	11
maple & brown sugar	1 pkg	160	32	3	13
oats 'n' fiber					
apple & bran	1 pkg	130	26	3	na
plain	1 pkg	110	18	3	0
raisin & bran	1 pkg	150	32	3	16
raisins & spice	1 pkg	150	33	3	16
sweet 'n' mellow	1 pkg	150	30	3	14
regular					
gourmet	⅓ cup	100	18	3	0
quick	½ cup	150	27	4	0
(Health Valley) hot cereal cups					
Amazing Apple	1 cup	210	41	4	9
Banana Gone Nuts	1 cup	240	45	4	9
Maple Madness! w/raisins	1 cup	240	47	4	19
(KETO) Carb Counters..all styles	2 scoops	150	12	9	0
(Krusteaz) dry					
Grain Gourmet Cracked Wheat Bulgur	¼ cup	150	32	6	0
Zoom/100% whole wheat	⅓ cup	120	23	6	0
(Malt-O-Meal)					
hot wheat cereal					
chocolate	1 serving	120	27	1	7
maple & brown sugar	1 serving	120	28	1	11

Food and Description	Amount	Total Calories	Total Carbs	Fiber	Sugars
original	1 serving	120	26	2	0
instant oatmeal/big bowl					
apples & cinnamon	1 serving	190	41	5	7
cinnamon & spice	1 serving	250	54	5	24
cinnamon roll	1 serving	240	49	4	19
deluxe variety	1 serving	225	46	4	21
fruit & creamy/variety	1 serving	195	25	1	14
maple & brown sugar	1 serving	230	49	5	20
regular	1 serving	110	24	2	11
(Maypo)					
instant maple	½ cup	210	36	3	0
Vermont-style	⅓ cup	180	33	3	0
(Mother's) dry					
barley	⅓ cup	170	37	5	0
multigrain	½ cup	130	29	5	0
oat bran	½ cup	150	25	6	0
oatmeal/instant	½ cup	150	27	4	1
rolled oats	½ cup	150	27	4	1
wheat germ	2 Tbs	50	6	2	1
whole wheat/100% natural	½ cup	130	30	4	0
(Post) instant					
Cream of Rice/dry	1 serving	170	38	0	0
Cream of Wheat/dry..plain..all styles	1 serving	120	25	1	0
Cream of Wheat/flavored					
apples 'n' cinnamon	1 pkt	130	29	1	16
cinnamon swirl	1 pkt	130	29	1	12
maple brown sugar	1 pkt	120	27	1	13
original	1 pkt	90	17	1	0
peaches 'n' cream	1 pkt	130	28	1	13
strawberries 'n' cream	1 pkt	130	28	1	24
(Quaker)					
farina..enriched					
cinnamon	¼ cup	150	33	2	0
quick-cooking	¼ cup	150	33	1	0
Nutrition for Women					
apple cinnamon	1 pkt	170	35	3	16
golden brown sugar	1 pkt	160	32	3	12
vanilla cinnamon	1 pkt	160	32	3	13
oat bran	½ cup	150	25	6	1
oatmeal					
Express Cups					
baked apple	1 cup	200	42	4	19
cinnamon roll	1 cup	210	41	4	17
golden brown sugar	1 cup	200	42	3	18
oatmeal..instant					
apple & cinnamon	1 pkt	130	27	3	12
apple crisp	1 pkt	150	31	3	14
banana bread	1 pkt	150	31	3	12
bananas & cream	1 pkt	140	26	2	11

Food and Description	Amount	Total Calories	Total Carbs	Fiber	Sugars
blueberries & cream	1 pkt	140	26	2	11
cinnamon & spice	1 pkt	170	35	3	16
cinnamon roll	1 pkt	160	33	3	13
double raisin Danish	1 pkt	170	36	3	16
French toast	1 pkt	160	33	3	14
honey nut	1 pkt	170	31	3	13
maple & brown sugar	1 pkt	160	33	3	13
peaches & cream	1 pkt	140	27	2	12
raisin & spice	1 pkt	150	33	3	16
raisins, dates & walnuts	1 pkt	140	27	2	13
regular	1 pkt	100	19	3	0
strawberries & cream	1 pkt	140	27	2	12
oatmeal..instant..Oatmeal Supreme					
apple raisin	1 pkt	150	32	3	13
banana walnut	1 pkt	150	28	3	9
cinnamon pecan	1 pkt	180	34	3	14
oatmeal..instant..reduced-sugar					
apple cinnamon	1 pkt	110	22	3	6
maple & brown sugar	1 pkt	120	24	3	4
oats/dry..all styles	⅓ cup	150	27	4	1
unprocessed bran	⅓ cup	35	11	8	1
whole wheat hot..natural cereal	½ cup	130	30	4	0
(Ralston) 3-Minute Brand					
instant hot Ralston	⅓ cup	150	31	5	0
instant oatmeal					
cinnamon roll	1 pkg	160	33	3	13
maple & brown sugar	1 pkg	160	33	3	13
oats/100% natural					
old-fashioned	1 serving	150	27	5	2
plus oat bran	1 serving	150	27	5	2
quick	1 serving	140	26	4	0
regular flavor	1 pkg	100	19	3	0
variety pack	1 pkg	130	27	3	12
(Skinners)..oat bran	1 serving	100	18	5	<1
(Stone-Buhr)					
4-grain cereal mates	⅓ cup	140	31	5	0
7-grain cereal	⅓ cup	140	31	4	0
oat bran	½ cup	150	25	6	1
oats					
rolled old-fashioned	¼ cup	150	28	5	<1
Scotch	¼ cup	150	28	4	0
CEREAL BAR (*See* BREAKFAST/CEREAL BAR; GRANOLA/GRANOLA-TYPE BAR)					
CERVELAT (*See* SAUSAGE)					
CHAMPAGNE (*See* WINE)					
CHARD/fresh					
cooked	½ cup	18	4	2	0
raw/chopped	½ cup	3	1	2	<1
CHAYOTE/fresh					
boiled	½ cup	19	4	2	0

Food and Description	Amount	Total Calories	Total Carbs	Fiber	Sugars
raw/whole	1 medium	50	11	6	<1

CHEESE (*See also* CHEESE ALTERNATIVE/IMITATION; CHEESE SPREAD; COTTAGE CHEESE; CREAM CHEESE)

■ **(4C Foods)**
100% IMPORTED

Italian Pecorino..home-style/grated	2 tsp	25	0	0	0
Parmesan..grated	2 tsp	20	0	0	0
Parmesan & Romano..grated	2 tsp	25	0	0	0
Romano..sharp	2 tsp	25	0	0	0

REGULAR

Italian Pecorino Romano..sharp/grated	2 tsp	25	0	0	0
Parmesan & Romano	2 tsp	25	0	0	0

■ **(Alouette)**

baby Brie..all styles	1 oz	110	2	0	2
baby Swiss					
light	1 oz	90	1	0	0
regular or smoked	1 oz	110	1	0	0
baked Brie in pastry kit	2 oz	220	15	1	5

MONTRACHET

goat cheese..all styles & flavors	1 oz	70	1	0	0

■ **(Alpine Lace)**
DELI SELF-SERVICE/chunk cheese
  reduced-fat

American	1 oz	80	2	0	1
cheddar	1 oz	90	0	0	0
feta	1 oz	50	1	0	0
hot pepper	1 oz	90	1	0	<1
provolone	1 oz	90	1	0	0
Swiss	1 oz	110	0	0	0

PRESLICED SELF-SERVICE DELI CHEESES
  reduced-fat

cheddar	1 oz	90	0	0	0
Co-Jack semisoft	1 oz	90	1	0	0
mozzarella/low-moisture	1 oz	70	1	0	1
Swiss	1 oz	110	0	0	0

  reduced-fat/reduced-sodium
    American

hot pepper	1 oz	90	1	0	<1
white	1 oz	90	1	0	<1
yellow	1 oz	90	1	0	<1
provolone	1 oz	90	1	0	1

  reduced-sodium

Muenster	1 oz	110	1	0	0

■ **(Athenos)**
feta..crumbled

basil & tomato	1 oz	80	<1	0	0
mild	1 oz	80	<1	0	0

Food and Description	Amount	Total Calories	Total Carbs	Fiber	Sugars
traditional					
reduced-fat	1 oz	60	<1	0	0
regular	1 oz	80	<1	0	0
■ (Boar's Head)					
American..all styles	1 oz	100	1	0	0
blue cheese..creamy	1 oz	90	0	0	0
butter kase	1 oz	100	0	0	0
cheddar					
Canadian	1 oz	110	0	0	0
horseradish	1 oz	110	2	0	0
sharp..all types	1 oz	110	<1	0	0
Vermont..all types	1 oz	110	0	0	0
Colby..longhorn	1 oz	110	<1	0	0
Edam	1 oz	90	0	0	0
feta	1 oz	60	1	0	0
Gloucester..double..yellow	1 oz	110	0	0	0
Gouda	1 oz	110	0	0	0
Havarti..all styles & flavors	1 oz	110	0	0	0
Monterey Jack..all types	1 oz	100	0	0	0
mozzarella/low-moisture	1 oz	90	<1	0	0
Muenster..all types	1 oz	100	0	0	0
provolone..all types	1 oz	100	1	0	0
Swiss					
baby Swiss	1 oz	110	<1	0	0
Gold Label/imported	1 oz	110	<1	0	0
lacy	1 oz	90	0	0	0
■ BONBEL (See (Laughing Cow) in this section)					
■ (Borden)					
Processed					
American..singles					
16 slices	1 oz	70	2	0	1
24 slices	⅔ oz	60	3	0	2
Big Bread size	? oz	80	2	0	1
fat-free	1 slice	30	2	0	1
California					
cheddar..all styles	1 oz	110	1	0	1
Monterey Jack	1 oz	100	1	0	1
mozzarella/Light Line	1 oz	50	1	0	0
Swiss					
American	1 oz	100	<1	0	0
sliced	1 oz	100	1	0	0
■ (Cabot)					
cheddar					
aged w/horseradish brick	1 oz	110	1	0	0
5-peppercorn/brick	1 oz	110	1	0	0
light	1 oz	70	1	0	0
mild/brick	1 oz	110	1	0	0
mild/slices	1 oz	110	1	0	0
pepper jack/brick	1 oz	110	1	0	1

Food and Description	Amount	Total Calories	Total Carbs	Fiber	Sugars
pepper jack/slices	1 oz	110	1	0	1
sharp..all styles & flavors	1 oz	110	1	0	0
Vermont..cheddar light..all types	1 oz	70	1	0	0
Monterey Jack..shredded	1 oz	110	1	0	1
mozzarella..fancy blend..shredded	1 oz	100	1	0	1
■ (Chavrie)					
goat's milk cheese..all styles & flavors	1.1 oz	50	1	0	1
■ (Churny)					
Maybud					
Edam/reduced-fat	1 oz	100	0	0	0
farmers	1 oz	90	1	0	0
Gouda/reduced-fat	1 oz	80	0	0	0
regular..port wine..diet snack	1 oz	70	1	0	0
■ (Cornville)					
Brie	1 oz	90	0	0	0
Camembert	1 oz	90	0	0	0
■ (County Line)					
Crackerbackers..all styles	1 oz	110	1	0	0
Regular					
American/sliced..16-count pkg	1 slice	70	1	0	0
cheddar					
extra sharp	1 oz	120	1	0	0
finely shredded	¼ cup	110	1	0	0
medium sharp	1 oz	110	1	0	0
mild	1 oz	110	1	0	0
sharp					
chunk	1 oz	110	1	0	0
shredded	¼ cup	110	1	0	0
Colby..all styles	1 oz	110	1	0	0
Monterey Jack	1 oz	110	1	0	0
mozzarella..all styles	¼ cup	80	1	0	0
Muenster	1 oz	110	0	0	0
Swiss, Old World	1 oz	110	0	0	0
taco/shredded	¼ cup	110	1	0	0
■ CRACKER BARREL (See (Kraft) in this section)					
■ (Di Giorno)					
Parmesan					
chunk	2 tsp	25	0	0	0
grated	2 tsp	20	0	0	0
shredded	2 tsp	20	0	0	0
Romano					
chunk	2 tsp	25	0	0	0
grated	2 tsp	25	0	0	0
shredded	2 tsp	20	0	0	0
■ (Dorman's)					
natural					
blue					
Castello/70%	1 oz	135	0	0	0
Danablu					

Food and Description	Amount	Total Calories	Total Carbs	Fiber	Sugars
40%	1 oz	100	0	0	0
60%	1 oz	110	0	0	0
brick	1 oz	110	1	0	0
Brie	1 oz	80	0	0	0
Camembert/50%	1 oz	90	0	0	0
Cheda-Jack					
reduced-fat/low-sodium	1 oz	80	1	0	0
regular	1 oz	90	1	0	0
cheddar					
reduced-fat/low-sodium	1 oz	80	1	0	0
regular	1 oz	110	1	0	0
Edam	1 oz	100	1	0	0
feta/45%	1 oz	90	0	0	0
Gouda	1 oz	100	0	0	0
Havarti					
45%	1 oz	90	0	0	0
60%	1 oz	120	0	0	0
Parmesan..grated	1 oz	130	1	0	0
provolone					
reduced-fat/low-sodium	1 oz	90	1	0	0
regular	1 oz	100	1	0	0
Romano	1 oz	100	1	0	0
Swiss					
no salt added	1 oz	100	0	0	0
reduced-fat/low-sodium	1 oz	90	0	0	0
regular	1 oz	100	0	0	0
tybo/45%	1 oz	100	0	0	0
■ (Dragone)					
Parmesan					
chunk	1 oz	110	1	0	0
grated	1 oz	110	1	0	0
shredded	¼ cup	100	1	<1	1
wedges	1 oz	100	<1	0	<1
ricotta					
part-skim	¼ cup	90	4	0	3
whole milk	¼ cup	100	5	0	3
■ (Finlandia)					
imported					
Gouda stick	1 oz	100	<1	0	0
Havarti stick	1 oz	100	<1	0	0
Muenster					
loaf	1 oz	100	<1	0	0
stick	1 oz	110	<1	0	0
Swiss					
Heavenly Light					
loaf	1 oz	80	<1	0	0
stick	1 oz	100	<1	0	0
high-cut loaf	1 oz	110	<1	0	0
regular stick	1 oz	110	<1	0	0

Food and Description	Amount	Total Calories	Total Carbs	Fiber	Sugars
■ (Friendship)					
farmer	2 Tbs	50	0	0	<1
hoop	2 Tbs	20	0	0	0
■ (Frigo)					
Cheese Heads/100% natural mini bars					
all styles	¾ oz	80	<1	0	0
Cheese Heads/100% natural string cheese					
cheddar swirls	1 oz	80	1	0	0
light natural	1 oz	60	3	0	0
mozzarella & cheddar swirls	1 oz	80	1	0	0
mozzarella					
part-skim/low-moisture	1 oz	80	1	0	0
shredded/all-natural	¼ cup	80	1	0	0
Parmesan					
chunk	1 oz	110	1	0	0
grated	1 oz	110	1	0	0
shredded	¼ cup	100	1	1	1
Parmesan & Romano					
grated	2 tsp	20	0	0	0
grated/dry	¼ cup	110	1	0	0
shredded Parmesan	¼ cup	100	1	<1	1
shredded Romano	¼ cup	70	<1	<1	<1
ricotta					
low-salt	¼ cup	110	2	0	2
part-skim	¼ cup	90	2	0	2
whole milk	¼ cup	110	2	0	2
Romano					
grated	1 oz	110	1	0	0
grated/dry	1 oz	130	1	0	0
shredded	¼ cup	100	1	1	1
whole	1 oz	110	1	0	0
■ (Hickory Farms)					
Neufchâtel					
chocolate	1 oz	110	8	0	na
orange	1 oz	100	4	0	na
peach	1 oz	90	3	0	na
pineapple	1 oz	90	2	0	na
rum date nut	1 oz	100	4	0	na
strawberry	1 oz	90	3	0	na
■ (Kaukauna)					
Deli-style					
cheese balls					
cheddar					
extra sharp..w/almonds	1 oz	100	4	1	4
garden vegetable..w/almonds	1 oz	120	5	1	5
horseradish..w/almonds	1 oz	90	4	1	4
port wine..w/almonds	1 oz	90	4	1	4
sharp cheddar					
w/almonds & hazelnuts	1 oz	90	4	1	4
smoky bacon w/almonds	1 oz	90	4	1	4

Food and Description	Amount	Total Calories	Total Carbs	Fiber	Sugars
cheese logs					
cheddar					
double sharp..w/almonds	1 oz	90	4	1	4
garlic & herb..w/almonds	1 oz	120	5	1	5
port wine..w/almonds	1 oz	90	4	1	4
sharp w/almonds & hazelnuts	1 oz	90	4	1	4
sharp hickory smoke..w/almonds	1 oz	90	4	1	4
■ (Kraft)					
100% PARMESAN CHEESES					
grated					
Parmesan or Romano..all styles	2 tsp	20	0	0	0
Parmesan-style..reduced-fat	2 tsp	20	2	0	0
shredded					
Parmesan	1 oz	110	1	0	0
Parmesan, Romano & Asiago	1 oz	110	1	0	0
CRACKER BARREL—Natural Cheeses					
baby Swiss	1 oz	110	0	0	0
cheddar..all styles	1 oz	120	0	0	0
extra-sharp white..reduced-fat	1 oz	90	0	0	0
sharp	1 oz	120	0	0	0
sharp/slices	~1 oz	90	0	0	0
sharp 2% milk..reduced-fat	1 oz	90	1	0	0
Vermont sharp cheese cuts	1 oz	120	0	0	0
white	1 oz	110	1	0	0
KRAFT DELI DELUXE CHEESES					
American slices..16-count pkg	¾ oz	80	1	0	0
cheddar					
sharp/slices..20-count pkg	~1 oz	90	0	0	0
Colby Jack slices..10-count pkg	~1 oz	90	0	0	0
mozzarella/low-moisture slices..					
10 count	¾ oz	60	0	0	0
pepper jack spicy slices..					
10-count pkg	~1 oz	90	0	0	0
Swiss slices..16-count pkg	½ oz	70	0	0	0
KRAFT (Nabisco) EASY CHEESES					
American...all flavors	~1 oz	90	2	0	2
cheddar	~1 oz	90	2	0	2
bacon	~1 oz	90	2	0	1
sharp	~1 oz	90	2	0	2
nacho cheese	~1 oz	90	3	0	2
NATURAL BRICK CHEESES					
cheddar & Monterey Jack					
bacon	1 oz	90	2	0	1
cube cheese	1 oz	120	0	0	0
extra-sharp	1 oz	110	1	0	0
marbled	1 oz	110	1	0	0
medium..8-oz brick	1 oz	110	1	0	0
mild					
2% milk reduced-fat	1 oz	80	0	0	0
cube cheese	1 oz	130	0	0	0

Food and Description	Amount	Total Calories	Total Carbs	Fiber	Sugars
longhorn	1 oz	110	0	0	0
regular..all styles	1 oz	110	1	0	0
sharp					
2% milk reduced-fat	1 oz	80	0	0	0
cube cheese	1 oz	130	0	0	0
regular/16-oz brick	1 oz	120	0	0	0
shredded	1 oz	110	1	0	0
fat-free	1 oz	40	1	0	0
finely	1 oz	120	1	0	0
shredded	1 oz	100	1	0	0
Colby	1 oz	110	1	0	0
2% milk reduced-fat	1 oz	80	0	0	0
cube cheese	1 oz	120	0	0	0
longhorn-style	1 oz	110	0	0	0
marbled	1 oz	110	1	0	0
midget	1 oz	110	0	0	0
& Monterey Jack	1 oz	110	1	0	0
Monterey Jack	1 oz	100	0	0	0
2% milk reduced-fat	1 oz	80	1	0	0
KRAFT NATURAL SHREDDED CHEESES					
cheese Italian-style					
classic garlic..w/seasonings	1 oz	100	2	1	0
mozzarella & Parmesan..shredded	1 oz	100	2	1	0
cheese Mexican-style/finely shredded					
cheddar jack	1 oz	110	1	0	0
w/jalapeño peppers	1 oz	110	1	0	0
taco	¼ cup	110	2	0	0
Classic Melts					
cheddar & American	1 oz	120	1	0	0
cheddar jack & American	1 oz	120	1	0	0
4-cheese	1 oz	120	1	0	0
Italian-style 5-cheese	1 oz	90	1	0	0
Mexican-style 4-cheese	1 oz	100	1	0	0
mild cheddar 2% milk					
finely shredded..8-oz bag	1 oz	80	1	0	0
Monterey jack	1 oz	100	1	0	0
mozzarella					
2% milk reduced-fat	1 oz	70	1	0	0
fat-free	1 oz	45	3	0	0
low-moisture					
finely shredded	1 oz	70	1	0	0
regular shredded	1 oz	80	1	0	0
pizza mozzarella & provolone	1 oz	90	1	0	1
Swiss	1 oz	110	1	0	0
KRAFT SINGLES					
American					
2% milk reduced-fat	1 slice	50	1	0	1
cheddar/sharp..2% reduced-fat	1 slice	50	1	0	1
regular/yellow	1 slice	60	1	0	1
Manchego singles	1 slice	70	1	0	1

Food and Description	Amount	Total Calories	Total Carbs	Fiber	Sugars
mozzarella					
2% milk reduced-fat	1 slice	50	1	0	1
regular 96-count box	1 slice	60	1	0	1
pepper jack..2% milk reduced-fat	1 slice	50	1	0	1
Swiss 2% milk reduced-fat	1 slice	50	1	0	1
POLLY-O					
bite-size balls	1.5 oz	120	0	0	0
cherry-size balls	1 oz	80	0	0	0
shredded					
fat-free	¼ cup	40	1	1	1
light	¼ cup	60	1	0	1
part skim	¼ cup	80	1	0	0
whole milk..8-oz bag	¼ cup	90	0	0	0
mozzarella w/Parmesan	¼ cup	90	1	0	0
Parmesan..grated	2 tsp	20	0	0	0
Parmesan & Romano..grated	2 tsp	20	0	0	0
ricotta					
fat-free	¼ cup	50	3	0	0
part-skim	¼ cup	80	3	0	0
whole milk	¼ cup	110	2	0	2
String-Ums & Polly-O..mozzarella					
reduced-fat	1 oz	80	1	0	0
regular	1 oz	80	1	0	0
Twistums..mozzarella* cheddar					
12-count	1 stick	60	0	0	0
super long..Polly-O	1 stick	90	1	0	0
VELVEETA					
light loaf	1 oz	60	3	0	2
Mexican loaf					
hot	1 oz	90	3	0	2
mild					
loaf	1 oz	90	3	0	2
shredded	¼ cup	130	3	0	3
original					
16-oz box/loaf	1 oz	90	3	0	3
shredded	¼ cup	130	3	0	3
slices/16-count pkg	¾ oz	60	1	0	1
■ (Land O' Lakes)					
DELI CHEESES/Chunk					
cheddar	1 oz	110	<1	0	<1
cheddar white	1 oz	110	<1	0	<1
Co-Jack semisoft	1 oz	110	<1	0	0
Havarti	1 oz	110	<1	0	<1
pepper jack	1 oz	110	<1	0	<1
NATURAL CHEESES					
American					
2-lb loaf	1 oz	110	1	0	<1
Golden Velvet	1 oz	80	2	0	0
brick	1 oz	100	<1	0	0
Cheddarella	1 oz	100	0	0	0

Food and Description	Amount	Total Calories	Total Carbs	Fiber	Sugars
presliced	1 slice	110	<1	0	0
semisoft	1 oz	100	0	0	0
cheddar..all styles	1 oz	110	<1	0	<1
Co-Jack					
chunk	1 oz	110	<1	0	0
presliced	1 slice	110	<1	0	0
Colby	1 oz	110	<1	0	0
presliced	1 slice	110	<1	0	0
Havarti..all styles	1 oz	110	<1	0	<1
Monterey Jack..all styles	1 oz	110	<1	0	0
mozzarella/pasteurized..part-skim	1 oz	80	<1	0	0
Muenster/presliced	1 slice	100	0	0	0
pepper jack/presliced	1 slice	110	0	0	0
provolone w/smoke flavor/sliced	1 slice	100	<1	0	0
Swiss/..all styles	1 oz	110	<1	0	0
PROCESSED CHEESES					
American..presliced pasteurized....					
all types	1 slice	110	<1	0	<1
jalapeño peppers..presliced	1 slice	90	2	0	2
■ (Laughing Cow)					
NATURAL CHEESE					
Babybel/mini					
Bonbel	1 piece	70	0	0	0
gouda	1 piece	80	0	0	0
light original	1 piece	50	0	0	0
mild cheddar	1 piece	70	0	0	0
regular	1 piece	70	0	0	0
PROCESSED CHEESE					
Cheezbits	6 pieces	70	2	0	2
Gourmet Cheese & Baguettes	1 unit	75	5	0	1.5
Wedges					
creamy Swiss					
light creamy..all flavors	1 wedge	35	1	0	1
original creamy Swiss	1 wedge	50	1	0	1
■ (Miceli's)					
SPECIALTY & IMPORTED CHEESES					
cheddar/mild..classic cut	1 oz	110	1	0	0
mozzarella/fresh					
ciliegini..classic cut	1 oz	80	1	0	0
ovoline	1 oz	70	1	0	0
sliced	1 oz	80	1	0	0
Parmesan..wedge	1 oz	100	1	0	1
pizza..classic cut/shredded	1 oz	80	1	0	0
ricotta					
Chicago-style	2 oz	90	3	0	3
fat-free	2 oz	45	3	0	2
light/low-fat	~2 oz	60	3	0	3
part-skim	2 oz	80	2	0	3
traditional	~2 oz	90	3	0	3

Food and Description	Amount	Total Calories	Total Carbs	Fiber	Sugars
■ **(MONTRACHET)** (*See* (Alouette) in this section)					
■ **(Nikos)** feta cheese..crumbles	1 oz	80	1	0	0
■ **(Polly-O)** (*See* (Kraft) in this section)					
■ **(Saladena)**					
SPECIALTY & IMPORTED					
blue crumbles	1 oz	100	1	0	0
feta crumbles	1 oz	90	1	0	0
goat crumbles	1 oz	90	1	0	0
Gorgonzola crumbles	1 oz	100	1	0	0
Mediterranean	1 oz	90	1	0	0
Provencal	1 oz	80	0	0	0
■ **(Sargento)**					
DELI-STYLE/SLICED CHEESES					
American Burger Cheese	1 slice	70	<1	0	0
cheddar..all styles	1 slice	80	0	0	0
Colby	1 slice	80	<1	0	0
Jarlsberg	1 slice	80	<1	0	0
Monterey Jack	1 slice	80	0	0	0
mozzarella	1 slice	60	1	0	0
Muenster	1 slice	80	0	0	0
provolone					
reduced-fat	1 slice	50	0	0	0
regular	1 slice	100	0	0	0
Swiss..8-oz brick					
aged	1 slice	70	0	0	0
reduced-fat	1 slice	60	1	0	0
thick	1 slice	110	1	0	0
thin	1 slice	70	0	0	0
OTHER FINE CHEESES					
blue cheese/crumbled	¼ cup	100	1	0	0
Parmesan/grated	2 tsp	25	0	0	0
Parmesan & Romano	2 tsp	25	0	0	0
ricotta					
fat-free	¼ cup	50	5	0	2
light	¼ cup	60	3	0	3
part-skim	¼ cup	70	3	0	3
whole milk	¼ cup	90	3	0	3
SHREDDED CHEESES					
cheese blends					
4-cheese Mexican	¼ cup	110	1	0	0
6-cheese Italian	¼ cup	90	1	0	0
angel hair Parmesan, mozzarella & Romano	¼ cup	100	1	0	0
cheddar jack					
regular	¼ cup	110	1	0	0
w/jalapeño	¼ cup	110	1	0	0
Italian w/garlic	¼ cup	100	1	0	0
mozzarella & provolone	¼ cup	90	0	0	0
pepper jack w/habañeros	¼ cup	90	0	0	0
nacho & taco	¼ cup	110	1	0	0

Food and Description	Amount	Total Calories	Total Carbs	Fiber	Sugars
Parmesan & Romano	2 tsp	20	0	0	0
pizza double cheese	¼ cup	90	1	0	0
taco	¼ cup	110	1	0	0
chef-style..all types	¼ cup	110	1	0	0
mozzarella	¼ cup	90	1	0	0
fancy					
Asiago/extra fine	2 tsp	20	0	0	0
cheddar..all types	¼ cup	110	1	0	0
Colby Jack	¼ cup	110	1	0	0
Monterey Jack	¼ cup	110	1	0	0
mozzarella	¼ cup	80	1	0	0
Parmesan	2 tsp	20	0	0	0
Swiss	¼ cup	110	<1	0	0
reduced-fat					
4-cheese Italian	¼ cup	80	1	0	0
4-cheese Mexican	¼ cup	80	<1	0	0
cheddar/mild	¼ cup	80	<1	0	1
mozzarella	¼ cup	80	<1	0	0
SNACK CHEESES					
sticks					
cheddar..mild					
6-count pkg	1 piece	100	0	0	0
singles	1 piece	110	1	0	0
Colby Jack					
6-count pkg	1 stick	80	<1	0	0
singles	1 piece	110	<1	0	0
■ (Stella)					
BLENDS					
3-cheese					
European	¼ cup	100	<1	<1	0
Italian	¼ cup	100	1	<1	<1
Mediterranean	¼ cup	90	1	<1	<1
Parmesan & Romano	¼ cup	100	<1	<1	<1
OTHER CHEESES					
Asiago/shredded	1 Tbs	30	0	0	1
blue/crumbled	¼ cup	100	0	0	0
feta/crumbled	¼ cup	70	1	<1	0
fontinella	1 oz	110	<1	0	<1
Gorgonzola	¼ cup	100	<1	<1	0
Kasseri	1 oz	110	<1	0	<1
Parmesan/shredded	¼ cup	100	1	1	1
Romano	¼ cup	100	<1	<1	<1
Swiss/natural	1 oz	100	0	0	0
■ (Weight Watchers)					
American/white or yellow fat-free					
all styles	¾ oz	30	3	0	2
cheddar					
fat-free..all styles	¾ oz	30	3	0	2
low-fat..all styles	1 oz	80	1	0	0
Parmesan/fat-free..grated	1 Tbs	15	2	0	1

Food and Description	Amount	Total Calories	Total Carbs	Fiber	Sugars
Swiss/fat-free..sliced	¾ oz	30	2	0	2
CHEESE, COTTAGE (*See* COTTAGE CHEESE)					
CHEESE, CREAM (*See* CREAM CHEESE)					
CHEESE ALTERNATIVE/IMITATION					
■ **(Cemac) Nu Tofu**					
fat-free..all styles	1 oz	40	2	0	0
regular					
cheddar					
low-sodium	1 oz	70	1	0	0
regular	1 oz	70	1	0	0
Monterey Jack	1 oz	70	2	0	0
mozzarella	1 oz	70	2	0	0
■ **(Dorman's) Lo-Chol**					
cheddar	1 oz	100	1	0	0
Colby	1 oz	110	1	0	0
mozzarella	1 oz	90	1	0	0
Muenster	1 oz	100	0	0	0
Swiss	1 oz	100	0	0	0
■ **(Formagg)**					
American/sliced					
classic	1 slice	60	1	0	0
white	1 slice	60	<1	0	0
yellow	1 slice	60	<1	0	0
zesty jalapeño	1 oz	60	1	0	0
cheddar					
shredded	1 oz	60	<1	0	0
sliced	1 slice	60	1	0	0
provolone/Vintage	1 oz	60	1	0	0
mozzarella/shredded	1 oz	60	1	0	0
ricotta/fat-free	½ cup	40	1	0	0
Swiss/sliced	1 oz	60	1	0	0
■ **(Frigo)**					
cheddar	1 oz	110	1	0	0
mozzarella	1 oz	90	1	0	0
■ **(Galaxy) soy cheese..all styles**					
and flavors	1 oz	60	2	0	<1
■ **(SMART BEAT) lactose-free..all styles**	1 slice	25	3	0	0
■ **(Soya Kaas) tofu**					
American cheddar/mild	1 oz	70	2	0	0
garlic & herb	1 oz	70	2	0	0
hickory-smoked cheddar	1 oz	80	2	0	0
mozzarella					
fat-free	1 oz	40	3	0	0
regular	1 oz	70	2	0	0
■ **(Tofutti)**					
Better Than Cream Cheese..all flavors	2 Tbs	80	1	0	0
soy cheese slices					
American	1 slice	70	2	0	0
mozzarella	1 slice	70	2	0	0
roasted garlic	1 slice	70	2	0	0

Food and Description	Amount	Total Calories	Total Carbs	Fiber	Sugars
■ (Yves) The Good Slice					
American	1 slice	35	0	0	0
cheddar	1 slice	35	0	0	0
jalapeño jack	1 slice	35	0	0	0
Swiss	1 slice	35	0	0	0
CHEESE DIP (*See* DIP)					
CHEESE SNACK (*See* SNACKS)					
CHEESE SPREAD (*See also* CHEESE ALTERNATIVE/IMITATION; CREAM CHEESE)					
■ (Alouette)					
crème de brie					
fines herbs	1 oz	220	1	0	0
original	1 oz	220	1	0	0
crème fraîche..cooking & topping	1 oz	100	1	0	1
gourmet layered/elegante					
roasted garlic & pesto	1 oz	100	2	0	1
roasted sweet peppers & olives	1 oz	90	2	0	1
sun-dried tomato/garlic	1 oz	100	2	0	1
spreadable cheeses					
cucumber dill/light	1 oz	50	2	0	2
garlic & herbs					
light	1 oz	50	1	0	1
regular	1 oz	70	1	0	1
peppercorn Parmesan	1 oz	80	1	0	1
savory vegetable	1 oz	60	1	0	1
spinach artichoke	1 oz	60	1	0	1
sun-dried tomato	1 oz	70	1	0	1
triple onion	1 oz	70	1	0	1
■ (Chavrie) goat cheese spread	2 Tbs	50	1	0	1
■ **CHEEZ WHIZ** (*See* (Kraft) in this section)					
■ (Connoisseur)					
aged English cheddar	2 Tbs	100	2	2	2
apple cinnamon wheel	2 Tbs	110	10	0	5
Asiago	2 Tbs	90	2	0	2
Brie	2 Tbs	90	2	0	2
cranberry	2 Tbs	100	5	1	3
Gorgonzola	2 Tbs	90	2	0	2
mango peach	2 Tbs	110	10	0	5
Swiss	2 Tbs	90	2	0	2
■ (Fleur de Lait)					
light					
crunchy garden vegetable	2 Tbs	60	2	0	1
garlic & herb/minced	2 Tbs	60	3	0	3
Mediterranean olive	2 Tbs	60	2	0	2
red ripe strawberry	2 Tbs	70	3	0	3
spinach artichoke	2 Tbs	60	2	0	2
Vidalia sweet onion	2 Tbs	60	3	0	3
Neufchâtel spread					
Bermuda onion	2 Tbs	90	2	0	1
date nut rum	2 Tbs	90	4	0	4
garlic & spice	2 Tbs	90	2	0	1

Food and Description	Amount	Total Calories	Total Carbs	Fiber	Sugars
herb & spice	2 Tbs	90	2	0	1
lemon	2 Tbs	90	5	0	5
lox/smoked salmon	2 Tbs	90	1	0	1
mandarin orange	2 Tbs	90	4	0	4
peach	2 Tbs	90	4	0	4
pineapple	2 Tbs	90	4	0	4
strawberry	2 Tbs	90	4	0	4
toasted onion	2 Tbs	90	2	0	1
wildberry	2 Tbs	90	4	0	4
■ (Kaukauna)					
cheese balls					
cheddar					
extra sharp..w/almonds	1 oz	100	4	1	4
garden vegetable..w/almonds	1 oz	120	5	1	5
horseradish..w/almonds	1 oz	90	4	1	4
port wine..w/almonds	1 oz	90	4	1	4
sharp cheddar w/almonds					
& hazelnuts	1 oz	90	4	1	4
smoky bacon w/almonds	1 oz	90	4	1	4
cheese logs					
cheddar					
double sharp.. w/almonds	1 oz	90	4	1	4
garlic & herb..w/almonds	1 oz	120	5	1	5
port wine..w/almonds	1 oz	90	4	1	4
sharp w/almonds & hazelnuts	1 oz	90	4	1	4
sharp hickory smoke..w/almonds	1 oz	90	4	1	4
COLD PACK CUPS					
light 50..all types and flavors	2 Tbs	70	5	0	5
original..all types and flavors	2 Tbs	90	3	0	3
■ (Kraft)					
Cheez Whiz					
jarred					
light	2 Tbs	80	6	0	4
original	2 Tbs	90	4	0	3
salsa con queso	2 Tbs	90	4	0	3
squeezable/plain	2 Tbs	100	4	0	1
Cracker Barrel whipped spreadables					
cheddar & cream cheese all styles	2 Tbs	80	<1	0	0
Old English brand..sharp spread					
regular Kraft jarred spreads	2 Tbs	90	1	0	0
bacon	2 Tbs	90	1	0	0
jalapeño pepper loaf	1 oz	80	3	0	2
olive & pimiento	2 Tbs	70	3	0	2
pimiento	2 Tbs	80	3	0	2
pineapple	2 Tbs	70	4	0	4
Roka/blue cheese spread	2 Tbs	80	2	0	1
Velveeta spread/Mexican					
all styles and flavors	1 oz	90	3	0	2
■ (Laughing Cow) spreadable cheeses					
Babybel/mini spreadable					

Food and Description	Amount	Total Calories	Total Carbs	Fiber	Sugars
cheddar	1 oz	70	1	0	0
original	1 oz	70	0	0	0
original spreadable..light	1 oz	30	0	0	0
■ (Nabisco) easy cheese spread					
all styles	2 Tbs	90	2	0	2
other..cheddar 'n' bacon	2 Tbs	90	2	0	1
■ (New Holland)					
garlic	1 oz	90	<1	0	0
jalapeño	1 oz	80	0	0	0
mild & creamy Danish-style	1 oz	110	1	0	0
natural vegetable	1 oz	80	2	0	0
plain	1 oz	90	0	0	0
sun-dried tomato..reduced-fat	1 oz	90	2	0	0
■ (Owl's Nest)					
bacon	2 Tbs	110	4	0	3
cheddary					
ranch	2 Tbs	100	3	0	2
w/sharp cheddar cheese	2 Tbs	110	4	0	3
garlic	2 Tbs	100	3	0	2
horseradish					
w/sharp cheddar cheese	2 Tbs	100	4	0	3
peppers galore	2 Tbs	100	3	0	2
port wine	2 Tbs	100	3	0	2
port wine...light..50% less fat	2 Tbs	70	5	0	5
Swiss almond	2 Tbs	100	3	0	2
Vermont/sharp white cheddar	2 Tbs	100	3	0	2
Vermont/sharp white cheddar..light	2 Tbs	70	5	0	5
■ ROKA (See (Kraft) in this section)					
■ VELVEETA (See (Kraft) in this section)					
■ (Wispride)					
COLD PACKS					
cheddar					
light 50..all types & flavors	2 Tbs	70	5	0	5
regular..all types & flavors	2 Tbs	90	3	0	3
DELI-STYLE					
cheese balls					
cheddar					
& cream w/almonds	1 oz	100	3	1	3
extra sharp w/almonds	1 oz	100	4	1	4
sharp cheddar					
w/almonds	1 oz	90	4	1	4
w/almonds & hazelnuts	1 oz	90	4	1	4
garden vegetable w/almonds	1 oz	120	5	1	4
garlic & herb	1 oz	120	5	1	4
horseradish w/almonds	1 oz	90	4	1	4
port wine w/almonds	1 oz	90	4	1	4
smoky bacon w/almonds	1 oz	90	4	1	4
Swiss w/almonds	1 oz	80	2	1	2

CHEESE SUBSTITUTE (See CHEESE ALTERNATIVE/IMITATION)
CHERIMOYA

Food and Description	Amount	Total Calories	Total Carbs	Fiber	Sugars
raw/whole/medium	2 lbs	515	130	13	na
CHERRY					
CANNED or JARRED					
(C&S) maraschino..w/stems	1 large	10	2	0	1
(Del Monte)..dark..sweet					
in heavy syrup	½ cup	100	24	<1	24
(Musselman's)					
cherries jubilee	2.3 oz	80	20	1	20
red tart..pitted	4.2 oz	50	12	1	8
(S&W)					
dark..sweet..in heavy syrup	½ cup	140	34	1	26
maraschino..all colors	1 cherry	10	2	0	1
Royal Anne..in heavy syrup	½ cup	110	26	1	23
DRIED					
(Chukar)					
bing	1 serving	130	33	3	29
Cherry Medley	1 serving	115	27	2	20
Rainier	1 serving	130	33	3	29
tart	1 serving	129	37	4	18
tart 'n' sweet	1 serving	180	24	2	19
(Sonoma)..bing..sweet tart	¼ cup	140	34	2	25
(Traverse Bay) cherry snacks					
chocolate-covered	1.3 oz	70	26	2	23
yogurt-covered	1.2 oz	150	25	1	20
red tart..premium	1.5 oz	130	31	2	28
FRESH					
(Dole)	1 cup	90	20	3	17
sour red	1 cup	51	12	1	12
sweet	10 medium	49	11	1.5	10
FROZEN					
(Big Valley)..dark sweet	¾ cup	60	20	3	17
(Cascadian Farm)..dark sweet	1 cup	72	17	2	15
GLACÉ					
(S&W) green or red cherries	5 pieces	80	20	0	20
(Seneca)..cherries..all colors	6 pieces	90	23	0	23
cherry pineapple mix	2 Tbs	100	24	0	24
CHERRY JUICE/JUICE BLEND/JUICE DRINK					
BOTTLED, BOXED, or CANNED					
(After The Fall) cherry blend	8 fl oz	100	26	0	0
(Capri Sun) wild cherry	6.75 fl oz	110	30	0	30
(Dole) mountain cherry	8 fl oz	120	30	0	30
(Hi-C) wild cherry	8 fl oz	120	30	0	30
(Libby's) Juicy Juice	8 fl oz	140	33	0	33
(Welch's) 100% juice/pourable					
Cherry Sensation	8 fl oz	130	32	0	30
(Tropicana Twister)					
black cherry	8 fl oz	140	35	0	34
cherry raspberry	8 fl oz	130	31	0	28
(R. W. Knudsen)					
black	11 fl oz	180	43	0	32

Food and Description	Amount	Total Calories	Total Carbs	Fiber	Sugars
celebratory/sparkling..organic	8 fl oz	110	28	0	23
cider	8 fl oz	130	33	0	30
fruit juice spritzer cherry cola	12 fl oz	170	42	0	34
FROZEN/PREPARED					
(Cascadian Farm) mountain					
concentrate	2 oz	120	30	0	28
from concentrate	8 fl oz	120	30	0	28
(Dole) mountain cherry	8 fl oz	140	34	0	32
(Welch's) Welchade	8 fl oz	130	31	0	30
CHERVIL..dried	1 tsp	1	0	0	0
CHESTNUT					
Chinese					
boiled or steamed	1 oz	44	10	<1	0
dried	1 oz	103	23	<1	0
roasted	1 oz	68	15	0.5	0
European					
boiled or steamed	1 oz	37	8	<1	0
dried	1 oz	106	22	<1	0
roasted	1 oz	70	15	4	0
Japanese					
boiled or steamed	1 oz	16	3.5	<1	0
dried	1 oz	102	23	<1	0
roasted	1 oz	57	13	<1	0
CHESTNUT FLOUR (*See* FLOUR)					
CHEWING GUM (*See* GUM)					
CHICKEN (*See* LUNCHEON MEAT; VEGETARIAN FOODS)					
■ **CHICKEN & CHICKEN PARTS/FRESH**					
broiler/fryer					
dark meat					
meat & skin					
batter-dipped & fried	4 oz	338	11	0	0
flour-coated & fried	4 oz	323	4.5	0	0
roasted	4 oz	287	0	0	0
stewed	4 oz	264	0	0	0
meat only					
fried	~5 oz	334	3.5	0	0
roasted	~5 oz	286	0	0	0
stewed	~5 oz	269	0	0	0
giblets/organs					
giblets/chopped or diced					
flour-coated & fried	1 cup	402	6	0	0
simmered	1 cup	228	1.5	0	0
gizzard/simmered	1 cup	222	1.5	0	0
roaster..chopped or diced	1 cup	222	1.5	0	0
heart/simmered	4 oz	210	0	0	0
chopped or diced	1 cup	268	0	0	0
liver/simmered	~5 oz	220	1	0	0
broiler/fryer...chopped	1 cup	220	1	0	0
light meat					
meat & skin					

Food and Description	Amount	Total Calories	Total Carbs	Fiber	Sugars
batter-dipped & fried	4 oz	312	11	<1	0
flour-coated & fried	4 oz	279	2	<1	0
roasted	4 oz	250	0	0	0
stewed	4 oz	228	0	0	0
meat only					
fried	4 oz	135	<1	0	0
roasted	4 oz	195	0	0	0
stewed	4 oz	180	0	0	0
parts					
backs					
meat & skin					
flour-coated & fried	4 oz	375	7	0	0
roasted	4 oz	340	0	0	0
meat only..roasted	4 oz	271	0	0	0
breast					
meat & skin					
batter-dipped & fried	4 oz	295	10	<1	0
flour-coated & fried	4 oz	252	2	0	0
roasted	4 oz	223	0	0	0
stewed	4 oz	29	0	0	0
meat only					
roasted	4 oz	187	0	0	0
stewed	4 oz	171	0	0	0
drumstick					
meat & skin					
batter-dipped & fried	4 oz	304	9	0	0
flour-coated & fried	4 oz	278	2	0	0
roasted	4 oz	245	0	0	0
meat only..roasted	4 oz	195	0	0	0
half chicken					
roaster..meat w/skin & bone	1.5 lbs	1,071	0	0	0
roaster..meat..w/skin..no bone	1.5 lbs	253	0	0	0
stewing chicken					
w/skin & bone	13.5 oz	744	0	0	0
w/meat & skin..no bone	9.2 oz	253	0	0	0
stewing chicken..meat only	9.2 oz	270	0	0	0
chopped or diced	1 cup	332	0	0	0
leg					
meat & skin					
batter-dipped & fried	4 oz	310	10	<1	0
flour-coated & fried	4 oz	285	3	<1	0
meat only..roasted	4 oz	217	0	0	0
thigh					
meat & skin					
batter-dipped & fried	4 oz	314	10	<1	0
flour-coated & fried	4 oz	297	4	<1	0
roasted	4 oz	279	0	0	0
meat only..roasted	4 oz	237	0	0	0
wing					

Food and Description	Amount	Total Calories	Total Carbs	Fiber	Sugars
meat & skin					
batter-dipped & fried	4 oz	367	12.5	<1	0
flour-coated & fried	4 oz	365	3	<1	0
roasted	4 oz	330	0	0	0
meat only..roasted	4 oz	230	0	0	0
roaster/roasted					
dark meat/meat only					
chopped or diced	1 cup	270	0	0	0
sliced	4 oz	205	0	0	0
light meat/meat only					
chopped or diced	1 cup	214	0	0	0
sliced	4 oz	175	0	0	0
whole/meat & skin	4 oz	253	0	0	0
stewing chicken/stewed					
dark meat/meat only					
chopped or diced	1 cup	298	0	0	0
sliced	4 oz	242	0	0	0
dark meat/meat & skin	4 oz	264	0	0	0
light meat/meat only					
chopped or diced	1 cup	300	0	0	0
sliced	4 oz	240	0	0	0
light meat..meat & skin	4 oz	228	0	0	0

■ CHICKEN & CHICKEN PARTS/FRESH OR FROZEN/BRAND NAME

(Butterball)
FRESH/RAW

Food and Description	Amount	Total Calories	Total Carbs	Fiber	Sugars
Best of the Fryer	4 oz	180	0	0	0
breast fillet/skinless & boneless					
seasoned..all flavors	1 fillet	110	1	0	0
thin	1 fillet	110	0	0	0
drumsticks	4 oz	160	0	0	0
thighs/family pack					
regular	1 4 oz	210	0	0	0
skinless	1 4 oz	120	0	0	0
whole chicken/seasoned					
BBQ	4 oz	220	1	0	0
herb garlic	4 oz	220	1	0	0
regular..whole	4 oz	210	1	0	0
wings					
drummettes	3 pieces	170	0	0	0
regular	4 oz	220	0	0	0

(Perdue)
FRESH/UNCOOKED (unless otherwise noted)

Food and Description	Amount	Total Calories	Total Carbs	Fiber	Sugars
breast					
skinless & boneless/individually frozen	5.9 oz	160	0	0	0
thin-sliced/skinless & boneless	2.8 oz	80	0	0	0
breast tenderloins/individually frozen	4 oz	110	0	0	0
Fit 'n' Easy..breast					
skinless & boneless	4 oz	110	0	0	0

Food and Description	Amount	Total Calories	Total Carbs	Fiber	Sugars
tenderloins	4 oz	120	0	0	0
ground					
breast	4 oz	100	0	0	0
regular	4 oz	180	0	0	0
regular burger patties	4 oz	170	0	0	0
Oven Stuffers..roaster breast/ skinless & boneless	4 oz	130	0	0	0
Ovenables/boneless/seasoned					
home-style	4 oz	100	0	0	0
Italian-style	4 oz	130	2	0	1
lemon pepper	4 oz	110	2	0	2
teriyaki	4 oz	110	4	0	0
roasting chicken/seasoned					
honey-flavored					
dark	4 oz	260	4	0	3
white	4 oz	190	4	0	3
toasted garlic					
dark	4 oz	260	1	0	0
white	4 oz	180	1	0	0
(Tyson)					
FRESH UNCOOKED					
breast					
boneless & skinless	4 oz	110	0	0	0
skinless split w/ribs	4 oz	110	0	0	0
split w/ribs	4 oz	180	0	0	0
Tasty Selections/boneless & skinless					
Italian	4 oz	110	2	0	1
lemon herb	4 oz	100	2	0	0
Tenders	4 oz	100	0	0	0
drumsticks	4 oz	160	0	0	0
ground	4 oz	150	0	0	0
skinless	4 oz	120	0	0	0
leg					
quarters	4 oz	190	0	0	0
whole	4 oz	230	1	0	0
thigh	4 oz	220	0	0	0
boneless & skinless cutlets	4 oz	110	0	0	0
whole chicken					
cut-up	4 oz	220	0	0	0
family roaster	4 oz	210	0	0	0
wings	4 pieces	240	0	0	0
FRESH INDIVIDUALLY FROZEN					
breast					
boneless & skinless..half..w/rib meat	4 oz	170	0	0	0
half	4 oz	230	0	0	0
Cornish game hen..w/o giblets	4 oz	200	0	0	0
drumsticks	2 pieces	140	0	0	<1
tenderloins, boneless..skinless	2 pieces	80	0	0	0
thighs..boneless..skinless	1 piece	170	0	0	0
wings	4 pieces	240	0	0	0

Food and Description	Amount	Total Calories	Total Carbs	Fiber	Sugars
CHICKEN ENTRÉE/DINNER (See also ASIAN FOOD; FROZEN ENTRÉE/DINNER; MEXICAN FOOD; PASTA ENTRÉE/DINNER; RICE DISH)					
(Banquet)					
FROZEN					
breast tenders Buffalo-style					
original	5 tenders	250	15	<1	1
seasoned	5 tenders	230	16	0	2
nuggets/breaded original	7 nuggets	280	19	1	3
patties..breaded..grilled	2.7 oz	110	3	1	0
popcorn chicken..breast fritters	3 oz	190	18	1	2
wings/breaded honey BBQ	3 oz	220	4	0	3
(Betty Crocker)					
BOX MIX					
Chicken Helper/prepared as directed					
cheddar & broccoli	1 cup	310	26	0	5
cheddar & mozzarella	1 cup	340	32	1	3
chicken fried rice	1 cup	260	22	1	1
chicken & herb rice	1 cup	260	24	2	0
chicken & mashed potatoes	1 cup	250	22	1	2
chicken potato au gratin	1 cup	270	25	1	4
chicken & stuffing	1 cup	290	27	1	3
creamy chicken & rice	1 cup	220	32	0	2
creamy roasted garlic	1 cup	280	26	2	3
fettuccini Alfredo	1 cup	300	27	1	4
4-cheese	1 cup	310	26	1	5
Parmesan pasta	1 cup	290	30	1	6
Southwestern	⅔ cup	240	27	1	2
Complete Meals/prepared as directed					
chicken & buttermilk biscuits	⅓ pkg	320	41	2	4
home-style dumplings & chicken	⅕ pkg	250	33	2	3
(Boar's Head)					
COOKED/READY-TO-COOK					
breasts					
aroastica-seasoned	1 oz	60	0	0	0
BBQ sauce–basted	2 oz	60	3	0	1
Blazing Buffalo–Style..all flavors	2 oz	60	0	0	0
(Dinty Moore)					
CANNED/MICROWAVEABLE					
canned stew					
chicken & dumplings	1 cup	230	27	0	1
chicken stew	1 cup	220	16	2	3
microwaveable American classics					
chicken & dumplings	1 bowl	280	35	3	2
chicken & noodles	1 bowl	260	28	2	3
chicken & rice	1 bowl	250	20	3	3
chicken w/mashed potatoes	1 bowl	220	27	2	2
microwave cup					
chicken & dumplings	1 cup	200	25	1	1
noodles & chicken	1 cup	190	19	1	2
(Green Giant)					

Food and Description	Amount	Total Calories	Total Carbs	Fiber	Sugars
FROZEN					
Create a Meal!/as packaged					
chicken Alfredo	2 cups	230	33	3	6
garlic herb	2⅓ cups	230	30	3	3
lemon pepper	1½ cups	140	30	5	7
Parmesan herb	1¾ cups	160	29	5	3
stir-fry					
garlic	1⅔ cups	130	25	4	14
lo mein	2⅓ cups	170	33	3	9
teriyaki	1¾ cups	100	20	4	12
(Hormel)					
CANNED..IN BROTH					
America's Choice..chunk chicken	2 oz	50	0	0	0
breast of chicken					
no salt	2 oz	50	0	0	0
regular	2 oz	50	0	0	0
chunk chicken	2 oz	60	0	0	0
lemon	2 oz	50	1	0	0
Southwest	2 oz	50	2	0	0
tomato basil w/garlic	2 oz	50	2	0	2
FULLY COOKED ENTRÉES					
Always Tender..boneless					
boneless chicken breast	1 breast	150	2	0	0
Italian	1 breast	170	3	0	1
lemon pepper	1 breast	180	5	0	4
teriyaki	1 breast	180	8	0	6
chicken breast					
& gravy..family pack	1 breast	130	4	0	2
w/gravy	1 breast	130	4	0	2
w/teriyaki..family pack	1 breast	230	30	0	28
(Louis Rich)					
READY-TO-COOK/REFRIGERATED					
breast cuts..all types	3 oz	130	1	0	1
breast strips..all types	3 oz	110	1	0	0
(Mrs. Fearnow's)					
Brunswick chicken stew..canned	8 oz	160	20	1	3
(Perdue)					
FULLY COOKED					
breast					
cutlets					
home-style	1 patty	120	10	0	0
Italian-style/white	1 patty	130	11	2	2
original	3 oz	190	0	0	0
tenderloins/white	3 oz	140	0	0	0
FRESH/COOKED					
Cornish hen					
dark	3 oz	200	0	0	0
white	3 oz	160	0	0	0
drumsticks/roasted	1 piece	110	0	0	0
ground	3 oz	170	0	0	0

Food and Description	Amount	Total Calories	Total Carbs	Fiber	Sugars
leg quarters	3 oz	220	0	0	0
soup & stew baking chicken					
dark	3 oz	210	0	0	0
white	3 oz	170	0	0	0
thighs/roasted	1 thigh	240	0	0	0
thin-sliced/skinless & boneless	2 oz	80	0	0	0
whole chicken/cooked					
dark	3 oz	210	0	0	0
white	3 oz	170	0	0	0
wings/roasted	2 wings	210	0	0	0
INDIVIDUALLY FROZEN/FULLY COOKED					
breast/skinless & boneless	4.2 oz	140	0	0	0
hot & spicy wings	3 oz	180	1	0	0
nuggets/breast	3.4 oz	250	15	1	1
tenderloins/breast	3 oz	200	13	0	1
skinless & boneless	3 oz	100	0	0	0
thighs/skinless & boneless	1 thigh	180	0	0	0
Short Cuts/Chicken Breast					
roasted & carved					
honey-roasted	½ cup	90	2	0	0
Italian-style	½ cup	90	3	0	1
lemon pepper	½ cup	100	2	0	0
original	½ cup	90	2	0	0
Southwestern-seasoned	½ cup	100	2	0	1
strips/carved					
in barbecue sauce	6 oz	200	24	0	23
in garlic & herb sauce	5 oz	100	4	2	1
in marinara sauce	5 oz	120	5	0	1
in teriyaki sauce	5 oz	190	26	0	22
Wingettes..fresh wings..cooked	3 oz	210	0	0	0
(Schwan's)					
FROZEN/PARTIALLY OR FULLY COOKED UNLESS OTHERWISE STATED					
Chicken Express/meal kit					
chicken & broccoli	1 bowl	500	68	2	2
teriyaki	1 bowl	360	66	3	10
w/fried rice	¼ bag	320	56	2	15
Chicken/other meal kits					
breast fajita	2 fajitas	290	33	4	3
Southwestern-style	¼ pkg	200	28	3	8
stir-fry meal kit	¼ bag	260	45	3	13
Cordon Bleu	5 oz	290	13	1	1
wings					
barbecue	4 pieces	170	1	0	1
Buffalo-style boneless	4 pieces	210	15	1	0
hot	4 pieces	170	1	0	0
teriyaki	4 pieces	250	22	1	8
(Swanson)					
CANNED					
chicken & dumplings	1 cup	230	26	2	2
chicken à la king	1 cup	320	20	2	3

Food and Description	Amount	Total Calories	Total Carbs	Fiber	Sugars
Mixin' Chicken in broth..premium	2 oz	100	<1	<1	0
chicken breast	2 oz	60	1	0	0
chunk chicken	2 oz	70	<1	<1	0
(Tyson)					
BOXED/BAGGED ITEMS/FULLY COOKED					
bites/box	13 pieces	180	11	0	0
breast/diced..box	3 oz	120	1	0	0
breast fillets..bag					
mesquite	1 piece	130	1	0	1
regular	1 piece	290	21	2	0
teriyaki	1 piece	170	7	0	4
breast strips					
fajita-style	3 oz	120	1	0	1
grilled/box	3 oz	110	2	0	2
Italian-style/box	3 oz	120	2	0	1
lemon/box	3 oz	120	1	0	0
Southwest/bag	3 oz	120	1	0	0
meatballs/bag	3 oz	180	6	2	1
nuggets	3 oz	90	0	0	0
breast nuggets/box	5 pieces	280	21	0	1
patties					
regular	1 patty	180	12	1	1
Southwestern-style	1 patty	240	10	1	0
popcorn chicken..bites	6 pieces	210	17	2	1
strips/bag					
Buffalo-style	2 pieces	230	21	1	1
crispy	2 pieces	200	13	1	0
tenderloins/breast/box	1 piece	150	12	1	1
Southern-style	1 piece	150	12	1	1
spicy	1 piece	160	13	1	1
tenders					
breast/box..honey batter	5 pieces	220	13	2	3
wings					
BBQ-style/box	3 pieces	200	7	0	7
Buffalo/bag	4 pieces	220	1	0	0
honey BBQ/box	3 pieces	250	13	1	4
hot 'n' spicy/box	3 pieces	180	1	0	0
hot 'n' spicy/box	4 pieces	220	1	0	0
Wings of Fire/box	3 pieces	260	14	2	1
(Weaver)					
FROZEN/BONELESS					
breast strips					
Buffalo	2 pieces	220	13	1	1
crispy	2 pieces	220	13	2	1
low-fat	3 pieces	120	14	0	4
regular	3 pieces	230	14	1	1
breast tenders					
honey batter	5 pieces	220	13	2	3
regular	5 pieces	240	15	0	0

Food and Description	Amount	Total Calories	Total Carbs	Fiber	Sugars
croquettes					
w/ ¼ cup gravy	2 pieces	230	15	0	2
w/o gravy	3 pieces	340	27	2	5
mini-drums/crispy	5 pieces	250	14	1	2
nuggets	4 pieces	210	9	1	0
patties					
breast	1 patty	170	10	1	1
Italian	1 patty	210	12	1	1
original	1 patty	180	10	1	1
popcorn chicken/Buffalo	1 serving	230	13	1	1
Buffalo-style hot	3 pieces	190	0	0	0
honey BBQ	3 pieces	200	7	0	2
CHICKEN SEASONING (*See* SEASONINGS)					
CHICKEN SUBSTITUTES (*See* VEGETARIAN FOODS)					
CHICKPEA/GARBANZO BEAN					
CANNED					
(Bush's Best)					
16-oz can	4.5 oz	130	22	9	1
20-oz can	4.5 oz	120	20	4	4
(Eden) garbanzo	½ cup	120	20	4	4
(Fermano's)	4.5 oz	110	18	8	3
(Goya) Spanish-style	7.5 oz	150	32	9	0
(Progresso)					
chickpeas	½ cup	120	20	5	3
garbanzo beans	½ cup	100	16	4	3
(S&W) all styles	½ cup	80	28	7	2
(Sun Vista) frijoles garbanzos	½ cup	110	17	6	1
DRY/RAW					
(Arrowhead Mills)	¼ cup	170	29	6	0
(Best Yet)	¼ cup	110	29	14	1
CHILI/CHILI BEANS (*See also* MEXICAN FOOD)					
CANNED					
(Armour)					
hot Western-style w/beans	7.5 oz	280	27	11	4
w/beans	7.5 oz	320	27	13	4
(Bush's Best) Chili Magic					
chili starter					
Louisiana hot	4.4 oz	110	21	5	3
Texas medium	4.4 oz	120	20	5	3
traditional mild	4.4 oz	110	19	5	2
(Chili Man)					
w/beans	7.5 oz	330	28	10	2
w/o beans	7.5 oz	380	16	6	2
(Dennison's)					
chili..w/beans 99% fat-free					
beef	1 cup	210	29	8	2
turkey	1 cup	210	29	7	3
con carne					
chunky	1 cup	300	32	9	2

Food and Description	Amount	Total Calories	Total Carbs	Fiber	Sugars
hot					
w/beans	1 cup	370	32	9	2
w/o beans	1 cup	330	20	3	1
hot & chunky	1 cup	350	36	11	2
original	1 cup	360	30	11	2
w/mild green chilis	1 cup	360	38	11	3
vegetarian..99% fat-free	1 cup	220	35	9	6
(Eden) organic chili beans	½ cup	130	21	7	1
(Health Valley)..99% fat-free					
medium turkey	1 cup	220	34	8	8
vegetarian					
burrito flavor	1 cup	160	30	11	8
lentil	1 cup	160	28	11	9
mild	1 cup	160	30	11	9
spicy	1 cup	160	30	11	9
(Hormel)					
w/beans	7.5 oz	270	34	7	5
chunky	7.5 oz	270	34	7	5
hot	7.5 oz	270	34	7	5
less salt	7.5 oz	340	30	9	3
turkey	7.5 oz	200	26	5	6
vegetarian	7.5 oz	200	38	7	6
w/o beans	7.5 oz	270	34	7	5
hot	7.5 oz	210	17	3	3
hot & spicy	7.5 oz	210	17	3	3
less salt	7.5 oz	210	17	3	3
turkey	7.5 oz	190	17	3	4
(S&W)					
chili beans					
original..w/zesty sauce	4.4 oz	110	23	6	1
w/chipotle peppers	4.4 oz	90	21	6	1
Chili Makin's					
black bean	4.3 oz	90	19	6	9
home-style	4.3 oz	90	19	6	9
original	4.3 oz	90	19	6	9
(Skyline)					
original recipe	3 oz	150	3	1	na
family-size/tub	8.5 oz	270	5	2	na
for chili dogs	1.7 oz	45	1	0	na
(Stagg)					
Chili Laredo	1 cup	320	27	6	3
Chunkeroo	1 cup	300	26	5	6
Classic	1 cup	330	28	5	7
Country Brand	1 cup	320	29	5	6
Dynamite Hot	1 cup	320	27	6	3
Ranch House	1 cup	290	32	6	6
Rio Blanco	1 cup	250	19	4	5
Silverado/beef	1 cup	230	33	6	7
Steakhouse	1 cup	330	16	2	5
Turkey Ranchero	1 cup	240	31	6	6

Food and Description	Amount	Total Calories	Total Carbs	Fiber	Sugars
Vegetable Garden	1 cup	200	37	7	9
JARRED					
(Bush's Best)					
home-style chili..no-beans original w/beans	7.5 oz	240	15	3	5
chunky	7.5 oz	260	26	9	5
hot	7.5 oz	250	26	8	5
MICROWAVEABLE					
(The Allens) Mexican chili beans					
frijoles enchiladas	4.4 oz	130	21	8	1
(Fantastic Foods)					
Cha Cha Chili	1 cup	220	37	11	6
3-bean	1 cup	180	28	5	5
vegetarian	¼ pkg	100	17	4	4
(Health Valley) chili cups..all flavors	1/3 cup	120	21	6	3
(Stagg) Chili Smart Pak/shelf-staple					
Chili Laredo	1 cup	320	27	6	3
Chunkeroo	1 cup	300	26	5	6
Classic	1 cup	330	28	5	7
Country Brand	1 cup	320	29	5	6
Dynamite Hot	1 cup	320	27	6	3
Fiesta Grill	1 cup	240	25	5	8
Ranch House	1 cup	290	32	6	6
Rio Blanco	1 cup	250	19	4	5
Silverado/beef	1 cup	230	33	6	7
Steakhouse	1 cup	330	16	2	5
Turkey Ranchero	1 cup	240	31	6	6
Vegetable Garden	1 cup	200	37	7	9
MIX..dry mix only					
(Fantastic Foods)					
Cha Cha Chili	1 cup	220	37	11	6
3-bean	1 cup	180	28	5	5
vegetarian	¼ pkg	100	17	4	4
(McCormick)					
hot	¼ pkt	35	4	2	0
mild	¼ pkt	30	5	1	0
original	¼ pkt	30	5	2	0
(Old El Paso) chili mix	1 Tbs	15	3	<1	0
CHINESE FOOD (*See* ASIAN FOOD, also FROZEN ENTRÉE/DINNER)					
CHINESE PARSLEY (*See* CILANTRO)					
CHIVES					
freeze-dried	1 Tbs	1	0	0	0
raw	1 Tbs	1	0	0	0
	¼ cup	2	0.5	0	0
CHOCOLATE (*See* BAKING BARS, BITS, CHIPS, CHUNKS & PIECES; CANDY)					
CHOCOLATE, HOT (*See* COCOA; MILK MIX)					
CHOCOLATE SYRUP (*See* ICE CREAM TOPPING; MILK MIX)					
CHUB (*See* CISCO)					
CHUTNEY					
(Crosse & Blackwell)					

Food and Description	Amount	Total Calories	Total Carbs	Fiber	Sugars
apple curry	1 Tbs	25	7	0	5
apricot chardonnay	1 Tbs	25	7	0	5
cranberry	1 Tbs	40	10	0	9
Major Grey's mango..all styles	1 Tbs	60	14	0	14
peach zinfandel	1 Tbs	25	6	0	5
pear cardamom	1 Tbs	25	6	0	5
(Patak's) original					
hot mango spice	1 Tbs	60	14	0	14
mango pickle..hot	1 Tbs	45	3	1	0
sweet mango	1 Tbs	60	14	0	14
CIDER					
BOTTLED or BOXED					
(Alpenglow) apple/sparkling	8 fl oz	120	30	0	30
(Indian Summer)..all flavors	8 fl oz	120	30	0	26
(Knudsen) Thirst Quencher					
cider & spice	8 fl oz	120	30	0	30
(Martinelli's) sparkling apple cider	8 fl oz	140	35	0	31
single-serve	8.4 fl oz	150	37	0	33
(Musselman's)..sparkling	8 fl oz	150	36	0	31
(Odwalla) harvest apple	8 fl oz	130	28	0	27
MIX					
(Alpine) apple cider drink/prepared					
original or spiced	8 fl oz	80	20	0	20
sugar-free	8 fl oz	15	4	0	0
CILANTRO/CHINESE PARSLEY/CORIANDER LEAF					
dried	1 tsp	2	0	0	0
	1 Tbs	5	0	0	0
fresh	1 tsp	2	0	0	0
	1 Tbs	5	0	0	0
CINNAMON/ground	1 tsp	10	2	0	0
CISCO/CHUB meat only..smoked	2 oz	100	0	0	0
CITRUS JUICE/JUICE DRINK (*See also* FRUIT PUNCH)					
BOTTLED, BOXED, or CANNED					
(Five Alive)..citrus..41% juice	8 fl oz	120	30	0	28
FROZEN or REFRIGERATED..prepared					
(Hanson's)..citrus orange	8 fl oz	130	30	0	29
CLAM (*See also* SEAFOOD ENTRÉE/DINNER)					
CANNED					
(3 Diamonds) whole	2 oz	45	0	0	0
(Bumble Bee)..baby..fancy whole	3.33 oz	50	2	0	0
(Chicken of the Sea)					
baby whole	2.22 oz	35	1	0	0
chopped or minced	⅓ cup	30	2	0	1
smoked baby	1 can	200	2	0	0
whole	2 oz	30	1	0	0
(Crown Prince)..baby					
boiled	⅓ cup	40	2	0	0
natural	⅓ cup	40	1	0	0
(Doxsee) solids & liquid					
chopped or minced	1.85 oz	25	2	0	<1

Food and Description	Amount	Total Calories	Total Carbs	Fiber	Sugars
(Geisha)					
baby					
chopped	2.16 oz	30	1	0	0
fancy smoked/in cottonseed	1.875 oz	130	4	1	0
whole	3.33 oz	50	2	0	0
FRESH					
raw	3 oz	63	2	0	0
steamed	3 oz	126	4	0	0
FROZEN					
(Matlaw's)					
casino	1.3 oz	60	7	1	na
stuffed..box	3.7 oz	180	21	3	na
CLAM CHOWDER (*See* SOUP)					
CLAM JUICE					
(Crown Prince)	1 Tbs	5	1	0	<1
(Doxsee) Natural	1 Tbs	5	0	0	0
CLAM SAUCE (*See* SAUCE)					
CLOVES/ground	1 tsp	7	1	0	0
CLUB SODA (*See* COCKTAIL MIXER; SOFT DRINK)					
COBBLER (*See* PIE & COBBLER)					
COCKTAIL/COCKTAIL MIXER (*See also* LIQUEUR; LIQUOR, DISTILLED; WINE)					
generic and brands..(mixed drinks are from standard recipe)					
amaretto..56-proof	1 fl oz	110	9	0	0
(Bacardi)..frozen					
prepared w/rum					
banana	7 fl oz	210	35	0	33
peach	7 fl oz	200	33	0	31
prepared w/water					
banana	7 fl oz	150	35	0	33
peach	7 fl oz	130	33	0	31
(Bailey's) Irish Cream					
34 proof	1 fl oz	95	5	0	0
30 proof..light	1 fl oz	75	7	0	0
Bloody Mary	1 drink	95	16	0	na
brandy..cherry blend..48-proof	1 fl oz	80	9	0	0
coffee liqueur..53-proof	1 fl oz	115	16	0	0
cosmopolitan	1 drink	215	12	0	na
crème de cacao..54-proof	1 fl oz	100	15	0	0
crème de menthe..60-proof	1 fl oz	120	14	0	0
daiquiri..canned	1 fl oz	40	5	0	0
Galliano..80-proof	1 fl oz	100	8	0	0
Grand Marnier..80-proof	1 fl oz	100	7	0	0
Harvey Wallbanger	1 drink	200	17	0	na
Kahlúa..53-proof	1 fl oz	90	11	0	0
mudslide..w/milk	1 drink	150	10	0	na
kirsch..68-proof	1 fl oz	80	6	0	0
mai tai	1 drink	225	16	0	14
Manhattan	2.5 fl oz	128	3	0	na
margarita	~3 fl oz	170	4	0	4
(Bacardi)..frozen					

Food and Description	Amount	Total Calories	Total Carbs	Fiber	Sugars
prepared w/rum	7 fl oz	160	25	0	25
prepared w/water	7 fl oz	90	24	0	24
martini	2.5 fl oz	156	0	0	0
mint julep	10 fl oz	215	4	0	na
Pernod..80-proof	1 fl oz	75	2	0	0
piña colada/canned (Bacardi)..frozen	6.8 fl oz	525	60	0	na
prepared w/rum	7 fl oz	260	37	0	35
prepared w/water	7 fl oz	200	37	0	35
sambuca..84-proof	1 fl oz	100	7	0	0
schnapps..80-proof	1 fl oz	100	7	0	0
screwdriver	1 drink	174	14	0	14
tequila sunrise	6.8 fl oz	230	24	0	24
Tia Maria..64-proof	1 fl oz	90	9	0	0
Tom Collins	1 drink	210	12	0	na
triple sec..60-proof	1 fl oz	80	7	0	0
whiskey sour..canned	6.8 fl oz	250	28	0	na
white Russian	3.5 fl oz	268	16	0	na
COCKTAIL MIXER (*See also* COCKTAIL; SOFT DRINK; WATER; individual fruit juice listings)					
(Bacardi) frozen..prepared w/water					
fruit mixers w/o alcohol					
margarita	7 fl oz	90	25	0	23
piña colada	7 fl oz	170	37	0	34
rum runner	7 fl oz	140	33	0	32
strawberry daiquiri	7 fl oz	120	32	0	30
(Baja Bob's) bottled mix					
Bloody Mary					
lean & mean	4 oz	20	4	0	3
margarita					
original	4 oz	10	<1	0	0
sweet & sour	4 oz	10	<1	0	0
wild strawberry	3 oz	10	3	0	0
piña colada	4 oz	30	4	1	3
(Canada Dry)					
club soda..all types	8 fl oz	0	0	0	0
Collins	8 fl oz	100	30		30
ginger ale					
cherry					
diet	8 fl oz	0	0	0	0
regular	8 fl oz	90	21	0	21
cranberry					
diet	8 fl oz	5	<1	0	<1
regular	8 fl oz	140	37	0	37
golden					
diet	8 fl oz	0	0	0	0
regular	8 fl oz	100	24	0	24
plain					
diet	8 fl oz	0	0	0	0
regular	8 fl oz	120	33	0	33

Food and Description	Amount	Total Calories	Total Carbs	Fiber	Sugars
seltzer/sparkling water	8 fl oz	0	0	0	0
whiskey sour mix/wild cherry	8 fl oz	90	22	0	22
(Holland House)					
Bloody Mary/bottled					
smooth & spicy	4 fl oz	15	4	0	na
daiquiri					
raspberry..bottled	4 fl oz	140	36	0	36
regular/dry mix	1 pkg	65	16	0	16
strawberry..bottled	4 fl oz	180	46	0	44
mai tai/dry mix	1 pkg	64	16	0	16
margarita					
regular..bottled	4 oz	100	26	0	25
regular..dry mix	1 pkg	57	14	0	14
strawberry..bottled	4 fl oz	180	46	0	44
old-fashioned..bottled	4 fl oz	90	23	0	22
piña colada..dry mix	1 pkg	82	12	0	12
sweet & sour..bottled	4 fl oz	130	31	0	31
Tom Collins..dry mix	1 pkg	65	15	0	15
whiskey sour..bottled	4 fl oz	130	31	0	31
whiskey sour..dry mix	1 pkg	65	16	0	16
(Jero) bottled mixes					
Bloody Mary					
regular	1 serving	170	10	0	10
spicy jalapeño	1 serving	45	10	0	10
cherry bar mix	1 serving	45	14	0	13
grenadine	1 serving	90	22	0	21
Manhattan	1 serving	60	16	0	16
margarita	1 serving	190	47	0	47
old-fashioned	1 serving	130	32	0	32
pina colada	1 serving	290	64	0	64
strawberry					
daiquiri	1 serving	310	78	0	78
margarita	1 serving	310	78	0	78
sweet & sour	1 oz	150	38	0	38
triple sec	1 oz	40	10	0	10
(Major Peters') bottled mixes					
Bloody Mary					
hot & spicy	1 serving	45	11	0	7
original	1 serving	45	11	0	7
salsa-style	1 serving	45	11	0	7
The Works	1 serving	45	11	0	7
grenadine	1 serving	80	20	0	20
mai tai	1 serving	200	42	0	40
margarita	1 serving	200	50	0	50
old-fashioned	1 serving	150	39	0	39
piña colada					
⅓ bottle	1 serving	260	67	0	64
½ bottle	1 serving	320	79	0	74
strawberry					
daiquiri	1 serving	200	51	0	51

Food and Description	Amount	Total Calories	Total Carbs	Fiber	Sugars
margarita	1 serving	200	50	0	50
sweet & sour	1 serving	200	51	0	51
triple sec	1 serving	35	9	0	9
(Mr. & Mrs. T) bottled					
Bloody Mary					
regular	4.5 fl oz	20	4	0	4
rich & spicy	4.5 fl oz	30	6	0	6
margarita					
regular	3 fl oz	80	20	0	20
strawberry	3.5 fl oz	100	24	0	24
piña colada	4 fl oz	150	39	0	39
sweet & sour	3 fl oz	70	17	0	17
(Rose's) grenadine syrup	1 fl oz	65	16	0	16
(Schweppes)					
bitter lemon	6 fl oz	110	20	0	20
club soda..all types..unflavored	8 fl oz	0	0	0	0
Collins mixer	6 fl oz	90	19	0	19
ginger ale					
diet	8 fl oz	0	0	0	0
dry grape	6 fl oz	90	23	0	23
regular	6 fl oz	65	15	0	15
seltzer/sparkling water	8 fl oz	0	0	0	0
tonic water..plain					
diet	8 fl oz	0	0	0	0
regular	6 fl oz	65	15	0	15
(Tabasco) Bloody Mary	8 fl oz	60	22	2	8
COCOA (*See also* MILK MIX)					
(Ghirardelli) sweet ground chocolate					
& cocoa	3 Tbs	100	24	2	20
unsweetened	1 Tbs	20	4	2	0
(Hershey) all styles	1 Tbs	20	3	1	0
(Nestlé)	1 Tbs	15	3	1	0
COCONUT					
(Baker's) Angel Flake..all styles	2 Tbs	70	6	1	5
(Griffin's)	2 Tbs	70	9	1	9
(Let's Do Organic)					
flakes	2 Tbs	100	1	0	0
shredded					
light	2 Tbs	60	<1	0	0
regular	2 Tbs	100	1	0	0
COCONUT CREAM					
canned..sweetened					
(Coco Lopez)	2 Tbs	120	20	0	18
(Goya) Cocoa Cream of Coconut	2 Tbs	140	22	0	19
COCONUT MILK					
canned					
(A Taste of Thai) unsweetened					
light	⅓ cup	45	3	0	0
original	⅓ cup	140	3	0	0
(Goya)	1 Tbs	50	1	0	0

Food and Description	Amount	Total Calories	Total Carbs	Fiber	Sugars
COCONUT WATER (Goya)	12 fl oz	150	31	10	0
COD (*See also* COD ROE; SEAFOOD ENTRÉE/DINNER)					
Atlantic & Pacific					
canned	3 oz	89	0	0	0
cooked—dry heat	3 oz	89	0	0	0
dried	3 oz	246	0	0	0
raw	3 oz	70	0	0	0
COFFEE/COFFEE-LIKE BEVERAGE					
FLAVORED					
bottled/carton					
(Folger's)..Jakada..coffee latte					
French roast	10.5 oz	170	30	0	29
mocha	10.5 oz	190	35	0	34
vanilla	10.5 oz	170	32	0	31
(Nescafé Frothe)					
Chocolate Mocha	8.47 oz	80	19	0	18
Divinely Mocha	8.47 oz	90	13	0	11
Enchanting Vanilla	8.47 oz	90	13	0	0
(Silk) by White Wave					
soy latte/bottle	11 oz	220	39	0	31
soy latte coffee..carton	1 cup	170	25	1	23
INSTANT					
(General Foods)					
International Coffee					
cappuccino/prepared					
Café Mocha/decaf	1 cup	60	9	0	7
Café Vienna					
decaf/sugar-free/fat-free	1 cup	30	5	0	0
regular	1 cup	70	11	0	9
Cappuccino Coolers					
chocolate	1 cup	60	16	1	14
French vanilla	1 cup	60	15	0	15
hazelnut	1 cup	60	15	0	14
French vanilla café					
decaffeinated	1 cup	60	10	0	7
fat-free	1 cup	25	5	0	0
fat-free/sugar-free	1 cup	5	5	0	0
regular	1 cup	60	10	0	7
sugar-free	1 cup	25	5	0	0
hazelnut	1 cup	60	9	1	7
Irish cream café	1 cup	60	10	0	7
Italian cappuccino	1 cup	60	9	0	7
orange cappuccino					
regular	1 cup	60	9	0	7
sugar-free	1 cup	30	5	0	0
Suisse Mocha					
decaffeinated	1 cup	60	9	0	7
fat-free	1 cup	25	5	0	0
fat-free/sugar-free	1 cup	5	5	0	0
regular	1 cup	60	9	0	7

Food and Description	Amount	Total Calories	Total Carbs	Fiber	Sugars
sugar-free	1 cup	25	5	0	0
Swiss white chocolate	1 cup	70	12	0	9
Viennese chocolate café	1 cup	50	10	0	9
(Hills Brothers) prepared					
cinnamon roll	1 serving	120	20	<1	15
double mocha	1 serving	120	19	1	15
English toffee	1 serving	120	19	1	13
French vanilla					
decaf	1 serving	120	19	1	13
regular	1 serving	120	19	1	13
hazelnut	1 serving	120	19	1	13
pecan coffee cake	1 serving	120	21	<1	15
(Land O' Lakes) Cappuccino Classics/mix					
amaretto	1 pkt	130	23	0	22
Chocolate Supreme	1 pkt	150	25	1	20
French vanilla	1 pkt	130	23	0	22
Suisse Mocha	1 pkt	140	25	1	22
Suprema	1 pkt	140	25	0	22
NONFLAVORED (prepared unless otherwise noted)					
(Brim)					
decaf	6 fl oz	2	1	0	0
regular	6 fl oz	4	1	0	0
(Flavia)					
decaf					
French roast	1 cup	<1	0	0	0
gourmet..all styles	1 cup	<1	0	0	0
hazelnut	1 cup	3	1	0	0
(Folger's) ground					
decaf or regular	6 fl oz	4	1	0	0
(Kava) mix only	1 tsp	2	1	0	0
(Maxwell House) decaf	6 fl oz	2	1	0	0
(Nescafé) instant/all styles	6 fl oz	4	1	0	0
(Pero) hot beverage drink..prepared					
w/malt & barley/no caffeine	6 fl oz	4	1	0	0
(Postum) coffee-flavored grain					
beverage prepared w/water	8 fl oz	10	2	0	0
(Sanka)					
decaf	6 fl oz	2	1	0	0
instant	6 fl oz	2	<1	0	0
(Taster's Choice)..all types	6 fl oz	4	1	0	0
(Worthington) Natural Touch					
Kaffree Roma/mix only	1 tsp	10	2	0	0
(Yuban)					
espresso	2 fl oz	1	<1	0	0
regular	6 fl oz	4	1	0	0

COFFEE CREAMER (*See* CREAM; CREAMER, NONDAIRY)
COLD CUTS (*See* LUNCHEON MEAT)
COLLARDS
CANNED

(Allens) seasoned Southern-style	½ cup	35	5	1	1

Food and Description	Amount	Total Calories	Total Carbs	Fiber	Sugars
verduras collards picadas/chopped ½ cup (Allens Sunshine) seasoned	½ cup	30	3	3	1
Southern-style	½ cup	35	5	1	1
(Glory Foods) seasoned	½ cup	50	7	3	0
FROZEN/CHOPPED					
(McKenzie's)	3.2 oz	30	2	2	1
(Pictsweet)	3.3 oz	25	2	2	1

CONDIMENTS (*See* ASIAN FOOD; MEXICAN FOOD; SAUCE; SEASONINGS; individual listings)

COOKIE (*See also* BROWNIE/BROWNIE-LIKE BARS; CAKE, SNACK CRACKER)

■ **(Archway)**

Food and Description	Amount	Total Calories	Total Carbs	Fiber	Sugars
ABC sugar cookies	12 cookies	130	21	0	8
almond crescent	2 cookies	100	17	1	6
apple raisin	1 cookie	110	17	<1	9
apple-filled oatmeal	1 cookie	90	15	0	7
apricot-filled oatmeal	1 cookie	90	15	0	7
Aunt Mary's sugar cookies	1 cookie	130	22	0	11
Bells & Stars	3 cookies	150	19	<1	8
cashew nougat	3 cookie	170	16	0	9
cherry-filled	1 cookie	90	15	0	7
chocolate brownie cookie	1 cookie	140	21	<1	12
chocolate chip					
bag	5 cookies	160	22	<1	11
brownie	1 cookie	140	22	<1	12
drop	1 cookie	90	25	0	7
icebox	1 cookie	110	14	0	7
semisweet	1 cookie	140	19	<1	12
sugar-free	1 cookie	110	16	0	0
w/walnuts	1 cookie	140	19	<1	11
coconut macaroon					
original	1 cookie	100	14	1	10
striped	1 cookie	100	14	0	11
cookie jar hermits	1 cookie	90	32	<1	16
dark molasses	1 cookie	120	20	0	10
date-filled oatmeal	1 cookie	90	15	<1	8
devil's food/fat-free	1 cookie	60	15	0	0
Dutch apple	1 cookie	110	17	<1	8
Dutch cocoa	1 cookie	100	18	0	10
frosty lemon	1 cookie	100	16	0	10
fruit & honey bar	1 bar	190	33	<1	18
fruitcake cookies	3 cookies	140	22	1	10
ginger snap..reduced-fat	5 cookies	140	25	0	12
gingerbread cookies	3 cookies	140	22	0	9
iced molasses	1 cookie	120	20	0	10
iced oatmeal..10-oz pkg	1 cookie	120	19	<1	10
lemon					
malted nutty nougat	3 cookies	160	17	2	11
molasses..old-fashioned	1 cookie	100	18	0	10
nutty nougat	3 cookies	170	16	<1	9
oatmeal					

Food and Description	Amount	Total Calories	Total Carbs	Fiber	Sugars
date-filled	1 cookie	100	17	<1	9
pecan	1 cookie	140	16	<1	7
raisin	1 cookie	120	20	<1	11
raisin bran..original	1 cookie	110	18	<1	10
raspberry/fat-free	1 cookie	100	23	1	13
peanut butter..home-style	1 cookie	140	17	<1	9
pecan ice box	1 cookie	110	14	0	6
pfeffernusse	2 cookies	100	23	<1	5
raspberry-filled	1 cookie	90	15	0	7
rocky road..original	1 cookie	130	18	<1	10
Ruth's golden oatmeal	1 cookie	120	18	1	9
strawberry-filled	1 cookie	90	15	0	7
sugar	1 cookie	100	17	0	8
sugar drop cookies	1 cookie	80	13	0	7
wedding cake	3 cookies	160	20	0	9
windmill/old-fashioned	1 cookie	90	14	<1	6
■ (Bakery Wagon)					
cobbler/fat-free					
apple	1 cookie	100	17	1	8
cranberry apple	1 cookie	70	16	1	10
raspberry	1 cookie	90	16	1	7
cookie/low-fat					
date-filled oat	1 cookie	90	15	1	5
iced molasses..regular	1 cookie	100	18	1	9
raspberry-filled oat	1 cookie	90	16	1	7
soft oatmeal	1 cookie	100	15	1	10
gingersnap	5 cookies	160	22	1	10
■ (Barbara's Bakery)					
animal cookies/vanilla	8 cookies	120	18	<1	5
crisp cookies					
chocolate chip	1 cookie	80	9	<1	5
double Dutch chocolate	1 cookie	80	9	<1	4
old-fashioned oatmeal	1 cookie	60	8	<1	5
traditional shortbread	1 cookie	80	9	<1	3
fig bars..low-fat traditional					
blueberry	1 bar	60	15	0	9
fig/traditional	1 bar	60	14	0	8
Snackimals					
chocolate chip	10 cookies	120	19	0	8
oatmeal/wheat-free	10 cookies	110	18	1	6
vanilla	10 cookies	110	17	0	5
■ (Betty Crocker)					
mix/prepared					
bar & cookie mixes					
Sunkist lemon bar	1 bar	140	24	0	18
cookie mixes					
chocolate					
chip	2 cookies	160	21	0	14
chunk	2 cookies	150	21	1	13
double chocolate chunk	2 cookies	150	21	1	13

Food and Description	Amount	Total Calories	Total Carbs	Fiber	Sugars
peanut butter chip	2 cookies	150	7	1	12
oatmeal	2 cookies	150	22	<1	12
oatmeal chocolate chip	2 cookies	150	21	0	13
peanut butter	2 cookies	160	20	0	12
rainbow	2 cookies	110	22	0	13
sugar cookie	3 cookies	160	22	0	13
gingerbread cake/cookie mix..					
prepared	1 cookie	230	39	0	18
■ CAMEO (*See* (Nabisco) in this section)					
■ (Carr's)					
biscuits for tea					
dark chocolate	2 biscuits	130	20	1	5
milk chocolate	2 biscuits	130	14	1	10
plain	2 biscuits	140	20	1	5
Imperials					
dark chocolate	2 cookies	150	19	2	11
milk chocolate	2 cookies	140	18	1	11
milk chocolate & cream	2 cookies	130	14	1	10
ginger lemon creams	2 cookies	140	19	1	11
Hob-Nobs	2 cookies	140	19	1	7
Sweet Graham cookies	2 pieces	140	20	<1	5
■ CHIPS AHOY (*See* (Nabisco); (Pillsbury) in this section)					
■ CHIPS DELUXE (*See* (Keebler) in this section)					
■ (Dare)					
Breaktime					
chocolate chip	1 cookie	150	21	21	9
coconut	1 cookie	150	22	1	11
ginger	1 cookie	140	23	0	10
oatmeal	1 cookie	140	22	0	10
Dare					
blueberry cheesecake	1 cookie	90	11	<1	6.5
butter cream	1 cookie	85	11	0.5	3.5
café mocha	1/11 pkg	150	20	0	10
carrot cake	1 cookie	92	11	<1	6.5
chocolate chip	1 cookie	76	10	<1	6
chocolate fudge	1 cookie	100	13	1	8
cinnamon Danish	1/8 pkg	350	30	2	4
coconut cream	1 cookie	100	13	0	7
French cream	1 cookie	80	8	<1	4
Harvest of the Rain Forest	1 cookie	69	7	0	3
lemon cream	1 cookie	100	14	0	7
maple leaf cream	1 cookie	80	12	0	7
milk chocolate fudge	1 cookie	97	12	<1	5
Sun Maid					
raisin	1 cookie	52	7.5	<1	4.5
whippet					
original pure chocolate	1/8 pkg	130	21	0	8
raspberry pure chocolate	1/8 pkg	150	21	0	9
■ (Drake's)					
chocolate chip	2 cookies	140	19	1	11

Food and Description	Amount	Total Calories	Total Carbs	Fiber	Sugars
chocolate chocolate chip	2 cookies	130	20	2	11
coconut	2 cookies	140	19	1	10
coconut macaroon	1 cookie	135	19	1	10
lemon	2 cookies	130	20	0	10
oatmeal	2 cookies	130	20	2	9
■ (Entenmann's) soft-baked					
Chewy Snack Barz					
brownie chip	1 bar	170	25	1	14
original recipe..chocolate chip	1 bar	180	25	1	14
rainbow chip	1 bar	180	26	1	12
chocolate chip..pouch					
cookie bites	1.5 oz	220	29	1	17
cookie bites...original	⅛ pouch	210	28	1	16
devil's food/low-fat cookie cake	1 cookie	60	13	0	8
Happy Valentine's Day	~1 oz	130	16	0	6
holiday butter	2 cookies	130	16	0	6
oatmeal raisin bites	⅛ pouch	190	30	2	17
oatmeal raisin cookie bites..1.5-oz pkg	⅛ pkg	190	30	2	17
soft-baked chocolate chip					
chocolate chip..original	1 oz	150	20	1	12
milk chocolate chip	3 cookies	150	20	1	12
■ (Estee)					
chocolate chip..original	4 cookies	150	21	1	5
chocolate sandwich	3 cookies	160	24	1	9
coconut..original	4 cookies	140	19	<1	5
fig bar..low-fat	2 bars	100	23	3	13
fudge	4 cookies	150	19	1	5
lemon thins	4 cookies	140	19	<1	5
oatmeal raisin	4 cookies	130	19	1	6
original sandwich	3 cookies	160	24	1	10
peanut butter sandwich	3 cookies	160	22	1	7
shortbread	4 cookies	130	22	<1	5
sugar wafer					
chocolate cream	7 cookies	160	21	<1	9
double-decker lemon cream	5 cookies	170	23	0	10
triple-decker banana, chocolate &					
strawberry cream	3 cookies	140	18	0	8
vanilla cream	7 cookies	160	22	0	9
vanilla & strawberry cream	5 cookies	170	23	0	10
vanilla sandwich	3 cookies	160	25	<1	7
vanilla thins	4 cookies	140	19	<1	5
■ (Famous Amos)					
chocolate chip	4 cookies	150	20	<1	10
individual pkg..12 cookies	1 pkg	200	27	1	14
chocolate chip & pecan	4 cookies	150	19	<1	10
chocolate cream sandwich	3 cookies	150	24	<1	13
low-fat/iced/individual pkg					
gingersnaps	1 pkg	200	41	1	17
lemon snaps	1 pkg	200	42	<1	18
oatmeal chocolate chip & walnut	4 cookies	150	19	1	10

Food and Description	Amount	Total Calories	Total Carbs	Fiber	Sugars
raisin	4 cookies	140	21	<1	11
■ (Fifty/50)					
LOW-FAT/fructose-sweetened					
apple cinnamon cookie bar	1 bar	120	23	1	12
fudge brownie bar	1 bar	110	23	1	12
sandwich					
chocolate	3 cookies	160	26	<1	10
duplex	3 cookies	160	26	<1	10
vanilla	3 cookies	170	23	0	0
SUGAR-FREE/fructose-sweetened					
butter	4 cookies	160	20	<1	7
chocolate chip	4 cookies	170	17	<1	7
coconut	4 cookies	160	18	1	6
fudge brownie	4 cookies	160	19	<1	8
oatmeal/hearty	4 cookies	140	20	<1	7
peanut butter	4 cookies	160	19	<1	8
wafers					
chocolate	6 wafers	150	20	<1	0
chocolate raspberry	6 wafers	150	20	<1	0
strawberry vanilla	6 wafers	150	20	<1	0
vanilla	6 wafers	150	20	<1	0
SUGAR-FREE/sweetened w/Maltitol					
chocolate chip	4 cookies	140	22	<1	0
lemon cream	3 cookies	150	22	0	0
oatmeal	4 cookies	140	22	<1	0
shortbread	8 cookies	160	21	0	0
■ (Frookie)					
animal..circus	9 cookies	130	21	1	7
sandwich creams/50% less fat					
chocolate	3 cookies	130	24	0	12
French vanilla almond	3 cookies	130	24	0	12
lemon chiffon	3 cookies	130	24	0	12
vanilla wafers/fat-free	8 cookies	110	26	0	18
■ (Grandma's)					
home-style/big cookies					
chocolate chip	1 cookie	200	28	1	14
fudge chocolate chip	1 cookie	190	18	1	16
molasses	1 cookie	160	29	<1	18
oatmeal raisin	1 cookie	180	30	1	15
peanut butter	1 cookie	200	24	1	13
rich & chewy..chocolate chip..soft	1 pkg	270	39	1	23
sandwich cream..regular size					
peanut butter	5 cookies	210	28	1	13
vanilla	5 cookies	210	30	<1	15
■ (Health Valley)					
Café Creations					
chocolate chip	1 cookie	100	13	2	5
chocolate chocolate chip	1 cookie	100	13	2	5
raisin oatmeal	1 cookie	90	15	1	7
chocolate					

Food and Description	Amount	Total Calories	Total Carbs	Fiber	Sugars
chip oatmeal	1 cookie	100	14	1	7
chunk	1 cookie	120	15	1	8
Cookie Cremes sandwich cookies					
chocolate	2 cookies	120	19	0	11
chocolate mint	2 cookies	120	19	0	11
double chocolate	2 cookies	120	18	0	11
vanilla-flavored	2 cookies	120	19	0	10
double chocolate chunk	1 cookie	120	15	1	7
fat-free cookies					
apple spice	3 cookies	100	24	3	11
apricot delight	3 cookies	100	24	3	11
raisin oatmeal	3 cookies	100	24	3	11
fat-free healthy chips					
double chocolate	3 cookies	100	24	3	11
old-fashioned	3 cookies	100	24	3	11
original-style	3 cookies	100	24	3	11
low-fat biscotti-style					
amaretto	2 cookies	120	23	3	7
chocolate	2 cookies	120	23	3	7
oatmeal					
peanut	1 cookie	100	14	1	6
raisin	1 cookie	90	14	1	7
white chocolate chunk	1 cookie	140	16	9	10
■ **HONEY MAID** (*See* (Nabisco) in this section)					
■ **(Keebler)**					
Chips Deluxe					
Carb Sensible Cookies					
chocolate chip	1 cookie	70	9	2	2
w/pecans	1 cookie	70	8	2	0
chocolate chocolate chip					
peanut butter	1 cookie	70	9	2	1
Regular Cookies					
chocolate chip					
mini	4 cookies	150	19	0	9
original	1 cookie	80	10	<1	5
chocolate lovers	1 cookie	80	10	0	6
coconut	1 cookie	80	9	0	4
rainbow					
mini	4 cookies	150	20	0	9
regular	1 cookie	80	10	0	5
soft & chewy	1 cookie	70	10	0	5
w/peanut butter cups	1 cookie	90	10	0	5
E. L. Fudge sandwich cookies					
butter fudge sandwich	2 cookies	130	18	1	9
w/fudge cream filling	2 cookies	120	18	<1	9
Butterfinger blasted	2 cookies	180	23	<1	13
fudge w/fudge cream filling	2 cookies	129	18	<1	9
mini fudge cream filling	7 cookies	130	21	0	10
peanut butter double-stuffed	2 cookies	180	21	<1	13
Fudge Shoppe cookies					

Food and Description	Amount	Total Calories	Total Carbs	Fiber	Sugars
Deluxe Grahams	3 cookies	140	19	<1	10
Fudge Lover's Fudge Sticks	3 pieces	160	17	<1	15
Fudge Sticks	3 pieces	150	19	0	14
Fudge Stripes					
original	3 cookies	150	20	1	9
reduced-fat	3 cookies	150	20	<1	9
Grasshopper	4 cookies	150	19	<1	12
Grahams					
chocolate	8 crackers	140	23	1	9
cinnamon crisp					
low-fat	8 crackers	110	23	1	10
regular	8 crackers	130	23	1	9
honey Graham					
low-fat	9 crackers	120	25	1	9
regular	8 cookies	140	23	0	7
original	8 cookies	130	22	1	7
KEEBLER					
original cookies					
animal cookies..Ernie's	10 pieces	130	22	1	7
frosted	8 pieces	150	21	0	12
country-style oatmeal	2 cookies	130	18	<1	8
Danish wedding	4 cookies	130	19	1	11
vanilla wafers					
mini	18 cookies	140	21	<1	9
original	8 cookies	150	22	1	10
Sandies					
caramel pecan	1 cookie	80	9	0	3
chocolate chip & pecan	1 cookie	80	9	0	4
cinnamon	1 cookie	80	9	0	3
Fruit Delights					
apple cobbler	1 cookie	80	11	<1	6
strawberry cheesecake cookie	1 cookie	80	11	<1	6
original					
w/almonds	1 cookie	90	9	0	3
w/pecans	1 cookie	80	9	0	4
pecan	1 cookie	90	9	0	3
mini	4 cookies	160	17	<1	7
reduced-fat (25%) w/pecans	1 cookie	80	10	0	3
Simply Shortbread	1 cookie	80	10	0	3
Soft Batch cookies..chocolate chip	1 cookie	80	10	<1	6
Sugar Wafers					
peanut butter	4 wafers	160	18	<1	11
vanilla	3 wafers	130	19	0	13
Vienna Fingers					
fudge thins	4 cookies	160	22	<1	10
mint fudge thins	4 cookies	160	22	<1	10
original	2 cookies	150	21	0	10
reduced-fat (25%)	2 cookies	140	23	0	11
■ {Krinos} Viennese wafers					
coffee	4 wafers	170	22	1	15

Food and Description	Amount	Total Calories	Total Carbs	Fiber	Sugars
hazelnut	4 wafers	170	24	<1	16
peanut butter	4 wafers	170	23	<1	14
sesame cream	4 wafers	170	21	1	14
vanilla	4 wafers	170	24	<1	15
■ (Lance)					
Choc-O-Lunch	1.5-oz pkg	200	31	2	13
chocolate chip mini cookies..1-oz pkg	½ pkg	130	21	<1	6
Lem-O-Lunch	5 cookies	210	29	1	10
oatmeal creams	1 cookie	240	36	1	20
On a Nekot cookie					
peanut butter	6 cookies	250	29	1	13
s'mores	6 cookies	250	32	<1	16
strawberry cookies	5 cookies	210	30	<1	12
sugar wafers	4 cookies	150	18	0	14
Van-O-Lunch	6 cookies	210	31	0	13
vanilla	4 wafers	150	18	0	14
(Lil Dutch Maid))					
Almond Windmill	2 cookies	110	18	1	5
Chip Delight	4 cookies	150	22	0	9
chocolate cream	3 cookies	130	23	0	13
coconut macaroon	2 cookies	130	20	1	7
duplex cream	3 cookies	150	23	0	13
oatmeal	4 cookies	140	24	1	13
vanilla cream	3 cookies	150	23	0	1
■ (Little Debbie)					
BARS					
caramel cookie bar	1 bar	160	22	9	16
Cosmic crispy bar	1 bar	200	33	0	19
holiday crispy bar	1 bar	190	33	0	20
marshmallow crispy bars	1 bar	140	26	0	13
big packs	1 bar	190	35	1	18
nutty bar wafer bar					
big packs	1 pkg	330	32	1	22
boxed	1 pkg	290	31	1	20
individual pkg	2 oz	310	32	2	20
peanut butter crunch bar..boxed	1 pkg	280	32	1	19
COOKIES					
Apple Flips	1 pkg	150	24	<1	13
chocolate chip	1.35 oz	190	24	<1	12
cookie wreaths	1 pkg	100	12	0	7
Easter puffs	1 pkg	150	24	0	18
fig bars	1 pkg	150	31	1	20
fudge round					
boxed	1 pkg	150	23	<1	14
individual pkg	2.5 oz	310	48	1	30
German chocolate cookie ring	1 cookie	140	18	1	11
ginger	1 pkg	90	15	0	8
oatmeal raisin..individual pkg	1 cookie	170	25	<1	14
PB&J oatmeal pie	1 pkg	140	22	<1	12
peanut cluster	1 pkg	200	23	<1	16

Food and Description	Amount	Total Calories	Total Carbs	Fiber	Sugars
Pumpkin Delight	1 pkg	150	24	0	13
Star Crunch Cosmic Snack	1 pkg	290	44	<1	26
MARSHMALLOW PIES					
banana..individual pkg	1.5 oz	180	30	0	18
chocolate..boxed	1 pkg	160	28	0	15
marshmallow supremes..boxed	1 pkg	140	22	<1	15
■ (Manischewitz) macaroon	2 cookies	90	15	4	6
■ (Mother's)					
ABC					
cinnamon Grahams	12 cookies	140	20	0	8
sugar cookies	12 cookies	130	21	0	8
almond shortbread	3 cookies	190	20	<1	7
Animal Parade	9 pieces	135	20	0	9
Candy Blasters	2 cookies	120	17	<1	10
candy chip	4 cookies	150	21	<1	12
checkerboard wafer	4 wafers	150	17	0	11
choco peanut butter	2 cookies	190	25	<1	13
chocolate chip					
angel	3 cookies	190	21	<1	9
small	5 cookies	160	21	<1	10
chocolate cream	2 cookies	190	26	<1	14
chocolate marble cream	2 cookies	190	27	1	2
circus animal	6 cookies	150	21	0	13
classic assortment	2 cookies	140	17	<1	9
Cocadas Coconut	5 cookies	160	21	<1	9
coffee cream sandwich	2 cookies	180	26	1	12
Cookie Parade	4 cookies	140	19	<1	9
Dinosaur Grahams	2 cookies	140	23	0	8
double fudge sandwich	2 cookies	180	24	2	12
English tea sandwich	2 cookies	180	28	<1	13
fig bar	1 bar	80	16	<1	9
Flaky Flix					
fudge wafer	2 cookies	140	18	2	12
vanilla wafer	2 cookies	140	17	1	14
fudge circus animal	6 cookies	140	20	0	14
fudge graham	2 cookies	150	21	<1	12
gingerbread man	6 cookies	140	21	1	7
iced/old-fashioned					
chocolate	2 cookies	160	22	<1	12
lemonade	2 cookies	160	22	0	11
iced raisin	2 cookies	170	24	0	16
macaroons/old-fashioned	2 cookies	170	17	<1	9
Marias	3 cookies	170	28	<1	9
Marie Lu	3 cookies	160	27	0	9
mint square	2 cookies	150	21	<1	14
oatmeal					
butterscotch	2 cookies	120	19	1	9
chocolate chip	2 cookies	120	19	1	9
cream sandwich old-fashioned	2 cookies	190	26	1	15

Food and Description	Amount	Total Calories	Total Carbs	Fiber	Sugars
oatmeal	2 cookies	130	22	1	13
oatmeal & raisin	2 cookies	140	19	<1	8
raisin	5 cookies	150	20	2	9
peanut butter..old-fashioned	2 cookies	150	15	0	8
rainbow wafer	4 wafers	140	18	0	9
striped shortbread	3 cookies	170	22	1	8
sugar	2 cookies	140	19	1	8
sugar-free					
checkerboard wafers	6 wafers	140	18	0	0
chocolate chip	4 cookies	140	22	<1	0
chocolate cream	3 cookies	150	23	<1	0
lemon-flavored cream	3 cookies	150	23	0	0
oatmeal	4 cookies	140	22	<1	0
peanut butter	4 cookies	160	19	1	0
pecan shortbread	4 cookies	170	17	<1	0
shortbread	8 cookies	160	21	0	0
vanilla cream	3 cookies	150	23	0	0
sugared lemon-flavor..old-fashioned	2 cookies	150	19	<1	10
taffy sandwich	2 cookies	190	27	<1	16
triplet assortment	2 cookies	160	20	<1	10
vanilla..123 artificially flavored	12 cookies	130	21	0	8
vanilla cream sandwiches	2 cookies	180	26	1	12
vanilla wafer	8 cookies	140	22	0	11
■ (Mrs. Fields) (*See* FAST FOOD)					
■ (Murray)					
REGULAR COOKIES					
chocolate chip	2 cookies	150	19	0	9
coconut	2 cookies	150	19	<1	9
coconut macaroon	3 cookies	120	16	<1	6
lemon cream sandwich	3 cookies	140	22	0	11
oatmeal/old-fashioned					
iced	2 cookies	140	20	1	10
Southen kitchen	2 cookies	140	20	1	9
sugar wafers/duplex	5 cookies	140	20	0	12
windmill..Dutch	3 cookies	140	22	0	9
SUGAR-FREE COOKIES					
chocolate chip	3 cookies	150	20	<1	0
& pecan	3 cookies	160	19	<1	0
creams	3 cookies	120	19	1	0
chocolate	3 cookies	120	18	<1	0
double fudge	3 cookies	140	23	2	0
fudge-dipped					
shortbread	5 cookies	130	20	<1	0
wafers	4 cookies	140	19	<1	0
gingersnap	7 cookies	130	23	0	0
lemon					
sandwich	3 cookies	120	19	<1	0
sugar wafers	4 cookies	130	19	0	0
oatmeal	5 cookies	150	21	7	0
peanut butter	3 cookies	150	16	1	9

Food and Description	Amount	Total Calories	Total Carbs	Fiber	Sugars
shortbread	8 cookies	120	22	1	0
pecan	3 cookies	170	18	<1	0
vanilla sugar wafer	4 cookies	130	19	0	0
■ (Nabisco)					
CHIPS AHOY/Chocolate Chip Cookies					
Candy Blasts	½ oz	80	10	0	5
caramel/6-count	1 cookie	180	23	1	17
chocolate					
chewy	1.2 oz	150	22	1	13
chewy real chocolate chips	1.2 oz	170	24	1	14
chip/4 cookies	1.4 oz	200	27	1	13
chunky	1 cookie	80	10	0	5
white fudge	½ oz	80	10	0	6
Cremewiches					
chocolate					
w/chocolate cream	1 oz	150	22	1	14
w/peanut butter	1 oz	150	20	1	11
w/vanilla cream	1 oz	150	22	1	14
real chocolate chip	3 cookies	160	21	1	10
1.4-oz package	1 pkg	200	27	1	13
reduced-fat	1 cookie	140	22	1	9
HONEY MAID GRAHAMS					
chocolate	1 oz	130	24	1	9
sticks	1 oz	130	24	1	9
cinnamon	8 cookies	130	25	1	11
low-fat	8 cookies	120	26	1	12
sticks	1 oz	120	23	1	8
Go-Pak	1 oz	130	25	1	9
honey/original	1 oz	140	24	1	8
low-fat	8 cookies	120	26	1	8
sticks	1 oz	130	23	1	8
oatmeal crunch	1 oz	130	24	1	8
NABISCO FAMILY FAVORITES					
Barnum's Animals					
box/2.125 oz	½ box	130	23	1	7
Snak Saks/bag	1 oz	130	23	1	7
Biscos sugar wafer	8 cookies	140	21	0	13
Cameo creme sandwich	2 cookies	130	21	0	10
Famous wafers..chocolate	~1 oz	140	24	1	11
gingersnap..old-fashioned	4 cookies	120	22	0	9
grahams..original	8 cookies	130	24	1	7
Imperio/combination..Combinato	1.25 oz	170	25	1	11
Lorna Doone shortbread	4 cookies	140	19	1	6
Mallomars..pure chocolate	2 cookies	120	17	1	12
marshmallow fudge twirls	1 piece	130	20	0	14
Morelianas..orange Naranja	1 oz	130	19	0	9
National Arrowroot Biscuit	1 cookie	20	4	0	1
oatmeal..iced	1 cookie	80	12	0	6
Pecanz..pecan shortbread	½ oz	90	9	0	3
Social Tea biscuits	6 cookies	120	20	1	7

Food and Description	Amount	Total Calories	Total Carbs	Fiber	Sugars
zwieback	1 piece	35	6	0	1
NEWTONS					
cobblers					
apple	2 cookies	90	22	1	12
caramel apple	2 cookies	130	26	0	13
cinnamon	2 cookies	90	22	1	12
Cherries 'n' Cheescake snackable fig	1.3 oz	120	25	0	15
2-count	2 oz	200	39	3	22
fat-free..2-GO!..12-pack	2 cookies	90	22	1	12
regular	2 cookies	110	22	1	14
peach apricot	2 cookies	70	17	0	10
raspberry	2 cookies	90	22	1	12
& yogurt	2 cookies	130	26	1	13
strawberry	2 cookies	90	21	0	10
& yogurt	2 cookies	130	26	1	14
kiwi	1 oz	100	29	9	11
Snackable Dessert shortcake	1.3 oz	130	25	1	14
NILLA VANILLA WAFER					
chocolate reduced-fat	1 oz	110	23	1	12
original	1 oz	140	21	0	11
reduced-fat	1 oz	120	24	0	12
NUTTER BUTTER					
4-count pack	1 pkg	260	37	1	16
Bites/1.25-oz package	1 pkg	170	23	1	11
Bites/Snak Saks	1 oz	140	20	1	9
peanut butter cream patty	5 cookies	170	18	1	8
peanut butter sandwich	2 cookies	130	18	1	8
OREO					
chocolate	1.32 oz	160	24	1	13
cream/4-count	1.12 oz	150	21	1	13
football	1.2 oz	160	24	1	13
fudge-covered	~1 oz	90	13	1	9
fudge mint-covered	1 oz	90	12	1	8
reduced-fat	1.2 oz	140	26	1	14
Cookie Barz					
8-count	1 bar	150	18	1	13
individual	1.23 oz	180	23	1	15
Double Delight Chocolate					
Coffee 'n' cream	1 oz	150	21	1	13
mint 'n' cream	1 oz	140	20	1	13
Double-Stuff Chocolate	1 oz	140	20	1	13
1.5-oz package	1 pkg	210	29	1	20
mini					
chocolate	1.25 oz	170	25	1	14
12-count	1 pkg	200	13	1	9
bite-size/3-oz pkg	⅓ pkg	140	21	1	11
cream	1.25 oz	170	25	1	13
Go-Pak Cup/bite-size	¼ cup	140	21	1	11
Go-Pak/chocolate	1 pkg	210	29	1	20
Oreo & mini Chips Ahoy..20-pack	1 pkg	170	25	1	14

Food and Description	Amount	Total Calories	Total Carbs	Fiber	Sugars
red & white cream	1 oz	140	21	1	11
Snak Saks..chocolate	1 pkg	140	21	1	11
Uh-Oh w/chocolate cream	1.2 oz	170	25	1	12
white fudge–covered	¾ oz	110	14	0	10
Winter 4 Fun shapes..w/red cream	1 oz	140	29	1	13
SNACKWELL's					
BITE-SIZE					
chocolate chip	~1 oz	130	22	1	10
double chocolate chip	~1 oz	130	22	1	10
peanut butter chip	~1 oz	120	20	1	9
CARBWELL					
fudge brownie cookie	1 serving	90	17	0	0
fudge-striped shortbread	1 serving	150	24	1	0
FAT-FREE..DEVIL'S FOOD COFFEE CAKE	1 cookie	50	12	0	7
ORIGINAL					
coconut creme	2 cookies	110	19	1	13
golden devil's food	1 cookie	50	11	0	7
mint creme	2 cookies	110	19	1	13
peanut butter..bite-size	13 cookies	120	29	1	8
SUGAR-FREE					
chocolate chip	1 oz	150	23	1	0
chocolate sandwich	1 oz	130	23	1	0
cream sandwich	1 oz	130	23	1	0
fudge-covered grahams	1 serving	150	24	1	0
fudge-striped shortbread	~1 oz	110	16	1	0
lemon creme sandwich	1 oz	130	24	0	0
oatmeal	~1 oz	90	17	1	0
shortbread	1 oz	130	22	1	0
TEDDY GRAHAMS					
Graham Snacks					
Bob the Builder	1 oz	120	21	1	8
cinnamon	1 oz	120	24	1	7
chocolate	1 oz	130	22	1	8
honey & cinnamon sticks.. 20-count	1.25 oz	150	26	1	10
cinnamon	1 oz	130	23	1	8
1.25-oz pkg	1 pkg	160	27	1	9
Clifford the Big Red Dog	1 oz	130	23	1	7
honey	1 oz	130	23	1	8
1.25-oz package	1 pkg	150	26	1	0
Dora the Explorer	1 oz	130	22	1	7
honey/chocolate	1.25 oz	150	26	1	9
mini chocolatey chip Snak Saks	1 oz	140	22	1	8
■ **(Nestlé) Toll House**					
REFRIGERATED/READY-TO-BAKE					
Break & Bake					
chocolate chip	1 cookie	110	16	1	9
& caramel	1 cookie	100	15	1	10
& fudge	1 cookie	110	15	1	9
& peanut butter	1 cookie	100	13	<1	7

Food and Description	Amount	Total Calories	Total Carbs	Fiber	Sugars
walnut chocolate	1 cookie	110	14	0	8
chocolate chunk	1 cookie	110	15	1	9
sugar	1 cookie	110	15	<1	8
rolled cookies					
chocolate chip..original	1 cookie	140	20	0	13
Ultimates					
chip & chunks	1 cookie	200	23	1	14
chocolate almond fudge	1 cookie	190	24	1	16
chocolate chip lovers	1 cookie	200	25	1	16
macadamia white fudge	1 cookie	200	23	<1	16
turtles	1 cookie	190	24	1	16
■ **(Nonni's)**					
biscotti					
chocolate	1 piece	130	19	1	11
Decadence	1 piece	130	19	1	11
original	1 piece	100	15	1	8
Paradise	1 piece	130	19	1	11
Cio	1 piece	130	19	1	11
Noci Cio	1 piece	150	21	1	12
■ **OREO** (*See* (Nabisco) in this section)					
■ **(Otis Spunkmeyer)**					
(NOTE: frozen cookie dough = baked cookies)					
Supreme Indulgence Super Premium/2-oz size					
chocolate chunk	1 cookie	250	35	1	21
oatmeal raisin	1 cookie	230	35	2	21
peanut butter chocolate chip	1 cookie	260	32	1	19
white chunk macadamia nut	1 cookie	270	31	<1	20
Sweet Discovery/1.3-oz medium size					
butter sugar	1 cookie	160	23	<1	14
buttercrunch toffee	1 cookie	170	23	0	15
Café Vienna	1 cookie	170	23	0	14
Carnival	1 cookie	160	23	<1	14
chocolate w/Reese's Pieces	1 cookie	170	23	<1	14
chocolate chip					
double	1 cookie	180	23	<1	17
milk chocolate chunk	1 cookie	170	22	<1	13
regular	1 cookie	170	24	0	16
w/pecans	1 cookie	170	22	<1	14
w/walnuts	1 cookie	180	22	<1	14
oatmeal					
cranberry	1 cookie	150	24	2	15
raisin	1 cookie	160	23	1	13
peanut butter	1 cookie	180	20	1	11
chocolate chunk	1 cookie	180	23	<1	16
Sweet Discovery/4-oz./old-fashioned size					
butter sugar	½ cookie	250	35	1	21
buttercrunch toffee	½ cookie	250	35	<1	22
Carnival	½ cookie	250	36	1	22
chocolate chip					
double chocolate	½ cookie	270	35	1	26

Food and Description	Amount	Total Calories	Total Carbs	Fiber	Sugars
regular	½ cookie	250	36	<1	21
oatmeal raisin	½ cookie	230	34	2	19
peanut butter					
chocolate chunk	½ cookie	240	35	1	23
regular	½ cookie	270	31	2	17
turtle	½ cookie	250	33	1	21
white chocolate macadamia nut	½ cookie	280	33	<1	21
Sweet Discovery/3-oz cookies					
chocolate chip	1 cookie	370	53	2	32
oatmeal raisin	1 cookie	350	51	3	29
peanut butter	1 cookie	390	45	2	25
white chocolate macadamia nut	1 cookie	390	50	1	32
Traditional Recipe/1.5-oz cookies					
Carnival	1 cookie	180	27	<1	16
chocolate chip					
double chocolate	1 cookie	180	26	1	17
regular	1 cookie	180	27	<1	16
oatmeal raisin	1 cookie	180	26	1	14
peanut butter	1 cookie	190	22	<1	12
Ranger	1 cookie	190	24	1	12
sugar	1 cookie	180	26	0	14
white chocolate macadamia nut	1 cookie	190	26	<1	15
Traditional Recipe/2.5-oz cookies					
Carnival	1 cookie	310	44	1	27
chocolate chip	1 cookie	310	45	1	27
double chocolate	1 cookie	310	43	2	28
oatmeal raisin	1 cookie	300	43	2	24
peanut butter	1 cookie	320	37	1	21
Ranger	1 cookie	310	41	2	19
sugar	1 cookie	310	44	<1	23
Otis Spunkmeyer Express/2-oz cookies					
chocolate chunk	1 cookie	250	36	1	21
double chocolate chip	1 cookie	250	34	2	21
oatmeal raisin	1 cookie	240	37	2	22
peanut butter	1 cookie	270	29	2	16
white chunk macadamia nut	1 cookie	270	35	<1	22
■ (Pamela's)					
BISCOTTI					
almond anise	2 pieces	170	26	1	8
chocolate walnut	2 pieces	170	25	1	8
lemon almond	2 pieces	170	26	1	8
CARB-CONSCIOUS					
chocolate chip walnut	1 cookie	60	9	<2	1
coconut	1 cookie	60	7	<1	0
peanut butter	1 cookie	50	8	<2	0
ORGANIC COOKIES					
chocolate chunk pecan shortbread	2 cookies	190	22	1	6
dark chocolate chocolate chunk	2 cookies	160	22	1	12
espresso chocolate chunk oatmeal	2 cookies	160	22	1	12

Food and Description	Amount	Total Calories	Total Carbs	Fiber	Sugars
chocolate chunk	2 cookies	170	21	1	11
raisin walnut	2 cookies	100	12	<1	6
spicy ginger	2 cookies	160	24	1	14
TRADITIONAL COOKIES/wheat- and gluten-free					
butter shortbread	1 cookie	120	15	<1	3
carob hazelnut	1 cookie	120	15	0	5
chocolate chip					
chunky	1 cookie	120	16	<1	8
walnut	1 cookie	130	14	<1	6
ginger w/sliced almonds	1 cookie	110	14	<1	4
peanut butter	1 cookie	90	10	<1	7
shortbread					
lemon	1 cookie	120	15	0	5
pecan	1 cookie	130	15	<1	4
swirl	1 cookie	120	16	<1	5
■ (Peak Freans)					
arrowroot	4 biscuits	150	26	1	7
coffee cream	2 biscuits	140	19	0	9
cream/assorted	1 oz	140	19	0	9
fruit cream	2 biscuits	130	20	0	10
ginger crisp	~1 oz	4.5	27	1	12
Nice biscuits	4 biscuits	160	25	1	9
petit beurre	1 oz	130	22	1	5
shortcake	3 cookies	140	18	0	5
■ (Pepperidge Farm)					
CHOCOLATE CHUNK/CRISPY COOKIES					
Chesapeake/dark chocolate pecan	1 cookie	140	15	0	7
Nantucket/dark chocolate chunk	1 cookie	140	16	0	9
Sanibel/milk chocolate almond	1 cookie	140	16	1	7
Sausalito/milk chocolate macadamia	1 cookie	140	16	0	9
Sedona/dark chocolate toffee pecan	1 cookie	130	17	1	10
Tahoe/white chocolate macadamia	1 cookie	130	17	1	6
DISTINCTIVE COOKIES					
Bordeaux..original	4 cookies	130	19	1	12
Brussels..mint	3 cookies	190	22	1	13
Chantilly..raspberry	3 cookies	120	23	1	11
Chessmen					
butter pecan	3 cookies	130	18	1	6
butterscotch	3 cookies	120	18	0	7
Geneva	3 cookies	160	18	1	8
Lido	1 cookie	90	10	0	5
Salzburg	2 cookies	150	21	5	9
Verona					
apricot raspberry	3 cookies	140	22	1	10
strawberry	3 cookies	140	22	1	10
MILANO COOKIES					
French vanilla	2 cookies	130	16	<1	8
mint	3 cookies	170	21	<1	13
orange	2 cookies	130	16	<1	8

Food and Description	Amount	Total Calories	Total Carbs	Fiber	Sugars
raspberry	2 cookies	130	16	<1	8
regular	2 cookies	180	21	<1	11
Mini Cookies					
Brussels	8 cookies	150	18	1	11
Chessmen	9 cookies	140	21	1	6
chocolate chunk	4 cookies	160	17	9	19
Milano	6 cookies	160	18	<1	9
mint	6 cookies	120	20	1	11
Nantucket	4 cookies	150	20	0	10
OLD-FASHIONED HOME-STYLE COOKIES					
ginger man	4 cookies	130	21	1	11
lemon nut	3 cookies	170	18	2	7
sugar	3 cookies	140	20	<1	10
PIROUETTE					
chocolate hazelnut	2 cookies	130	19	<1	11
chocolate mint	2 cookies	130	20	0	14
French vanilla	2 cookies	140	18	0	10
SOFT-BAKED COOKIES					
Augusta	1 cookie	130	15	1	9
Laredo..oatmeal dark chocolate	1 cookie	140	21	1	12
milk chocolate caramel..chewy	1 cookie	140	21	1	13
Nantucket/dark chocolate chunk	1 cookie	140	16	0	9
Santa Cruz/oatmeal raisin	1 cookie	140	21	1	11
Sausalito/milk chocolate macadamia	1 cookie	140	16	0	9
■ (Pillsbury)					
READY-TO-BAKE/REFRIGERATED COOKIE DOUGH					
chocolate chip	1 cookie	120	15	<1	9
w/walnuts	1 cookie	120	14	<1	8
sugar	1 cookie	120	15	0	8
REFRIGERATED COOKIE DOUGH					
chocolate chip					
double & chunk	1 cookie	140	17	1	10
home-baked classics	1 cookie	160	20	<1	12
reduced-fat	1 cookie	110	19	<1	12
roll	1 cookie	140	17	<1	10
tub	1 cookie	140	17	<1	10
w/walnuts	1 cookie	130	16	<1	9
chocolate chunk	1 cookie	140	17	<1	10
M&M's	2 cookies	150	18	<1	11
holiday	1 cookie	150	18	<1	11
oatmeal chocolate chip	1 cookie	120	16	<1	10
peanut butter	1 cookie	130	16	<1	9
shaped					
Christmas tree	2 cookies	160	19	0	9
ghost	2 cookies	160	18	1	10
gingerbread	2 cookies	140	18	0	9
Linus/Great Pumpkin	2 cookies	160	19	0	9
Peter Cottontail	2 cookies	160	19	0	9
Rudolph	2 cookies	160	19	0	10

Food and Description	Amount	Total Calories	Total Carbs	Fiber	Sugars
Shamrock	2 cookies	160	19	0	9
Snoopy valentine	2 cookies	160	19	0	9
sugar	2 cookies	130	18	9	19
holiday	2 cookies	130	17	9	19
white chocolate chunk	2 cookies	130	17	6	11
■ SNACKWELL'S (*See* (Nabisco) in this section)					
■ (Spaans Cookie Co.)					
LOW-FAT COOKIES					
banana	2 cookies	100	19	1	10
chocolate chip	2 cookies	110	20	1	12
fudge 'n' chips	2 cookies	100	20	1	12
oat bran 'n' chips	2 cookies	100	19	1	10
REGULAR COOKIES					
butter melt	2 cookies	130	17	0	8
chocolate chip	2 cookies	120	17	1	10
cinnamon bears	1 cookie	100	14	0	6
cocoa bears	1 cookie	100	14	0	6
coconut krispies	2 cookies	120	18	1	11
date oatmeal	2 cookies	120	19	1	10
fruit 'n' honey	2 cookies	110	18	1	9
fudge brownie	2 cookies	120	18	0	10
fudge 'n' chips..w/walnuts	2 cookies	120	17	0	10
harvest	2 cookies	130	18	0	9
holiday	2 cookies	130	18	0	9
oat bran 'n' raisin	1 cookie	110	18	1	9
peanut butter	2 cookies	130	15	1	7
shortbread	2 cookies	120	18	0	8
soft oatmeal	2 cookies	110	18	1	9
speculaas/windmills	2 cookies	130	18	1	7
sugar bear	1 cookie	100	14	0	6
toasted almond	2 cookies	130	16	0	6
SUGAR-FREE COOKIES					
cherry crisps	3 cookies	110	16	0	0
chocolate chip swirls	3 cookies	110	17	1	0
crunchy vanilla	3 cookies	120	17	0	0
Dutch chocolate	3 cookies	110	16	0	0
lemon coconut	3 cookies	120	16	1	0
peanut butter	3 cookies	120	16	0	0
spiced windmill	3 cookies	110	16	1	0
■ (Stella D'Oro)					
Biscotti					
almond	~½ oz	100	13	1	5
chocolate almond	~½ oz	90	13	1	7
chocolate chunk	~½ oz	90	14	0	8
French vanilla	~½ oz	90	15	0	7
Breakfast Treats					
chocolate	¾ oz	90	15	1	8
original	¾ oz	90	15	0	6
mini	1 oz	120	21	9	9

Food and Description	Amount	Total Calories	Total Carbs	Fiber	Sugars
Viennese cinnamon	¾ oz	90	16	0	8
Coffee Treats/toast					
almond	1 oz	110	19	1	9
angel wings	~1 oz	170	14	0	1
anisette	1 oz	130	27	0	13
mini	1 oz	130	27	0	13
sponge..low-fat	~1 oz	90	19	1	9
sponge..original	~1 oz	90	18	0	9
banana walnut	~1 oz	100	19	0	9
blueberry	~1 oz	100	20	0	10
cinnamon raisin	~1 oz	100	20	0	10
Roman egg biscuits	1 oz	130	21	0	8
Cookies					
almond					
delight	1 oz	160	17	1	6
toast	1 oz	110	21	1	19
anginetti	1 oz	130	22	0	17
egg jumbo	~1 oz	120	26	0	13
Lady Stella assortment	1 oz	130	29	1	9
Margherite					
combination	1 oz	130	20	1	8
original	1 oz	130	29	9	8
Swiss fudge	~1 oz	170	15	0	7
■ **TOLL HOUSE** (*See* (Nestlé) in this section)					
■ **(Tree of Life)**					
Creme Supremes					
mint	2 cookies	120	18	1	10
original	2 cookies	120	18	1	10
fruit bars					
apple spice	2 cookies	120	22	2	9
fig	2 cookies	120	21	3	10
peach apricot	2 cookies	120	22	2	11
honey-sweet					
Colossal Carrot Cake	1 cookie	110	16	1	5
Lemon Burst	1 cookie	110	15	1	5
Oh-So-Oatmeal	1 cookie	110	14	1	4
Pecans-a-Plenty	1 cookie	125	14	1	4
Monster Fat-Free					
gingerbread	¼ cookie	80	19	2	0
maple pecan	¼ cookie	90	20	2	10
Royal Vanilla	2 cookies	120	17	0	10
Small World					
animal grahams	7 pieces	120	21	3	8
chocolate chip	7 cookies	120	20	3	6
soft-baked					
chocolate chip	1 cookie	125	15	1	5
double fudge	1 cookie	110	16	2	5
Maui macaroon	1 cookie	135	12	2	4
oatmeal	1 cookie	115	16	2	5

Food and Description	Amount	Total Calories	Total Carbs	Fiber	Sugars
peanut butter	1 cookie	125	13	1	4
wheat-free					
American oatmeal	1 cookie	90	11	1	3
California carob	1 cookie	105	14	6	4
Georgia peanut butter	1 cookie	95	8	1	3
Mountain maple walnut	1 cookie	100	9	6	4
■ (Umeya)					
fortune cookies	4 cookies	110	25	<1	13
■ (Voortman)					
almonette	1 cookie	100	12	0	4
chocolate chip	1 cookie	100	14	0	7
chocolate chip..sugar-free	1 cookie	100	13	0	<1
chocolate wafer..sugar-free	3 cookies	160	18	0	<1
chunky chocolate chip	1 cookie	230	32	<1	17
Coconut Delight	1 cookie	90	10	0	6
Dutch creme	1 cookie	110	16	0	9
fudge-striped oatmeal	1 cookie	130	18	<1	10
fudge swirl	1 cookie	90	12	0	6
Gingerboy	1 cookie	90	14	0	6
jumbo chocolate chip	1 cookie	230	32	<1	17
jumbo oatmeal raisin	1 cookie	270	41	1	19
jumbo peanut delight	1 cookie	240	34	1	12
maple creme sandwich	1 cookie	110	15	0	8
oatmeal apple	1 cookie	270	41	1	19
Peanut Delight	1 cookie	120	14	<1	6
shortbread					
regular	1 cookie	110	13	0	4
swirl	1 cookie	110	13	0	4
sugar	1 cookie	90	13	0	6
vanilla wafers	3 cookies	170	21	0	13
windmill	1 cookie	90	12	0	6
(World Classics)					
chocolate chunk	1 cookie	120	16	1	9
espresso chocolate chunk	1 cookie	120	16	1	9
oatmeal raisin	1 cookie	120	18	1	9
COOKIE CRUMBS (See also CRACKER CRUMBS & MEAL)					
(Nabisco)					
Oreo					
cookie crumbs	2 Tbs	90	13	1	7
crunchies	~½ oz	50	8	0	4
COOKING SPRAY					
(Crisco)					
natural blend oil	⅓-sec spray	120	0	0	0
natural butter..no-stick	⅓-sec spray	0	0	0	0
original w/canola oil	⅓-sec spray	120	0	0	0
pure all-natural oil..100% extra-virgin	⅓-sec spray	120	0	0	0
(Mazola) all types	2-sec spray	0	0	0	0
(Pam) all flavors & types	⅓-sec spray	0	0	0	0
(Weight Watchers) all types	1-sec spray	0	0	0	0
CORIANDER LEAF (See CILANTRO)					

Food and Description	Amount	Total Calories	Total Carbs	Fiber	Sugars
CORIANDER SEED					
whole	1 tsp	5	1	0	0
	1 Tbs	15	3	2	0
CORN					
CANNED/JARRED					
(Blue Boy)					
cream-style..sweet	½ cup	90	20	2	6
whole kernel..sweet	½ cup	70	12	2	5
(Del Monte)					
corn 'n' butter	½ cup	90	14	<1	5
cream-style..golden					
regular	½ cup	90	18	3	6
supersweet	½ cup	60	14	2	7
Santa Fe..in hearty sauce	½ cup	70	16	1	1
sweet/summer crisp	½ cup	70	13	3	4
white	½ cup	60	11	3	7
whole kernel					
fiesta	½ cup	50	12	2	5
gold & white	½ cup	80	18	2	6
golden					
regular	½ cup	90	18	3	6
supersweet..no sugar added	½ cup	60	11	3	7
(Fancifood) baby corn	6 pieces	25	3	2	3
(Green Giant)					
Mexicorn	⅓ cup	60	14	1	4
Niblets					
white shoepeg	⅓ cup	80	16	1	3
yellow					
extra sweet					
plain	½ cup	80	16	<1	5
regular	⅓ cup	50	10	2	4
no salt or sugar added	⅓ cup	60	13	2	3
super sweet..yellow & white	⅓ cup	50	11	1	3
whole kernel/sweet	½ cup	80	17	2	4
(KA-ME) baby cocktail corn	½ cup	20	3	2	3
(Libby's)					
sweet cream-style	½ cup	90	20	2	6
vacuum-packed	⅓ cup	70	12	2	5
whole kernel	½ cup	90	18	2	7
(S&W)					
cream-style..traditional					
home-style	½ cup	60	14	2	7
w/starch	½ cup	100	24	1	6
whole kernel					
sweet 'n' crisp	⅓ cup	70	12	2	6
young/sweet/tender	½ cup	90	14	2	5
FROZEN					
(Birds Eye)					
corn on the cob					
big ears	1 ear	140	34	2	3

Food and Description	Amount	Total Calories	Total Carbs	Fiber	Sugars
corn blend..gold & white	½ cup	60	11	2	2
little ears	1 ear	80	18	1	4
sweet/corn on the cob	2 ears	110	26	3	5
kernels					
baby gold & white	½ cup	80	15	2	6
baby white	⅔ cup	60	11	2	4
baby whole	½ cup	100	20	3	2
cut kernels	⅓ cup	70	17	3	5
sweet, young & tender	½ cup	80	19	1	5
(C&W) all styles	⅔ cup	80	19	1	5
(Cascadian Farm) corn on the cob	2 cobs	120	28	3	3
(Green Giant)					
corn on the cob					
extra sweet	1 ear	120	22	3	13
Nibblers/6-ear pkg	1 ear	70	14	1	2
Niblets/4-ear pkg	1 ear	150	32	3	6
cream-style					
boil-in-bag	½ cup	110	23	2	6
sweet	½ cup	90	19	1	7
kernels..niblets					
boil-in-bag					
corn & butter	⅔ cup	110	22	2	5
extra sweet	⅔ cup	70	13	2	6
no sauce	⅔ cup	80	17	3	3
shoepeg white/boil-in-bag					
no sauce	½ cup	70	14	2	3
white corn & butter	¾ cup	110	21	3	3
(McKenzie's) Southern					
white corn Silver Queen–style	½ cup	80	19	1	5
white creamed Silver Queen–style	½ cup	100	24	3	6
(Ore-Ida) corn on the cob..mini	1 ear	80	16	2	2

CORN BREAD (*See* BREAD)
CORN CAKE (*See* RICE CAKES)
CORN CHIPS (*See* TORTILLA CHIPS)
CORN CHOWDER (*See* SOUP)
CORN DISH (*See also* FROZEN ENTRÉE/DINNER; VEGETABLES, MIXED)
CANNED or JARRED

(Aunt Nellie's) corn relish	1 Tbs	20	5	0	2
(Del Monte) Savory Sensations					
Santa Fe corn in hearty sauce	½ cup	70	16	1	1
(Green Giant) corn relish	1 Tbs	20	5	0	2

FROZEN

(Mrs. Paul's) corn fritter	1 fritter	130	15	1	4

CORN DOG (*See also* FRANKFURTER)

(State Fair) w/Ball Park					
cheese corn dog	3.25 oz	250	12	0	7
beef..jumbo	4 oz	300	36	10	9
cheeseburger flavor stickwich	4 oz	270	20	<1	3
chicken..jumbo	4 oz	260	31	0	9
classic					

Food and Description	Amount	Total Calories	Total Carbs	Fiber	Sugars
all meat	2.67 oz	210	25	2	6
jumbo	4 oz	340	40	2	19
large	3.2 oz	270	32	1	15
fiesta jalapeño cheese	3.2 oz	230	21	2	4
meat	2.7 oz	220	26	3	7
turkey					
classic	2.67 oz	190	26	1	7
jumbo	4 oz	280	32	2	8
large	3.2 oz	220	26	1	6
light	4 oz	210	28	3	10
mini	4 oz	310	31	2	6
CORN GRITS (*See also* CEREAL)					
(Albers) quick hominy..white or					
yellow..dry	¼ cup	140	31	1	0
(Arrowhead Mills) dry					
white	¼ cup	150	33	1	0
yellow	¼ cup	130	30	1	0
(Aunt Jemima)					
quick..dry	1 pkt	130	29	2	0
regular/old-fashioned	1 pkt	140	32	2	0
(Jim Dandy) enriched..dry					
quick or regular	1.6 oz	160	35	1	0
(Quaker)					
instant/dry					
American cheese	1 pkt	100	21	1	0
country bacon	1 pkt	100	21	1	0
4-cheese cheddar blend	1 pkt	100	21	1	0
ham 'n' cheese	1 pkt	100	20	1	0
original	1 pkt	100	21	1	0
real					
butter flavor	1 pkt	100	21	1	0
cheddar cheese	1 pkt	100	20	1	0
red eye & country gravy	1 pkt	100	21	1	0
quick/dry					
golden grits	¼ cup	120	29	2	0
regular	¼ cup	130	29	2	0
regular-old-fashioned/white hominy	¼ cup	140	32	2	0
(Spice Hunter) microwaveable cups					
butter & cheddar	1 cup	180	34	0	2
ham & cheddar	1 cup	180	34	0	1
CORN NUT (*See* SNACKS)					
CORN PONE (*See* BREAD)					
CORN PUDDING (*See* PUDDING & MOUSSE)					
CORN SYRUP (*See* PANCAKE & WAFFLE SYRUP)					
CORNED BEEF (*See* BEEF; LUNCHEON MEAT)					
CORNED BEEF HASH (*See* BEEF DISH/ENTRÉE)					
CORNFLAKE CRUMBS (Kellogg's)	2 Tbs	40	9	0	1
CORNISH GAME HEN (*See* CHICKEN)					
CORNMEAL/dry					
(Arrowhead Mills)					

Food and Description	Amount	Total Calories	Total Carbs	Fiber	Sugars
blue	¼ cup	130	25	3	0
yellow	¼ cup	120	27	3	0
(Aunt Jemima) self-rising					
white..enriched..bolted	3 Tbs	90	24	1	0
yellow..degermed	3 Tbs	90	24	2	0
(Martha White) enriched..yellow	3 Tbs	120	25	2	1
(Quaker) dry					
masa harina	¼ cup	110	24	3	0
preparada para tortillas	⅓ cup	160	27	1	1
white..enriched	3 Tbs	90	21	1	0
yellow..enriched	3 Tbs	90	21	1	0
CORNMEAL MIX (*See also* BAKE & FRY MIX; CORNMEAL)					
(Aunt Jemima) self-rising					
buttermilk white	3 Tbs	80	24	1	1
white/bolted	3 Tbs	80	24	1	1
yellow	3 Tbs	140	24	1	1
(Martha White) dry..self-rising..enriched					
white	3 Tbs	110	22	2	0
yellow	3 Tbs	110	23	2	1
(Miracle Maize) mix only					
country-style	3 Tbs	130	29	1	10
sweet	3 Tbs	100	22	1	2
CORNSTARCH					
(Argo)	1 Tbs	30	7	0	0
(Cream) 100% pure	1 Tbs	30	7	0	0
(Maizena)					
caramel flavor	1 Tbs	35	9	0	0
regular flavor	1 Tbs	30	7	0	0
vanilla flavor	1 Tbs	35	8	0	0
COTTAGE CHEESE (*See also* CHEESE)					
(Borden) creamed					
2% fat	½ cup	90	4	0	4
4% fat	½ cup	120	4	0	4
dry curd/5% fat	½ cup	80	3	0	3
(Breakstone)..creamed					
2% fat..large or small curd	½ cup	90	4	0	3
4% fat..large or small curd	½ cup	120	5	0	4
fat-free	½ cup	120	7	0	3
(Crowley) creamed					
1% fat					
calcium-fortified	½ cup	90	3	0	2
plain	½ cup	90	3	0	2
w/pineapple	½ cup	110	15	0	14
4% fat					
plain	½ cup	120	4	0	4
w/peaches	½ cup	140	17	0	15
w/pineapple	½ cup	140	15	0	14
(Hood)					
1% low-fat					
black pepper & herbs	½ cup	80	6	0	4

Food and Description	Amount	Total Calories	Total Carbs	Fiber	Sugars
chive & toasted onion	½ cup	80	6	0	4
no salt added	½ cup	80	6	0	5
pineapple cherry	½ cup	110	16	0	12
plain	½ cup	80	6	0	4
w/peaches	½ cup	110	18	0	13
w/strawberries	½ cup	120	19	0	15
4% fat					
chive					
country-style	½ cup	110	5	0	4
large curd	½ cup	110	5	0	4
pineapple	½ cup	130	15	0	12
fat-free					
pineapple	½ cup	100	16	0	12
plain	½ cup	80	7	0	4
(Knudsen) creamed					
1.5% fat "On the Go"					
peach	½ cup	110	13	0	12
pineapple	½ cup	120	14	0	12
strawberry	½ cup	110	13	0	12
tropical fruit	½ cup	110	13	0	11
2% low-fat					
single-serve/4-count	1 cup	90	3	0	3
small curd	½ cup	100	5	0	4
4% fat					
large curd	½ cup	130	4	0	3
small curd	½ cup	120	4	0	3
nonfat/free..regular	½ cup	80	4	0	3
(Light 'n' Lively) creamed					
1% fat..plain	½ cup	80	5	0	4
nonfat	½ cup	80	7	0	5
(Nordica)					
low-fat	½ cup	80	5	0	5
small curd/4% milk	½ cup	100	4	0	4
(Weight Watchers) creamed					
1% fat	½ cup	90	4	0	4
2% fat	½ cup	100	4	0	4
COUSCOUS (*See also* PASTA; SOUP/DEHYDRATED)					
(Casbah) mix only					
almond chicken vegetarian	1 pkg	160	29	<1	3
asparagus au gratin..organic	1 pkg	150	28	1	3
cheddar broccoli	1 pkg	130	23	<1	3
Hearty Harvest	1 pkg	180	36	2	3
(Marrakesh Express) dry mix					
mango salsa	2 oz	190	38	1	8
Parmesan cheese	2 oz	200	42	1	2
plain	2 scoops	220	45	1	2
roasted chicken..w/vegetables	2 oz	190	39	2	3
sun-dried tomato & herb	2 oz	190	39	2	3
wild mushroom	2 oz	190	39	1	4
(Near East) mix..prepared					

Food and Description	Amount	Total Calories	Total Carbs	Fiber	Sugars
broccoli	1 cup	210	42	3	3
herbed chicken	1 cup	220	42	3	2
Mediterranean curry	1 cup	220	42	3	3
original/plain	1 cup	230	46	2	1
Parmesan	1 cup	220	41	2	3
roasted garlic & olive oil	1 cup	230	41	2	1
toasted pine nut	1 cup	230	40	2	2
tomato lentil	1 cup	220	42	3	3
wild mushroom herb	1 cup	230	42	3	2
COWPEA (*See* BLACK-EYED PEA)					
CRAB (*See also* CRAB, IMITATION; CRAB DISH; SEAFOOD ENTRÉE/DINNER)					
CANNED/meat only					
(3 Diamonds)					
fancy w/leg meat	3 oz	40	2	0	0
fancy white	3 oz	45	0	0	0
lump	2 oz	45	1	0	0
(Bumble Bee) Orleans					
fancy lump crabmeat..all styles	2 oz	40	0	0	0
(Chicken of the Sea) drained					
crabmeat	2 oz	40	2	0	1
fancy	2 oz	40	2	0	0
jumbo lump	2 oz	35	1	0	1
pink or white	2 oz	30	1	0	1
(Geisha)					
lump	2 oz	45	1	0	0
snow	2 oz	35	1	0	0
white	2 oz	50	1	0	1
(Phillips) backfin..pasteurized.. hand-picked	2 oz	45	0	0	0
(S&W) Dungeness	⅓ cup	80	0	0	0
FRESH/REFRIGERATED MEAT ONLY					
brand-specific					
(Phillips) tub..pasteurized backfin or claw	2 oz	45	0	0	0
nonbrand					
Alaska..Alaskan King					
cooked—moist heat..leg	3 oz	82	0	0	0
	1 medium	129	0	0	0
blue..cooked—moist heat	3 oz	90	0	0	0
Dungeness..cooked—moist heat	3 oz	95	1	0	0
soft shell..cooked—moist heat	4 oz	115	0	0	0
FROZEN					
(Phillips) restaurant-style cocktail crab claws	2 oz	45	0	0	0
CRAB, IMITATION					
(Louis Kemp)					
Crab Delights/fat-free					
chunks	3.2 oz	80	11	0	3
flake-style	3.2 oz	80	11	0	3
leg-style	3.2 oz	80	11	0	2

Food and Description	Amount	Total Calories	Total Carbs	Fiber	Sugars
shreds	3.2 oz	80	13	0	2
CRAB DISH (*See also* SEAFOOD ENTRÉE/DINNER)					
FROZEN					
(Dining In)					
crab cakes..Maryland-style	3 oz	150	6	0	0
crab Rangoon..homemade	2 oz	160	18	0	2
(Mrs. Paul's)..deviled crab cake	1 cake	190	23	0	4
(Nancy's) seafood..crab cakes	6 oz	350	28	2	10
(Phillips)					
crab cake..Boardwalk Maryland	2.75 oz	250	8	1	1
Crab Slammers..jalapeño	2 oz	160	14	1	2
MIX					
(Zatarain's)					
crab cake mix..New Orleans–style.. mix only	1.15 oz	100	24	0	0
CRAB APPLE					
(Frieda's) fresh/raw/w/skin..whole	5 oz	110	28	0	0
CRACKER (*See also* COOKIE; SNACKS)					
■ (Adrienne's)					
Courtney's English Water Crackers.. all flavors	4 crackers	60	10	0	0
Gourmet Lavosh Hawaii flatbread					
bite-size	1 oz	120	19	1	1
caraway & rye	1 oz	115	20	1	1
Classic Island	1 oz	120	19	1	1
mini-bite snack	1 oz	120	19	1	1
peppercorn	1 oz	115	20	1	1
portion-control pkgs	1 oz	120	19	1	1
rosemary garlic	1 oz	125	19	1	1
Slightly Onion	1 oz	120	19	1	1
ten-grain	1 oz	110	19	3	2
■ (Ak-Mak)					
100% whole wheat	5 crackers	116	19	4	2
cracker bread					
Armenian					
regular	1 sheet	100	19	2	2
whole wheat	1 sheet	116	19	4	2
round					
no seeds	1 cracker	100	20	2	2
seeded	1 cracker	100	19	2	2
whole wheat	1 cracker	116	19	4	2
■ (Austin)					
snack pack/individual packages					
cheddar on wheat..sandwich					
reduced-fat	1 pkg	170	25	1	5
regular	1 pkg	200	24	<1	5
cheese Dolphins & Friends	1 pkg	200	16	<1	<1
cheese & peanut butter..reduced-fat	1 pkg	170	24	1	5
cheese on cheese	1 pkg	200	24	<1	5
grilled cheese sandwich	1 pkg	200	23	<1	5

Food and Description	Amount	Total Calories	Total Carbs	Fiber	Sugars
PB&J sandwich crackers	1 pkg	200	24	<1	6
peanut butter on cheese sandwich crackers					
original	1 pkg	200	23	1	4
50% more peanut butter	1 pkg	250	25	2	5
toast sandwich					
reduced-fat	1 pkg	170	25	1	5
regular	1 pkg	200	23	1	5
zoo animal crackers	16 pieces	130	25	<1	7
■ (Barbara's Bakery)					
Cheese Bites	22 crackers	120	20	<1	1
Go-Go Grahams/organic					
chocolate	8 crackers	130	23	1	9
cinnamon	8 crackers	130	23	<1	9
honey	8 crackers	130	22	<1	7
lemon ginger	8 crackers	130	22	<1	7
Rite Light Rounds					
original	5 crackers	60	11	0	<1
savory poppy seed	5 crackers	60	11	0	<1
tamari sesame	5 crackers	70	10	0	<1
Wheatines/all natural					
cracked pepper	4 crackers	50	11	1	1
original	4 crackers	60	11	<1	<1
■ (Blue Diamond)					
Nut-Thins					
almond	~16 crackers	120	20	<1	0
hazelnut	~16 crackers	120	21	<1	0
pecan	~16 crackers	120	21	0	0
smokehouse	~16 crackers	120	20	<1	0
■ BRETON (*See* (Dare) in this section)					
■ (Campbell's) soup & oyster	32 pieces	70	9	0	0
■ (Carr's)					
Assortments					
biscuits for cheese	3 biscuits	83	13	<1	<1
distinctive flavor assortment	3 crackers	70	10	0	1
Entertainers					
cheddar	3 crackers	80	9	1	1
croissant	3 crackers	70	10	0	1
poppy & sesame	4 crackers	80	9	1	0
Wheatolo English biscuits	1 biscuit	70	10	0	1
whole wheat	2 crackers	80	11	1	3
Monterey Crackers					
hearty wheat	3 crackers	50	9	<1	1
roasted vegetable	3 crackers	50	8	0	1
savory wheat	3 crackers	60	9	1	2
sesame onion	3 crackers	60	9	1	2
rosemary	7 crackers	130	18	<1	1
stoned wheat	3 crackers	60	10	<1	0
Table Water Crackers	5 crackers	70	13	1	0
w/cracked pepper	5 crackers	70	13	1	0
w/roasted garlic & herbs	5 crackers	70	13	<1	0

Food and Description	Amount	Total Calories	Total Carbs	Fiber	Sugars
w/toasted sesame seeds	5 crackers	70	13	1	0
■ COMBOS (*See* (M&M* Mars) in this section)					
■ (Dare)					
BREMER					
crackers					
caraway	1 oz	130	21	2	1
soup & chili	½ oz	60	11	0	0
wafers					
cracked wheat/box	½ oz	66	11	0.5	0
low-sodium/box	½ oz	70	12	0	0
original/can	½ oz	70	11	0	0
sesame	½ oz	68	11	0.5	0
BRETON					
mini crackers					
cheddar	20 crackers	87	11	0	<1
French onion	19 crackers	100	13	1	1
garden vegetable	20 crackers	87	12	<1	1.5
wheat	20 crackers	90	11	1	1.5
regular crackers					
Cabaret crisp & cream	1 cracker	20	3	0	<1
multigrain..thin wheat	1 cracker	23	2.5	0	<1
original thin wheat	1 cracker	21	2.5	0	0
sesame thin wheat	1 cracker	21	2.5	0	0
Vinta	1 cracker	30	4	<1	0.5
Vivant Zesty Vegetable	1 cracker	22	3	0	<1
■ (Devonsheer)					
melba rounds					
organic..regular or unsalted					
garlic	5 pieces	60	11	1	0
plain	5 pieces	50	12	1	0
sesame	5 pieces	60	10	1	0
regular					
other					
honey bran	5 pieces	50	12	1	0
onion	5 pieces	50	11	1	0
savory herb	5 pieces	50	11	1	0
12-grain	5 pieces	50	12	1	0
vegetable	5 pieces	50	12	1	0
melba toast					
garlic	3 pieces	50	11	1	0
plain					
rye	3 pieces	50	11	1	0
sesame					
regular	3 pieces	50	10	1	0
unsalted	3 pieces	50	11	1	0
12-grain	3 pieces	50	11	1	0
vegetable	3 pieces	50	11	1	0
wheat					
■ (Eden)					
rice crackers					

Food and Description	Amount	Total Calories	Total Carbs	Fiber	Sugars
brown rice	1 oz	120	22	2	1
nori maki	15 crackers	110	24	2	0
■ **(Edward & Sons)**					
brown rice snaps					
toasted onion	8 crackers	60	13	<1	<1
vegetable	8 crackers	60	11	1	<1
■ **(Finn)** Crispbread..dark..all styles	2 pieces	40	9	2	0
■ **(Frito-Lay)**					
Cheetos					
bacon cheddar	1 pkg	190	25	1	3
cheddar cheese	1 pkg	210	23	1	5
golden toast & cheddar	1 pkg	240	25	1	5
Doritos					
jalapeño & cheddar	1 pkg	230	26	1	5
nacho cheesier	1 pkg	240	25	1	6
Peanut Pan					
cheese peanut butter	1 pkg	210	23	1	3
toast peanut butter	1 pkg	210	23	<1	3
■ **(Frookie)** snack..all styles	13 crackers	120	18	2	0
■ **(Hain)**					
bites..cheddar					
golden	22 pieces	120	23	1	na
white	22 pieces	120	23	1	na
other crackers..regular or no salt added					
original	11 pieces	110	23	1	0
saltines	5 pieces	60	13	0	0
sesame	11 pieces	140	19	1	0
soup/oyster	35 pieces	60	13	0	0
vegetable	11 pieces	140	19	1	0
whole wheat..rich	11 pieces	130	18	1	0
■ **(Health Valley)**					
LOW-FAT					
bruschetta vegetable	6 crackers	60	10	1	1
cracked pepper	5 crackers	60	10	1	1
French onion	10 crackers	60	10	1	1
garden herb	6 crackers	60	10	1	1
sesame	5 crackers	60	10	1	1
stoned wheat	5 crackers	60	10	1	1
whole wheat	6 crackers	60	10	2	1
ORIGINAL					
amaranth graham	6 crackers	120	22	3	4
oat bran graham	6 crackers	120	22	3	3
rice bran	6 crackers	110	19	3	4
OTHER corn bread crackers..all flavors	4 crackers	60	11	1	2
■ **(J. J. Flats)**					
breadflats					
Flavorall	1 piece	60	9	1	0
garlic	1 piece	60	10	1	0
multigrain	1 piece	60	10	1	0
onion	1 piece	60	10	1	0

Food and Description	Amount	Total Calories	Total Carbs	Fiber	Sugars
plain	1 piece	60	10	1	0
poppy	1 piece	60	10	1	0
sesame	1 piece	50	9	1	0
■ (KA-ME)					
rice crunch crackers..all styles	16 pieces	110	22	0	<1
■ (Kashi)					
Tasty Little Crackers					
7-grain	15 crackers	130	22	2	3
country cheddar	18 crackers	130	21	0	1
honey sesame	15 crackers	130	22	2	5
natural ranch	18 crackers	130	22	2	3
■ (Kavli)					
Norwegian crispbread					
crispy thin	2 slices	40	8	6	<1
hearty thick	1 slice	35	8	2	<1
■ (Keebler)					
CRACKER SANDWICHES					
cheese & peanut butter	1 pkg	190	22	<1	4
club & cheddar	1 pkg	260	31	1	6
original	1 pkg	180	21	<1	1
toast & peanut butter	1 pkg	200	23	1	5
wheat & cheddar	1 pkg	200	24	<1	5
KRISPY CRACKERS					
saltines					
fat-free	5 crackers	60	13	0	0
mild cheddar	5 crackers	60	10	1	0
original	5 crackers	60	12	<1	<1
soup & oyster	17 crackers	70	12	0	1
whole wheat	5 crackers	60	12	1	1
MUNCH 'EMS/baked					
cheddar	39 crackers	140	19	1	1
original/seasoned	41 crackers	140	21	1	2
ranch	40 crackers	140	20	1	1
sour cream & onion	39 crackers	140	20	1	1
OTHER CRACKERS					
Club Crackers					
33% reduced-fat	4 crackers	70	12	0	2
50% reduced-sodium	5 crackers	70	9	0	1
original	4 crackers	70	9	0	1
Rumbly Grahams					
chocolate chip	23 pieces	140	22	<1	8
cinnamon	20 pieces	140	22	<1	8
honey	20 pieces	140	22	<1	8
Toasteds					
buttercrisp	5 crackers	80	10	0	1
onion	5 crackers	80	10	0	2
sesame	5 crackers	80	10	<1	1
wheat	5 crackers	80	10	1	2
Wheatables					
honey wheat	17 crackers	140	20	1	5

Food and Description	Amount	Total Calories	Total Carbs	Fiber	Sugars
original					
reduced-fat	19 crackers	140	22	2	4
regular	16 crackers	140	20	1	4
7-grain	17 crackers	140	20	1	4
Zesta saltines					
export sodas	3 crackers	60	10	<1	0
fat-free	5 crackers	60	13	0	0
original	5 crackers	60	11	0	0
soup & oyster	45 crackers	70	9	0	1
SUNSHINE					
Cheez-It					
cheddar jack	26 crackers	160	18	0	1
chili cheese	25 crackers	160	17	<1	0
hot & spicy	26 crackers	150	17	<1	1
juniors	44 crackers	140	13	<1	0
original	26 crackers	160	17	<1	0
Parmesan garlic	26 crackers	150	19	0	1
party mix	½ cup	130	19	1	1
reduced-fat	30 crackers	140	20	<1	0
white cheddar	26 crackers	150	18	<1	<1
HiHo					
original	5 crackers	80	10	0	1
reduced-fat	5 crackers	70	11	1	1
Twisterz..all flavors	17 crackers	140	19	<1	1
TOWN HOUSE					
Bistro Crackers					
corn bread	2 crackers	80	11	1	2
multigrain	2 crackers	80	11	1	2
rye	2 crackers	80	10	1	1
regular					
original	5 crackers	80	9	1	1
reduced-fat	6 crackers	70	11	1	2
wheat	5 crackers	80	9	1	2
■ (Lance)					
Captain's Wafers					
cream cheese & chives	6 crackers	200	23	<1	6
grilled cheese	6 crackers	200	22	1	6
peanut butter w/honey	6 crackers	190	23	1	5
smokehouse chedddar	6 crackers	180	27	2	5
cheese on wheat	6 crackers	200	22	2	4
malt/peanut butter on crispy malt	6 crackers	190	18	1	2
Nipchee/cheddar cheese on cheese	6 crackers	200	21	1	3
peanut butter on wheat	6 crackers	200	21	1	4
Toastchee..sandwich					
peanut butter & cheese	6 crackers	220	23	2	3
reduced-fat	6 crackers	180	27	2	5
toasty/peanut butter/buttery	6 crackers	190	17	1	3
■ (Little Debbie)					
cheddar on cheese	1-oz pkg	130	16	1	3
peanut butter cheese	1-oz pkg	130	16	<1	2

Food and Description	Amount	Total Calories	Total Carbs	Fiber	Sugars
	1.39-oz pkg	190	23	1	3
peanut butter toasty crackers	1-oz pkg	130	16	<1	3
■ (M&M* Mars) (See also PRETZELS)					
Combos snack					
cheddar cheese	1 oz	140	18	0	4
	1.7-oz pkg	240	31	1	7
pepperoni pizza	1 oz	140	17	1	3
	1.7-oz pkg	240	31	1	6
■ (Manischewitz)					
matzo					
egg & onion	1 matzo	110	23	0	0
everything	1 matzo	110	22	1	0
Passover egg	~ 1 oz	130	27	0	0
saltine	1 matzo	110	24	0	0
savory garlic	1 matzo	100	23	1	0
thin					
original	1 matzo	100	22	0	0
tea	1 matzo	100	22	0	0
unsalted	1 matzo	110	24	0	0
whole wheat	1 oz	110	22	4	0
Tam Tams					
everything	1 oz	110	22	1	0
garlic	1 oz	110	22	1	0
no salt	1 oz	140	18	0	0
onion	10 pieces	150	18	0	0
original	10 pieces	145	17	0	0
■ (Nabisco)					
NABISCO					
Barnum's animal crackers	1 oz	130	23	1	7
Better Cheddars/baked					
original	1 oz	150	17	1	0
reduced-fat	1 oz	140	19	1	0
Cheese Nips					
cheddar	1 oz	150	19	1	0
jalapeño cheddar	1 oz	150	19	1	1
mini	1 oz	150	19	1	0
packs 2 Go!..1.65-oz pkg	1 pkg	230	29	1	1
reduced-fat	1 oz	130	21	1	0
salsa & cheddar doubles	1 oz	150	19	1	1
thin crisps/100-calorie	~1 oz pkg	100	15	1	0
Chicken in a Biskit	1 oz	170	18	1	2
Flavor Crisps/bacon-baked	1 oz	160	19	1	2
Sociables/baked..savory	1 oz	70	9	0	1
Swiss cheese/baked	1 oz	140	18	1	2
Twigs sesame & cheese sticks	1 oz	150	18	1	1
vegetable thins/baked	1 oz	160	19	1	2
OTHER CRACKERS					
Grahams & Teddy Grahams..Nabisco brand					
chocolate crackers	1 oz	130	24	1	9
	1.25 oz	150	26	1	10

Food and Description	Amount	Total Calories	Total Carbs	Fiber	Sugars
mini snak saks	1 oz	140	22	1	8
sticks	1 oz	130	24	1	9
cinnamon cracker	1 oz	120	23	1	8
	1.25 oz	160	27	1	9
Bob the Builder	1 oz	130	22	1	7
Go-Paks	⅓ pkg	130	25	1	9
low-fat	1 oz	120	26	1	12
sticks	1 oz	120	25	1	11
Dora the Explorer	1 oz	130	23	1	8
honey cracker	1 oz	140	24	1	8
	1.25-oz pkg	150	26	1	9
Bearwiches	1 oz	130	19	0	9
Go-Paks	⅓ pkg	130	23	1	8
low-fat	1 oz	120	26	1	8
sticks	1 oz	130	24	1	9
original graham crackers	1 oz	130	24	1	7
Harvest Crisps..Wheat Thins					
5-grain	1 oz	140	23	1	4
garden vegetable	1 oz	130	22	1	4
Honey Maid Graham Crackers					
apple cinnamon sticks	~1 oz	130	25	1	9
chocolate	1 oz	130	24	1	9
sticks	1 oz	130	24	1	9
cinnamon	1 oz	130	25	1	11
Go-Pak	⅓ pkg	130	25	1	9
low-fat	~1 oz	120	26	1	12
sticks	1 oz	120	23	1	8
honey	1.22 oz	140	24	1	8
low-fat	~1 oz	120	26	1	8
sticks	~1 oz	130	24	1	9
oatmeal crunch	1 oz	130	24	1	8
Premium saltines					
fat-free	½ oz	60	12	0	0
gold	½ oz	70	10	0	1
multigrain	½ oz	60	10	1	0
original	½ oz	60	11	0	0
soup & oyster	½ oz	60	11	0	0
unsalted tops	½ oz	70	11	0	0
Social Tea biscuits	1 oz	120	20	1	7
Teddy Cheddy..baked	1 oz	150	19	1	0
Toast Crackers					
w/cheddar cheese	1.4 oz pkg	200	22	1	4
w/peanut butter	1.38 oz pkg	190	24	1	5
Wheatsworth stone-ground wheat	~½ oz	80	10	1	0
RED OVAL FARMS					
Stoned Wheat Thins					
mini	~1 oz	130	21	1	1
regular or lower-sodium	½ oz	60	10	1	0
RITZ					
Bits					

Food and Description	Amount	Total Calories	Total Carbs	Fiber	Sugars
cracker sandwiches					
cheese	1 oz	150	16	0	4
Go-Pak	⅓ pkg	160	18	0	4
Packs 2 Go!	1.5-oz pkg	230	23	1	6
graham cracker s'mores	1 oz	150	22	1	11
	1.25-oz pkg	170	25	1	12
jalapeño cheddar	1 oz	160	18	1	4
peanut butter	1.25-oz pkg	180	21	1	4
	1.5-oz pkg	230	23	1	6
fun-size holiday	1 oz	140	20	1	10
Go-Pak	⅓ pkg	160	19	1	4
Packs 2 Go!	1.5-oz pkg	210	24	1	5
peanut butter fudge	1 oz	150	19	1	5
chips					
oven-toasted/crunch..all flavors	1 oz	140	20	1	1
crisp crackers..crispy baked	1 oz	140	22	1	3
OTHER RITZ CRACKERS					
assortment/cheese, cracked pepper & wheat	~½ oz	80	10	0	1
assortment/cracked pepper & wheat	~½ oz	80	10	0	1
bite-size/original	1.3-oz pkg	190	23	1	3
garlic butter/4-count	~½ oz	80	10	0	1
original	~½ oz	80	10	0	1
reduced-fat/4-count	~½ oz	70	11	0	2
peanut butter	1.4 oz	190	24	1	5
snack/cheddar-baked mix	1.5 pkg	200	28	2	3
mixers/Snak Saks	1.14 oz	150	20	1	2
sticks	1 oz	150	19	1	2
w/peanut butter	1.38-oz pkg	190	24	1	5
w/real cheese/8-count	1.38-oz pkg	200	22	1	4
w/whole wheat	~½ oz	70	11	1	1
SNACKWELL'S reduced-fat					
cracked pepper	½ oz	60	10	0	1
wheat	½ oz	70	11	1	2
zesty cheddar	1 oz	130	23	<1	2
TRISCUIT					
cheddar	1 oz	120	20	3	1
low-sodium	1 oz	140	22	4	0
original	1 oz	140	21	4	0
reduced-fat	1 oz	120	21	3	0
roasted garlic	1 oz	140	22	4	0
WHEAT THINS					
big	1 oz	140	20	1	3
honey	1 oz	150	21	1	5
low-salt	1 oz	150	21	1	3
multigrain	1 oz	140	21	2	4
original	1 oz	150	21	1	3
original..baked	1 oz	150	21	1	3
ranch	1 oz	140	19	1	3
reduced-fat	1 oz	130	21	1	3

Food and Description	Amount	Total Calories	Total Carbs	Fiber	Sugars
reduced-fat..baked	1 oz	130	21	1	3
snack					
baked original	1 oz	150	21	1	3
minis..100-calorie pkg	1 pkg	100	16	1	3
zwieback toast	2 pieces	35	6	0	1
■ (Old London)					
FLATBREAD CRACKERS					
everything	2 pieces	60	9	1	0
sesame	2 pieces	60	9	1	0
MELBA SNACK					
bacon	5 pieces	60	11	2	0
garlic	5 pieces	60	11	2	0
Mexicali corn	5 pieces	60	10	2	0
nacho	5 pieces	70	9	2	0
onion	5 pieces	60	12	1	0
rye	5 pieces	60	12	2	0
sesame	5 pieces	60	9	1	0
white	5 pieces	60	12	2	0
whole grain	5 pieces	60	12	2	0
MELBA TOAST					
garlic	3 pieces	50	11	2	0
onion	3 pieces	45	11	2	0
rye	3 pieces	45	11	2	0
sesame	3 pieces	50	10	2	0
wheat	3 pieces	50	11	2	0
white	3 pieces	50	11	2	0
whole grain	3 pieces	45	11	2	0
■ (Pepperidge Farm)					
ENTERTAINING CRACKERS					
Butter Thins	4 crackers	70	10	0	1
Country Cheese	2 crackers	80	8	0	0
Hearty Wheat	3 crackers	80	10	1	2
Quartet Assortment	3 crackers	70	10	1	1
Trio Collection	4 crackers	70	10	1	<1
GOLDFISH CRACKERS					
cheddar cheese–blasted					
Burstin' BBQ	51 pieces	140	19	<1	<1
Extra Cheddar	51 pieces	140	18	1	<1
Nothing but Nacho	51 pieces	140	20	4	0
X-plosive Pizza	51 pieces	140	19	1	<1
crisps					
cheddar jack	1 oz	150	17	1	1
cheesy sour cream onion	1 oz	150	17	1	1
4-cheese	1 oz	150	18	1	1
Liberty w/real cheese	1 oz	140	10	1	1
SANDWICH SNACKERS					
cheddar w/peanut butter filling	1 oz	140	18	<1	3
original					
w/cheese filling	1 oz	150	18	<1	4

Food and Description	Amount	Total Calories	Total Carbs	Fiber	Sugars
w/peanut butter filling	1 oz	140	19	<1	4
white cheddar	1 oz	150	18	<1	4
SNACK STICKS					
pretzel	12 sticks	120	26	1	2
pumpernickel	12 sticks	120	22	2	2
3-cheese	12 sticks	150	20	1	0
wheat	12 sticks	130	22	1	4
WATER BISCUITS..all flavors	5 crackers	60	11	1	0
■ **(Pritikin)**					
brown rice crackers	7 crackers	60	13	0	0
low-sodium onion & garlic	8 crackers	60	13	0	0
unsalted	7 crackers	60	13	0	0
■ **RED OVAL FARMS** (*See* (Nabisco) in this section)					
■ **RITZ** (*See* (Nabisco) in this section)					
■ **(Ry-Krisp)**					
fat-free	2 crackers	60	8	4	0
hearty rye	1 slice	50	10	3	0
light rye	2 slices	50	7	3	0
natural	2 crackers	40	7	4	0
seasoned	2 crackers	60	10	3	0
sesame	2 crackers	60	11	3	0
■ **(Ryvita)**					
breaks	1 slice	48	10	2	3
crispbread					
Allinson Organic					
wholemeal	1 slice	17	3	<1	0
dark	1 slice	28	6	2	<1
dark rye..plain	1 slice	28	6	2	<1
multi-grain	1 slice	37	6.5	2	<1
original wheat	1 slice	28	6	1.5	<1
crackerbread					
high-fiber	1 slice	16	3	1	0
original	1 slice	19	4	0	0
wholemeal	1 slice	18	3.5	<1	<1
■ **(Sesmark)**					
rice thins					
brown	15 pieces	120	25	<1	0
cheddar	15 pieces	130	26	<1	0
original sesame	15 pieces	130	24	<1	0
teriyaki-flavored	13 pieces	130	24	<1	0
savory rice minis					
chili cheese	35 pieces	120	24	<1	0
lightly salted	40 pieces	120	25	0	0
nacho corn	35 pieces	120	23	<1	1
sesame garlic	37 pieces	120	24	<1	0
savory thins					
cracked wheat	15 pieces	100	21	<1	0
original	15 pieces	120	24	<1	0
teriyaki	13 pieces	130	24	0	0

Food and Description	Amount	Total Calories	Total Carbs	Fiber	Sugars
toasted onion & garlic	15 pieces	110	24	1	0
sesame thins					
cheddar	9 pieces	150	15	1	0
garlic	9 pieces	150	15	1	0
original	9 pieces	150	15	1	0
unsalted	11 pieces	160	15	1	0
■ **SNACKWELL'S** (*See* (Nabisco) in this section)					
■ **SUNSHINE** (*See* (Nabisco) in this section)					
■ **TRISCUIT** (*See* (Nabisco) in this section)					
■ **(Valley Lahvosh)**					
cracker bread					
hearts					
cinnamon	7 crackers	110	24	<1	7
original	8 crackers	120	23	<1	3
rounds					
2" dia	7 crackers	110	23	<1	3
3" dia	4 crackers	110	22	2	3
5" dia	1 cracker	70	14	0	2
15" dia	⅛ cracker	110	23	<1	3
deli	7 crackers	120	22	<1	3
Sweetheart Crispies	7 crackers	120	22	<1	3
wheat rounds					
3" dia	4 crackers	110	22	2	3
5" dia	1 cracker	70	14	0	2
15" dia	⅛ cracker	110	23	<1	3
wraps..15" dia					
cracked wheat	5-1" slices	160	28	2	3
original	5-1" slices	160	28	1	3
spinach	5-1" slices	160	28	1	3
tomato	5-1" slices	160	28	2	3
■ **(Venus)**					
bran wafers	5 crackers	60	11	2	0
cracked wheat wafers	5 crackers	60	11	0	0
cracker bread					
Armenian thin	2 pieces	100	19	0	0
original	5 pieces	60	11	0	0
hors d'oeuvre	3 pieces	60	11	0	0
oat bran wafers	5 crackers	60	11	2	0
Old Brussels Waferettes					
cheddar	5 pieces	80	7	0	0
jalapeño	5 pieces	80	7	1	0
rye wafers/low-salt	5 pieces	60	11	0	0
stoned wheat..wafers..bite-size	7 crackers	60	11	0	0
water crackers/fat-free	5 crackers	55	11	0	0
■ **(Wasa)**					
crispbread					
delikatess rye	1 slice	26	5	1	0
fiber rye	1 slice	30	5	2.5	0
hearty rye	1 slice	40	8	2	0
multigrain	1 slice	45	8	2	0

Food and Description	Amount	Total Calories	Total Carbs	Fiber	Sugars
organic rye	1 slice	35	8	2	0
sesame					
No'e'	1 slice	30	5	2.5	0
Runda	1 slice	55	9	1	<1
rye					
light	1 slice	25	5	1	0
original	1 slice	35	7	1	0
sodium-free	1 slice	30	7	2	0
sourdough	1 slice	35	7	1	<1
wheat doré	1 slice	50	9	1	<1
■ (Westbrae)					
natural rice wafers					
5-spice	7 crackers	50	11	0	0
no salt	7 crackers	50	11	0	0
sesame	7 crackers	50	11	0	0
tamari	7 crackers	50	11	0	0
CRACKER CRUMBS/MEAL (*See also* MATZO MEAL & MIX)					
(Golden Dipt)					
Cracker meal..no salt..all styles	¼ cup	145	31	1	<1
Modern Maid..matzoh meal	¼ cup	145	31	1	<1
(Manischewitz) matzo	¼ cup	130	28	1	<1
(Nabisco) cracker meal..baking topping	¼ cup	110	22	1	0
CRANBERRY					
DRIED					
(Ann's House of Nuts)	⅓ cup	130	34	2	31
(Ocean Spray) Craisins..all flavors	⅓ cup	130	33	2	27
(Sonoma)	⅓ cup	120	29	2	26
(Sun Maid)	⅓ cup	140	34	2	31
(Traverse Bay)					
cranberries	⅓ cup	140	31	2	28
cranberries, berry & cherry	⅓ cup	150	35	2	25
FRESH					
chopped	½ cup	27	7	2	5
(Ocean Spray)	2 oz	30	7	2	5
whole..w/o stems	1 cup	46	12	4	10
CRANBERRY JUICE/JUICE BLEND/JUICE DRINK					
BOTTLED, BOXED, or CANNED					
(After The Fall)					
Cape Cod Cranberry	8 fl oz	100	24	0	21
Naturally Cranberry	8 fl oz	120	30	0	26
(Dole) cranberry cocktail	8 fl oz	140	34	0	34
	11.5 fl oz	200	49	0	49
(Knudsen)					
cranberry nectar	8 fl oz	140	34	0	31
Just Juice	8 fl oz	60	14	0	7
sparkling cranberry	8 fl oz	130	30	0	30
(Langer's)					
cranberry cocktail	8 fl oz	140	35	0	35
cranberry drink/diet	8 fl oz	30	9	0	9
cranberry raspberry drink blend					

Food and Description	Amount	Total Calories	Total Carbs	Fiber	Sugars
diet	8 fl oz	30	9	0	<1
regular	8 fl oz	150	36	0	36
cranberry juice	8 fl oz	140	35	0	35
(Ocean Spray)					
Cravin' Less Sugar juice drink					
cranberry wildberry	8 fl oz	80	20	0	17
juice & tea					
cranberry	8 fl oz	100	24	0	24
white cranberry–peach	8 fl oz	100	25	0	25
light-style					
juice cocktail	8 fl oz	40	10	0	10
juice drink	8 fl oz	40	10	0	10
premium 100% juice blends					
cranberry					
& Concord grape	8 fl oz	150	37	0	37
& Georgia peach	8 fl oz	140	34	0	34
& mixed berry	8 fl oz	150	38	0	38
& Pacific raspberry	8 fl oz	140	34	0	34
cranberry blend	8 fl oz	140	35	0	35
regular juice cocktail					
apple	8 fl oz	160	40	0	40
cranberry	8 fl oz	130	33	0	33
raspberry	8 fl oz	140	34	0	34
strawberry	8 fl oz	140	37	0	37
regular juice drink					
Crancherry	8 fl oz	150	39	0	39
Crangrape	8 fl oz	160	40	0	40
Cranmango	8 fl oz	130	35	0	0
Cranraspberry	8 fl oz	140	34	0	34
Cranstrawberry	8 fl oz	140	37	0	37
spritzer..cranberry	11.75 oz	160	40	0	40
(Old Orchard) low-carb					
apple cranberry	8 fl oz	26	6	0	4
cranberry	8 fl oz	29	6	0	4
cranberry raspberry	8 fl oz	23	6	0	5
white cranberry	8 fl oz	39	6	0	6
(Tropicana)					
cranberry apple	10 fl oz	170	42	0	42
cranberry cocktail	8 fl oz	140	34	0	34
cranberry grape	8 fl oz	170	41	0	41
cranberry raspberry	8 fl oz	140	35	0	35
(Welch's)					
cranberry cocktail drink	5.5 fl oz	100	25	0	23
	10 fl oz	140	35	0	34
juice cocktail	5.5 fl oz	100	24	0	23
	8 fl oz	120			
	10 fl oz	140	36	0	35
juice cocktail drink	11.5 fl oz	200	51	0	50
	8.45 fl oz	180	45	0	44

Food and Description	Amount	Total Calories	Total Carbs	Fiber	Sugars
sparkling juice..Celebration	8 fl oz	160	49	9	38
Welch's pourable cranberry					
apple	8 fl oz	120	41	0	40
grape	8 fl oz	170	42	0	40
raspberry	8 fl oz	150	37	0	36
FROZEN..prepared, unless noted otherwise					
(Old Orchard)					
apple cranberry	8 fl oz	120	31	0	29
cranberry raspberry	8 fl oz	130	31	0	29
(Welch's)					
100% juice blend concentrate	2 oz	150	36	0	35
juice cocktail					
cranberry					
light	8 fl oz	50	13	0	12
regular	8 fl oz	140	36	0	35
cranberry apple	8 fl oz	160	40	0	39
cranberry raspberry					
light	8 fl oz	50	13	0	12
regular	8 fl oz	150	37	0	36
CRANBERRY SAUCE					
canned					
(Ocean Spray)					
cranberries	2 oz	30	7	0	5
Cran-Fruit cranberry crushed fruit					
orange	¼ cup	120	29	0	28
raspberry	¼ cup	120	29	0	27
strawberry	¼ cup	120	29	0	27
jellied	¼ cup	110	25	0	21
whole berry	¼ cup	110	27	0	22
(S&W) jellied or whole berry	¼ cup	100	26	0	22
CRANBERRY ORANGE RELISH					
can or jar	¼ cup	120	29	0	28
CRAYFISH/mixed species..farmed					
cooked—moist heat	3 oz	75	0	0	0
raw	3 oz	60	0	0	0
CREAM (*See also* CREAMER, NONDAIRY; SOUR CREAM; SOUR CREAM SUBSTITUTE; WHIPPED TOPPING)					
(Alouette) crème fraîche cooking					
& topping cream	1 oz	100	11	0	1
(Devon Cream Company)					
clotted cream	2 Tbs	140	<1	0	<1
w/brandy	2 Tbs	140	3	0	3
w/Drambuie	2 Tbs	130	3	0	3
w/Grand Marnier	2 Tbs	130	3	0	3
w/strawberries	2 Tbs	100	4	0	4
double Devon cream	2 Tbs	130	<1	0	<1
(Hood)					
half-and-half	2 Tbs	40	1	0	1
heavy	1 Tbs	50	0	0	0

Food and Description	Amount	Total Calories	Total Carbs	Fiber	Sugars
light	1 Tbs	30	<1	0	<1
(Land O' Lakes)					
half-and-half	2 Tbs	35	1	0	1
fat-free	2 Tbs	20	3	0	2
light	1 Tbs	20	3	0	2
gourmet	2 Tbs	40	1	0	0
heavy gourmet whipping	1 Tbs	50	1	0	1
(Rockview Farms) whipping cream					
heavy..grade A	1 Tbs	50	1	0	1
(Umpqua) whipping cream					
old-fashioned heavy	1 Tbs	60	1	0	1
CREAM CHEESE (*See also* CHEESE ALTERNATIVE/IMITATION; CHEESE SPREAD)					
(Breakstone) Temp-Tee..whipped	3 Tbs	80	<1	0	<1
(Connoisseur)					
apple cinnamon	1 oz	110	10	0	5
cranberry	1 oz	100	5	1	3
mango peach	1 oz	110	10	0	5
(Dorman's)					
65% fat	2 Tbs	90	1	0	0
70% fat	2 Tbs	100	1	0	0
(Fleur de Lait)					
light					
crunchy garden vegetable	2 Tbs	60	2	0	1
garlic & herb/minced	2 Tbs	60	3	0	3
Mediterranean olive	2 Tbs	60	2	0	2
red ripe strawberry	2 Tbs	70	3	0	3
spinach artichoke	2 Tbs	60	2	0	2
Vidalia sweet onion	2 Tbs	60	3	0	3
Neufchâtel spread					
Bermuda onion	2 Tbs	90	2	0	1
date nut rum	2 Tbs	90	4	0	4
garlic & spice	2 Tbs	90	2	0	1
herb & spice	2 Tbs	90	2	0	1
lemon	2 Tbs	90	5	0	5
lox/smoked salmon	2 Tbs	90	1	0	1
mandarin orange	2 Tbs	90	4	0	4
peach	2 Tbs	90	4	0	4
pineapple	2 Tbs	90	4	0	4
strawberry	2 Tbs	90	4	0	4
toasted onion	2 Tbs	90	2	0	1
wildberry	2 Tbs	90	4	0	4
(Fresh Cut)					
bacon & horseradish	2 Tbs	90	1	0	<1
Bermuda onion & chives	2 Tbs	90	2	0	2
date nut & rum	2 Tbs	90	4	0	4
garlic & spice	2 Tbs	90	1	0	<1
herb & spice	2 Tbs	90	2	0	1
lox	2 Tbs	90	1	0	<1
peaches & cream	2 Tbs	90	3	0	3

Food and Description	Amount	Total Calories	Total Carbs	Fiber	Sugars
strawberry	2 Tbs	90	3	0	3
(Kraft)					
Philadelphia brand					
brick					
fat-free	1 oz	30	2	0	1
Neufchâtel					
⅓ less fat	1 oz	70	1	0	1
original	1 oz	100	1	0	1
regular/soft					
fat-free					
plain	2 Tbs	30	1	0	1
light	2 Tbs	60	2	0	2
original	2 Tbs	100	1	0	1
whipped					
regular	2 Tbs	70	1	0	1
w/chives	2 Tbs	70	3	0	3
w/mixed berries	2 Tbs	70	3	0	3
Philly's flavors/soft					
blueberry	2 Tbs	100	5	0	5
garden vegetable					
fat-free	2 Tbs	30	2	0	1
regular	2 Tbs	90	2	0	1
honey nut	2 Tbs	110	4	0	3
pineapple	2 Tbs	100	4	0	4
raspberry	2 Tbs	100	5	0	4
strawberry					
fat-free	2 Tbs	30	2	0	1
light	2 Tbs	70	1	0	1
regular	2 Tbs	90	4	0	4
(Weight Watchers) light	2 Tbs	40	1	0	1
CREAMER, NONDAIRY (*See also* CREAM)					
LIQUID					
(International Delight)					
amaretto					
fat-free	1 Tbs	30	7	0	6
original	1 Tbs	45	6	0	6
reduced-calorie	1 Tbs	30	3	0	3
chocolate cream	1 Tbs	40	7	0	5
cinnamon hazelnut					
fat-free	1 Tbs	30	7	0	6
regular	1 Tbs	40	7	0	6
French vanilla royal					
fat-free	1 Tbs	30	7	0	6
original	1 Tbs	45	6	0	6
hazelnut					
original	1 Tbs	45	6	0	6
reduced-calorie	1 Tbs	30	3	0	3
Irish cream					
fat-free	1 Tbs	30	7	0	5

Food and Description	Amount	Total Calories	Total Carbs	Fiber	Sugars
original	1 Tbs	45	7	0	6
Southern pecan	1 Tbs	40	7	0	5
vanilla hazelnut..original	1 Tbs	45	6	0	6
vanilla toffee caramel	1 Tbs	40	7	0	5
(Mocha Mix)					
fat-free	1 Tbs	10	1	0	0
light	1 Tbs	10	<1	0	<1
original	1 Tbs	20	1	0	0
(Nestlé)					
Coffee-mate					
amaretto	1 Tbs	40	5	0	5
café mocha					
fat-free	1 Tbs	25	2	0	0
regular	1 Tbs	40	5	0	5
chocolate raspberry	1 Tbs	40	5	0	5
cinnamon vanilla	1 Tbs	40	5	0	5
cinnamon vanilla cream	1 Tbs	40	5	0	5
eggnog	4 Tbs	60	9	0	7
French vanilla	1 Tbs	40	5	0	5
fat-free	1 Tbs	10	2	0	0
gingerbread	4 Tbs	60	9	0	7
hazelnut					
Carb-select	1 tbs	15	2	0	1
fat-free	1 Tbs	25	2	0	0
regular	1 Tbs	40	5	0	5
Irish cream					
fat-free	1 Tbs	25	2	0	0
regular	1 Tbs	40	5	0	5
original					
fat-free	1 Tbs	10	2	0	0
low-fat	1 Tbs	10	1	0	0
regular	1 Tbs	20	2	0	0
vanilla Carb-select	1 Tbs	15	2	0	1
Coffee-mate half-and-half					
hazelnut	1 Tbs	70	8	0	8
original	1 Tbs	40	1	0	1
vanilla	1 Tbs	60	7	0	7
POWDERED					
(Dean Foods)					
Cremora					
fat-free	1 tsp	10	2	0	0
light	1 tsp	10	2	0	0
original	1 tsp	15	2	0	0
Royale	1 tsp	15	1	0	0
(Nestlé)					
Coffee-mate					
cinnamon vanilla cream	4 tsp	60	9	0	7
French vanilla	4 tsp	60	9	0	7
fat-free	4 tsp	50	11	0	6
hazelnut	4 tsp	60	9	0	7

Food and Description	Amount	Total Calories	Total Carbs	Fiber	Sugars
fat-free	4 tsp	50	11	0	6
original					
fat-free	1 tsp	10	2	0	0
light	1 tsp	10	2	0	0
regular	1 tsp	10	1	0	0
half-and-half					
hazelnut	2 Tbs	60	8	0	8
original	2 Tbs	40	1	0	1
vanilla	2 Tbs	60	7	0	7
Latte Creations					
classic	2 Tbs	100	12	0	4
mocha	2 Tbs	90	14	0	9
vanilla	2 Tbs	90	14	0	9
CREPE					
READY-TO-SERVE					
(Frieda's) French bistro–style	1 crepe	30	5	0	2
(French Style) 7 crepes	1 crepe	30	5	0	2
CRISPBREAD (*See* CRACKER)					
CROAKER					
breaded & fried	3 oz	188	6	0	0
raw	3 oz	89	0	0	0
CROISSANT					
READY-TO-SERVE					
(Awrey's)					
butter	1 oz	110	12	0	1
sandwich..sliced	1.5 oz	160	19	<1	2
sliced	3 oz	330	37	1	4
unsliced	3 oz	330	37	1	4
tip-to-tip croissant	2 oz	220	25	<1	3
(Sara Lee)					
FOOD SERVICE					
100% vegetable shortening					
sliced	2 oz	220	25	1	12
	3 oz	320	38	2	14
butter..sliced	2 oz	220	24	1	4
	3 oz	330	37	2	6
natural butter-flavored..sliced	2 oz	240	23	1	3
	2.5 oz	270	32	<1	6
	3 oz	360	36	2	5
1½-oz croissant	1 croissant	170	19	0	3
2-oz croissant	1 croissant	220	26	<1	4
3-oz sandwich croissant	1 croissant	320	38	2	14
*RETAIL/*frozen..French-style					
petite	2 croissants	230	26	1	0
plain	1 croissant	170	20	1	0
CROUTONS					
(Arnold) crispy					
classic					
Italian	5 croutons	30	4	1	0
seasoned	5 croutons	30	5	1	0

Food and Description	Amount	Total Calories	Total Carbs	Fiber	Sugars
home-style/larger..garlic herb (Brownberry)	5 croutons	30	5	1	0
classic					
Italian	5 croutons	30	4	1	3
seasoned	5 croutons	30	5	1	0
home-style/larger..garlic herb (Cardini)	5 croutons	30	5	0	1
Caesar	2 Tbs	35	4	0	0
garlic & butter	2 Tbs	35	4	0	0
Italian	2 Tbs	30	4	0	0
(Chatam Village)					
Caesar	2 Tbs	35	4	0	0
cheese & garlic	2 Tbs	40	4	0	0
garden herb	2 Tbs	35	4	0	0
garlic & butter	2 Tbs	35	4	0	0
garlic & onion..fat-free	2 Tbs	30	4	0	0
(Devonsheer) all flavors	2 Tbs	30	4	0	0
(Edward & Sons) Organic/Vegan					
Italian herbs	2 Tbs	28	5	0	0
lightly salted	2 Tbs	30	5	0	0
onion garlic	2 Tbs	30	5	0	0
(Old London)					
RESTAURANT-STYLE..all flavors	2 Tbs	30	5	1	0
TOASTETTES/round..all flavors	10 croutons	25	3	0	0
(Pepperidge Farm)					
CLASSIC CUT					
fat-free..all flavors	6 croutons	30	5	0	<1
regular					
cheese garlic	11 croutons	35	5	0	<1
onion garlic	11 croutons	30	5	0	<1
seasoned	11 croutons	30	5	0	<1
GENEROUS CUT					
buttermilk ranch	6 croutons	30	5	0	<1
classic Caesar	6 croutons	35	4	0	<1
cracked pepper & Parmesan	6 croutons	35	4	0	<1
sourdough cheese	6 croutons	30	4	0	<1
zesty Italian	6 croutons	35	4	0	0
CROWDER PEA					
canned					
(Luck's) seasoned w/pork	7.5 oz	200	21	6	1
(The Allens)..crowder peas	4.4 oz	110	19	8	0
dried..(Lowe's) 16-oz bag	3 oz	120	22	4	1
CRUMPET					
(Wolferman's)					
blueberry	1 crumpet	90	20	<1	4
cinnamon sugar	1 crumpet	90	18	<1	3
classic	1 crumpet	90	18	0	2
raspberry	1 crumpet	90	19	<1	4
CUCUMBER (*See also* PICKLE)					
raw..sliced	½ cup	7	3	1	0

Food and Description	Amount	Total Calories	Total Carbs	Fiber	Sugars
whole..peeled	1 medium	20	4	1	0
CUCUMBER DISH (*See* PICKLE; PICKLE RELISH)					
CUMIN SEED/whole	1 tsp	8	1	0	0
CUPCAKE (*See* CAKE, SNACK)					
CURD TOPPING					
(Wolferman's)					
Elizabethan curd					
lemon	1 Tbs	60	12	0	12
raspberry	1 Tbs	60	12	0	12
CURRANT					
black..raw	½ cup	36	8	0	6
red or white/raw	½ cup	31	8	5	6
Zante/dried					
(S&W) canned	¼ cup	130	31	2	29
CURRY (*See also* SAUCE)					
(Patak's)					
PASTES					
biryani	2 Tbs	180	6	3	0
extra-hot	2 Tbs	160	4	0	0
garam masala	2 Tbs	130	4	0	1
madras	2 Tbs	160	4	0	0
mild	2 Tbs	170	5	0	0
tandoori	2 Tbs	30	5	1	2
tikka	2 Tbs	160	4	0	0
vindaloo	2 Tbs	160	4	0	0
SAUCES					
dopiaza cooking sauce	½ cup	90	11	0	8
korma	½ cup	220	12	1	7
korma cooking sauce	½ cup	240	13	1	9
rogan josh	½ cup	190	12	1	5
tikka masala cooking sauce	½ cup	120	12	0	6
tikka masala sauce	½ cup	220	14	1	9
vindaloo	½ cup	320	14	1	6
(A Taste of Thai)					
BASES					
green	1 tsp	15	1	1	0
Panang	1 tsp	25	2	0	1
red	1 tsp	20	1	0	0
yellow	1 tsp	30	1	0	0
CURRY POWDER/ground	1 tsp	6	1	<1	<1
CUSK					
raw	3 oz	75	0	0	0
steamed	3 oz	95	0	0	0
CUSTARD (*See* PIE; PUDDING & MOUSSE)					
CUTTLEFISH..cooked—moist heat	3 oz	135	1	0	0

D

Food and Description	Amount	Total Calories	Total Carbs	Fiber	Sugars
DANDELION GREENS/fresh					
cooked	1 cup	35	7	3	0
raw/chopped	1 cup	25	5	2	0
DANISH (*See* PASTRY)					
DATE					
(Amport) diced	¼ cup	130	36	4	36
(Del Monte)					
chopped	¼ cup	120	31	3	29
whole..pitted..medium	5–6 dates	120	31	3	29
(Dole)					
chopped	1 oz	120	33	3	28
dried..ground	1 oz	110	26	2	13
whole..pitted..medium	4–6 dates	120	31	3	29
(Frieda's) Medjool	2–3 dates	120	31	3	29
(Sun-Maid) chopped..all types	1.3 oz	120	33	3	28
DEER (*See* VENISON)					
DESSERT TOPPING (*See* CREAM; ICE CREAM TOPPING; WHIPPED TOPPING)					
DILL SEED..whole	1 tsp	6	1	<1	0
DINNER (*See* ASIAN FOOD; BEEF DISH/ENTRÉE; EGG DISH/MEAL; FAST FOOD; FROZEN ENTRÉE/DINNER; MEXICAN FOOD; PASTA ENTRÉE/DINNER; PIZZA; PORK ENTRÉE/DINNER; RICE DISH; SEAFOOD ENTRÉE/DINNER; VEGETARIAN FOODS; individual listings)					
DIP (*See also* SALAD DRESSING; SAUCE; SEASONINGS)					
FROZEN					
(Calavo) Mexican-style avocado guacamole..medium or mild	2 Tbs	50	4	2	2
(Heinz) T.G.I Friday's..spinach, cheese & artichoke	2 Tbs	45	2	2	1
MIX					
(NOTE: Unless otherwise stated, data are for dry mix only.)					
(Frito-Lay) prepared					
Ruffles dip mixes					
French onion					
naturally & artificially flavored	2 Tbs	70	3	<1	1
ranch	2 Tbs	70	3	<1	<1
(Hidden Valley) prepared					
Fiesta	2 Tbs	70	3	<1	<1
French onion	2 Tbs	70	3	<1	<1
garden vegetable	2 Tbs	70	3	<1	<1
original ranch..regular recipe w/sour					

Food and Description	Amount	Total Calories	Total Carbs	Fiber	Sugars
cream party dip..prepared	2 Tbs	70	3	0	>1
(Knorr)					
DIP MIX					
cracked pepper ranch	½ tsp	5	0	0	0
garden dill	½ tsp	5	0	0	0
onion chive	½ tsp	5	<1	0	0
RECIPE CLASSICS/soup, dip & recipe mix					
French onion	⅓ box	35	6	0	1
roasted garlic herb	⅓ box	80	13	0	2
vegetable	¼ box	30	6	1	2
(Lipton)					
DIP MIX..onion	1/16 pkg	5	1	0	0
RECIPE SECRETS/soup & dip mix					
beefy onion	⅛ pkg	25	5	0	0
onion mushroom	⅕ pkg	30	5	0	0
ranch	⅙ pkg	30	6	0	0
savory herb w/garlic	⅛ pkg	30	5	0	1
vegetable	⅕ pkg	30	6	1	2
(McCormick/Schilling) Dip Classics					
country herb	1 tsp	10	1	0	0
French onion	¾ tsp	5	1	0	0
garlic & pepper	¾ tsp	5	1	0	0
ranch	¾ tsp	5	1	0	0
spinach	½ tsp	10	1	0	0
spring onion	½ tsp	5	1	0	0
vegetable	½ tsp	5	1	0	0
■ **READY-TO-SERVE**					
(Armour)					
bacon cheddar cheese	2 Tbs	40	2	0	0
bean	2 Tbs	40	6	2	1
cheddar/jalapeño	2 Tbs	35	4	0	0
cheese/chili	2 Tbs	30	3	0	0
nacho bean	2 Tbs	40	6	2	1
(Athenos) hummus					
artichoke & garlic	2 Tbs	45	4	<1	0
black olive	2 Tbs	50	5	1	0
cucumber dill	2 Tbs	60	5	1	0
Greek-style	2 Tbs	60	5	1	0
original	2 Tbs	60	5	1	0
pesto	2 Tbs	50	6	2	0
roasted					
eggplant	2 Tbs	45	4	1	0
garlic	2 Tbs	50	4	1	0
red pepper	2 Tbs	60	6	2	0
scallion	2 Tbs	50	6	2	0
3-pepper/spicy	2 Tbs	60	5	1	<1
(Calavo) guacamole					
medium	2 Tbs	50	4	2	1
mild	2 Tbs	50	4	2	1
spicy	2 Tbs	50	3	2	1

Food and Description	Amount	Total Calories	Total Carbs	Fiber	Sugars
(Dean's)					
bacon & horseradish	2 Tbs	60	2	0	2
creamy dill	2 Tbs	50	2	0	2
creamy taco	2 Tbs	50	2	0	2
French onion					
w/bacon	2 Tbs	60	3	0	2
fat-free	2 Tbs	25	3	0	1
light	2 Tbs	35	3	0	2
original	2 Tbs	60	3	0	1
green onion	2 Tbs	60	3	0	2
guacamole					
regular	2 Tbs	80	1	0	1
zesty	2 Tbs	90	2	0	1
ranch	2 Tbs	60	2	0	2
veggie	2 Tbs	60	2	0	2
(Frito-Lay)					
DIP KITS					
Doritos nacho cheese & spicy queso	1 kit	610	70	5	5
Fiesta cheese dip & scoops	1 kit	450	42	3	1
Frito-Lay brand..French onion	2 Tbs	60	4	0	1
Fritos chili cheese & scoops	1 kit	510	49	2	3
Ruffles & French onion	1 kit	460	32	3	4
Tostitos & cheese	1 kit	430	34	2	<1
PARTY BOWL DIPS					
Southwestern salsa	1 serving	10	2	<1	1
spicy queso	1 serving	40	4	0	1
thick 'n' chunky salsa	1 serving	15	3	1	1
zesty bean & cheese	1 serving	40	4	<1	<1
REGULAR FRITOS TUB DIPS					
bean..hot or original	2 Tbs	40	5	1	0
black bean	2 Tbs	30	6	2	<1
cheddar cheese..mild	2 Tbs	60	4	0	2
chili cheese	2 Tbs	45	3	0	1
French onion	2 Tbs	60	3	0	<1
jalapeño cheese	2 Tbs	50	4	0	2
TOSTITOS DIPS					
all-natural salsa					
hot	2 Tbs	15	3	1	2
medium	2 Tbs	15	3	1	2
mild	2 Tbs	15	3	1	2
fire-roasted tomato salsa	2 Tbs	15	2	1	1
queso supreme	2 Tbs	45	4	<1	<1
restaurant-style con queso	2 Tbs	45	4	<1	<1
roasted garlic–flavored					
(Heinz) T.G.I Friday's					
spinach, cheese & artichoke	2 Tbs	45	2	2	1
(Kaukauna)					
chili con queso deli..medium	2 Tbs	70	5	0	4
French onion	2 Tbs	50	4	0	1
nacho cheese/medium	2 Tbs	80	3	0	3

Food and Description	Amount	Total Calories	Total Carbs	Fiber	Sugars
salsa con queso deli..medium	2 Tbs	70	5	0	4
veggie ranch	2 Tbs	50	3	0	1
(Kraft)					
CHEEZ WHIZ					
Cheezin 'n' Squeezing	2 Tbs	100	4	0	1
light	2 Tbs	80	6	0	4
original	2 Tbs	90	4	0	3
salsa con queso	2 Tbs	90	4	0	3
HANDI-SNACKS					
cheese dip					
& breadsticks	⅓ pkg	110	13	0	3
& crackers	⅓ pkg	100	10	9	2
& Mr. Salty pretzels	⅓ pkg	100	12	0	1
& Ritz crackers	¼ pkg	100	10	0	2
OTHER DIPS..all flavors	2 Tbs	60	3	0	1
(Litehouse)					
FOR FRUIT					
caramel					
fat-free	2 Tbs	110	28	0	16
Hershey's chocolate	2 Tbs	120	24	0	14
toffee..Heath	2 Tbs	120	27	0	16
caramel apple					
fat-free	2 Tbs	120	27	0	19
light	2 Tbs	110	28	0	17
premium	2 Tbs	150	23	0	21
chocolate fat-free	2 Tbs	70	19	<1	12
cinnamon vanilla	2 Tbs	90	9	0	7
strawberry cream	2 Tbs	90	9	0	7
vanilla cream	2 Tbs	90	9	0	7
GLAZES					
apple cinnamon	3 Tbs	70	17	0	0
blueberry	3 Tbs	70	18	0	10
peach	3 Tbs	70	18	0	10
strawberry					
regular	3 Tbs	100	26	0	15
sugar-free	3 Tbs	35	8	0	0
FOR VEGETABLES					
avocado	2 Tbs	140	2	0	1
dill	2 Tbs	150	2	0	1
jalapeño cheddar	2 Tbs	150	1	0	1
onion	2 Tbs	110	2	0	1
ranch	2 Tbs	120	2	0	1
salsa	2 Tbs	60	2	0	2
(Marie's)					
dill	2 Tbs	80	2	0	2
French onion	2 Tbs	80	3	0	2
ranch..home-style	2 Tbs	80	3	0	2
spinach	2 Tbs	85	3	0	2
(Marzetti)					
FOR FRUIT					

Food and Description	Amount	Total Calories	Total Carbs	Fiber	Sugars
caramel apple					
fat-free	2 Tbs	120	27	0	19
light	2 Tbs	110	26	0	14
old-fashioned	2 Tbs	150	23	0	21
chocolate-flavored					
fat-free	2 Tbs	100	25	0	20
natural	2 Tbs	120	21	0	20
cream cheese	2 Tbs	70	10	0	9
peanut butter caramel	2 Tbs	130	16	1	11
FOR VEGETABLES					
bacon ranch	2 Tbs	120	2	0	1
blue cheese	2 oz	180	1	0	0
celery & carrot	1.5 oz	220	2	0	2
dill					
fat-free veggie	2 Tbs	30	6	0	2
light	2 Tbs	60	2	0	1
regular	2 Tbs	140	2	0	1
French onion					
light	2 Tbs	70	3	0	2
regular	2 Tbs	130	2	0	1
guacamole	2 Tbs	120	2	0	1
ranch					
fat-free	2 Tbs	35	6	0	2
garlic..roasted	2 Tbs	140	2	0	1
light	2 Tbs	80	6	0	3
organic	2 Tbs	130	2	0	1
sour cream & onion..fat-free	2 Tbs	35	6	0	2
Southwestern	2 Tbs	30	6	0	2
spinach	2 Tbs	140	1	0	1
veggie					
light	2 Tbs	70	3	0	2
original	2 Tbs	140	2	0	1
singles	2 Tbs	130	2	0	1
(Old El Paso)					
black bean	2 Tbs	25	5	1	<1
cheese 'n' salsa..all styles	2 Tbs	40	3	0	<1
jalapeño	2 Tbs	30	4	2	0
(Phillips) seafood dip..crab & spinach					
original	2 Tbs	60	1	0	0
restaurant recipe	2 Tbs	60	1	0	0
(Skyline Chili)..all styles	2 Tbs	120	2	0	0
(T. Marzetti's)					
FOR FRUIT					
apple dip					
caramel					
fat-free	2 Tbs	150	23	0	21
light	2 Tbs	110	26	0	14
peanut butter	2 Tbs	130	16	1	11
old-fashioned	2 oz	210	35	0	28

Food and Description	Amount	Total Calories	Total Carbs	Fiber	Sugars
chocolate-flavored	2 Tbs	110	23	1	19
FOR VEGETABLES					
blue cheese	2 Tbs	180	1	0	0
dill	2 Tbs	140	2	0	1
ranch					
bacon	2 Tbs	120	2	0	1
fat-free	2 Tbs	35	6	0	2
light	2 Tbs	70	3	0	2
organic	2 Tbs	130	2	0	1
original	2 Tbs	140	1	0	1
Southwestern ranch	2 Tbs	120	2	0	1
spinach	2 Tbs	140	1	0	1
(Tribe of Two Sheiks) hummus					
classic	2 Tbs	50	4	1	<1
dill	2 Tbs	50	4	1	<1
Forty Spice	2 Tbs	50	4	1	<1
jalapeño	2 Tbs	50	4	1	<1
roasted garlic	2 Tbs	50	4	1	<1
scallion	2 Tbs	50	4	1	<1
DISTILLED LIQUOR (*See* LIQUOR, DISTILLED)					
DOCK					
cooked..drained	4 oz	25	3	<1	0
raw..chopped	1 cup	30	4	4	0
DOLPHIN FISH (*See also* MAHI MAHI)					
raw	3 oz	75	0	0	0
DONUT (*See also* BAGEL; COOKIE; PASTRY)					
(Awrey's)					
Dunkers					
almond	2 donuts	240	32	0	17
glazed					
regular	2 donuts	240	32	0	17
rings..4"	1 donut	270	30	1	12
sour cream	1 donut	380	51	0	30
plain..2¼ oz	2 donuts	330	38	0	14
powdered sugar jelly Bismark..4"	1 donut	270	33	1	14
(Dolly Madison)..Gems					
frosted	1 donut	280	30	1	18
powdered sugar	1 donut	250	32	0	15
(Entenmann's)					
Donut Holes..glazed Little Bites	4 pieces	220	28	1	17
Donuts					
classic					
frosted devil's food	1 donut	320	34	2	24
rich frosted/8-count	1 donut	280	27	1	15
ultimate chocolate lover's	1 donut	310	34	2	23
Donut Shoppe					
Popems					
cinnamon	4 pieces	250	32	1	22
glazed	4 pieces	210	29	1	19

Food and Description	Amount	Total Calories	Total Carbs	Fiber	Sugars
holiday	4 pieces	220	32	1	25
rich-frosted holiday	4 pieces	310	27	1	16
Popettes..softee powdered	4 pieces	240	30	1	15
(Hostess)					
Donets					
chocolate	1 donut	180	19	0	12
frosted	1 donut	180	20	1	12
glazed/old-fashioned	1 donut	260	39	1	14
plain	1 donut	140	16	<1	8
powdered	1 donut	150	19	<1	11
raspberry O's	1 donut	230	35	<1	17
(KrispyKreme)					
apple fritter	1 fritter	380	46	2	23
cake					
cinnamon sugar	1 donut	280	37	<1	18
pumpkin spice	1 donut	340	42	<1	27
traditional	1 donut	230	25	<1	9
Caramel Kreme Crunch	1 donut	350	43	<1	25
chocolate					
iced cream-filled	1 donut	350	39	<1	23
iced cruller	1 donut	290	37	<1	25
iced custard-filled	1 donut	300	35	<1	17
malted cream	1 donut	390	49	<1	30
cinnamon twist	1 twist	230	33	<1	19
coffee & cream	1 donut	360	43	<1	27
dulce de leche	1 donut	290	30	<1	12
glazed					
blueberry-filled	1 donut	290	35	<1	18
chocolate-iced	1 donut	250	33	<1	21
w/sprinkles	1 donut	260	38	<1	24
cruller	1 donut	240	26	<1	14
devil's food	1 donut	340	42	<1	27
lemon-filled	1 donut	290	34	<1	18
original	1 donut	200	22	<1	10
raspberry-filled	1 donut	300	39	<1	21
sour cream	1 donut	340	42	<1	27
strawberry-filled	1 donut	290	32	<1	14
twist	1 twist	210	28	<1	16
vanilla-iced	1 donut	240	32	<1	20
honey & oat	1 donut	340	42	<1	27
key lime pie	1 donut	330	40	<1	23
maple-iced	1 donut	240	32	<1	20
New York cheesecake	1 donut	330	36	<1	17
powdered					
cream-filled	1 donut	340	36	<1	19
raspberry	1 donut	300	36	<1	17
vanilla-iced					
cream-filled	1 donut	340	38	<1	23
raspberry-filled	1 donut	350	50	<1	31
w/sprinkles	1 donut	270	35	<1	19

Food and Description	Amount	Total Calories	Total Carbs	Fiber	Sugars
(Little Debbie)					
cake..glazed donut	1 pkg	450	53	0	31
donut sticks..box	1 pkg	230	25	0	16
mini donuts					
frosted	1 pkg	360	39	1	24
glazed	1 pkg	280	41	0	28
powdered/packaged	1.78 oz	210	27	0	15
	2.5 oz	310	38	<1	20
(TastyKake)					
apple fritter..Oxford	1.5 oz	170	21	1	7
Krispy Stix	1.5 oz	180	31	0	14
mini donuts					
bubble gum	6 donuts	250	37	<1	26
cinnamon	6 donuts	210	26	<1	11
plain glaze	6 donuts	270	38	<1	23
powdered sugar	6 donuts	290	37	<1	19
rich frosted	6 donuts	380	42	3	24
regular					
cinnamon	1 donut	210	26	<1	11
coated	1 donut	220	25	2	13
plain	1 donut	210	23	<1	8
premium-frosted	1 donut	250	31	2	17
sugar	1 donut	200	25	1	11
DRESSING (See MAYONNAISE/MAYONNAISE-TYPE DRESSING; SALAD DRESSING; STUFFING/DRESSING)					
DRUM/freshwater..baked	3 oz	130	0	0	0
DUCK					
domesticated					
raw					
liver	1.5 oz	60	0	0	0
roasted					
meat only..breast..boneless	3 oz	120	0	0	0
meat & skin..leg w/bone	3 oz	185	0	0	0
wild..raw					
meat only..breast..boneless	3 oz	105	0	0	0
meat & skin..½ duck	9.5 oz	570	0	0	0
DUMPLING (See also CHICKEN ENTRÉE/DINNER; FROZEN ENTRÉE/DINNER; PASTA ENTRÉE/DINNER; POTATO DISH/ENTRÉE; Potstickers entry in ASIAN FOOD; SOUP; VEGETARIAN FOODS)					
dry/pasta					
(Creamette) yolk-free dumplings	2 oz	210	41	1	2
(Skinner) dumplings	2 oz	210	42	2	2

E

Food and Description	Amount	Total Calories	Total Carbs	Fiber	Sugars
ÉCLAIR (*See* PASTRY)					
EEL					
cooked—dry heat	3 oz	200	0	0	0
raw	3 oz	156	0	0	0
EGG (*See also* EGG SUBSTITUTE; VEGETARIAN FOODS)					
GENERIC					
chicken..raw	1 large	70	1	0	0
duck..raw	1 large	130	1	0	0
goose..raw	1 large	265	2	0	0
quail..raw	1 large	14	0	0	0
turkey..raw	1 large	135	1	0	0
INDIVIDUAL BRANDS					
(Eggland's Best)					
extra-large	1 egg	90	<1	0	0
jumbo	1 egg	90	<1	<1	0
large	1 egg	40	<1	0	0
medium	1 egg	70	<1	<1	0
(Land O' Lakes)					
cage-free all-natural	1 egg	70	1	0	0
extra-large	1 egg	80	1	0	0
large	1 egg	70	1	0	–
(Papetti) refrigerated					
All Whites	~1 oz	25	0	0	0
Quick Eggs	2 oz	30	1	0	1
(Sauder) free-range..extra-large	1 egg	80	1	<1	0
(Wilcox)					
100% organic..brown..large	1 egg	70	1	0	0
Dino super jumbo	1 egg	100	1.5	0	0
Omega-3 fortified..brown egg	1 egg	70	1	0	0
EGG DISH/MEAL (*See also* BREAKFAST SANDWICH; EGG; EGG SUBSTITUTE; FROZEN ENTRÉE/DINNER; VEGETARIAN FOODS; individual FAST FOOD listings)					
FROZEN or REFRIGERATED					
(Chef's Omelet)					
ham & cheese	½ pkg	180	5	0	0
sausage & cheese	½ pkg	240	4	0	0
3-cheese	½ pkg	230	5	0	0
Western-style	½ pkg	150	6	0	0
(Hormel) Quick Meal..microwaveable					
Canadian-style bacon, egg & cheese muffin	4.5 oz	260	29	1	2

Food and Description	Amount	Total Calories	Total Carbs	Fiber	Sugars
sausage, egg & cheese muffin	5.1 oz	400	29	1	2
(Nancy's) quiche..microwaveable single servings					
broccoli cheddar	1 quiche	430	34	2	6
cheese trio bistro favorite	1 quiche	450	32	1	4
(Schwan's) Pour-a-Quiche					
broccoli & cheddar	4.3 oz	180	14	0.5	3
3-cheese	4.3 oz	200	16	4	3
JARRED					
(Penrose) pickled					
5.5-oz jar	1 egg	45	1	1	0
36-oz jar	1 egg	50	1	1	0
EGG ROLL (*See* ASIAN FOOD; FROZEN ENTRÉE/DINNER; SEAFOOD ENTRÉE/DINNER)					
EGG SUBSTITUTE					
(Con Agra) Egg Beaters					
frozen..fat-free	½ cup	30	1	0	1
refrigerated					
cheese & chive	½ cup	30	1	0	1
egg whites	½ cup	30	0	0	1
fat-free pour spout	½ cup	30	1	0	1
garden vegetable	½ cup	30	1	0	1
original	½ cup	30	1	0	<1
Southwestern	½ cup	30	1	0	0
(Just Whites)..dried egg whites	2 tsp	15	4	0	<1
(Morningstar Farms) frozen					
Better 'n' Eggs	¼ cup	20	0	0	0
Scramblers	¼ cup	35	2	0	2
(Papetti Foods)					
Better 'n' Eggs	2 oz	30	1	0	1
The Right Egg	2 oz	30	1	0	1
(Second Nature)					
no-cholesterol	2 fl oz	60	3	0	<1
no-fat	2 fl oz	35	1	0	1
(Tofutti) Egg Watchers	¼ cup	30	1	0	<1
(Wonderslim) fat & egg substitute	¼ cup	35	8	1	na
EGGNOG (*See also* MILK; MILK MIX)					
(Borden) premium/can	4 oz	160	17	0	13
(Dairyland)					
classic	4 oz	155	25	0	22
light	4 oz	108	20	0	18
original	4 oz	118	21	0	17
REFRIGERATED					
(HP Hood) Southern Comfort..nonalcoholic					
Carb Countdown	4 oz	120	9	2	4
fat-free/sugar-free	8 oz	110	18	0	12
golden	4 oz	180	22	0	20
light	4 oz	140	22	0	21
traditional	4 oz	190	24	0	21
vanilla	4 oz	180	22	0	21
vanilla spice	4 oz	210	29	0	22

Food and Description	Amount	Total Calories	Total Carbs	Fiber	Sugars
(Robert's)					
classic	8 oz	190	24	0	23
hometown holiday	8 oz	200	26	0	26
(Sinton's)					
Colorado	4 oz	170	21	0	15
old-fashioned	4 oz	170	21	0	15
EGGPLANT/fresh					
(Frieda's) Japanese..Chinese..raw	⅔ cup	20	5	2	3
(Patak's Original) relish/brinjal					
eggplant & tahini..sweet & spicy	½ oz	70	8	1	6
(Peloponnese) Baba Ganoush					
eggplant & tahini spread	1 oz	40	2	1	0
EGGPLANT DISH (See also FROZEN ENTRÉE/DINNER)					
FROZEN					
(Michael Angelo's) eggplant Parmesan	1 cup	280	23	4	5
(Mrs. Paul's) eggplant Parmesan	½ box	190	18	2	6
ELDERBERRY/raw	1 cup	105	27	10	0
ELK/meat only					
raw	1 oz	31	0	0	0
roasted	4 oz	165	0	0	0
ENCHILADA SAUCE (See MEXICAN FOOD; SAUCE)					
ENDIVE/raw..chopped	½ cup	4	1	1	0
ENGLISH MUFFIN (See MUFFIN)					
ESCARGOT (See SNAIL)					
ESCAROLE/raw	½ cup	4	1	1	0
ESCAROLE SOUP (See SOUP)					
EXTRACTS & FLAVORINGS					
(Durkee)					
almond extract	1 tsp	13	0	0	0
butter flavoring	1 tsp	3	0	0	0
cherry extract	1 tsp	3	0	0	0
chocolate flavoring	1 tsp	7	0	0	0
coconut flavoring	1 tsp	8	0	0	0
lemon extract	1 tsp	17	0	0	0
maple extract	1 tsp	6	0	0	0
orange extract	1 tsp	14	0	0	0
raspberry extract	1 tsp	10	0	0	0
rum flavoring	1 tsp	14	0	0	0
strawberry extract	1 tsp	12	0	0	0
vanilla extract..pure	1 tsp	12	1	0	0
(McCormick/Schilling)					
almond extract	1 tsp	10	0	0	0
anise extract	1 tsp	23	0	0	0
banana imitation extract	1 tsp	11	0	0	0
black walnut extract	1 tsp	12	0	0	0
brandy imitation extract	1 tsp	20	0	0	0
chocolate extract	1 tsp	8	0	0	0
coconut imitation extract	1 tsp	7	0	0	0
mint & peppermint extract	1 tsp	20	0	0	0
pineapple imitation extract	1 tsp	12	0	0	0
root beer concentrate	1 tsp	13	0	0	0
sherry extract	1 tsp	14	0	0	0

FIG 209

F

Food and Description	Amount	Total Calories	Total Carbs	Fiber	Sugars
FAJITA (*See* FROZEN ENTRÉE/DINNER; MEXICAN FOOD)					
FALAFEL..mix only, unless otherwise noted					
(Casbah) mix only	1.5 oz	160	20	2	0
(Fantastic Foods) Fantastic Falafel	¼ cup	120	21	6	3
(Near East) vegetarian					
chickpea/fava bean..prepared	1 cup	230	18	5	3
pita stuffers w/garbanzo beans	1.25 oz	120	21	6	3
FAST FOOD (*See* listings in separate section at end of book.)					
FAT (*See also* BEEF TALLOW; BUTTER; COOKING SPRAY; LARD; MARGARINE, MARGARINE SPREAD & SPRAY; OIL; PORK FAT; SHORTENING, VEGETABLE; SHORTENING SUBSTITUTE)					
bacon fat	1 Tbs	126	0	0	0
beef fat/separable/raw	1 Tbs	108	0	0	0
chicken fat	1 Tbs	115	0	0	0
duck fat	1 Tbs	115	0	0	0
goose fat	1 Tbs	115	0	0	0
pork backfat/raw	1 oz	230	0	0	0
FAT SUBSTITUTE (*See also* OIL; SHORTENING, VEGETABLE; SHORTENING SUBSTITUTE)					
(Wonderslim) fat & egg substitute	¼ cup	35	8	1	na
FAVA BEAN (Progresso) canned	½ cup	110	20	5	0
FENNEL LEAVES/raw..sliced	½ cup	3	1.5	1	0
FENNEL SEED	1 tsp	7	1	0	0
FENUGREEK SEED	1 tsp	12	2	1	0
FIELD PEA					
(Allens)					
regular	½ cup	120	21	6	1
tiny tender..w/snaps	½ cup	120	21	6	1
(Bush's Best) w/snaps	½ cup	110	17	5	0
(Glory Foods)					
regular	½ cup	70	12	5	2
w/snaps	½ cup	80	14	4	2
(Trappey's) flavored w/slab bacon					
tender	½ cup	90	15	5	0
w/snaps	½ cup	110	19	4	0
FIG					
CANNED					
(Oregon Fruit) Kadota..whole in heavy syrup	½ cup	130	30	3	16
DRIED					
(Blue Ribbon Orchard Choice)					

Food and Description	Amount	Total Calories	Total Carbs	Fiber	Sugars
Calimyrna	½ cup	120	28	5	21
Mission					
figlets	1.4 oz	120	28	5	21
figs	½ cup	120	28	5	21
(Krinos) Katanata	3 figs	100	26	4	21
(Sun-Maid) Calimyrna	¼ cup	120	28	5	21
FRESH	1 medium	37	10	2	na
FILBERT/HAZELNUT (*See also* HAZELNUT; HAZELNUT BUTTER/SPREAD)					
(Diamond) in the shell or shelled	1 oz	190	5	3	0
(Planters) chopped	2 oz	350	9	5	2
FILO DOUGH (*See* PASTRY DOUGH)					
FISH (*See* GEFILTE FISH; SEAFOOD ENTRÉE/DINNER; individual listings)					
FISH CHOWDER (*See* SOUP)					
FIVE-SPICE SEASONING (*See* SEASONINGS)					
FLAN (Con-Gelli)..mix..dry mix only					
caramel custard vanilla	⅛ pkg	60	19	0	15
FLATBREAD (*See* CRACKER)					
FLATFISH (*See also* FLOUNDER)					
cooked—dry heat	3 oz	100	0	0	0
FLAVORINGS (*See* EXTRACTS & FLAVORINGS)					
FLAXSEED (Arrowhead Mills)	3 Tbs	140	11	6	0
FLOUNDER (*See also* FLATFISH; SEAFOOD ENTRÉE/DINNER)					
cooked—dry heat	3 oz	100	0	0	0
FLOUR					
(Alma)					
coarse wheat	¼ cup	150	33	<1	<1
fine wheat	¼ cup	150	33	<1	<1
(Arrowhead Mills)					
amaranth	⅓ cup	120	20	2	<1
barley	⅓ cup	95	19	4	0
blue corn meal	⅓ cup	130	25	5	0
brown rice	⅓ cup	130	27	2	0
buckwheat	⅓ cup	115	20	6	<1
kamut	⅓ cup	130	25	4	0
millet	⅓ cup	130	26	3	0
oat	⅓ cup	120	21	3	0
pastry	⅓ cup	110	23	3	0
Perfect Harvest	¼ cup	130	24	4	0
rye	¼ cup	110	23	4	0
soy	¼ cup	100	9	4	0
spelt	⅓ cup	130	25	4	0
white					
rice	⅓ cup	120	28	<1	0
unbleached enriched	¼ cup	120	26	<1	0
yellow cornmeal	⅓ cup	120	27	3	0
(Aunt Jemima)..self-rising	¼ cup	100	24	0	0
(Eden Foods)..whole kamut flour	½ cup	200	37	3	0
(Gold Medal)					
all-purpose	¼ cup	100	22	<1	<1
better for bread	¼ cup	100	22	<1	0
better for wheat bread	¼ cup	100	21	1	0

Food and Description	Amount	Total Calories	Total Carbs	Fiber	Sugars
organic	¼ cup	100	22	<1	0
self-rising	¼ cup	100	22	<1	0
whole wheat	¼ cup	90	21	3	0
(Hodgson Mill)					
50/50 wheat	¼ cup	100	21	2	0
all-purpose..unbleached	¼ cup	100	23	1	0
best for bread	¼ cup	100	22	1	0
pastry whole wheat	¼ cup	110	22	3	0
white	¼ cup	100	21	3	0
whole wheat..graham	¼ cup	100	22	3	0
(Lundberg Family Farms)					
nutra-farmed brown rice	¼ cup	120	36	1	1
organic brown rice	¼ cup	110	22	2	1
(Pillsbury)					
bread	¼ cup	100	22	2	0
rye..medium	¼ cup	100	22	2	<1
Shake & Blend	¼ cup	100	23	<1	<1
white					
all-purpose					
bleached	¼ cup	110	23	0	0
self-rising bleached	¼ cup	100	22	<1	0
unbleached	¼ cup	100	22	<1	0
whole wheat	¼ cup	120	22	4	<1
(Robin Hood)					
best for blending	¼ cup	120	25	0	0
better for bread					
60% whole wheat	¼ cup	120	25	2	0
home-style white	¼ cup	120	25	0	0
multigrain blend	¼ cup	120	25	3	0
rye	¼ cup	122	25	2	0
whole wheat	¼ cup	120	24	4	0
(Softasilk) enriched bleached cake	¼ cup	100	23	1	0
(Wondra) flour	¼ cup	100	23	<1	0

FRANKFURTER (*See also* CORN DOG; FRANKFURTER, VEGETARIAN; SAUSAGE; VEGETARIAN FOODS; individual FAST FOOD listings)

(Armour) jumbo	2 oz	200	5	0	1
(Ball Park)					
Ball Park Franks					
beef	2 oz	180	15	1	4
Better for You					
fat-free					
beef	1.78 oz	55	7	0	2
regular	1.78 oz	50	6	0	2
light					
beef	1.78 oz	100	3	0	1
smoked white turkey..bun-size	1.78 oz	45	5	0	3
bun-size					
beef	2 oz	180	3	0	2
regular	2 oz	180	3	0	2
Grillmaster					

Food and Description	Amount	Total Calories	Total Carbs	Fiber	Sugars
beef	2.9 oz	240	3	0	1
Cajun	2.9 oz	260	4	0	1
garlic	2.9 oz	260	3	0	1
smoky	2.9 oz	260	3	0	2
Singles					
beef	1.6 oz	150	3	0	2
cheese	1.6 oz	150	2	0	2
regular	1.6 oz	150	2	0	2
Smokies	2 oz	180	2	0	1
(Boar's Head)					
beef					
cocktail	5 franks	170	0	0	0
light					
natural casing	1.6 oz	90	0	0	0
skinless	1.6 oz	90	0	0	0
natural casing	2 oz	160	1	0	0
skinless	1.6 oz	120	0	0	0
pork & beef					
natural casing	2 oz	150	0	0	0
skinless	2 oz	150	0	0	0
(Eckrich) jumbo					
cheese	1 frank	180	2	0	1
regular	1 frank	190	2	0	1
turkey, chicken & pork	1.6 oz	140	2	0	0
jumbo	2 oz	170	1	0	0
(Healthy Choice)					
bun-size					
low-fat	1 frank	70	7	0	2
meat	1 frank	70	6	0	1
deli-size	1 frank	100	7	0	2
(Hebrew National)					
franks					
¼-pound dinner	4 oz	350	1	0	0
97% fat-free	1 frank	45	3	0	0
beef					
7-count	1.75 oz	150	1	0	0
reduced-fat	1.7 oz	120	0	0	0
Franks in a Blanket	5 pieces	290	8	1	1
(Hillshire Farm)					
bun-size					
beef	2 oz	180	2	0	0
cheese	2 oz	180	2	0	0
regular	2 oz	180	2	0	0
Lit'l Beef	2 oz	170	2	0	2
Lit'l Smokies					
beef	6 pieces	170	2	0	2
meat	6 pieces	180	2	0	2
wieners					
bun-size	2 oz	180	2	0	0
Lit'l Wieners	6 pieces	170	2	0	2

Food and Description	Amount	Total Calories	Total Carbs	Fiber	Sugars
(Hormel)					
cocktail franks					
smokies	6 smokies	170	0	0	0
beef	6 smokies	180	2	0	2
w/cheese	6 smokies	170	1	0	1
	1-oz link	80	0	0	0
corn dogs	2.78 oz	240	24	1	8
hot dogs					
fat-free	1 frank	45	5	0	3
hot dogs/beef					
fat-free	1 frank	45	5	0	2
regular	2 oz	170	0	0	0
(Johnsonville)					
cocktail links/fully cooked					
beef links	6 links	180	2	0	0
Little Smokies	6 links	180	1	0	0
wieners	1.75 oz	150	1	0	0
(Oscar Mayer)					
corn dogs..5-count	3.25 oz	260	25	1	9
Little Smokies					
cheese	2 oz	180	2	0	1
regular	2 oz	170	1	0	1
Lunchables..All Star					
hot dogs	1 box	450	64	1	40
hot dogs w/cola	1 box	480	69	1	46
turkey franks..all styles	1 frank	100	2	0	1
XXL Hot Dogs					
deli-style beef franks	2.7 oz	230	1	0	0
original smoked hot dogs	2.7 oz	240	1	0	0
premium					
beef franks	2.7 oz	240	1	0	0
hot & spicy hot dogs	2.7 oz	210	1	0	1
(Shelton's) turkey franks	1.2 oz	60	1	0	0
(Wranglers)					
beef	1 frank	170	1	0	1
cheese	1 frank	170	1	0	1
jalapeño	1 frank	170	1	0	1
smoked	1 frank	170	1	0	1

FRANKFURTER, VEGETARIAN (See VEGETARIAN FOODS)
FRENCH FRIES (See FROZEN ENTRÉE/DINNER; POTATO; individual FAST FOOD listings)
FRENCH ONION SOUP (See SOUP)
FRENCH TOAST
bread

Food and Description	Amount	Total Calories	Total Carbs	Fiber	Sugars
(Arnold) cinnamon French toast	1 slice	100	15	1	4
(Pepperidge Farm) sweet bread					
brown sugar & cinnamon	1 slice	140	25	1	8
French vanilla	1 slice	140	23	<1	7
maple syrup & cinnamon	1 slice	130	25	2	7

frozen
(Aunt Jemima)

Food and Description	Amount	Total Calories	Total Carbs	Fiber	Sugars
SLICES					
cinnamon..12.5-oz box/6-count	2 slices	220	34	2	6
home-style	2 slices	240	39	2	6
STICKS					
cinnamon..12-count box	4 sticks	350	52	1	16
cinnamon sticks..w/syrup cups	6.6 oz	540	101	2	46
(Bob Evans) stuffed French toast					
w/apples & cream cheese	1 box	460	70	2	42
w/berries & cream cheese	1 box	360	68	3	39
(Eggo) French Toaster Sticks					
chocolate chip	2 slices	210	35	1	10
cinnamon	2 slices	220	37	1	15
original	2 slices	220	36	1	11
FRITTER (*See* CORN DISH; DONUT; PASTRY)					
FROG..legs..raw	3.5 oz	70	0	0	0
FROSTING (*See* CAKE FROSTING/ICING)					
FROZEN ENTRÉE/DINNER (*See also* ASIAN FOOD; BEEF DISH/ENTRÉE; CHICKEN ENTRÉE/DINNER; MEXICAN FOOD; PASTA ENTRÉE/DINNER; PIZZA; POTATO DISH/ENTRÉE; RICE DISH; VEGETARIAN FOODS)					
■ (Advance)					
ADVANCE FAST FIXIN'					
BBQ ribs	3 oz	120	8	0	3
beef					
fingers..12-oz tray	3 oz	260	15	2	1
meatballs					
12-oz tray	3 oz	250	5	2	0
28-oz tray	3 oz	260	6	2	2
Italian	3 oz	200	3	1	0
patties/breaded	3 oz	260	15	2	1
chicken breast					
nuggets	3 oz	200	13	2	0
nuggets/cheese	3 oz	200	18	1	0
patties	3 oz	200	13	2	0
popcorn chicken	3.3 oz	190	14	0	0
strips	3 oz	200	13	2	0
chuckwagon patties..beef & turkey	3 oz	260	15	2	1
RESTAURANT-STYLE..FAST FIXIN'					
beef					
burgers	3 oz	230	1	0	0
country-fried steak	4.55 oz	350	1	1	0
Philly beef steak	3.5 oz	80	3	1	1
steak fingers	3.25 oz	230	25	7	4
chicken					
breast tenders	2 oz	100	7	0	0
breasts					
chicken-fried	4.55 oz	330	24	0	0
fire-roasted	5 oz	180	3	0	1
tenders					
BBQ-style	4.8 oz	180	4	0	4
buffalo-style..20-oz bag	2 oz	210	13	1	0

Food and Description	Amount	Total Calories	Total Carbs	Fiber	Sugars
fajitas					
beef	3 oz	140	2	0	0
chicken					
breast	2.4 oz	100	1	0	0
thigh	3 oz	140	1	0	0
■ (Banquet)					
BONE-IN CHICKEN					
fried chicken pieces					
country fried..8 pieces	3 oz	280	7	0	1
honey BBQ..skinless..8 pieces	3 oz	220	4	0	3
hot & spicy..8 pieces	3 oz	280	7	0	1
original..8 pieces	3 oz	250	13	0	1
skinless..8 pieces	3 oz	240	11	0	1
Southern fried..8 pieces	3 oz	280	7	0	1
wings					
honey BBQ	3 oz	220	4	0	3
hot & spicy	3 oz	240	8	0	<1
BONELESS CHICKEN & MISCELLANEOUS					
nuggets					
breast	7 nuggets	280	13	1	2
fun..our original	4 nuggets	300	10	<1	3
mozzarella	6 nuggets	280	19	1	3
original	5 nuggets	290	14	1	1
plain	7 nuggets	280	13	1	2
Southern fried	6 nuggets	260	15	1	4
patties					
breast..grilled	1 patty	110	3	1	0
fat-free	1 patty	100	15	<1	3
original	1 patty	240	12	1	3
Southern fried	1 patty	230	16	0	2
popcorn chicken	11 pieces	190	18	1	2
tenders					
fat-free	3 tenders	120	16	<1	2
original	5 tenders	250	15	<1	1
Southern fried	5 tenders	260	16	1	<1
FAMILY-SERVE ENTRÉES					
gravy					
& charbroiled beef	1 patty	210	6	3	1
& meat loaf	1 serving	170	5	1	2
& Salisbury steak	1 serving	230	6	1	2
& sliced beef	1 serving	120	3	<1	2
& sliced turkey	1 serving	130	5	1	1
lasagna w/meat sauce	1 cup	230	6	1	2
macaroni & cheese	1 cup	200	30	2	6
noodles & beef	1 cup	150	16	2	1
HEARTY ONES					
chicken fried steak	1 meal	820	63	6	13
chicken fried steak meal	1 meal	630	42	8	8
fried chicken	1 meal	910	70	5	8
pot pies					

Food and Description	Amount	Total Calories	Total Carbs	Fiber	Sugars
chicken	½ pie	510	44	3	6
turkey	½ pie	510	44	3	6
pork rib	1 meal	720	62	7	18
Swiss steak	1 meal	740	37	7	7
turkey	1 meal	620	54	10	11
KID CUISINE					
beef patty w/cheese	1 meal	440	56	5	27
cheese pizza	1 meal	430	71	5	34
chicken nuggets meal	1 meal	460	62	4	32
chicken nuggets	1 meal	500	54	4	34
corn dog meal	1 meal	490	70	7	33
fish sticks	1 meal	330	45	4	23
fried chicken	1 meal	600	41	4	9
hamburger pizza	1 meal	400	61	5	32
macaroni & cheese	1 meal	370	58	4	24
taco roll-ups	1 meal	420	55	4	25
MEALS					
BBQ beef patty	1 meal	380	37	7	13
BBQ chicken	1 meal	330	37	2	18
BBQ pork rib	1 meal	400	37	4	22
beef enchilada	1 meal	370	55	8	8
beef patty	1 meal	310	22	2	5
cheese enchilada	1 meal	350	54	8	8
chicken & pasta marinara	1 meal	390	42	6	7
chicken enchilada	1 meal	350	54	9	7
chicken fingers w/brownie	1 meal	570	57	2	22
chicken fried steak	1 meal	420	39	4	9
chicken nuggets	1 meal	410	38	3	4
fish stick	1 meal	470	58	1	28
fried chicken	1 meal	310	22	2	5
fried chicken meal	1 meal	470	35	2	4
fried rice w/chicken	1 meal	330	51	5	3
home-style noodles w/chicken	1 meal	400	45	7	6
honey-roasted turkey	1 meal	230	30	5	5
lasagna w/meat sauce	1 meal	320	46	7	10
macaroni & cheese	1 meal	420	57	5	7
Mexican	1 meal	450	56	8	8
Mexican-style enchilada combo	1 meal	370	55	18	8
meat loaf	1 meal	240	20	4	6
pepperoni pizza	1 meal	480	56	5	30
pork cutlet	1 meal	430	38	6	10
Salisbury steak	1 meal	360	28	3	4
sliced beef	1 meal	270	19	4	12
Swedish meatballs	1 meal	400	33	5	0
turkey	1 meal	270	30	3	7
veal Parmesan w/pasta	1 meal	330	34	3	10
Yankee pot roast	1 meal	210	21	3	6
POT PIES					
beef	1 pie	430	38	2	5
chicken	1 pie	400	35	2	6

Food and Description	Amount	Total Calories	Total Carbs	Fiber	Sugars
chicken & broccoli	1 pie	350	32	2	9
macaroni & cheese	1 pie	210	34	1	10
turkey	1 pie	390	38	3	5
■ **(Barber Foods)**					
STUFFED CHICKEN BREASTS					
broccoli & cheese					
light	1 breast	220	15	1	3
regular	1 breast	330	20	2	2
Cordon Bleu					
w/cheese & ham	1 breast	360	14	1	1
light	1 breast	240	14	0	2
Kiev w/garlic butter & parsley	1 breast	420	16	1	1
w/crème brie & apples	1 breast	320	12	1	7
w/mashed potatoes	1 breast	340	21	1	2
w/scallops & lobster	1 breast	380	25	1	2
STUFFED CHICKEN NUGGETS					
w/cheddar & bacon..breaded	2.4 oz	190	8	0	1
■ **(Birds Eye)**					
EASY RECIPE CREATIONS/gourmet meal starter/as packaged					
basil herb primavera	2 cups	260	31	3	5
Oriental lo mein	2⅓ cups	200	36	2	15
roasted garlic Parmesan	1⅔ cups	240	27	2	6
sesame ginger teriyaki	2¼ cups	140	24	4	15
spicy Szechuan..w/cashews	1¾ cups	180	20	4	18
sweet & sour w/pineapple tidbits	1⅔ cups	200	45	3	41
tortellini parmigiana	2¼ cups	240	25	4	5
SIMPLY GRILLIN'/side dishes					
garden herb	¼ box	140	10	4	6
potatoes & onions	¼ box	180	25	3	1
roasted corn & potatoes	⅕ box	140	19	3	6
roasted garlic	⅕ box	120	17	3	5
VOILÀ! All-in-One Meal/as packaged (unless otherwise noted)					
beef					
steak/sirloin & garlic potatoes	5.7 oz	190	22	5	4
chicken					
Alfredo/prepared	1 cup	240	26	2	5
down-home chicken & vegetables	8.4 oz	180	17	4	5
fajitas	8.4 oz	150	13	3	7
garden herb	6.3 oz	280	30	3	9
garlic	7.3 oz	240	27	2	6
pesto primavera	6.3 oz	210	24	2	7
roasted garlic chicken & vegetables	8.8 oz	120	13	3	4
stir-fry	7.3 oz	160	22	2	13
teriyaki	7 oz	150	15	4	5
3-cheese	7.3 oz	210	44	2	12
Tuscan/chicken & sausage	8.4 oz	170	10	3	6
shrimp/garlic	6.3 oz	220	27	2	6
■ **(Boston Market)**					
BEEF					
filet of beef w/peppercorn					

Food and Description	Amount	Total Calories	Total Carbs	Fiber	Sugars
mustard sauce	1 meal	360	32	2	8
meat loaf w/gravy	1 meal	400	19	3	2
pot roast w/vegetables & mashed potatoes	1 meal	420	37	5	5
Salisbury steak w/mushroom gravy & macaroni	1 meal	750	44	4	4
Swedish meatballs in sauce w/noodles	½ box	440	34	4	7
CHICKEN					
country fried w/mashed potatoes	1 meal	620	43	5	10
glazed rotisserie white meat w/mashed potatoes, gravy & green beans	1 meal	440	28	4	10
home-style chicken w/noodles in creamy sauce w/carrots	1 meal	580	52	4	2
pimavera penne pasta & vegetables	1 meal	520	42	4	6
white meat w/teriyaki sauce	1 meal	460	63	4	17
POT PIES					
chicken	½ box	570	41	2	3
chicken, broccoli & cheese	½ box	630	33	1	4
turkey	½ box	540	42	2	3
SIDE DISHES					
chili bowl	1 bowl	340	31	24	2
mini loaves	1 loaf	210	33	4	5
potatoes..new	½ box	130	18	1	1
soup bowl	1 bowl	200	23	1	2
TURKEY					
breast medallions w/dressing	1 meal	490	42	4	11
oven-roasted breast w/mashed potatoes & gravy	1 meal	420	28	4	8
■ **(Chef America)** stuffed sandwiches, etc.					
CROISSANT POCKET/singles					
chicken Alfredo	1 sdw	320	35	3	8
chicken, broccoli & cheddar	1 sdw	310	34	3	9
chicken Parmesan	1 sdw	370	36	3	10
egg, sausage & cheese	1 sdw	360	34	3	8
5-cheese pizza	1 sdw	390	37	3	10
ham & cheddar	1 sdw	340	36	3	14
meatballs & mozzarella	1 sdw	330	35	3	11
pepperoni pizza	1 sdw	390	39	3	8
Philly steak & cheese	1 sdw	360	33	3	11
turkey bacon club	1 sdw	320	30	3	7
HOT POCKETS/singles					
bacon, egg & cheese	1 sdw	170	20	1	4
barbecue sauce w/beef	1 sdw	340	47	3	12
beef & cheddar	1 sdw	360	39	3	8
beef taco	1 sdw	320	37	3	5
cheeseburger	1 sdw	340	40	3	14
chicken & cheddar w/broccoli	1 sdw	300	38	3	9
chicken fajita	1 sdw	290	36	3	9
chicken melt w/bacon	1 sdw	350	36	3	12

Food and Description	Amount	Total Calories	Total Carbs	Fiber	Sugars
4-cheese pizza	1 sdw	390	41	3	11
4-meat & 4-cheese pizza	1 sdw	360	35	3	5
ham, egg & cheese	1 sdw	150	17	1	4
ham 'n' cheese	1 sdw	310	33	3	7
Italian-style meat trio	1 sdw	350	39	3	7
jalapeño steak & cheese	1 sdw	320	39	3	8
meatballs w/mozzarella	1 sdw	330	39	3	11
pepperoni pizza	1 sdw	360	41	3	12
pepperoni & sausage	1 sdw	380	38	3	9
Philly steak & cheese	1 sdw	370	40	3	15
pizza minis					
double cheese	5 pieces	240	30	2	6
pepperoni	5 pieces	240	20	2	5
sausage & pepperoni	5 pieces	230	29	2	7
sausage, egg & cheese	1 sdw	170	19	1	4
sausage pizza	1 sdw	360	37	3	6
steak fajita	1 sdw	280	34	3	11
3-cheese & chicken quesadilla	1 sdw	320	38	3	7
turkey & ham w/cheese	1 sdw	300	34	3	8
LEAN POCKETS/singles					
barbecue sauce w/beef	1 sdw	290	47	3	11
cheeseburger	1 sdw	280	42	3	11
chicken broccoli & cheddar	1 sdw	260	39	3	9
chicken fajita	1 sdw	260	38	3	7
chicken Parmesan	1 sdw	280	43	3	5
ham & cheddar	1 sdw	280	40	3	7
ham & cheese..Ultra 12 grams					
net carbs	1 sdw	210	10	8	3
meatballs & mozzarella					
original	1 sdw	290	44	3	8
Ultra 12 grams net carbs	1 sdw	200	19	7	4
pepperoni pizza deluxe	1 sdw	280	42	3	6
Philly steak & cheese	1 sdw	280	40	3	6
sausage, egg & cheese	1 sdw	140	19	2	4
sausage & pepperoni pizza	1 sdw	280	41	3	9
steak fajita	1 sdw	260	39	3	10
supreme pizza..Ultra 12 grams					
net carbs	1 sdw	200	19	7	4
3-cheese & chicken quesadilla	1 sdw	280	41	3	8
turkey & ham w/cheddar	1 sdw	280	43	3	8
turkey, broccoli & cheese	1 sdw	270	39	3	8
LEAN POCKETS/value packs					
meatballs & mozzarella..12-count	1 piece	290	44	3	8
pepperoni pizza..12-count	1 piece	280	42	4	7
Philly steak & cheese..12-count	1 piece	280	40	3	6
POT PIE EXPRESS/singles					
chicken	1 pie	350	40	2	9
chicken & broccoli	1 pie	350	40	3	6
turkey	1 pie	340	35	3	4

Food and Description	Amount	Total Calories	Total Carbs	Fiber	Sugars
■ (Chef's Choice)					
BOWLS					
beef					
garlic beef & broccoli	1 bowl	360	10	5	<1
hearty beef stew	1 bowl	270	9	3	6
chicken					
cacciatore	1 bowl	310	12	3	5
fajita	1 bowl	330	9	3	5
primavera	1 bowl	330	10	4	6
pork					
Mexican-style	1 bowl	370	9	3	6
shrimp					
stir-fry	1 bowl	130	11	4	5
Toscana	1 bowl	370	10	1	5
CHICKEN					
Alfredo	1¼ cups	330	31	4	1
fried rice	1⅓ cups	270	40	2	9
garlic primavera	1½ cups	230	29	5	2
marinara	1⅔ cups	250	26	4	7
Santa Fe	1⅔ cups	270	33	4	6
stir-fry	1⅔ cups	220	23	5	18
SHRIMP					
shrimp Alfredo	1¼ cups	280	31	4	1
fried rice	1½ cups	230	37	3	12
linguini	1⅓ cups	190	33	4	3
stir-fry	1⅔ cups	160	23	4	18
■ (Delimex)					
taquitos					
beef	5 pieces	370	49	8	0
chicken	4.8 oz	370	47	8	0
3-cheese	5 pieces	400	50	6	2
■ (Dining In)					
seafood favorites					
catfish w/shrimp & 7 vegetables	1 pkg	120	4	1	0
stuffed green peppers..w/sauce	¼ pkg	200	19	1	6
■ (Ethnic Gourmet)					
INDIAN-STYLE					
chicken					
biryani	1 bowl	410	57	3	7
korma	1 meal	360	34	3	5
tandoori w/spinach	1 meal	330	39	5	3
tikka masala	1 meal	350	37	7	5
JAPANESE-STYLE					
teriyaki					
chicken	1 bowl	340	63	2	9
vegetarian	1 bowl	330	71	4	12
KOREAN-STYLE					
beef bulgogi..beef & vegetables	1 meal	350	36	2	10
SINGAPOREAN-STYLE					
Singapore noodles	1 bowl	290	44	8	4

Food and Description	Amount	Total Calories	Total Carbs	Fiber	Sugars
THAI-STYLE					
chicken massaman	1 meal	330	44	4	13
chicken pad Thai	1 meal	430	71	3	20
lemongrass & basil chicken	1 meal	400	53	4	11
pad Thai w/shrimp	1 bowl	350	64	3	13
VIETNAMESE-STYLE					
Thit Ga Kho Tieu..chicken & vegetables	1 meal	330	44	8	4
■ **(Freezer Queen)**					
COOK-IN-POUCH					
chicken à la king	1 pouch	60	5	3	2
creamed chipped beef	1 pouch	100	8	6	1
gravy					
& Salisbury steak	1 pouch	150	8	2	1
& sliced beef	1 pouch	60	5	1	1
& sliced turkey	1 pouch	70	6	1	1
DELUXE FAMILY ENTRÉES					
beef & peppers w/rice	1 pkg	230	38	1	3
cheesy chicken & broccoli w/rice	~⅓ pkg	260	35	2	3
chicken & biscuits	⅓ pkg	180	21	3	4
lasagna in meat sauce	8 oz	250	25	4	5
pork ribs in BBQ sauce..boneless	⅙ pkg	200	11	4	8
turkey & dressing w/gravy	8 oz	180	20	3	3
MEALS					
beef					
& peppers w/sauce & rice	1 meal	330	55	1	3
charbroiled patty w/gravy, mashed potatoes, peas & carrots	1 meal	280	16	6	2
sliced w/gravy & mashed potatoes	1 meal	200	16	4	5
chicken					
nuggets w/apple dessert	1 meal	340	30	4	5
patty w/mashed potatoes & corn	1 meal	360	33	5	4
sweet & sour w/rice	1 meal	300	56	5	4
fish sticks w/macaroni & cheese	1 meal	290	34	4	5
lasagna w/meat sauce	1 meal	380	47	4	7
meat loaf w/gravy & mashed potatoes	1 meal	250	20	5	5
pork/boneless rib-shaped patty w/BBQ sauce & vegetables	1 meal	340	27	5	12
pot roast w/gravy & vegetables	1 meal	220	20	4	5
Salisbury steak & gravy w/whipped potatoes	1 meal	280	23	5	4
turkey & gravy w/dressing	1 meal	260	31	1	5
veal parmigiana w/pasta in sauce	1 meal	350	33	9	3
■ **(Green Giant)**					
CREATE A MEAL!/prepared					
beefy noodle	1¼ cups	350	31	3	4
cheesy pasta & vegetables	1¼ cups	420	29	2	9
chicken Alfredo	1¼ cups	400	36	3	8
garlic herb chicken	1¼ cups	380	30	3	3
home-style stew	1 cup	340	24	3	4
lemon pepper chicken	1⅔ cups	310	30	5	7

Food and Description	Amount	Total Calories	Total Carbs	Fiber	Sugars
lo mein	1¾ cups	320	33	3	9
skillet lasagna	1¼ cups	340	31	3	10
stir-fry					
garlic & ginger	1½ cups	270	25	4	14
teriyaki	1¼ cups	230	18	4	10
sweet & sour	1¼ cups	340	43	3	31
Szechuan	1¼ cups	310	20	4	12
SKILLET MEALS/as packaged					
beef stew	¼ pkg	180	27	4	5
chicken Alfredo	¼ pkg	270	35	2	5
chicken lo mein	¼ pkg	200	30	3	7
chicken teriyaki	¼ pkg	180	27	4	5
chicken & cheesy pasta	¼ pkg	260	31	2	5
creamy chicken noodle	¼ pkg	290	42	3	11
garlic chicken pasta	¼ pkg	260	31	2	5
steak teriyaki	¼ pkg	250	45	3	8
sweet & sour chicken	¼ pkg	320	62	3	22
■ **(Healthy Choice)**					
DINNER MEALS					
beef pot roast	1 meal	320	30	6	24
beef Stroganoff	1 meal	320	39	6	14
beef tips portobello	1 meal	280	28	3	16
blackened chicken	1 meal	300	36	5	15
boneless beef ribs w/BBQ sauce	1 meal	360	47	8	18
charbroiled beef patty	1 meal	310	37	6	24
chicken broccoli Alfredo	1 meal	300	34	2	5
chicken enchiladas	1 meal	360	59	8	3
chicken parmigiana	1 meal	320	40	6	10
chicken teriyaki	1 meal	270	37	6	14
country-breaded chicken	1 meal	370	55	5	23
country herb chicken	1 meal	280	37	5	19
grilled turkey breast	1 meal	250	31	5	19
herb-baked fish	1 meal	360	51	6	12
honey-glazed chicken	1 meal	320	46	6	8
lemon pepper fish	1 meal	280	46	4	17
mesquite chicken BBQ	1 meal	300	44	5	14
oven-roasted beef	1 meal	280	33	5	7
roasted chicken breast	1 meal	280	32	7	8
Salisbury steak	1 meal	360	45	5	19
stuffed pasta shells	1 meal	290	40	5	10
sweet & sour chicken	1 meal	340	54	3	21
traditional meat loaf	1 meal	340	36	6	17
traditional turkey breast	1 meal	330	50	4	26
ENTRÉES & QUICK MEALS					
beef teriyaki	1 meal	310	44	5	17
breaded chicken breast strips					
w/macaroni & cheese	1 meal	290	35	3	5
cheddar broccoli potatoes	1 meal	270	41	7	7
cheesy rice & chicken	1 meal	250	28	4	8
chicken breast & vegetables	1 meal	260	32	2	4

Food and Description	Amount	Total Calories	Total Carbs	Fiber	Sugars
chicken carbonara	1 meal	290	32	2	4
chicken enchilada	1 meal	300	46	6	4
chicken fettuccini Alfredo	1 meal	290	32	3	3
chicken piccata	1 meal	260	36	2	5
country-glazed chicken	1 meal	230	28	3	3
fettuccini Alfredo	1 meal	280	40	3	5
grilled chicken breast					
& pasta	1 meal	250	225	4	6
w/mashed potatoes	1 meal	190	19	3	0
home-style chicken & pasta	1 meal	250	28	5	6
lasagna bake	1 meal	270	38	4	13
macaroni & cheese	1 meal	290	44	5	5
mandarin chicken	1 meal	250	36	4	10
manicotti w/3 cheeses	1 meal	280	44	4	16
Oriental-style chicken	1 meal	240	28	4	5
rigatoni w/broccoli & cheese	1 meal	270	29	5	4
roasted turkey breast	1 meal	220	23	3	1
Salisbury steak & red-skin potatoes	1 meal	200	20	4	5
sesame chicken	1 meal	260	34	4	9
slow-roasted turkey breast					
& mashed potatoes	1 meal	210	17	4	1
spaghetti & sauce w/seasoned beef	1 meal	310	48	7	8
tuna casserole	1 meal	270	31	5	4
FLAVOR ADVENTURES					
beef					
merlot	1 meal	240	25	6	6
Oriental-style	1 meal	310	33	5	4
steak/grilled					
in roasted garlic sauce	1 meal	220	22	5	8
in whiskey	1 meal	280	38	6	18
chicken					
creamy herb-roasted	1 meal	240	29	5	7
grilled basil	1 meal	330	37	5	4
grilled Caesar	1 meal	300	33	5	3
grilled marinara	1 meal	270	35	5	8
Margherita	1 meal	340	42	6	11
princess	1 meal	310	41	5	5
roasted chardonnay	1 meal	290	32	4	2
Tuscan	1 meal	340	39	4	4
MIXED GRILLS					
steak					
BBQ sauce	1 meal	420	59	7	24
w/teriyaki dip sauce	1 meal	350	39	11	23
w/zesty steak sauce	1 meal	350	44	8	16
■ **HOT POCKETS** (*See* (Chef America) in this section)					
■ **(Italian Village)**					
cavatelli/low-salt	3.5 oz	250	51	2	2
gnocchi/potato	4.6 oz	260	54	4	3
manicotti/cheese	3.3 oz	190	16	1	0
ravioli					

Food and Description	Amount	Total Calories	Total Carbs	Fiber	Sugars
beef square	4 oz	220	38	2	2
bite-size/cheese	4 oz	220	35	1	3
cheese					
garlic lover's square	4 oz	200	34	1	3
large round	4.8 oz	240	34	1	3
mini round	4 oz	220	35	1	3
square	3.7 oz	190	16	1	0
Villa Prima					
Florentine	4.5 oz	210	35	1	4
4-cheese	4.5 oz	260	33	1	3
garlic basil	4 oz	170	29	2	3
portobello mushroom	4 oz	170	29	2	3
tortellini					
cheese	3.5 oz	230	42	2	2
meat	3.5 oz	250	43	2	2
■ **KID CUISINE** (*See* (Banquet) in this section)					
■ (Lean Cuisine)					
CAFÉ CLASSICS/meals					
beef					
orange	1 meal	300	42	2	14
Oriental	1 meal	210	33	2	8
oven-roasted	1 meal	210	18	2	9
peppercorn	1 meal	220	25	3	8
portobello	1 meal	220	25	3	5
pot roast	1 meal	200	25	2	4
Southern beef tips	1 meal	250	37	3	12
bow tie pasta & chicken	1 meal	220	31	3	6
chicken					
w/almonds	1 meal	260	38	2	12
w/basil cream sauce	1 meal	260	30	2	4
carbonara	1 meal	270	31	2	5
fiesta-grilled	1 meal	260	31	3	6
glazed	1 meal	230	25	1	6
grilled	1 meal	160	15	4	4
herb-roasted	1 meal	190	23	3	5
honey mustard	1 meal	260	38	1	11
in peanut sauce	1 meal	280	32	2	6
marsala	1 meal	140	12	3	4
Mediterranean	1 meal	260	38	4	6
à l'orange	1 meal	230	35	2	10
Parmesan	1 meal	270	36	2	9
piccata	1 meal	270	41	1	8
w/roasted garlic	1 meal	230	28	1	2
sesame	1 meal	320	48	2	13
sweet & sour	1 meal	290	51	1	20
teriyaki	1 meal	280	42	0	11
& vegetables	1 meal	250	33	3	4
baked	1 meal	230	32	2	5
fish..baked	1 meal	290	32	2	5
meat loaf & whipped potatoes	1 meal	270	30	3	4

Food and Description	Amount	Total Calories	Total Carbs	Fiber	Sugars
pork..honey-roasted	1 meal	230	34	3	11
shrimp & angel hair pasta	1 meal	240	34	2	7
turkey					
glazed tenderloins	1 meal	270	39	4	19
roasted breast	1 meal	270	51	3	30
DINNERTIME SELECTIONS					
beef					
Salisbury steak	1 meal	320	35	6	9
steak tips Dijon	1 meal	310	44	5	11
chicken					
fettuccini	1 meal	380	51	5	9
Florentine	1 meal	370	53	6	9
glazed	1 meal	310	39	3	7
grilled w/penne pasta	1 meal	340	46	5	7
Oriental-glazed	1 meal	330	58	2	14
roasted	1 meal	320	48	4	7
Tuscan	1 meal	270	34	3	9
rigatoni..jumbo	1 meal	390	50	6	10
turkey breast..roasted	1 meal	340	50	6	13
EVERYDAY FAVORITES					
Alfredo pasta w/chicken & broccoli	1 meal	270	38	3	6
angel hair pasta	1 meal	260	48	4	10
cheddar potato, deluxe	1 meal	260	35	5	8
cheese					
cannelloni	1 meal	240	31	3	8
ravioli	1 meal	260	38	3	10
chicken					
chow mein	1 meal	230	35	2	3
enchilada suiza	1 meal	290	48	3	7
fettuccini	1 meal	270	34	2	6
honey Dijon grilled	1 meal	230	25	3	15
lasagna					
5-cheese	1 meal	310	44	4	11
Florentine	1 meal	270	37	3	9
w/meat sauce	1 meal	310	43	3	9
mandarin	1 meal	270	46	2	11
roasted	1 meal	260	33	2	3
fettuccini Alfredo	1 meal	280	40	2	7
hunan beef & broccoli	1 meal	230	36	1	9
lasagna					
cheese Florentine bake	1 meal	270	36	3	7
classic 5-cheese	1 meal	310	44	4	11
w/meat sauce	1 meal	310	43	3	9
macaroni & beef	1 meal	270	38	3	8
macaroni & cheese	1 meal	300	42	1	8
penne pasta	1 meal	270	50	5	13
potato					
cheddar deluxe	1 meal	260	35	5	8
roasted w/broccoli	1 meal	240	37	4	8
potstickers/Oriental-style	1 pkg	320	55	3	11

Food and Description	Amount	Total Calories	Total Carbs	Fiber	Sugars
Santa Fe rice & beans	1 meal	300	53	5	10
spaghetti					
w/meatballs	1 meal	260	37	3	7
w/meat sauce	1 meal	240	35	3	7
steak tips portobello	1 meal	130	13	3	5
stuffed cabbage	1 meal	190	26	4	6
Swedish meatballs	1 meal	290	36	2	5
teriyaki stir-fry	1 meal	300	49	3	11
3-bean chili w/rice	1 meal	270	43	8	11
turkey..roasted w/vegetables	1 meal	120	13	4	4
vegetable egg roll	1 meal	330	62	3	16
■ LEAN POCKETS (See (Chef America) in this section)					
■ (Marie Callender's)					
FAMILY-SERVE ENTRÉES					
country fried chicken & gravy	1 serving	460	39	2	11
escalloped noodles & chicken	1 cup	360	27	1	5
fettuccini Alfredo chicken & broccoli	1 serving	390	27	2	2
lasagna	1 cup	310	27	2	9
lasagna w/meat sauce	1 cup	310	18	2	6
meat loaf w/mashed potatoes	1 serving	250	17	2	4
Salisbury steak w/macaroni & cheese	1 serving	470	31	2	3
turkey w/mashed potatoes	1 serving	310	18	2	6
DINNERS					
beef stroganoff	1 meal	410	39	6	5
beef tips..sliced in gravy	1 meal	410	34	6	11
chicken fried steak	1 meal	640	46	7	9
chicken					
Cordon Bleu	1 meal	490	38	5	5
honey-roasted	1 meal	470	24	7	8
parmigiana	1 meal	580	24	6	5
Southwestern	1 meal	360	33	6	9
country fried chicken	1 meal	660	63	9	13
fish w/macaroni & cheese	1 meal	400	36	6	14
grilled chicken & mashed potatoes	1 meal	470	30	2	4
ham steak	1 meal	410	43	5	22
herb-roasted chicken &					
mashed potatoes	1 meal	580	24	6	5
meat loaf w/mashed potatoes	1 meal	510	34	5	10
pork chop dinner	1 meal	630	53	6	7
pot roast	1 meal	400	35	6	9
roast beef	1 meal	380	27	7	7
Salisbury steak	1 meal	440	34	6	14
sweet & sour chicken	1 meal	580	76	6	39
turkey w/gravy & dressing	1 meal	360	36	6	11
ONE-DISH CLASSICS					
cheese ravioli..marinara sauce	1 meal	610	80	10	23
cheesy chicken breast & rice	1 meal	470	39	3	11
chicken					
breast & rice w/cream sauce	1 meal	560	56	4	5

Food and Description	Amount	Total Calories	Total Carbs	Fiber	Sugars
carbonara	1 meal	520	57	3	5
chunky w/noodles	1 meal	650	54	3	5
teriyaki	1 meal	420	72	4	33
chili..w/corn bread	1 meal	480	49	11	15
country beef stew & corn bread	1 meal	430	69	5	8
fettuccini					
Alfredo	1 meal	900	73	6	5
w/broccoli & chicken	1 meal	730	49	3	5
primavera	1 meal	550	57	6	8
grilled chicken breast w/pasta	1 meal	570	64	3	6
lasagna bake w/meat sauce	1 meal	470	52	3	13
macaroni & cheese	1 cup	340	39	1	9
meat lasagna	1 cup	270	25	4	9
spaghetti & meat sauce	1 meal	690	86	11	14
stuffed pasta medley	1 meal	470	53	4	15
Swedish meatballs	1 meal	560	56	3	12
turkey breast medallions w/pasta	1 meal	630	58	4	5
POT PIES..9.5-oz					
beef	1 pie	650	50	2	7
chicken	1 pie	660	53	3	9
chicken & broccoli	1 pie	670	54	4	11
chicken au gratin	1 pie	660	43	3	9
turkey	1 pie	660	56	3	9
■ **(Michael Angelo's)**					
chicken Parmesan	1 meal	730	101	3	7
eggplant Parmesan	1 meal	280	23	4	5
fettuccini Alfredo/baked chicken breast	1 meal	740	95	2	4
Italian-style sausage w/classic sauce	1 meal	160	5	1	3
lasagna					
w/meat sauce	9 oz	290	26	4	5
vegetable	8 oz	230	23	3	1
Tre Bella Ravioli..spinach & pepperoni	1 meal	280	23	4	5
■ **(Michelina's)**					
AUTHENTICO					
black bean chili w/rice	1 pkg	400	76	10	3
chicken					
& vegetable stir-fry	1 pkg	200	29	3	4
fried	1 pkg	310	27	2	3
glazed w/rice	1 pkg	250	45	2	8
littles	1 pkg	300	31	2	0
pop'n chicken	1 pkg	350	38	3	0
primavera w/spirals	1 pkg	250	36	3	3
corn dawgs	1 dawg	320	37	2	5
fettuccini Alfredo	1 pkg	370	46	3	4
fettuccini primavera w/chicken	1 pkg	270	37	3	3
lasagna					
Alfredo	1 pkg	340	38	2	4
4-cheese	1 pkg	280	43	3	4
4-cheese layered	1 pkg	260	30	1	7

Food and Description	Amount	Total Calories	Total Carbs	Fiber	Sugars
w/meat sauce	1 pkg	280	40	3	7
linguini w/clams	1 pkg	290	50	2	2
macaroni					
& cheese	1 pkg	240	41	2	4
& cheese w/ham	1 pkg	310	34	2	5
& sharp cheddar cheese	1 pkg	400	50	3	5
meatballs & mashed potatoes	1 pkg	270	20	2	3
meat loaf	1 pkg	270	20	2	3
noodles					
w/chicken, peas & carrots	1 pkg	260	34	2	3
Romanoff w/meatballs	1 pkg	300	42	3	7
stroganoff	1 pkg	320	35	2	2
penne w/chicken	1 pkg	330	48	2	4
pepper steak w/rice	1 pkg	250	43	1	5
ravioli/cheese	1 pkg	390	42	2	5
rigatoni/cheese-stuffed	1 pkg	300	42	3	7
roast turkey	1 pkg	250	32	2	7
roasted sirloin supreme	1 pkg	230	30	2	2
Salisbury steak	1 pkg	290	22	2	3
spaghetti & meatballs	1 pkg	300	44	4	6
Swedish meatballs	1 pkg	390	41	3	4
teriyaki chicken w/rice	1 pkg	280	64	1	7
vegetable chicken stir-fry	1 pkg	200	29	3	4
LEAN GOURMET					
beef pepper steak w/rice	1 pkg	260	43	1	5
beef stroganoff	1 pkg	250	38	2	2
cheese manicotti	1 pkg	290	48	3	7
chicken					
Alfredo Florentine	1 pkg	250	41	2	4
French recipe	1 pkg	180	23	4	4
glazed	1 pkg	260	45	2	9
fettuccini Alfredo	1 pkg	270	38	2	5
lasagna..5-cheese	1 pkg	220	36	5	8
macaroni & cheese	1 pkg	300	51	3	5
meat loaf	1 pkg	210	22	2	3
pasta in wine & mushroom sauce	1 pkg	290	46	3	3
rigatoni/cheese-stuffed	1 pkg	260	37	3	8
roasted sirloin supreme	1 pkg	230	30	2	2
Salisbury steak	1 pkg	200	23	2	4
shrimp w/pasta & vegetables	1 pkg	260	37	2	5
spaghetti & meat sauce	1 pkg	280	45	4	6
Swedish meatballs	1 pkg	290	40	3	5
SIGNATURE MEALS					
beef pot roast	1 pkg	260	35	4	3
chicken Alfredo w/broccoli	1 pkg	400	36	3	4
Salisbury steak & gravy	1 pkg	410	35	2	5
shrimp Alfredo	1 pkg	290	31	2	3
■ (Mrs. Paul's) Bowls					
shrimp					

Food and Description	Amount	Total Calories	Total Carbs	Fiber	Sugars
Alfredo	1 bowl	300	39	2	3
fried rice	1 bowl	290	54	2	17
garlic butter	1 bowl	290	48	5	7
stir-fry	1 bowl	330	67	2	25
sweet & sour	1 bowl	310	65	1	16
Thai-style peanut	1 bowl	330	51	4	7
& tortellini	1 bowl	340	58	5	20
■ (Ore Ida)					
BAGEL BITES					
cheese & pepperoni	3.14 oz	210	29	2	5
cheese, sausage & pepperoni	3.14 oz	200	28	2	5
spicy nacho	3.14 oz	240	26	1	1
3-cheese	3.14 oz	200	28	2	3
BAGEL BITES/STUFFED					
pepperoni & cheese	3 oz	210	28	1	3
3-cheese	3 oz	210	26	2	4
ultra 5-cheese	3.14 oz	220	24	1	3
■ (Pagoda)					
ASIAN DELIGHTS					
chicken wings..BBQ seasoned.. 6.5-oz box	1 box	420	16	1	12
RICE POTS					
beef & broccoli	1 box	440	66	3	21
chicken					
sweet & sour	1 box	370	60	2	32
teriyaki	1 box	440	77	2	34
vegetable/teriyaki	1 box	370	78	4	37
WONTONS					
cream cheese	½ box	270	21	1	2
crispy pork	½ box	180	21	2	2
■ (Pepperidge Farm)					
pot pies					
beef	1 pie	490	47	2	4
chicken					
& broccoli	1 pie	490	42	2	9
chunky Parmesan	1 pie	520	57	2	7
creamy Alfredo w/broccoli	1 pie	600	46	4	3
primavera	1 pie	530	49	2	4
roasted	1 pie	410	43	3	7
white meat	1 pie	510	43	3	7
turkey..roasted	1 pie	500	38	2	6
■ (Popper's)					
BREADED					
mushrooms	⅓ box	140	19	2	1
zucchini	⅓ box	210	23	2	2
CHEESE					
crisps/nacho cheddar	4 oz	460	39	3	2
nuggets/mozzarella	⅙ box	90	8	0	0
sticks/mozzarella..8-oz box	⅙ box	90	6	1	1

Food and Description	Amount	Total Calories	Total Carbs	Fiber	Sugars
MINI TAQUITOS					
beef	3 oz	200	24	4	0
chicken	3 oz	210	27	5	0
POPCORN SHRIMP..bourbon-glazed	2.8 oz	210	19	0	1
STUFFED JALAPEÑOS					
cheddar cheese					
big-size	2.5 oz	220	15	1	3
8-oz box	2.66 oz	220	15	1	3
mild	3.5 oz	290	19	2	4
cream cheese	2.66 oz	240	15	2	4
3-cheese	~1 oz	80	6	1	1
■ (Schwan's)..Complete Meals					
baked potato w/broccoli & cheese	2 halves	370	50	4	7
beef					
& broccoli w/rice	1 cup	290	45	2	7
w/chunky mashed potatoes	¼ tray	320	20	8	2
cheese tortellini	1 cup	220	34	3	1
chicken					
& broccoli express	1 bowl	500	68	2	2
& dumplings meal kit	1 cup	200	20	2	3
fajita..meal kit	2 fajitas	290	33	4	3
lo mein express bowl	1 bowl	470	59	5	16
pot pie	1 pie	670	58	5	7
Southwestern-style meal kit	¼ pkg	200	28	3	8
lasagna..single-serve Italian-style	1 tray	340	28	1	12
traditional	1 tray	500	50	4	10
vegetable	1 tray	420	41	4	7
sausage penne Italiano meal kit	¼ pkg	270	26	5	9
shrimp meal kit					
& broccoli Alfredo	¼ pkg	270	23	4	2
stir-fry	¼ pkg	260	45	3	13
stuffed pasta shells	3 shells	320	31	2	1
■ (Stouffer's)					
ENTRÉES					
cheesy spaghetti bake..12 oz	1 meal	430	39	4	6
chicken					
à la king	1 meal	350	45	2	6
enchilada & Mexican rice	1 serving	220	33	2	5
pot pie..10-oz pkg	1 pie	740	56	4	8
creamed chipped beef	½ cup	150	9	0	5
fettuccini Alfredo	1 meal	520	51	4	6
5-cheese lasagna	1 meal	350	41	5	9
lasagna					
bake	1 meal	410	50	5	10
w/meat sauce..10-oz pkg	1 pkg	370	38	4	8
w/tomato sauce & Italian sausage	1 meal	410	44	3	11
macaroni					
& beef w/tomatoes	1 meal	330	42	3	13
& cheese..9-oz pkg	1 pkg	390	44	2	8

Food and Description	Amount	Total Calories	Total Carbs	Fiber	Sugars
& cheese..12-oz pkg	½ pkg	320	31	2	5
& cheese & broccoli	1 meal	350	38	4	4
w/ fish sticks	1 pkg	380	41	1	6
manicotti..3-cheese	1 meal	340	39	2	8
ravioli..roasted chicken..Italian-style	1 meal	360	42	2	7
rigatoni					
cheese-stuffed & ravioli	1 meal	470	51	2	7
Italian sausage-stuffed..Italian-style	1 meal	380	41	2	8
w/roasted white meat chicken	1 meal	430	47	3	3
spaghetti w/meatballs in sauce	1 pkg	380	46	4	8
stuffed green pepper..10-oz pkg	1 pkg	240	24	2	8
stuffed peppers w/beef & sauce	½ pkg	180	21	2	6
Swedish meatballs	1 pkg	510	43	3	4
tuna					
noodle casserole	1 meal	340	34	2	8
tetrazzini	1 meal	370	33	2	5
turkey pot pie..10-oz pkg	1 pie	740	52	4	8
vegetable lasagna	1 pkg	410	41	4	6
Welsh rarebit	~¼ pkg	120	6	1	2
HOME-STYLE					
beef					
green pepper steak	1 meal	280	35	1	5
meat loaf	1 meal	340	28	2	3
pot roast	1 meal	250	28	2	3
Stroganoff	1 meal	350	32	3	3
chicken					
breast					
baked	1 meal	270	21	2	2
fried	1 meal	380	38	1	2
in mushroom gravy	1 meal	370	28	2	6
tenders in BBQ sauce	1 meal	460	40	3	19
fettuccini	1 meal	370	39	3	7
Monterey	1 meal	530	58	4	24
parmigiana	1 meal	440	53	4	10
roasted w/stuffing	1 meal	460	38	3	8
Southwestern-style					
grilled lime	1 meal	490	67	9	9
mesquite-flavored	1 meal	440	50	8	9
fish fillet w/macaroni & cheese	1 meal	410	45	1	7
meat loaf	1 meal	560	46	6	12
pork..roasted	1 meal	320	39	3	18
Salisbury steak	1 meal	350	28	1	5
turkey breast..roasted	1 meal	280	33	2	5
veal parmigiana	1 meal	430	49	5	11
■ **LEAN CUISINE** (*See* (Lean Cuisine) in this section)					
SIDE DISHES					
cheddar potato bake	½ pkg	250	19	1	2
corn soufflé	1 serving	180	21	2	7
creamed spinach	½ pkg	230	8	2	3
harvest apples	½ pkg	210	43	3	36

Food and Description	Amount	Total Calories	Total Carbs	Fiber	Sugars
potatoes au gratin	1 serving	150	20	3	3
spinach soufflé	⅓ pkg	130	10	1	4
whipped potatoes & gravy	~½ pkg	150	16	1	3
■ (Swanson)					
HUNGRY MAN DINNERS					
Angus beef					
meat loaf XXL w/mashed potatoes	1 pkg	860	70	4	7
Salisbury steak w/onion gravy	1 pkg	470	26	4	6
boneless chicken..Southern fried	1 pkg	1010	85	6	2
cheeseburger sandwiches..hero	1 sdw	730	56	4	10
chopped beef steak	1 pkg	640	41	2	5
■ (T.G.I. Friday's)					
chicken					
crispy baked breast strips	⅓ pkg	190	15	1	2
popcorn..bourbon-glazed	⅓ pkg	180	16	1	9
quesadilla rolls	⅓ pkg	100	9	0	0
wings					
BBQ..honey	½ pkg	180	7	1	0
buffalo	⅓ pkg	100	0	0	0
Cheese Teasers..mozzarella	~1 oz	100	9	1	1
dip..spinach, cheese & artichoke	2 Tbs	45	2	2	1
egg rolls..Southwestern	⅓ box	190	20	1	1
pizzas..mini deep-dish					
buffalo-style chicken	⅓ pizza	140	2	0	1
chicken w/honey BBQ sauce	⅓ pizza	150	5	0	4
potato skins					
bacon & cheddar	2.2 oz	160	10	2	1
stuffed					
broccoli & cheddar	⅓ pkg	140	16	4	1
cheddar & bacon	⅓ pkg	170	16	3	1
4-cheese & pepperoni	⅓ pkg	160	16	3	1
■ (Tyson)					
MEAL KITS					
beef					
fajita strips w/vegetables & flour tortillas	½ bag	160	21	1	2
chicken					
fajitas..white meat w/vegetables & flour tortillas	½ bag	130	17	2	3
fried rice w/vegetable blend	½ bag	440	69	5	15
quesadilla w/four tortillas	¼ bag	250	26	3	2
stir-fry w/white rice Oriental-style	½ bag	430	73	5	24
■ (Weight Watchers)					
MAIN STREET BISTRO SELECTIONS/bowls					
beef & vegetable rice	1 bowl	260	40	3	17
chicken stir-fry	1 bowl	300	45	4	6
seafood linguini	1 bowl	290	45	4	3
Southwestern-style chicken	1 bowl	230	35	6	9
teriyaki chicken	1 bowl	280	48	3	5

Food and Description	Amount	Total Calories	Total Carbs	Fiber	Sugars
SMART ONES/meals					
angel hair pasta	1 meal	240	42	4	5
baked potato, broccoli & cheese	1 meal	260	39	6	9
beef pot roast	1 meal	220	9	2	4
broccoli & cheddar & roasted potatoes	1 meal	250	33	4	7
chicken					
enchilada suiza	1 meal	340	38	3	5
fajita supreme	1 meal	260	33	3	4
fiesta	1 meal	210	35	5	5
fire-grilled w/vegetables	1 meal	280	45	2	12
glazed	1 meal	260	45	5	3
golden-baked w/garlic	1 meal	270	42	2	5
honey Dijon	1 meal	210	38	2	9
lemon herb piccata	1 meal	250	36	2	3
marsala	1 meal	170	12	3	4
Mirabella	1 meal	180	30	4	4
Oriental	1 meal	230	34	3	3
oven-roasted	1 meal	260	37	2	2
Santa Fe	1 meal	230	10	3	6
tenderloins w/BBQ sauce	1 meal	300	32	3	10
Thai w/noodles	1 meal	290	39	2	12
fettuccini Alfredo	1 meal	270	39	3	7
lasagna					
Bolognese	1 meal	240	43	4	5
Florentine	1 meal	290	36	5	3
traditional w/meat sauce	1 meal	300	38	3	10
macaroni & cheese..3-cheese	1 meal	290	45	2	2
meat loaf w/gravy	1 meal	260	22	5	1
pepper steak	1 meal	230	32	4	4
peppercorn fillet of beef	1 meal	220	19	3	14
radiatore Romano	1 meal	280	40	4	7
ravioli Florentine	1 meal	220	34	3	7
rigatoni/creamy w/broccoli & chicken	1 meal	240	39	4	7
roast beef w/gravy	1 meal	230	24	4	3
Salisbury steak	1 meal	260	25	4	4
shrimp marinara	1 meal	180	28	4	4
spaghetti					
Bolognese	1 meal	280	43	5	4
marinara	1 meal	280	46	4	7
spicy Szechuan-style chicken w/veg	1 meal	220	34	4	7
Swedish meatballs	1 meal	280	34	3	2
tuna noodle gratin	1 meal	270	38	3	6
turkey..roasted medallions	1 meal	200	33	2	3
turkey..stuffed breast	1 meal	270	37	5	14
ziti..3-cheese marinara	1 meal	290	47	5	5
SMART ONES/Smartwiches					
garden veggies & mozzarella	1 sdw	270	38	3	4
ham & cheddar	1 sdw	270	38	1	6
pepperoni pizza	1 sdw	270	39	2	5

Food and Description	Amount	Total Calories	Total Carbs	Fiber	Sugars
■ **(WOLFGANG PUCK)** (*See also* PIZZA)					
canneiloni..ricotta	1 meal	420	37	13	8
lasagna					
4-cheese	1 meal	480	43	10	3
Italian vegetable	1 meal	410	49	9	8
mushroom	1 meal	440	53	9	4
spicy chicken	1 meal	470	45	13	4
Parmesan..eggplant	1 plate	300	17	6	9
pasta wrap..chicken & spinach	1 container	460	68	6	9
ravioli					
4-cheese	1 meal	330	16	2	5
mushroom & spinach	1 meal	260	15	3	3
sweet potato	1 meal	360	35	4	2
tortellini					
mushroom	1 meal	430	54	6	3
spicy chicken	1 meal	490	51	6	4
■ **YU SING** (*See* ASIAN FOOD)					
FROZEN NONDAIRY DESSERT (*See* FRUIT ICES, BARS & POPS; ICE CREAM & ICE CREAM-LIKE FROZEN DESSERTS; RICE FROZEN DESSERT; SHERBET; TOFU FROZEN DESSERT)					
FRUCTOSE (*See* SUGAR SUBSTITUTE)					
FRUIT (*See* FRUIT, MIXED; individual listings)					
FRUIT, MIXED (*See also* SNACKS)					
CANDIED/GLACÉ					
(S&W)					
cake mix	2 Tbs	90	25	2	20
cherries..all colors	5 pieces	80	20	0	16
citron	39 pieces	90	23	1	17
ginger	39 pieces	90	23	1	17
lemon peel	58 pieces	80	23	2	18
orange peel	58 pieces	80	23	2	18
pineapple					
green, red & natural	1 slice	180	46	0	43
wedges..all styles	5 pieces	80	21	0	20
(Seneca)					
cake mix	2 Tbs	70	18	0	10
cherries..all colors	6 pieces	90	23	0	14
citron	2 Tbs	70	18	<1	10
lemon peel	2 Tbs	70	18	0	10
orange peel	2 Tbs	70	18	0	10
pineapple	2 Tbs	90	21	0	12
CANNED or JARRED					
(Del Monte)					
cherry mixed..Very Cherry	½ cup	90	22	<1	19
chunky mixed					
in extra-light syrup/light	½ cup	60	15	0	14
in heavy syrup	½ cup	100	24	1	23
in 100% juice	½ cup	60	15	0	14
fruit cocktail	½ cup	100	24	1	23

Food and Description	Amount	Total Calories	Total Carbs	Fiber	Sugars
in 100% juice	½ cup	60	15	1	14
individual pull-top can	½ cup	100	24	1	23
light	½ cup	60	15	0	14
mixed fruit					
pull-top can	½ cup	80	20	<1	19
light	½ cup	50	22	<1	19
in 100% juice	½ cup	50	13	<1	12
tropical fruit..individual pull-top can	4.5 oz	80	21	1	20
(S&W)					
fruit cocktail..orchard ripe in heavy syrup	½ cup	90	22	1	20
mixed fruit..natural-style..chunky	½ cup	80	20	1	18
DRIED					
(Del Monte)	½ cup	110	30	5	17
(Sun-Maid)					
fruit bits	1.4 oz	120	29	2	24
goldens & cherries	1.5 oz	130	31	2	27
mixed fruit	1.4 oz	100	25	3	17
tropical trio	1.4 oz	130	34	1	27
(Traverse Bay) fruit medley	1.5 oz	110	26	2	12
FRESH/REFRIGERATED					
(Del Monte)					
Fruit Naturals..tropical medley	½ cup	70	18	<1	16
Orchard Select..premium..mixed	½ cup	80	20	<1	18
Sunfresh papaya/extra-light syrup	½ cup	70	17	1	16
Sunfresh tropical fruit salad					
in light syrup	½ cup	80	20	1	16
in pineapple/passion fruit juices	½ cup	80	21	1	20
(Dole) tropical fruit salad bowls	1 bowl	80	19	1	17
FROZEN (C&W)	1 cup	60	14	2	12
FRUIT & NUT MIX (*See* SNACKS)					
FRUIT COCKTAIL (*See* FRUIT, MIXED)					
FRUIT/FRUIT JUICE DRINK (*See also* FRUIT PUNCH; LEMONADE/LEMONADE-FLAVORED DRINK; SOFT DRINK; SOFT DRINK MIX; TEA; individual listings)					
BOTTLED, BOXED, CANNED, or POUCH					
(After The Fall) bottle..spritzers					
banana Casablanca..83% juice	12 oz	100	19	0	19
black cherry..83% juice	12 oz	180	45	0	36
Key West lime cooler..83% juice	12 oz	100	25	0	24
Mango Montage..90% juice	12 oz	110	27	0	23
(Capri Sun) juice drink..6.75-oz pouch					
grape	1 pouch	100	25	0	25
Mountain Cooler	1 pouch	90	23	0	23
Surfer Cooler	1 pouch	100	27	0	27
(Dole) Paradise Blend	8 fl oz	120	30	1	29
(Fuze) Healthy Infusions/bottle					
cranberry raspberry	9 oz	10	2	0	1
Slenderize	9 oz	10	2	0	1

Food and Description	Amount	Total Calories	Total Carbs	Fiber	Sugars
(Minute Maid)					
bottles					
berry kiwi	12 oz	160	43	0	42
Strawberry Passion	12 oz	170	46	0	44
tropical citrus	12 oz	160	44	0	42
Hi-C Blast/box..Boppin' Strawberry	6.75 oz	100	26	0	25
Hi-C Sour Blast/pouch					
green apples	6.75 oz	100	26	0	25
wild cherry	6.75 oz	110	29	0	28
(R. W. Knudsen) fruit juice spritzers/can					
black cherry	12 oz	170	42	0	34
boysenberry	12 oz	160	40	0	38
cranberry	12 oz	190	45	0	45
kiwi lime	12 oz	130	32	0	28
lemon lime	12 oz	170	41	0	38
Mandango Fandango	12 oz	190	45	0	45
mandarin lime	12 oz	170	42	0	41
orange passionfruit	12 oz	160	40	0	38
red raspberry	12 oz	170	38	0	32
strawberry	12 oz	170	42	0	38
tangerine	12 oz	170	40	0	35
vanilla cream	12 oz	160	35	0	34
(Tropicana) smoothies..fruit flavors	11 oz	250	59	5	46
(V8 Splash) juice drink					
regular					
berry blend	8 oz	110	27	0	27
citrus blend	8 oz	110	27	0	27
fruit medley	8 oz	110	27	0	27
guava passion fruit	8 oz	110	27	0	25
mango peach	8 oz	110	27	0	27
orange pineapple	8 oz	110	27	0	27
peach lemonade	8 oz	110	27	0	27
raspberry lemonade	8 oz	100	26	0	26
strawberry kiwi	8 oz	110	27	0	27
smoothies					
orange cream	8 oz	130	29	1	25
peach mango	8 oz	120	27	0	27
strawberry banana	8 oz	130	30	0	29
tropical colada	8 oz	130	30	1	28
wild berry cream	8 oz	130	30	0	29
(Welch's)					
Harvest Blend	8 fl oz	140	35	0	34
Mango Passion	8 fl oz	180	45	0	44
Mountain Berry Blackberry	8 fl oz	140	34	0	33
orange pineapple apple	8 fl oz	140	35	0	34
sparkling cocktail..all flavors	8 fl oz	160	40	0	38
FROZEN/PREPARED					
(Welch's) from concentrate					
Screaming Wild Berry	8 fl oz	130	34	0	33
Strawberry Breeze	8 fl oz	140	34	0	33

Food and Description	Amount	Total Calories	Total Carbs	Fiber	Sugars
FRUIT ICES, BARS & POPS (*See also* SHERBET)					
(Baskin-Robbins) ices..all flavors	4-oz scoop	130	34	0	34
(Blue Bunny)					
REGULAR TREATS					
banana pops	1 bar	35	8	0	7
Chamoy & Chili	1 bar	70	17	0	13
Chillin' Juice Pops..all flavors	1 pop	40	10	0	8
citrus snacks	1 bar	50	12	0	10
Mickey Shimmy pops	1 pop	50	13	0	10
Peluca's Tamarina & Chili	1 bar	80	18	0	14
Polar pops..24 pack..all flavors	1 pop	40	10	0	8
root beer pops	1 pop	40	10	0	8
Slush pops	1 pop	45	11	0	9
Stitch Bomb pops	1 pop	50	11	0	9
SUGAR-FREE POPS	1 pop	25	7	0	0
(Dreyer's)					
fruit bars					
creamy coconut	1 bar	120	21	0	16
lemonade	1 bar	80	20	0	19
lime	1 bar	80	20	0	19
peach	1 bar	90	23	0	21
strawberry	1 bar	80	21	0	20
tropical	1 bar	100	26	0	26
wild berry	1 bar	80	20	0	18
(Edy's)					
fruit bars					
creamy coconut	1 bar	120	21	0	16
lemonade	1 bar	80	20	0	19
lime	1 bar	80	20	0	19
peach	1 bar	90	23	0	21
strawberry	1 bar	80	21	0	20
tangerine	1 bar	80	20	0	19
tropical	1 bar	100	26	0	26
(Häagen-Dazs) sorbet					
bars..chocolate	1 bar	80	20	1	14
pints					
chocolate	½ cup	120	28	2	20
mango	½ cup	120	30	1	24
orange	½ cup	120	30	1	24
Orchard Peach	½ cup	120	33	1	29
raspberry	½ cup	120	30	2	26
strawberry	½ cup	120	30	1	27
Zesty Lemon	½ cup	120	31	1	27
(Hendrie's)					
ice pops					
citrus stix..all flavors	1 pop	45	11	0	11
kids' karnival stix..all flavors	1 pop	70	15	0	15
mix stix..all flavors	1 pop	40	9	0	8
pop stix..all flavors	1 pop	40	9	0	9
(Hood)					

Food and Description	Amount	Total Calories	Total Carbs	Fiber	Sugars
Hawaiian Punch					
Arctic Surfers..all flavors	1 pop	50	12	0	8
(LifeSavers) pops					
no sugar added..all flavors	1 pop	10	2	0	2
regular..all flavors	1 pop	40	10	0	10
Red, White & Blue pops	1 pop	70	15	0	10
(Kemps)					
fruit bars..12-count box..all flavors	1 pop	50	13	0	12
ice pops.. All American	1 pop	80	10	0	8
Pop Jr.'s..24-count box					
tropical variety	1 pop	80	10	0	8
all other flavors	1 pop	180	20	0	16
(Kool-Aid) Kool-pops..all flavors	1 pop	50	13	0	13
(Luigi's) real Italian ice cups					
cherry	6 oz	110	27	0	22
chocolate fudge	6 oz	160	40	1	31
lemon	6 oz	100	26	0	20
lemon & strawberry	6 oz	110	27	0	20
strawberry	6 oz	120	31	2	24
(Minute Maid) fruit juice bars..					
all flavors	1 bar	60	15	0	14
(Nestlé USA) Ice Screamers					
Bug Pops..all flavors	1 pop	90	23	0	2
Itzakadoozie..all pop flavors	1 pop	90	23	0	17
Tiger Ice..orange & grape striped	1 pop	60	15	0	12
FRUIT JUICE DRINK (*See* FRUIT/FRUIT JUICE DRINK; FRUIT PUNCH; individual listings)					
FRUIT PECTIN					
(Certo)	1 Tbs	2	1	0	0
(Sure-Jell)	¼ tsp	5	1	0	1
FRUIT PROTECTOR (*See also* FRUIT PECTIN)					
(Sure-Jell) Ever-Fresh	¼ tsp	5	<1	0	0
FRUIT PUNCH (*See also* FRUIT/FRUIT JUICE DRINK; SOFT DRINK; SOFT DRINK MIX)					
BOTTLED, BOXED, CANNED, or POUCH					
(Capri Sun)					
fruit/all-natural	6.75 fl oz	100	25	0	20
Mountain Cooler	6.75 fl oz	90	23	0	23
Pacific Cooler	6.75 fl oz	100	25	0	25
Super Cooler	6.75 fl oz	100	27	0	27
Tropical Punch	6.75 fl oz	90	25	0	25
(Hawaiian Punch)					
light	8 oz	45	11	0	11
regular					
Bodacious Berry	8 oz	110	29	0	28
Fruit Juicy Red	8 oz	120	29	0	29
Greenberry Rush	8 oz	120	30	0	29
Mazin' Melon Mix	8 oz	110	29	0	28
Orange Ocean	8 oz	120	29	0	29
Tropical Vibe	8 oz	110	29	0	28
(Hi-C) Hi-C Blast..box..fruit	6.75 oz	100	26	0	25

Food and Description	Amount	Total Calories	Total Carbs	Fiber	Sugars
(Kool-Aid)					
Bursts..tropical	6.75 oz	100	24	0	24
Crystal Light..low-calorie	8 fl oz	5	0	0	0
Splash..all flavors	8 fl oz	120	31	0	31
(Minute Maid) can..fruit/natural	12 oz	150	41	0	40
(Ocean Spray) fruit punch	8 oz	130	32	0	32
(Tropicana)					
citrus	8 fl oz	140	36	0	32
fruit	8 fl oz	130	32	0	32
fruit punch..light	8 fl oz	60	15	0	15
tropical	8 fl oz	130	33	0	30
(Welch's)					
fruit	11.5 fl oz	180	45	0	44
Fruit Harvest	8.45 fl oz	140	34	0	33
Juice Cocktail..fruit punch	8 fl oz	130	31	0	30
(Welchade)					
Screaming Wild Berry	8 fl oz	130	31	0	30
Strawberry Punch	8 fl oz	140	35	0	34
FROZEN OR REFRIGERATED/prepared					
(Minute Maid)					
berry	8 fl oz	110	31	0	30
citrus	8 fl oz	110	30	0	29
FRUIT SALAD (*See* FRUIT, MIXED)					
FRUIT SNACK (*See also* CANDY; individual fruit listings)					
(Betty Crocker)					
Fruit-by-the-Foot..all flavors	1 roll	80	21	0	14
Fruit Roll-Ups..all flavors	1 roll	50	12	0	7
Fruit Snacks..all flavors	1 pouch	80	21	0	14
Fruit String Thing..all flavors	1 pouch	80	21	0	14
Gushers..all flavors	1 pouch	90	20	0	13
(Nabisco)					
Capri fruit rolls..fruit punch	1 pkg	80	16	0	11
fruit snacks					
Blue's Clues/assorted	1 pkg	60	14	0	10
Dora the Explorer	1 pkg	60	14	0	10
Jimmy Neutron/assorted	1 pkg	80	19	0	14
Rugrats/assorted	1 pkg	80	18	0	14
SpongeBob Squarepants.. all flavors	1 pkg	80	19	0	15
FRUIT SPREAD (*See* JAM/JELLY/PRESERVES)					

G

Food and Description	Amount	Total Calories	Total Carbs	Fiber	Sugars
GARBANZO BEAN (*See* CHICKPEA)					
GARLIC (*See also* SEASONINGS)					
FRESH/RAW					
(Frieda's Elephant)	1 Tbs	5	1	0	0
minced	1 clove	4	1	0	0
whole	1 clove	5	1	0	0
JARRED					
(Christopher Ranch)					
crushed/minced	1 tsp	10	4	0	0
roasted	2 cloves	10	2	0	0
(Frieda's) marinated	1 oz	30	7	0	0
POWDERED (*See* SEASONINGS)					
GARLIC SALT (*See also* SEASONINGS)	¼ tsp	0	0	0	0
GAZPACHO (*See* SOUP)					
GEFILTE FISH					
(Manischewitz)					
jelled broth..fish only	1 piece	70	3	<1	<1
non-jelled	1 piece	70	1	<1	<1
sweet..2.5-oz piece	1 piece	50	4	<1	1
whitefish & pike..jelled broth					
fish only	1 piece	50	3	<1	<1
w/jell	1 piece	70	3	<1	<1
(Mother's)					
all whitefish					
jelled..1.5-oz piece	1 piece	45	3	0	<1
in liquid..1.5-oz piece	1 piece	55	5	0	<1
d'oeuvres..in liquid broth	5 balls	60	4	0	<1
fish d'oeuvres..liquid broth	5 balls	60	4	0	<1
Old World					
regular	1 ball	70	7	0	<1
sweet	1 ball	55	5	0	1
unsalted	1 ball	45	2	0	<1
(Rokeach) Old Vienna	3 oz	80	9	0	<1
GELATIN					
DRY					
(Knox) unflavored	1 pkt	25	0	0	0
MIX (NOTE: Unless stated otherwise, mix only = ½ cup prepared.)					
(Con-Gelli)					
rompope	⅛ pkg	100	21	0	21
strawberry	⅛ pkg	100	20	0	20

Food and Description	Amount	Total Calories	Total Carbs	Fiber	Sugars
(Hain) SuperFruits dessert..mix only					
cherry	2 Tbs	70	20	1	19
orange	2 Tbs	70	20	1	19
raspberry	2 Tbs	70	20	<1	19
strawberry	2 Tbs	90	20	1	19
(Hunt's) Snack Pack..mix only..all flavors	¼ pkg	100	24	0	22
(Jell-O) mix only					
Mystery Magical..all flavors	⅛ pkg	80	19	0	19
regular..all flavors	⅛ pkg	80	19	0	19
sugar-free/low-cal..all flavors	⅛ pkg	10	0	0	0
READY-TO-SERVE					
(Hunt's) Snack Pack					
juicy gels/cups..regular..all flavors	1 cup	100	25	0	24
(Jell-O)					
snack cups					
regular..all flavors	1 cup	70	17	0	17
sugar-free/low-cal..all flavors	1 cup	10	0	0	0
sticks..all flavors	1 stick	60	16	0	15
GINGER ROOT					
candied	1 oz	95	25	<1	15
fresh/raw/sliced	5 slices	8	2	0	0
	¼ cup	17	3.5	0.5	0
powdered..ground	1 tsp	6	1	0	0
GINGERBREAD (*See* BREAD; CAKE)					
GINKGO					
canned	1 oz	32	6	2.5	0
raw	1 oz	52	11	<1	0
GIZZARD (*See* CHICKEN; GOOSE; TURKEY)					
GOAT/boneless					
raw	4 oz	125	0	0	0
roasted	3 oz	122	0	0	0
GOOSE					
domesticated/roasted					
gizzard..raw	3 oz	119	0	0	0
liver..raw	3 oz	114	0	0	0
meat & skin	4 oz	346	0	0	0
meat only	4 oz	270	0	0	0
GOULASH (*See* BEEF DISH/ENTRÉE; FROZEN ENTRÉE/DINNER)					
GOURD					
boiled-drained/chopped	1 cup	100	26	na	0
boiled-drained/sliced	½ cup	50	13	na	0
raw/chopped	½ cup	10	2	na	0
GRAHAM CRACKER (*See* COOKIE; CRACKER)					
GRAHAM CRACKER CRUMBS (*See* CRACKER CRUMBS/MEAL)					
GRANADILLA (*See* PASSION FRUIT)					
GRANOLA (*See* CEREAL)					
GRANOLA/GRANOLA-TYPE BAR (*See* also BREAKFAST/CEREAL BAR)					
(Atkins)					
Advantage bars					
almond brownie chocolate	1 bar	230	2.6	2	0

Food and Description	Amount	Total Calories	Total Carbs	Fiber	Sugars
coconut	1 bar	250	2	1	0
cookies 'n' cream	1 bar	220	22	11	0
mocha crunch	1 bar	220	22	10	0
peanut butter	1 bar	218	2.6	1.2	0
(Biochem Ultimate) Lo-Carb 2					
chocolate brownie	1 bar	240	2	0	1
chocolate peanut butter & jelly	1 bar	250	3	0	1
chocolate s'mores	1 bar	230	3	0	0
coconut almond delight	1 bar	240	8	3	1
cool cappuccino	1 bar	230	2	0	1
creamy peanut butter	1 bar	270	2	0	1
lemon meringue	1 bar	230	3	0	3
raspberry swirl	1 bar	230	3	0	1
(EAS) AdvantEdge Carb Control					
apple cinnamon	1 bar	210	19	2	1
chocolate chip brownie	1 bar	210	20	2	1
chocolate cream pie	1 bar	220	18	2	1
chocolate peanut butter	1 bar	220	18	2	1
cookies 'n' cream	1 bar	210	18	2	1
lemon cheesecake	1 bar	210	19	2	1
(GeniSoy)					
GeniSoy Xtreme..1.6-oz bars					
Carrot Cake Quake	1 bar	190	24	1	18
crunch					
low-carb					
chocolate	1 bar	160	18	3	0
lemon	1 bar	150	19	2	1
peanut butter	1 bar	160	18	2	1
raspberry	1 bar	150	19	2	1
regular					
Island Blast	1 bar	160	29	2	19
Lemon Shot	1 bar	170	27	2	17
Peanut Butter Fix	1 bar	200	23	2	16
Razpberry Rush	1 bar	190	24	2	18
Rocky Road Trip	1 bar	190	23	2	16
Rugged Trails	1 bar	170	27	2	16
Summit Smash	1 bar	160	27	2	17
GeniSoy Soy Protein..2.2-oz bars					
Arctic Frost Crispy Chocolate Mint	1 bar	240	37	2	23
NY-style blueberry cheesecake	1 bar	220	34	1	28
Obsession Fudge cookies 'n' cream	1 bar	240	35	1	27
pure honey creamy peanut butter	1 bar	230	33	1	28
Southern-style chunky PB fudge	1 bar	240	34	2	22
Ultimate chocolate fudge brownie	1 bar	230	33	2	27
MLO Bio Protein Bars..2.85-oz bars					
chocolate peanut butter	1 bar	320	43	2	33
double chocolate	1 bar	310	43	3	35
honey peanut butter	1 bar	320	43	1	37
lemon	1 bar	300	43	1	36

Food and Description	Amount	Total Calories	Total Carbs	Fiber	Sugars
(Golden Temple) Wha Guru Chew snack bars					
almond ginger	1 bar	150	16	1	11
cashew					
almond	1 bar	160	9	1	8
vanilla	1 bar	150	16	0	9
peanut cashew	1 bar	160	11	<1	10
sesame almond	1 bar	160	10	2	10
(Health Valley)					
bakes..fat-free					
apple	1 bar	70	19	3	11
date	1 bar	70	18	3	11
raisin	1 bar	70	18	3	11
Café Creations					
chocolate					
espresso	1 bar	130	27	2	17
raspberry	1 bar	130	27	2	16
cinnamon Danish	1 bar	130	27	2	17
granola bars/fat-free..all flavors	1 bar	140	35	3	14
moist & chewy					
Dutch apple	1 bar	100	22	2	10
peanut crunch	1 bar	110	19	2	10
wild berry	1 bar	100	22	2	10
(Kashi) GoLean bars..high protein/fiber					
chocolate almond toffee	1 bar	290	45	6	31
cookies 'n' cream	1 bar	290	50	6	35
frosted spice cake	1 bar	290	49	6	33
honey vanilla yogurt	1 bar	290	49	6	32
malted chocolate crisp	1 bar	290	49	6	35
mocha java	1 bar	290	50	6	35
oatmeal raisin cookie	1 bar	280	49	6	33
peanut butter & chocolate	1 bar	290	48	6	31
strawberries 'n' cream	1 bar	290	50	6	33
(Kellogg's)					
Krave bars..all flavors	1 bar	200	29	2	21
Nutri-Grain					
bars..~1 oz					
chocolate chips	1 bar	100	17	<1	7
honey, oat & raisin	1 bar	110	18	1	9
chewy bites					
caramel nut crunch	1 bar	130	18	1	7
chocolate chip	1 bar	120	20	1	9
(Kudos) whole-grain bars					
chocolate chip	1 bar	120	20	1	13
chocolate fudge	1 bar	120	20	1	13
milk chocolate					
chocolate chip	1 bar	130	20	1	13
fruit & nut	1 bar	90	15	1	8
M&M's milk chocolate minis	1 bar	100	17	0	10
peanut butter	1 bar	130	18	1	13

Food and Description	Amount	Total Calories	Total Carbs	Fiber	Sugars
Snickers Bar	1 bar	100	16	9	19
(Luna)					
Glow snack bars..low-carb					
chocolate peanut crunch	1 bar	140	15	1	<1
fudge almond brownie	1 bar	140	15	2	<1
strawberry caramel sundae	1 bar	140	15	2	<1
Nutrition Bar for Women					
caramel apple	1 bar	180	29	3	17
cherry-covered chocolate	1 bar	180	28	2	14
chocolate peppermint stick	1 bar	180	29	2	15
chocolate pecan pie	1 bar	180	24	2	12
dulce de leche	1 bar	180	29	3	17
lemon zest	1 bar	180	26	2	14
Nutz Over Chocolate	1 bar	180	24	2	12
Orange Bliss	1 bar	180	29	2	15
peanut butter 'n' jelly	1 bar	170	28	2	13
s'mores	1 bar	180	26	2	12
sesame raisin crunch	1 bar	170	26	2	13
toasted nuts 'n' cranberry	1 bar	180	26	2	12
(Nature Valley)					
granola bar					
banana nut	2 bars	190	28	2	12
cinnamon	2 bars	180	29	2	12
maple brown sugar	2 bars	180	29	2	12
oats 'n' honey	2 bars	180	29	2	12
peanut butter	2 bars	180	29	2	12
roasted almond	2 bars	190	29	2	12
trail mix bar					
apple cinnamon	1 bar	150	24	1	13
fruit & nut	1 bar	140	24	2	12
(Odwalla) Odwalla Bar Caddys					
carrot	1 bar	220	45	4	26
chocolate	1 bar	240	40	5	21
chocolate chip peanut	1 bar	250	38	4	19
Cranberry C Monster	1 bar	220	47	4	25
peanut crunch	1 bar	260	40	3	17
super protein	1 bar	240	31	3	20
superfood	1 bar	230	41	5	22
(PowerBar)					
PowerBar Performance bar					
apple cinnamon	1 bar	230	45	3	20
banana	1 bar	230	45	3	20
cappuccino	1 bar	230	45	3	18
chocolate	1 bar	230	45	3	20
chocolate peanut butter	1 bar	240	45	3	20
malt nuts	1 bar	230	45	3	18
oatmeal raisin	1 bar	230	45	3	20
peanut butter	1 bar	240	45	3	16
raspberry 'n' cream stripes	1 bar	230	45	2	20
vanilla crisp	1 bar	230	45	3	20

Food and Description	Amount	Total Calories	Total Carbs	Fiber	Sugars
wild berry	1 bar	230	45	3	20
Pria					
Carbselect triple-layer nutrition bar					
caramel nut brownie	1 bar	170	21	2	1
cookies 'n' caramel	1 bar	170	22	2	1
peanut butter caramel nut	1 bar	170	21	2	1
(Quaker)					
CHEWY					
dips					
caramel nut	1 bar	140	21	1	10
chocolate chip	1 bar	150	21	1	13
peanut butter	1 bar	150	18	1	12
FRUIT 'N' CRUNCH BARS/all flavors	1 bar	160	31	2	14
granola bars					
Blastin' Chocolate	1 bar	110	22	1	10
chocolate chip	1 bar	120	21	1	8
chocolate chunk	1 bar	110	22	1	10
cookies 'n' cream..low-fat	1 bar	110	22	1	10
Graham Slam	1 bar	110	22	1	9
oatmeal raisin	1 bar	110	22	1	10
peanut butter	1 bar	110	18	1	8
& chocolate chunk	1 bar	120	29	1	8
PIECES					
Butterfinger	1 oz	120	23	1	10
Nestlé Crunch	1 oz	120	21	1	11
WHOLESOME					
baked apple	1 bar	110	22	1	10
cinnamon sugar	1 bar	110	22	1	9
oatmeal raisin	1 bar	110	22	1	10
(Slim-Fast)					
CARB OPTIONS/MEAL BARS					
chocolate					
chip brownie	1 bar	200	17	1	0
delight	1 bar	200	17	0	0
peanut	1 bar	200	17	1	1
cinnamon delight	1 bar	200	17	0	0
MEAL OPTIONS/MEAL GRANOLA BARS					
chewy..1.97-oz bars					
chocolate chip	1 bar	330	35	1	6
cranberry apple	1 bar	220	35	1	18
mixed berry	1 bar	220	35	1	19
peanut butter	1 bar	220	35	1	15
SLIM-FAST SUCCEED LOW-CARB					
snack bars..all flavors	1 bar	120	18	1	0
SNACK BARS/low-carb					
caramel nut	1 bar	120	19	1	1
chocolate peanut	1 bar	120	18	1	0
coconut almond	1 bar	120	15	2	<1
peanut butter crunch	1 bar	120	21	1	1
rocky road	1 bar	130	15	2	0

Food and Description	Amount	Total Calories	Total Carbs	Fiber	Sugars
GRAPE					
CANNED or PLASTIC CONTAINER					
(Oregon) fruit products..Thompson					
seedless grapes in light syrup	4.5 oz	100	23	1	21
FRESH/with or without seeds					
(Dole)	1½ cups	90	24	1	23
(Welch's) single-serve..all styles	1½ cups	90	24	1	23
GRAPE JUICE/JUICE BLEND/JUICE DRINK					
BOTTLED, BOXED, or CANNED					
(After The Fall)					
hearty grape	8 fl oz	150	37	0	37
sparkling grape juice	8 fl oz	130	31	0	31
Special Harvest Concord grape	8 fl oz	120	31	0	31
(Apple & Eve)					
Light & Fruitful..low-carb					
cranberry grape blend	8 fl oz	40	9	0	5
Sesame St...Grover's white grape	8 fl oz	130	38	0	38
(Libby's) Juicy Juice..100% grape	8 fl oz	130	31	0	28
(Minute Maid) 100% juice	6.75 fl oz	100	26	0	23
(R. W. Knudsen)					
Concord..Just Juice..organic	8 fl oz	160	40	0	38
grape fruit-juice spritzer	12 fl oz	170	41	0	37
(Welch's)					
Concord grape					
cranberry	8 fl oz	140	35	0	33
mango	8 fl oz	140	35	0	34
strawberry	8 fl oz	140	35	0	34
grape..juice drink	10 fl oz	210	53	0	52
lemonade	11.5 fl oz	190	47	0	46
grape apple	8 fl oz	150	36	0	35
purple grape	8 fl oz	170	41	0	40
red grape	8 fl oz	170	44	0	42
sparkling grape juice					
red	8 fl oz	160	41	0	39
white	8 fl oz	150	37	0	35
white grape					
berry	8 fl oz	140	35	0	33
cherry	8 fl oz	140	35	0	33
cranberry	8 fl oz	160	39	0	37
raspberry	8 fl oz	130	31	0	30
	11.5 oz	180	45	0	44
FROZEN/CHILLED/REFRIGERATED					
(Old Orchard)					
grape juice concentrate	8 fl oz	160	42	0	40
white grape juice	8 fl oz	160	38	0	38
(Welch's) prepared					
100% grape	8 fl oz	160	41	0	39
apple grape cherry	8 fl oz	150	38	0	37
purple grape..juice cocktail					
light	8 fl oz	50	13	0	12

Food and Description	Amount	Total Calories	Total Carbs	Fiber	Sugars
regular	8 fl oz	150	38	0	37
red grape	8 fl oz	170	44	0	42
white grape					
regular	8 fl oz	170	42	0	40
sweetened	8 fl oz	140	35	0	34
white grape–cranberry	8 fl oz	150	39	0	37

GRAPE LEAVES
CANNED or JARRED

(Alma)					
California	2 leaves	10	2	0	0
imported	2 leaves	10	2	0	0
(Krinos)	1 leaf	5	1	0	0
(Orlando California) drained	1 leaf	5	1	0	0
(Peloponnese) stuffed					
traditional Greek appetizer	3.3 oz	140	19	2	4

GRAPE SODA (*See* SOFT DRINK)

GRAPEFRUIT
CANNED, JARRED, or POUCH/sections

(Del Monte)					
Fruit Naturals..red grapefruit/pouch					
	½ cup	60	16	<1	13
red grapefruit..can	½ cup	90	21	1	17
Sunfresh..jar					
citrus salad	½ cup	45	9	2	8
red grapefruit	½ cup	80	19	2	9
in slightly sweetened fruit juice	½ cup	60	14	<1	11
white in real fruit juice	½ cup	80	19	<1	17

FRESH/whole

(Dole)	½ medium	60	16	6	0
(Ocean Spray) pink or white	½ medium	50	16	2	10

GRAPEFRUIT JUICE/JUICE BLEND/JUICE DRINK
BOTTLED, BOXED, or CANNED

(Dole) juice blend					
sunripe grapefruit..100%	8 fl oz	130	32	0	32
(Florida's Natural) premium..chilled	8 fl oz	100	24	0	23
grapefruit juice	8 fl oz	110	20	0	16
(Ocean Spray)					
premium 100% juice					
pink grapefruit juice	8 fl oz	110	28	0	25
ruby red	8 fl oz	130	32	0	29
white grapefruit juice	8 fl oz	100	24	0	21
ruby red juice drink	8 fl oz	120	30	0	30
ruby red juice drink..light	8 fl oz	40	10	0	10
(R. W. Knudsen) 100% juice..Rio Red	8 fl oz	140	35	0	29
(Tree Ripe) premium pink..no pulp	8 fl oz	100	24	0	23
(Tree Sweet)					
100% grapefruit					
original from concentrate	5.5 fl oz	60	14	0	17
	8 fl oz	90	21	0	12
pink grapefruit from concentrate	5.5 fl oz	70	17	0	16

Food and Description	Amount	Total Calories	Total Carbs	Fiber	Sugars
(Tropicana)					
Pure Premium					
plus calcium	8 fl oz	90	22	0	17
plus calcium & vitamin D	8 fl oz	110	26	0	22
Ruby Red	14 fl oz	160	39	0	30
sweet	8 fl oz	130	31	0	27
Twister..Ruby Red	10 fl oz	160	39	0	30
(V8 Splash) juice drink..citrus blend	8 fl oz	110	27	0	27
(Welch's) single-serve					
100% grapefruit juice	5.5 fl oz	70	17	0	16
	10 fl oz	130	32	0	30
FROZEN..prepared					
(Old Orchard) 100% juice					
ruby red concentrate	8 fl oz	110	29	0	27
GRAPEFRUIT PEEL/candied	1 oz	90	23	1	17
GRAVY (*See also* SAUCE; SEASONINGS)					
CANNED or JARRED/ready-to-serve					
(Franco-American)					
au jus	¼ cup	5	0	0	0
beef					
fat-free	¼ cup	15	3	0	0
slow-roasted	¼ cup	20	3	0	0
regular	¼ cup	25	3	0	1
w/onions	¼ cup	25	4	<1	2
w/roasted garlic	¼ cup	25	4	0	1
slow-roasted	¼ cup	25	3	0	0
brown w/ onions	¼ cup	25	4	<1	2
chicken					
fat-free					
slow-roasted	¼ cup	15	3	0	0
giblet	¼ cup	25	2	0	0
regular	¼ cup	35	4	0	1
w/roasted garlic	¼ cup	35	4	0	1
slow-roasted	¼ cup	25	3	0	0
country-style					
cream	¼ cup	35	3	0	1
sausage	¼ cup	70	6	0	1
mushroom..creamy or regular	¼ cup	20	3	0	1
pork/golden	¼ cup	40	3	0	1
turkey					
fat-free					
regular	¼ cup	20	4	0	0
slow-roasted	¼ cup	20	4	0	0
regular	¼ cup	25	3	0	1
slow-roasted	¼ cup	25	4	0	0
(Heinz)					
au jus..home-style	¼ cup	15	2	0	0
beef..home-style					
regular	¼ cup	25	3	0	0
w/onions	¼ cup	25	3	0	1

Food and Description	Amount	Total Calories	Total Carbs	Fiber	Sugars
brown..savory	¼ cup	25	3	0	1
chicken					
classic	¼ cup	30	4	0	1
fat-free	¼ cup	15	3	0	1
country..home-style	¼ cup	25	4	1	0
mushroom..home-style	¼ cup	25	3	0	0
pork..home-style	¼ cup	25	3	0	0
turkey					
fat-free	¼ cup	15	3	0	1
home-style	¼ cup	25	3	0	0
MIX (NOTE: Unless stated otherwise, 1 serving of mix = the amount in ¼ cup prepared.)					
(Knorr) mix only					
brown/classic	⅙ pkg	20	3	0	0
chicken/roasted	⅕ pkg	30	3	0	0
hunter mushroom/classics	⅕ pkg	25	4	0	1
turkey	⅕ pkg	25	4	0	0
(Lawry's)					
au jus	⅛ pkt	10	2	0	0
brown	¼ pkt	20	4	0	0
chicken	¼ pkt	25	4	0	0
turkey	¼ pkt	25	4	0	0
(McCormick/Schilling) mix only					
au jus	½ tsp	5	1	0	0
beef & herb	¼ pkg	30	3	0	1
brown..regular	1 Tbs	20	3	0	0
chicken	¼ pkg	35	4	2	1
chicken & herb /roasted	¼ pkg	25	3	0	2
country					
low-fat	⅛ pkg	40	5	0	2
original	⅛ pkg	50	4	0	2
sausage	⅛ pkg	45	4	0	2
home-style	1 Tbs	20	1	0	0
onion	2 tsp	20	3	0	0
pork	1 Tbs	20	4	0	1
turkey	⅙ pkg	20	3	0	1
(Pillsbury) mix only..all styles	¼ pkt	15	3	0	1
(Pioneer Brand)					
biscuit gravy	⅛ pkt	50	5	0	2
brown	⅛ pkt	20	4	0	0
Cajun brown w/Zatarain's seasoning	⅛ pkt	20	4	0	0
chicken	⅛ pkt	30	4	0	1
country	.31 oz	50	5	0	1
country sausage	⅛ pkt	40	5	0	2
peppered	⅛ pkt	50	5	0	1
turkey	⅛ pkt	25	4	0	1
FROZEN/REFRIGERATED					
(Bob Evans) original					
white gravy/pouch	8 oz	310	20	1	2
white w/pork sausage	9 oz	330	21	1	2

Food and Description	Amount	Total Calories	Total Carbs	Fiber	Sugars
GREAT NORTHERN BEAN					
CANNED					
(Bush's Best)	4.5 oz	110	18	7	0
(Eden)	½ cup	110	20	8	1
(Glory) seasoned	½ cup	90	15	3	0
(Luck's)					
& pinto beans..seasoned w/pork	½ cup	130	22	6	1
seasoned w/pork	½ cup	140	20	6	1
(Trappey's) flavored w/sausage	4.28 oz	110	24	7	1
DRIED (Best Yet) bag	1.2 oz	70	22	13	1
GREEK SOUP (*See* SOUP)					
GREEN BEAN/SNAP BEAN					
CANNED					
(The Allens)					
cut Italian..w/potatoes..Kentucky					
wonder–style	½ cup	45	7	2	2
seasoned..Southern-style	½ cup	45	8	3	2
(Allens Sunshine)					
cut Italian..Kentucky wonder–style	½ cup	35	7	3	2
w/potatoes	½ cup	35	7	2	2
(Blue Boy) all styles	½ cup	25	5	2	2
(Bush's Best) all styles	½ cup	20	5	2	2
(Del Monte)					
cut					
& potatoes w/ham-style flavor	3 oz	30	6	1	1
Blue Lake..all styles	½ cup	20	6	3	2
French-style..all types	1/2 cup	20	6	3	2
Italian cut	1/2 cup	30	6	3	2
Savory Sides green bean casserole	1/2 cup	70	11	2	3
Specialties..Blue Lake..seasoned	1/2 cup	20	4	2	2
(Green Giant)					
cut..all styles	½ cup	20	4	1	2
3-bean salad	½ cup	90	20	4	10
(Libby's) all styles	½ cup	25	5	2	2
(S&W) young & tender					
cut green & wax	½ cup	20	3	2	2
French-style..sliced	½ cup	20	4	2	2
(Stokely)					
French-style cut	½ cup	20	4	1	2
Italian flat cut	½ cup	20	4	2	2
shelly	½ cup	45	7	3	1
FROZEN					
(Birds Eye)					
green beans & spaetzle pasta					
w/bacon	9 oz	150	15	3	3
all cuts	½ cup	25	4	2	2
(Cascadian Farm)					
cut green beans	¾ cup	30	6	2	2
French green bean casserole	¾ cup	90	10	2	4

Food and Description	Amount	Total Calories	Total Carbs	Fiber	Sugars
green beans w/almonds (Green Giant)	¾ cup	70	10	4	4
cut	½ cup	20	4	2	2
green beans & almonds..boil-in-bag	⅔ cup	50	4	2	2
GREEN ONION (See SCALLION)					
GRENADINE SYRUP (Trader Vic's)	1 oz	90	22	0	na
GRITS (See CORN GRITS)					
GROUND CHERRY..raw	½ cup	37	8	2	na
GROUPER					
cooked—dry heat	3 oz	100	0	0	0
raw	3 oz	78	0	0	0
GUACAMOLE (See DIP; SEASONINGS)					
GUAVA					
canned (Herdez) whole in syrup	7 oz	190	32	5	30
fresh (Frieda's)	1 medium	45	10	5	5
GUAVA, STRAWBERRY/raw	1 cup	170	42	13	8
GUAVA JUICE/JUICE BLEND (See also FRUIT/FRUIT JUICE DRINK)					
(Jumex) nectar	8 fl oz	130	32	2	32
(Kern's) nectar	8 fl oz	150	37	0	33
(Knudsen) guava strawberry	8 fl oz	110	27	0	26
(Welch's) frozen, prepared	8 fl oz	140	34	0	33
GUAVA JUICE DRINK (See also FRUIT/FRUIT JUICE DRINK; FRUIT PUNCH; SOFT DRINK MIX)					
BOTTLED or CANNED					
(Minute Maid) guava citrus..light	12 fl oz	10	2	0	1
(V8 Splash) guava passionfruit	8 fl oz	110	27	0	25
GUAVA SAUCE/cooked	½ cup	43	27	0	25
GUINEA HEN/raw					
meat & skin	4 oz	180	0	0	0
meat only	4 oz	125	0	0	0
GUM					
(Bazooka)					
bubble	1 piece	15	4	0	4
soft..sugarless	1 piece	20	5	0	4
(Beech-Nut) regular..all flavors	1 piece	10	2	0	2
(Bubblicious) all flavors	1 piece	25	6	0	6
(Carefree) sugarless					
bubble gum	1 piece	10	2	0	2
cinnamon	1 piece	5	2	0	2
peppermint	1 piece	5	2	0	2
(Chiclets)					
regular..fruit	1 piece	10	2	0	2
sugarless	1 piece	5	2	0	0
(Dentyne) cinnamon	1 piece	10	2	0	2
(Dentyne Fire) sugarless..all flavors	1 piece	5	2	0	<1
(Extra)					
bubble gum..sugar-free..all flavors	1 piece	5	2	0	<1
regular..all flavors	1 piece	5	2	0	<1
(Freedent) all flavors	1 stick	10	2	0	2

Food and Description	Amount	Total Calories	Total Carbs	Fiber	Sugars
(Fruit Stripe) all flavors	1 piece	10	2	0	2
(Hubba Bubba) original					
regular	1 piece	20	6	0	6
sugar-free	1 piece	15	0	0	0
(Juicy Fruit) all flavors	1 piece	10	2	0	2
(Trident) all flavors	1 piece	5	1	0	<1
(Wrigley's) all styles and flavors	1 stick	10	2	0	2

GUMBO (See SEASONINGS; SOUP)

Food and Description	Amount	Total Calories	Total Carbs	Fiber	Sugars
HADDOCK (See also SEAFOOD ENTRÉE/DINNER)					
cooked—dry heat	3 oz	95	0	0	0
raw	3 oz	74	0	0	0
smoked	3 oz	99	0	0	0
HAKE (See WHITING)					
HALIBUT (See also SEAFOOD ENTRÉE/DINNER)					
Atlantic & Pacific..cooked—dry heat	3 oz	120	0	0	0
Greenland..raw	3 oz	160	0	0	0
HAM (See also LUNCHEON MEAT; PORK; TURKEY)					
(Alpine Lace)					
cooked or honey..95% fat-free	2 oz	60	2	0	1
(Boar's Head)					
Black Forest smoked	2 oz	60	2	0	2
branded deluxe	2 oz	60	2	0	2
Cappy brand	2 oz	60	3	0	2
gourmet pepper	2 oz	60	2	0	1
maple glazed honey coat	2 oz	60	3	0	3
pesto Parmesan..oven-roasted	2 oz	90	0	0	0
rosemary & sun-dried tomato	2 oz	70	2	0	0
seasoned fresh	2 oz	80	0	0	1
smoked Virginia	2 oz	60	2	0	2
Sweet Slice boneless smoked	2 oz	100	1	0	0
Virginia brand..pineapple-topped	2 oz	60	3	0	3
(Bryan)					
bone-in..Classic Perfection ham steak					
	8 oz	370	2	0	2
	5 oz	230	1	0	1

Food and Description	Amount	Total Calories	Total Carbs	Fiber	Sugars
natural juice..classic carving ham	3 oz	140	3	0	0
presliced					
hickory-smoked	2.5 oz	90	1	0	1
shaved honey	6 slices	100	1	0	1
smoked	3 oz	130	3	0	0
water added					
Classic Pit..double-smoked	3 oz	140	0	0	0
Hickory Gold Foil Wrap	3 oz	140	0	0	0
pit ham	3 oz	140	0	0	0
(DAK) Danish					
baked w/natural juices..fat-free	1 oz	30	0	0	0
canned ham	2 oz	100	1	0	1
chopped..canned	2 oz	170	1	0	1
chunk	2 oz	100	1	0	1
deli-sliced..smoked..97% fat-free	2 oz	60	0	0	0
honey ham w/natural juices	1 oz	30	0	0	0
imported slices..97% fat-free	1.6 oz	45	0	0	0
premium					
imported..97% fat-free	2 oz	50	0	0	0
slices..97% fat-free	1 oz	30	1	0	1
turkey ham..95% fat-free	1 oz	35	0	0	0
(Danola)					
baked brown sugar	2 oz	60	0	0	0
Black Forest..smoked	1.6 oz	60	0	0	0
hickory-smoked	2 oz	60	0	0	0
pepper-smoked..97% fat-free	1.8 oz	50	1	0	1
premium sliced..98% fat-free	1.8 oz	45	1	0	1
smoked					
maple-flavored honey	2 oz	70	2	0	2
pepper	2 oz	60	1	0	1
Virginia brand	2 oz	60	0	0	1
(Dubuque) Royal Buffet...extra-lean	3 oz	110	5	0	3
(Hillshire Farm)					
Bavarian-roasted..deli	2 oz	70	1	0	1
Black Oak	2 oz	90	1	0	1
ham					
bone-in & spiral-sliced					
brown sugar–cured	3 oz	120	6	1	0
honey-cured	3 oz	120	1	0	1
other..baked					
half..brown sugar–cured	2 oz	70	3	0	3
half..honey-cured	2 oz	60	2	0	2
ham patties	1 patty	180	<1	0	0
ham steak..bone-in	3 oz	130	3	0	3
Imperial Club ham	2 oz	70	<1	0	1
natural-juice ham					
Banjo ham	2 oz	70	0	0	0
Hearthstone ham	4 pieces	80	0	0	0
holiday ham..gift box	3 oz	120	2	0	2

Food and Description	Amount	Total Calories	Total Carbs	Fiber	Sugars
rolled & tied fresh ham	4 oz	200	5	0	2
(Hormel)..deli products					
Black Label..canned	3 oz	100	1	0	1
Black Forest..96% fat-free	2 oz	60	0	0	0
chunk..lean	2 oz	90	0	0	0
cooked..95% fat-free	2 oz	60	0	0	0
Cure 81					
bone-in..honey-glazed..spiral-sliced	3 oz	140	2	0	1
boneless..all styles	3 oz	100	0	0	0
Curemaster	3 oz	80	0	0	0
deviled	2 oz	150	2	1	2
double-smoked	2 oz	70	0	0	0
honey ham..sliced	2 oz	70	3	0	3
Light & Lean..cooked..97% fat-free	1 oz	25	0	0	0
patties..fully cooked					
ham	1 patty	180	1	0	1
ham & cheese	1 patty	180	0	0	0
(Louis Rich) Carving Board					
honey..thin-carved..97% fat-free	2.2 oz	70	2	0	2
(Louis Rich and Oscar Mayer) turkey ham					
50% less fat	1 oz	35	<1	0	0
smoked	1 oz	35	1	0	0
smoked..chopped	1 oz	35	1	0	0
(Oscar Mayer) deli-style					
brown sugar					
shaved	1.8 oz	60	3	0	3
thin-sliced	2 oz	70	4	0	4
honey..shaved	1.8 oz	50	2	0	2
smoked					
shaved	1.8 oz	45	0	0	0
thin-sliced	2 oz	50	0	0	0
(Plumrose) Danish					
baked					
96% fat-free	1 oz	35	0	0	0
brown sugar..97% fat free	1 oz	35	1	0	1
honey & brown sugar..97% fat-free	1 oz	35	1	0	1
ham steaks..smoked..97% fat-free	5.3 oz	150	3	0	2
honey..96% fat-free	1 oz	35	1.5	0	1.5
premium..canned	2 oz	60	0	0	0
95% fat-free	1 oz	35	0	0	0
97% fat-free	1 oz	30	0	0	0
smoked pepper	1.7 oz	50	1	0	1
Supreme					
Black Forest..smoked	2 oz	60	1	0	1
brown sugar..baked..97% fat-free	2 oz	60	1	0	1
imported..97% fat-free	2 oz	50	0	0	0
smoked..97% fat-free					
honey	2 oz	60	1	0	1

Food and Description	Amount	Total Calories	Total Carbs	Fiber	Sugars
maple-flavored honey	2 oz	70	2	0	0
Virginia	2 oz	60	0	0	0
Thin & Tasty..97% fat-free..all styles					
	2 oz	50	0	0	0
turkey ham	1 oz	35	0	0	0
(West Virginia Brand)					
fillets..boneless	3 oz	90	2	0	1
golden..boneless..97% fat-free	3 oz	90	2	0	1
lean original..semiboneless	3 oz	130	1	0	1

HAM SALAD (*See* LUNCHEON MEAT)

HAM SPREAD (*See* LUNCHEON MEAT SPREAD)

HAMBURGER (*See* BEEF; BEEF DISH/ENTRÉE; BUFFALO/BISON; FROZEN ENTRÉE/DINNER; TURKEY; VEGETARIAN FOODS; individual FAST FOOD listings)

HASH (*See* BEEF DISH/ENTRÉE; SAUSAGE DISH; TURKEY ENTRÉE/DINNER)

HAZELNUT (*See also* FILBERT)

Food and Description	Amount	Total Calories	Total Carbs	Fiber	Sugars
(Diamond of California)					
chopped	¼ cup	200	5	3	0
shelled 1 oz	~22 nuts	200	5	3	0
(Planters) hazelnuts..filberts	2 oz	350	9	5	2

HAZELNUT BUTTER/SPREAD

Food and Description	Amount	Total Calories	Total Carbs	Fiber	Sugars
(Ferrero) Nutella chocolate	1 Tbs	85	8	0	0
(Roaster Fresh) hazelnut butter	2 Tbs	184	6	0	0

HERBS (*See* SEASONINGS; individual listings)

HERRING (*See also* HERRING ROE)

Food and Description	Amount	Total Calories	Total Carbs	Fiber	Sugars
Atlantic					
cooked—dry heat	3 oz	172	0	0	0
kippered..no bone	1 oz	65	0	0	0
pickled..no bone	3 oz	220	1	0	na
raw	3 oz	134	0	0	0
(King Oscar)					
Kipper Snacks..fillets of herring	3.25 oz	190	0	0	0
kippered					
in mustard	¼ cup	100	0	0	0
in salsa picante	¼ cup	90	3	0	na
smoked	¼ cup	110	0	0	0
(Nathan's) snacks in wine sauce	¼ cup	90	7	0	na
Pacific					
cooked—dry heat	3 oz	215	0	0	0
raw	3 oz	166	0	0	0
(Vita Lunch) pickled..jarred	2 oz	130	5	0	5

HERRING ROE..raw | 3 oz | 120 | 1 | 0 | 0 |

HICKORY NUT dried..shelled | 1 oz | 187 | 5 | 2 | 0 |

HOLLANDAISE SAUCE (*See* SAUCE)

HOMINY (*See also* CORN GRITS)

Food and Description	Amount	Total Calories	Total Carbs	Fiber	Sugars
canned					
(Allens)					
golden	½ cup	120	27	4	1
maiz blanco para pozole.. Mexican..white	½ cup	100	22	4	1

Food and Description	Amount	Total Calories	Total Carbs	Fiber	Sugars
(Bush's Best)					
golden	½ cup	60	13	3	0
white	½ cup	70	14	4	0
(Springfield)					
fancy Mexican-style	½ cup	60	10	6	4
fancy white	½ cup	80	16	5	0
HOMINY GRITS (See CORN GRITS)					
HONEY					
(Aunt Sue's) raw..wild pure..squeeze	1 Tbs	60	17	0	16
(Knott's Berry Farm) pure	1 Tbs	60	16	0	16
(Sioux)	1 Tbs	60	16	0	16
HONEY BUTTER					
(Land O' Lakes) cinnamon or original	1 Tbs	90	4	0	3
HONEYDEW MELON fresh					
cut-up	1 cup	50	12	1	11
(Dole) whole	⅒ melon	50	13	1	12
HORSE/meat only..roasted	4 oz	200	0	0	0
HORSERADISH (See also SAUCE)					
jarred					
(Boar's Head)					
horseradish	1 tsp	0	0	0	0
horseradish sauce	1 tsp	15	1	0	0
(Gold's) hot, red, & white	1 tsp	4	1	0	0
(Hebrew National) red	1 Tbs	7	2	0	0
(Koop's) squeeze mustard horseradish	1 tsp	0	0	0	0
(Kraft)					
all styles	1 tsp	0	0	0	0
mustard	1 tsp	0	0	0	0
prepared	1 tsp	0	0	0	0
horseradish sauce	1 tsp	20	1	0	1
(Plochman's) premium spicy mustard	1 tsp	0	0	0	0
HOT CROSS BUN (See PASTRY)					
HOT DOG (See FRANKFURTER; individual FAST FOOD listings)					
HUMMUS (See also DIP)					
READY-TO-SERVE					
(Athenos) 14-oz tub					
black olive	2 Tbs	50	5	1	0
cucumber dill	2 Tbs	60	5	1	0
Greek	2 Tbs	50	5	<1	0
original	2 Tbs	60	5	1	0
pesto	2 Tbs	50	6	2	0
roasted eggplant	2 Tbs	45	4	1	0
roasted garlic	2 Tbs	60	5	1	0
roasted red pepper	2 Tbs	60	6	1	0
scallion	2 Tbs	50	6	2	0
spicy 3-pepper	2 Tbs	60	5	1	<1
(Athenos) Travelers (NOTE: 1 serving = 2 Tbs hummus w/2 pitas.)					
original	1 serving	130	17	1	<1
roasted eggplant	1 serving	120	16	2	1
roasted garlic	1 serving	130	17	1	<1

Food and Description	Amount	Total Calories	Total Carbs	Fiber	Sugars
roasted red pepper	1 serving	140	19	2	1
spicy 3-pepper	1 serving	130	17	2	2
HUNTER'S SOUP (*See* SOUP)					
HUSH PUPPY (*See* BREAD)					
HYACINTH BEAN..boiled..drained					
immature	½ cup	20	4	na	0
mature	½ cup	114	20	na	0

Food and Description	Amount	Total Calories	Total Carbs	Fiber	Sugars
ICE CREAM & ICE CREAM–LIKE FROZEN DESSERTS (*See also* FRUIT ICES, BARS & POPS; ICE CREAM BARS, SANDWICHES & FROZEN NOVELTIES; RICE FROZEN DESSERT; SHERBET; TOFU FROZEN DESSERT; YOGURT, FROZEN)					
■ (Alaskan Ice Cream)					
Bear Claw	½ cup	150	20	1	18
Caramel Caribou	½ cup	150	20	0	19
Extreme Moose Tracks	½ cup	170	19	1	16
Glacier Mint	½ cup	150	18	1	17
Moose Tracks	½ cup	170	18	1	17
The Mother Lode	½ cup	150	20	0	19
Otter Paws	½ cup	160	19	0	18
■ (Baskin-Robbins)					
CLASSIC FLAVORS					
banana nut	½ cup	260	27	1	26
black walnut	½ cup	280	25	1	23
chocolate	½ cup	260	33	0	31
chocolate almond	½ cup	310	32	1	29
chocolate chip	½ cup	270	28	1	26
chocolate chip cookie dough	½ cup	290	36	1	30
chocolate fudge	½ cup	270	35	0	32
chocolate ribbon	½ cup	240	31	0	31
French vanilla	½ cup	280	26	0	25
fudge brownie	½ cup	300	35	1	31
German chocolate cake	½ cup	300	36	1	35
Gold Medal Ribbon	½ cup	260	34	0	33
Jamoca	½ cup	240	26	0	24
Jamoca almond fudge	½ cup	270	31	1	28
nutty coconut ice cream	½ cup	300	28	1	27
old-fashioned butter pecan	½ cup	280	24	1	24
Oreo cookies 'n' cream	½ cup	280	32	1	27

Food and Description	Amount	Total Calories	Total Carbs	Fiber	Sugars
peanut butter 'n' chocolate	½ cup	320	31	1	28
pistachio almond	½ cup	290	25	1	23
pralines 'n' cream	½ cup	270	34	0	33
Reese's peanut butter	½ cup	300	31	0	28
rocky road	½ cup	290	36	1	32
vanilla	½ cup	260	26	0	26
very berry strawberry	½ cup	220	28	0	27
world-class chocolate	½ cup	270	33	0	32
ICE CREAM CAKES..SHEET					
chocolate chip w/devil's food cake	1 slice	330	38	1	29
mint chocolate chip w/devil's food cake	1 slice	290	33	1	26
Oreo Cookies 'n' cream w/white sponge cake	1 slice	300	40	1	28
pralines 'n' cream w/white sponge cake	1 slice	300	42	1	32
vanilla w/devil's food cake	1 slice	300	33	1	27
LOW-FAT..espresso 'n' cream	½ cup	180	32	1	29
LOW-FAT..NO SUGAR ADDED					
chocolate chip	½ cup	170	30	1	8
chocolate chocolate chip	½ cup	150	30	1	7
Mad About Chocolate	½ cup	170	33	1	8
pineapple coconut	½ cup	150	27	0	9
Tin Roof Sundae	½ cup	190	34	1	9
SEASONAL FLAVORS					
blueberry cheesecake	½ cup	270	32	0	30
Candy Cookie Commotion	½ cup	300	36	1	29
Chocoholic's Resolution	½ cup	300	38	0	35
Chocolate Mousse Royale	½ cup	300	37	1	34
Cinnamon Bun Swirl	½ cup	280	39	0	35
eggnog	½ cup	250	31	0	30
Jamoca Roca	½ cup	280	33	0	31
Key Lime Pie	½ cup	270	33	0	32
lemon custard	½ cup	260	30	0	30
Love Gone Sour	½ cup	270	32	0	31
macadamia nuts 'n' cream	½ cup	270	25	1	24
Mississippi Mud	½ cup	270	37	0	35
New York cheesecake	½ cup	280	31	0	27
Nutcracker Sweet	½ cup	300	41	1	28
oatmeal cookie	½ cup	270	37	0	31
peppermint	½ cup	270	32	0	31
pumpkin pie	½ cup	230	29	0	28
strawberry cheesecake	½ cup	270	32	0	30
Trick Oreo Treat	½ cup	300	36	1	29
Winter White Chocolate	½ cup	270	32	1	30
SUNDAES					
2-scoop hot fudge	1 serving	530	62	0	52
3-scoop hot fudge	1 serving	750	86	0	74
Banana Royale	1 serving	630	91	5	7

Food and Description	Amount	Total Calories	Total Carbs	Fiber	Sugars
banana split	1 serving	1030	168	7	140
Donkey Sundae	1 serving	530	78	3	63
■ (Ben & Jerry's)					
ORGANIC					
chocolate fudge brownie	½ cup	260	30	2	25
strawberry	½ cup	200	20	0	17
sweet cream & cookies	½ cup	240	23	0	18
vanilla	½ cup	220	18	0	16
ORIGINAL					
Brownie Batter	½ cup	310	32	1	26
butter pecan	½ cup	290	20	1	18
Cherry Garcia	½ cup	250	26	0	23
chocolate chip cookie dough	½ cup	280	31	0	24
chocolate chocolate cookie	½ cup	280	34	2	26
Chocolate for a Change	½ cup	270	36	2	23
Chocolate Fudge Brownie	½ cup	280	33	2	29
Chubby Hubby	½ cup	330	32	1	24
Chunky Monkey	½ cup	300	30	1	26
Coffee for a Change	½ cup	240	21	0	19
Coffee Heath Bar Crunch	½ cup	310	32	0	25
Everything but the...	½ cup	320	30	1	27
Fudge Central	½ cup	300	31	1	27
Half Baked	½ cup	280	34	1	31
Karamel Sutra	½ cup	290	33	1	27
Makin' Whoopie Pie	½ cup	270	33	2	24
mint chocolate cookie	½ cup	270	26	<1	22
New York Super Fudge Chunk	½ cup	310	30	2	25
oatmeal cookie chunk	½ cup	280	32	1	23
One Sweet Whirled	½ cup	280	33	1	17
peanut butter cup	½ cup	380	29	2	25
Phish Food	½ cup	280	37	2	23
Pistachio Pistachio	½ cup	280	21	0	18
Uncanny Cashew	½ cup	290	27	0	22
Vanilla for a Change	½ cup	240	21	0	19
Vanilla Heath Bar Crunch	½ cup	300	29	0	27
■ (Blue Bunny)					
CARB FREEDOM					
butter pecan	½ cup	110	11	4	2
chocolate almond fudge	½ cup	120	13	3	2
double strawberry	½ cup	100	13	3	2
mint chip	½ cup	110	11	4	2
vanilla bean	½ cup	100	10	4	2
NO SUGAR ADDED..FAT-FREE					
brownie sundae	½ cup	90	23	5	4
burgundy cherry	½ cup	90	22	4	4
caramel toffee crunch	½ cup	90	24	5	4
chocolate	½ cup	90	18	4	5
mint fudge swirl	½ cup	80	19	5	5
vanilla	½ cup	80	20	5	5
NO SUGAR ADDED..REDUCED-FAT					

Food and Description	Amount	Total Calories	Total Carbs	Fiber	Sugars
banana split	½ cup	120	20	2	3
Bunny Tracks	½ cup	150	20	3	4
butter pecan	½ cup	130	16	3	4
cherry vanilla	½ cup	120	18	2	4
double strawberry	½ cup	110	18	2	4
Exquisite Mint	½ cup	130	20	2	3
rocky road	½ cup	130	21	2	3
Tin Roof Sundae	½ cup	130	19	2	3
Turtle Sundae	½ cup	140	20	2	4
vanilla	½ cup	110	16	2	4
PREMIUM					
Chocolate Amore	½ cup	170	22	0	19
Chocolate Bunny Tracks	½ cup	200	24	<1	20
Bordeaux cherry chocolate	½ cup	160	20	0	17
Bunny Tracks	½ cup	190	21	1	19
butter pecan	½ cup	150	15	0	13
chocolate chip	½ cup	150	17	0	15
cookies 'n' cream	½ cup	150	19	0	15
double strawberry	½ cup	140	20	0	18
Exquisite Mint	½ cup	170	22	0	20
French vanilla	½ cup	150	17	0	15
homemade chocolate	½ cup	150	16	0	16
homemade turtle sundae	½ cup	180	21	0	19
homemade vanilla	½ cup	150	16	0	16
NASCAR Speedway Sundae	½ cup	190	22	0	18
Peanut Butter Panic	½ cup	200	19	<1	16
pistachio almond	½ cup	150	15	<1	13
praline pecan	½ cup	170	22	0	19
rocky road	½ cup	150	21	0	16
Super Fudge Brownie	½ cup	170	23	0	18
toasted almond fudge	½ cup	160	18	<1	14
Triple Raspberry Temptation	½ cup	150	21	0	18
■ (Breyers)					
ALL-NATURAL					
banana fudge chunk	½ cup	160	21	<1	18
butter almond	½ cup	160	14	<1	14
butter pecan	½ cup	170	14	0	14
calcium-rich natural vanilla	½ cup	130	14	0	14
caramel fudge	½ cup	160	20	0	18
caramel praline crunch	½ cup	170	22	0	21
cherry chocolate chip	½ cup	150	18	0	17
cherry vanilla	½ cup	140	17	0	16
chocolate	½ cup	150	17	<1	16
chocolate chip	½ cup	160	17	0	17
chocolate chip cookie dough	½ cup	170	20	0	17
coffee	½ cup	140	15	0	15
cookies & cream	½ cup	160	18	<1	16
dulce de leche	½ cup	140	20	0	19
French vanilla	½ cup	150	15	0	15
fresh banana	½ cup	140	20	0	18

Food and Description	Amount	Total Calories	Total Carbs	Fiber	Sugars
mint chocolate chip	½ cup	130	20	0	17
mocha almond fudge	½ cup	170	18	2	15
peach	½ cup	120	17	0	16
peanut butter & fudge	½ cup	170	17	<1	15
rocky road	½ cup	170	20	<1	18
strawberry	½ cup	120	15	0	15
vanilla	½ cup	140	15	0	15
homemade	½ cup	140	16	0	13
vanilla & chocolate fudge chunks	½ cup	170	19	0	17
vanilla fudge brownie	½ cup	160	19	<1	16
vanilla chocolate strawberry	½ cup	140	15	0	15
ALL-NATURAL..LIGHT					
French chocolate	½ cup	140	20	<1	16
French vanilla	½ cup	120	18	0	14
mint chocolate chip	½ cup	130	19	0	17
natural vanilla	½ cup	110	17	0	15
vanilla chocolate strawberry	½ cup	120	18	0	15
HOMEMADE					
butter pecan	½ cup	170	16	0	11
vanilla	½ cup	140	16	0	11
ICE CREAM PARLOR					
Almond Joy	½ cup	170	19	1	15
Creamsicle	½ cup	130	20	0	16
Fudgesicle chocolate fudge	½ cup	140	17	1	13
Heath English Toffee	½ cup	180	22	0	20
Hershey's chocolate w/almonds	½ cup	170	21	1	17
M&M'S					
mint	½ cup	170	19	0	17
vanilla fudge	½ cup	170	20	0	18
mint ice cream w/Oreo	½ cup	170	23	0	17
Oreo cookies & cream	½ cup	160	20	0	16
Reese's peanut butter cups	½ cup	180	22	0	18
Snickers	½ cup	160	20	0	17
Snickers Cruncher	½ cup	160	20	0	17
SpongeBob cookie dough	½ cup	160	21	0	17
strawberry shortcake	½ cup	160	23	0	18
Twix	½ cup	160	21	0	17
Twix..peanut butter	½ cup	170	18	<1	14
LIGHT & LOW-FAT TASTY ALTERNATIVES					
all-natural light					
French chocolate	½ cup	140	20	<1	16
French vanilla	½ cup	120	18	0	14
mint chocolate chip	½ cup	130	19	0	17
vanilla	½ cup	110	17	0	15
LOW-CARB					
CarbSmart					
butter pecan	½ cup	120	10	3	3
chocolate	½ cup	130	10	3	4
chocolate almond	½ cup	130	10	3	3
chocolate & vanilla	½ cup	70	9	2	0

Food and Description	Amount	Total Calories	Total Carbs	Fiber	Sugars
mint chocolate chip	½ cup	140	13	3	4
rocky road	½ cup	140	12	3	4
strawberry	½ cup	130	10	3	4
vanilla					
frozen dairy dessert	½ cup	130	9	3	0
ice cream	½ cup	130	10	3	4
NO SUGAR ADDED					
98% fat-free					
chocolate fudge brownie	½ cup	90	20	4	4
butter pecan	½ cup	120	15	4	4
chocolate caramel	½ cup	100	18	3	4
French vanilla	½ cup	100	19	3	4
vanilla	½ cup	100	14	3	5
vanilla fudge twirl	½ cup	110	19	3	4
vanilla chocolate strawberry	½ cup	90	15	3	4
■ (Carb Watchers)					
PREMIUM GOURMET					
butter pecan	½ cup	150	10	5	2
chocolate fudge swirl	½ cup	145	13	5	2
cookies & cream	½ cup	160	10	6	2
dulce de leche	½ cup	160	14	5	2
vanilla	½ cup	140	10	5	2
■ (Dreamery)					
banana split	½ cup	240	31	1	27
Black Raspberry Avalanche	½ cup	250	27	1	23
Blue Ribbon Berry Pie	½ cup	260	31	<1	25
brownie turtle sundae	½ cup	310	33	2	28
Caramel Toffee Bar Heaven	½ cup	270	32	0	29
Cashew Praline Parfait	½ cup	280	30	0	26
Cherry Chip Ba Da Bing	½ cup	280	33	1	28
Chocolate peanut butter chunk	½ cup	310	29	2	25
chocolate Truffle Explosion	½ cup	280	31	1	27
Coney Island Waffle	½ cup	310	32	1	28
deep dish apple pie	½ cup	280	34	0	28
Fortunate Vanilla	½ cup	300	33	1	26
Give Me S'mores	½ cup	280	39	1	25
Grandma's Cookie Dough	½ cup	290	32	0	23
hot fudge sundae	½ cup	310	29	<2	26
New York strawberry cheesecake	½ cup	260	28	0	23
Nuts About Malt	½ cup	290	29	1	24
raspberry brownie à la mode	½ cup	270	34	1	27
Strawberry Fields	½ cup	220	26	1	23
tiramisu..chunks	½ cup	260	31	0	24
triple butter pecan	½ cup	300	30	1	24
Ultimate Mudslide	½ cup	260	28	1	23
vanilla	½ cup	260	23	0	24
■ (Dreyer's..Edy's)					
GRAND					
CARB BENEFIT					
butter pecan	½ cup	170	13	6	2

Food and Description	Amount	Total Calories	Total Carbs	Fiber	Sugars
chocolate	½ cup	150	13	7	2
chocolate chip	½ cup	160	14	6	2
mint chocolate chip	½ cup	160	14	6	2
vanilla bean	½ cup	140	13	6	2
FAT-FREE..NO SUGAR					
chocolate fudge	½ cup	100	22	6	4
raspberry vanilla	½ cup	80	19	5	4
vanilla	½ cup	80	19	5	4
chocolate	½ cup	100	20	6	4
'n' caramel	½ cup	80	21	5	4
HOMEMADE					
chocolate	½ cup	150	19	0	15
Grovestand Peach	½ cup	120	17	0	15
mint chocolate chunk	½ cup	160	18	0	15
old-fashioned butter pecan	½ cup	150	15	0	11
strawberries & cream	½ cup	130	17	0	14
vanilla	½ cup	140	15	0	11
vanilla custard	½ cup	150	17	0	14
LIGHT					
butter pecan	½ cup	120	16	0	12
chocolate chip sandwich	½ cup	120	19	0	13
chocolate fudge chunk	½ cup	120	19	0	14
cookie dough	½ cup	130	19	0	13
cookies 'n' cream	½ cup	120	18	0	12
Crazy for Caramel	½ cup	110	18	0	15
espresso fudge chip	½ cup	120	18	0	13
French Silk	½ cup	120	19	0	14
Fudge Tracks	½ cup	120	18	0	13
Gingerbread Man	½ cup	120	19	0	14
Girl Scouts					
Tagalongs Cookie	½ cup	130	17	0	12
Thin Mint Cookie	½ cup	120	18	0	12
mint chocolate chip	½ cup	120	17	0	13
mocha almond fudge	½ cup	120	16	0	12
peppermint	½ cup	110	17	0	13
rocky road	½ cup	120	17	0	12
Strawberry Cheesecake Delight	½ cup	120	17	0	13
strawberry shortcake	½ cup	110	18	0	14
vanilla	½ cup	100	15	0	11
Vanillaberry Bar	½ cup	100	19	0	14
Vanilla Raspberry Escape	½ cup	120	19	0	15
LIGHT..SLOW-CHURNED RICH & CREAMY					
50/50 bar	½ cup	100	18	0	13
butter pecan	½ cup	120	16	0	12
chocolate	½ cup	110	16	0	11
Chocolate Chips!	½ cup	120	17	0	13
cookie dough	½ cup	130	19	0	13
cookies 'n' cream	½ cup	120	18	0	12
French Silk	½ cup	130	19	0	14
French vanilla	½ cup	100	15	0	11

Food and Description	Amount	Total Calories	Total Carbs	Fiber	Sugars
Fudge Tracks	½ cup	120	18	0	13
Mint Chocolate Chips!	½ cup	120	17	0	13
mocha almond fudge	½ cup	100	15	0	11
Neapolitan	½ cup	100	15	0	11
rocky road	½ cup	120	17	0	12
strawberry	½ cup	100	17	0	13
vanilla	½ cup	100	15	0	11
LIMITED EDITION					
50/50 Bar..Grand Light	½ cup	100	18	0	13
Drumstick Sundae..Nestlé	½ cup	180	19	0	15
Grovestand Peach	½ cup	120	17	0	14
NO SUGAR ADDED (See also Fat-Free in this section)					
butter pecan	½ cup	110	14	3	4
chips 'n' swirls	½ cup	90	16	3	3
chocolate	½ cup	90	13	0	3
cookie dough	½ cup	110	16	0	4
Mint Chocolate Chips!	½ cup	110	15	3	3
Neapolitan	½ cup	90	13	3	4
strawberry	½ cup	90	13	3	4
triple chocolate	½ cup	90	16	3	3
vanilla	½ cup	90	13	3	4
REGULAR					
almond praline	½ cup	170	21	0	16
America's vanilla	½ cup	150	13	0	11
Andes Cool Mint Amazing Flavor	½ cup	170	19	0	16
Blue Ribbon Chocolate Cake	½ cup	180	20	0	15
butter pecan	½ cup	170	16	0	13
chocolate	½ cup	150	16	0	15
chocolate caramel swirl	½ cup	170	19	0	16
Chocolate Chips!	½ cup	170	18	0	15
chocolate peanut butter	½ cup	200	17	0	13
coffee	½ cup	140	15	0	13
cookie dough	½ cup	180	31	0	15
cookies 'n' cream	½ cup	160	29	0	14
double fudge brownie	½ cup	170	19	0	15
eggnog	½ cup	140	18	0	15
French vanilla	½ cup	160	17	0	11
French vanilla fudge pie	½ cup	160	20	0	14
Fudge Tracks	½ cup	180	18	0	16
Galactic Chocolate	½ cup	160	22	0	17
Girl Scout					
Samoas Cookie	½ cup	170	21	0	17
Thin Mint Cookie	½ cup	170	18	0	13
Grovestand Peach	½ cup	120	17	0	14
Mint Chocolate Chips!	½ cup	170	18	0	15
mocha almond fudge	½ cup	160	17	0	14
Neapolitan	½ cup	140	16	0	14
Nestlé Toll House Cookie Swirl	½ cup	170	21	0	17
nutty cone crunch	½ cup	180	19	0	15
peanut butter					

Food and Description	Amount	Total Calories	Total Carbs	Fiber	Sugars
butter brownie	½ cup	200	18	0	14
cones	½ cup	160	19	0	14
cup	½ cup	180	19	0	15
peppermint	½ cup	150	17	0	12
pumpkin	½ cup	140	17	0	14
real strawberry	½ cup	130	16	0	15
rocky road	½ cup	170	17	0	13
spumoni	½ cup	150	16	0	13
strawberry cupcake	½ cup	140	19	0	15
Tin Roof Sundae	½ cup	170	18	0	15
toasted almond	½ cup	150	15	0	12
toffee bar	½ cup	170	19	0	18
Triple Chocolate Thunder	½ cup	160	18	0	15
Turtle Sundae	½ cup	160	18	0	14
Ultimate Caramel Cup	½ cup	170	22	0	19
vanilla	½ cup	150	14	0	11
bean	½ cup	140	15	0	14
chocolate	½ cup	150	16	0	14
Treasure	½ cup	160	19	0	16
■ (Godiva) super premium ice cream					
Belgian dark chocolate	½ cup	280	26	2	23
chocolate					
cheesecake	½ cup	310	36	1	30
raspberry truffle	½ cup	290	32	2	26
w/chocolate hearts	½ cup	330	32	2	29
chocolate-covered cookies 'n' cream	½ cup	300	32	<1	28
classic milk chocolate	½ cup	290	28	1	26
vanilla					
caramel pecan	½ cup	290	33	0	30
chocolate & chocolate					
caramel hearts	½ cup	310	32	1	29
white chocolate raspberry	½ cup	290	32	2	26
■ (Häagen-Dazs)					
ICE CREAM					
Bailey's Irish Cream	½ cup	270	23	0	22
bananas Foster	½ cup	260	28	0	24
black walnut	½ cup	300	21	0	19
butter pecan	½ cup	310	21	<1	18
café mocha	½ cup	310	30	<1	28
cherry vanilla	½ cup	240	23	0	22
chocolate	½ cup	270	22	1	21
chocolate					
chocolate chip	½ cup	300	26	2	24
mousse	½ cup	310	30	<1	27
peanut butter	½ cup	360	27	2	24
raspberry torte	½ cup	270	29	1	26
coffee	½ cup	270	21	0	21
cookies 'n' cream	½ cup	270	23	0	21
cookie dough chip	½ cup	310	29	0	24
crème brûlée	½ cup	280	23	0	22

Food and Description	Amount	Total Calories	Total Carbs	Fiber	Sugars
dulce de leche caramel	½ cup	290	28	0	28
French vanilla mousse	½ cup	310	29	0	28
macadamia brittle	½ cup	360	25	0	24
mango	½ cup	250	28	<1	27
mint chip	½ cup	300	26	<1	23
mocha almond fudge	½ cup	340	28	<1	26
peaches & cream	½ cup	240	29	0	27
peanut butter fudge chunk	½ cup	340	25	1	22
pineapple coconut	½ cup	230	25	0	24
pistachio	½ cup	290	22	<1	19
rocky road	½ cup	300	29	1	24
rum raisin	½ cup	270	22	0	21
strawberry	½ cup	250	23	<1	22
strawberry cheesecake	½ cup	270	28	0	26
tres leches	½ cup	270	26	0	24
vanilla	½ cup	270	21	0	21
caramel brownie	½ cup	300	30	0	25
chocolate chip	½ cup	310	26	<1	22
fudge	½ cup	290	26	0	24
Swiss almond	½ cup	300	24	<1	21
white chocolate raspberry truffle	½ cup	310	32	1	28
■ **(Healthy Choice)**					
Brownie Bliss	½ cup	130	24	1	16
butter pecan crunch	½ cup	100	18	2	4
cappuccino chocolate chunk	½ cup	120	20	<1	16
caramel fudge brownie	½ cup	120	21	1	17
Cherry Chocolate Mambo	½ cup	130	21	2	21
chocolate chocolate chunk	½ cup	120	21	1	17
cookies 'n' cream	½ cup	120	21	<1	16
Crazy Caramel	½ cup	120	23	<1	17
Double Karma	½ cup	140	28	<1	21
French Silk	½ cup	120	24	2	18
Happy Together	½ cup	150	29	1	21
Jumpin' Java	½ cup	130	25	<1	20
milk chocolate chip	½ cup	120	20	<1	16
peanut butter cup	½ cup	120	21	<1	17
praline & caramel	½ cup	120	23	1	19
rocky road	½ cup	130	25	1	17
Tin Roof Sundae	½ cup	120	21	1	16
Turtle Fudge Cake	½ cup	130	23	<1	21
vanilla	½ cup	110	19	<1	15
vanilla bean	½ cup	120	21	<1	16
■ **(Hood)**					
ALL-NATURAL..PEAK TREASURES					
Black Raspberry Ripple	½ cup	150	20	0	15
Caramel Cup Gold Mine	½ cup	170	22	0	17
Chocolate					
Brownie Mudslide	½ cup	170	23	1	16
Chip Canyon	½ cup	150	20	0	14
Peanut Butter Avalanche	½ cup	170	21	0	16

Food and Description	Amount	Total Calories	Total Carbs	Fiber	Sugars
Cookie Sandwich Snowstorm	½ cup	170	21	0	13
French Vanilla Vummit	½ cup	160	18	0	13
Fudge River Rapids	½ cup	150	20	0	15
Java Chip Trails	½ cup	160	19	0	14
Mint Cookie Caverns	½ cup	170	21	0	14
orange & vanilla swirls	½ cup	130	19	0	13
Triple Peaks	½ cup	140	16	0	13
Vanilla Snowdrift	½ cup	150	17	0	12
FAT-FREE					
apple crisp	½ cup	130	28	0	19
Chocolate Passion	½ cup	100	23	0	22
Chocolate Trio	½ cup	100	23	0	22
double brownie sundae	½ cup	120	27	0	25
Heavenly Mash	½ cup	120	27	0	25
Very Vanilla	½ cup	100	23	0	23
LIGHT					
Almond Praline Delight	½ cup	140	23	0	22
brownie sundae	½ cup	140	23	0	20
butter pecan	½ cup	140	19	0	19
Caribbean Coffee Royale	½ cup	110	18	0	17
chocolate almond chip	½ cup	140	22	0	20
choc. chocolate chip cookie dough	½ cup	140	21	0	21
Classic Trio	½ cup	110	18	0	18
cookies 'n' cream	½ cup	130	21	0	18
creamy vanilla	½ cup	110	18	0	18
Heavenly Hash	½ cup	130	22	0	21
Mud Pie Medley	½ cup	140	20	0	19
raspberry swirl	½ cup	120	22	0	20
Triple Nut Sundae	½ cup	140	22	0	19
TRADITIONAL					
Butterscotch Blast	½ cup	160	20	0	16
Chippedy Chocolatey	½ cup	150	8	0	14
chocolate	½ cup	140	17	0	12
Classic Trio	½ cup	140	17	0	13
Cookie Dough Delight	½ cup	160	20	0	14
cookies 'n' cream	½ cup	160	19	0	14
creamy coffee	½ cup	140	16	0	12
eggnog	½ cup	150	16	0	10
Fudge Twister	½ cup	140	20	0	15
Golden Vanilla	½ cup	140	16	0	13
grasshopper pie	½ cup	160	22	0	16
maple walnut	½ cup	150	27	0	13
natural vanilla bean	½ cup	140	16	0	13
Patchwork	½ cup	140	17	0	13
peppermint stick	½ cup	140	22	0	15
spumoni	½ cup	140	17	0	13
strawberry	½ cup	130	17	0	13
■ (Imagine)					
DREAM SUPREME					
Pralines 'n' Dream	½ cup	180	24	1	16

Food and Description	Amount	Total Calories	Total Carbs	Fiber	Sugars
NONDAIRY FROZEN DESSERTS					
cappuccino	½ cup	150	23	1	17
carob	½ cup	150	24	2	17
carob almond	½ cup	170	24	2	17
cocoa marble fudge	½ cup	150	25	2	15
cookies 'n' dream	½ cup	170	26	1	17
mint					
carob chip	½ cup	170	26	1	18
chocolate chip	½ cup	170	26	1	19
Neapolitan	½ cup	150	24	2	18
orange vanilla swirl	½ cup	150	24	1	18
strawberry	½ cup	140	24	1	19
vanilla	½ cup	150	23	1	17
vanilla Swiss almond	½ cup	180	25	1	18
■ (Kemp's)					
ROUND CONTAINER ICE CREAM					
all-natural vanilla	½ cup	150	17	0	13
apple pie	½ cup	160	19	0	13
Bear Tracks	½ cup	180	23	0	17
black raspberry	½ cup	150	18	0	14
butter pecan	½ cup	170	17	0	13
Caramel Cow Tracks	½ cup	170	23	0	17
Caramel Fudge Cow Tracks	½ cup	170	25	0	19
Caramel Invasion	½ cup	170	23	0	17
cherry fudge chunk	½ cup	160	20	0	16
chocolate chip	½ cup	160	19	0	15
cookies 'n' cream	½ cup	170	20	0	13
Deep Dark Secrets	½ cup	170	22	0	18
Double Fudge Moose Tracks	½ cup	180	22	<1	18
French vanilla	½ cup	150	19	0	14
homemade vanilla	½ cup	160	19	0	16
Jamaican Me Crazy	½ cup	160	22	0	16
Las Vegas Fudge Chunk	½ cup	190	20	0	17
maple nut	½ cup	160	17	0	13
Mint Cow Tracks	½ cup	190	21	0	17
Moose Tracks	½ cup	190	20	<1	18
New York strawberry cheesecake	½ cup	150	20	0	16
New York vanilla	½ cup	150	17	0	14
Northern Exposure	½ cup	190	21	0	17
Peanut Butter 'n' Fudge Cow Tracks	½ cup	190	19	0	15
Peanut Fudgester	½ cup	180	20	0	16
Pearson's					
mint patty	½ cup	160	19	0	15
nut goody	½ cup	170	20	0	16
Peppermint Bon Bon	½ cup	160	19	0	15
Raspberry Fudge Cow Tracks	½ cup	190	21	0	18
rocky road	½ cup	170	21	0	15
Seriously Chocolate	½ cup	190	24	0	20
Sneaker Doodles	½ cup	180	22	0	17
strawberries 'n' cream	½ cup	130	16	0	13

Food and Description	Amount	Total Calories	Total Carbs	Fiber	Sugars
toasted almond fudge	½ cup	170	18	0	15
Torch Truffle	½ cup	160	20	0	17
Twist and Shout	½ cup	200	18	0	13
vanilla	½ cup	150	17	0	14
vanilla custard	½ cup	160	19	0	16
white chocolate raspberry truffle	½ cup	160	21	0	16
SQUARE CONTAINER ICE CREAM					
Bear Creek Caramel	½ cup	150	21	0	16
Black Jack Cherry	½ cup	140	18	0	15
black walnut	½ cup	140	15	0	13
Blackberry Creek Swirl	½ cup	140	17	0	14
butter pecan	½ cup	150	15	0	12
candy cane	½ cup	140	18	0	15
caramel cashew crunch	½ cup	150	19	0	16
chocolate	½ cup	130	17	<1	15
chocolate almond cluster	½ cup	150	18	<1	15
chocolate chip	½ cup	140	17	0	14
chocolate chip cookie dough	½ cup	150	19	0	14
Chocolate Monster	½ cup	150	20	0	15
cinnamon	½ cup	130	16	0	13
cookies 'n' cream	½ cup	150	18	0	13
Cookies 'n' Scream	½ cup	140	18	0	14
cotton candy	½ cup	130	16	0	13
Dreaming of Mint	½ cup	150	21	0	18
dulce de leche	½ cup	140	18	0	15
French silk pie	½ cup	150	22	0	17
German chocolate cake	½ cup	150	20	<1	15
Gone Fishin'	½ cup	160	21	<1	18
Holiday Dazzle	½ cup	150	18	0	15
holiday mint cookie	½ cup	150	18	0	15
holiday mint fudge	½ cup	140	19	0	14
homemade vanilla	½ cup	140	17	0	15
key lime	½ cup	150	20	0	16
mango	½ cup	120	16	0	13
maple nut	½ cup	140	16	0	12
mint chocolate chip	½ cup	140	17	0	14
Moose Lake Fudge	½ cup	170	19	0	16
Neapolitan	½ cup	130	18	0	14
New York vanilla	½ cup	130	16	0	13
Nuts to You	½ cup	150	17	0	15
Orange Cream Dream	½ cup	130	23	0	18
peanut butter pie	½ cup	180	18	0	13
Pecan Turtle Trail	½ cup	160	20	0	15
pineapple coconut	½ cup	140	20	0	17
pink peppermint	½ cup	140	18	0	15
rocky road	½ cup	150	20	<1	14
strawberry	½ cup	120	16	0	13
Timber Lodge Mint	½ cup	170	19	0	17
Tin Roof Sundae	½ cup	140	19	0	14
tres leches	½ cup	150	21	0	15

Food and Description	Amount	Total Calories	Total Carbs	Fiber	Sugars
Turtle Tracks	½ cup	150	22	0	17
Under the Stars	½ cup	180	18	<1	14
vanilla	½ cup	130	16	0	13
vanilla chocolate	½ cup	130	16	0	14
■ (M&M's Brand)					
brownie chocolate	½ cup	180	22	0	18
mint	½ cup	190	20	0	18
vanilla	½ cup	180	22	0	18
■ (Pet)					
CARB LIMIT					
butter pecan	½ cup	120	13	4	3
chocolate	½ cup	110	13	4	3
Neapolitan	½ cup	110	13	4	3
HOMEMADE					
banana split	½ cup	160	24	0	21
Butter Pecan Madness	½ cup	180	19	0	16
peach cobbler	½ cup	150	20	0	15
vanilla	½ cup	150	18	0	15
SIGNATURE COLLECTIONS					
hot fudge sundae	½ cup	180	19	1	17
Moose Tracks	½ cup	190	19	1	16
Nuttin' But Turtles	½ cup	160	20	0	18
Oozle Doozle	½ cup	150	22	0	19
pistachio almond	½ cup	160	15	1	13
vanilla bean	½ cup	140	16	0	14
TRADITIONAL					
black walnut	½ cup	150	15	0	13
butter pecan	½ cup	160	15	0	13
cherry vanilla	½ cup	140	16	0	14
chocolate	½ cup	120	13	0	12
cookies 'n' cream	½ cup	160	19	0	15
French vanilla	½ cup	150	17	0	15
heavenly hash	½ cup	130	16	0	13
Neapolitan	½ cup	130	15	0	13
Nutty Buddy Chocolate Nut Sundae Cone	½ cup	160	20	0	15
strawberry	½ cup	130	17	0	15
vanilla	½ cup	140	16	0	14
■ (Schwan's)					
CARBS					
Carb Comfort					
butter pecan	½ cup	130	15	6	4
chocolate	½ cup	110	15	6	4
PREMIUM..PREMIUM PLUS					
chocolate double fudge brownie	½ cup	160	22	0	15
Chunky Chocolate Peanut Butter Binge	½ cup	190	19	0	14
Raspberry Rumble	½ cup	160	21	0	17
strawberry cheesecake	½ cup	150	20	0	16

Food and Description	Amount	Total Calories	Total Carbs	Fiber	Sugars
TRADITIONAL					
banana nut	½ cup	150	16	0	13
black raspberry	½ cup	130	16	0	12
butter pecan	½ cup	150	15	0	11
chip & mint	½ cup	150	17	0	13
chocolate	½ cup	140	17	0	12
almond	½ cup	150	17	1	12
chip	½ cup	150	17	0	13
chip cookie dough	½ cup	150	19	0	13
fudge ripple	½ cup	140	18	0	13
malt twist	½ cup	160	20	0	14
marshmallow ripple	½ cup	140	20	0	15
coffee	½ cup	140	16	0	11
cookies 'n' cream	½ cup	160	17	0	13
dark sweet cherry	½ cup	140	17	0	13
dulce de leche	½ cup	150	19	0	16
maple nut	½ cup	150	16	0	13
peaches 'n' cream	½ cup	130	20	0	16
Pecan Caramel Quake	½ cup	180	20	0	15
pecan praline sundae	½ cup	150	19	0	15
Race Trax	½ cup	160	20	0	15
rocky road	½ cup	150	21	0	15
strawberry	½ cup	130	16	0	12
Summer's Dream	½ cup	130	19	0	14
vanilla	½ cup	140	16	0	12
■ (Starbuck's)					
classic coffee	½ cup	270	22	1	21
coffee almond fudge	½ cup	270	22	1	21
Java chip	½ cup	270	22	1	21
■ (Tofutti) nondairy pints					
CHEESECAKE SUPREME					
blueberry	½ cup	200	20	0	15
chocolate	½ cup	200	20	0	15
strawberry	½ cup	200	20	0	15
LOW-FAT SUPREME					
chocolate fudge	½ cup	145	25	0	18
coffee marshmallow swirl	½ cup	120	24	0	14
vanilla fudge	½ cup	130	24	0	16
PREMIUM					
butter pecan	½ cup	210	22	0	17
chocolate cookie crunch	½ cup	210	26	0	13
chocolate supreme	½ cup	180	18	0	8
mint chocolate chip	½ cup	210	21	0	16
vanilla	½ cup	190	20	0	15
almond bark	½ cup	210	21	0	16
fudge	½ cup	190	25	0	18
Wildberry Supreme	½ cup	190	24	0	19
SUPER SOY SUPREME					
Bella Vanilla	½ cup	160	20	0	13
Cool Cappuccino	½ cup	170	21	0	14

Food and Description	Amount	Total Calories	Total Carbs	Fiber	Sugars
Plum Crazy	½ cup	160	26	0	18
NY NY Chocolate	½ cup	170	22	0	15
■ (Turkey Hill)					
CARB IQ					
butter pecan	½ cup	140	15	5	3
TRADITIONAL					
black cherry	½ cup	140	15	5	3
choco-malt chip	½ cup	170	22	0	20
Denali Original Moose Tracks	½ cup	190	21	1	16
Eagles Touchdown Sundae	½ cup	190	19	0	17
Neapolitan	½ cup	150	18	0	17
Peanut Butter Kandy Kake	½ cup	230	21	0	15
Philadelphia-style vanilla bean	½ cup	160	15	0	13
Phillies Graham Slam	½ cup	190	21	0	6
■ (Weight Watchers)					
low-fat..vanilla/chocolate giant sundae cups	1 cup	150	39	7	24
reduced-fat..no sugar added					
butter pecan	½ cup	110	15	5	4
crunchy peanut butter cup	½ cup	110	17	5	4
Moose Tracks	½ cup	130	18	4	4
Neapolitan	½ cup	90	16	5	4
vanilla	½ cup	90	15	5	5

ICE CREAM BARS, CONES & CUPS, SANDWICHES & FROZEN NOVELTIES (*See also* FRUIT ICES, BARS, & POPS; RICE FROZEN DESSERT; SHERBET; TOFU FROZEN DESSERT)

Food and Description	Amount	Total Calories	Total Carbs	Fiber	Sugars
■ (Atkins) Endulge					
BARS..Novelties					
caramel turtle sundae	1 bar	180	12	4	1
chocolate fudge	1 bar	130	12	5	1
peanut butter swirl	1 bar	180	12	4	1
vanilla fudge swirl	1 bar	180	12	4	1
SANDWICHES..Novelties					
chocolate	1 sdw	150	16	5	1
peanut butter	1 sdw	150	15	4	1
vanilla	1 sdw	150	15	4	1
■ (Ben & Jerry's) Peace Pops					
Cherry Garcia	1 pop	280	29	1	24
cookie dough	1 pop	380	41	<1	31
One Sweet Whirled	1 pop	270	28	1	24
vanilla	1 pop	300	26	<1	24
w/Heath toffee	1 pop	320	30	<1	28
■ (Blue Bunny)					
BARS..Novelties					
4-pack					
NASCAR Speedway Sundae	1 bar	300	25	<1	21
6-pack					
black raspberry	1 bar	230	20	1	16
crunch	1 bar	190	17	0	14
fudge	1 bar	110	15	0	12

Food and Description	Amount	Total Calories	Total Carbs	Fiber	Sugars
Goin' Bananas	1 bar	110	21	0	16
Heath	1 bar	190	16	0	13
root beer float	1 bar	90	15	0	12
Star Bars..reduced-fat	1 bar	130	13	0	11
Sundae Crunch					
chocolate	1 bar	170	22	0	14
Neapolitan	1 bar	190	19	0	12
strawberry	1 bar	170	22	0	14
12-pack					
English toffee	1 bar	130	12	0	9
homemade vanilla	1 bar	150	13	0	12
Krunch	1 bar	150	14	0	11
Star Bars..reduced-fat	1 bar	110	11	0	9
CONES..Novelties..The Champ!..6-Pack					
chocolate lovers	1 cone	300	38	1	28
caramel	1 cone	350	41	1	30
vanilla	1 cone	320	35	1	25
vanilla nutty sundae	1 cone	240	34	1	22
CUPS..Novelties..malt..4-pack	1 cup	220	35	0	28
DISNEY..Novelties					
Buzz Lightyear S'wiches	1 sdw	110	16	0	8
Mickey S'wiches	1 sdw	100	17	0	9
Mud'n Fudge Bars	1 bar	80	15	0	12
Power Ranger Cool Tubes	1 tube	80	18	0	15
Tigger Cookie-rrific	1 cookie	120	20	0	15
Winnie the Pooh Cool Tubes	1 tube	80	18	0	15
HEALTH SMART..raspberry & orange	1 bar	70	17	4	2
SANDWICHES..Novelties..10-pack					
homemade vanilla	1 sdw	180	25	0	16
Mississippi mud	1 sdw	190	27	1	14
strawberry cheesecake	1 sdw	180	28	0	16
vanilla	1 sdw	170	24	0	12
SWEET FREEDOM..Novelties..12-pack					
light..white chocolate almond	1 bar	100	10	2	2
sandwiches					
double vanilla	1 sdw	150	32	5	4
vanilla..low-fat	1 sdw	140	32	4	5
sundae cone..vanilla	1 cone	240	30	3	4
■ (Breyers) Hershey's almond bar	1 bar	270	20	<1	18
■ CARNATION (*See* (Nestlé) in this section)					
■ (Dove)					
BARS					
almond					
multipack	1 bar	270	23	1	20
singles	1 bar	340	28	1	24
milk chocolate caramel toffee crunch					
multipack	1 bar	270	29	1	26
singles	1 bar	330	35	1	31
original chocolate w/chocolate ice cream					
multipack	1 bar	260	27	3	22

Food and Description	Amount	Total Calories	Total Carbs	Fiber	Sugars
singles	1 bar	320	34	3	27
vanilla w/chocolate coating					
multipack	1 bar	260	26	2	21
singles	1 bar	320	32	2	26
vanilla w/milk chocolate coating					
multipack	1 bar	260	25	1	22
singles	1 bar	330	31	1	28
LIMITED EDITION DOVE BAR					
Crunchy Cookies w/Cream	1 bar	280	28	1	23
MINIATURES					
Flavor Collection	5 pieces	310	32	2	25
milk chocolate					
w/French vanilla ice cream	5 pieces	320	32	2	26
w/vanilla ice cream	5 pieces	320	30	1	27
■ **DRUMSTICK** (*See* (Nestlé) in this section)					
■ **(Eskimo Pie)**					
BARS					
chocolate éclair	1 bar	220	20	<1	18
Frosty the Snowman	1 bar	100	11	0	7
ice cream bar w/dark chocolate coat	2.5-oz bar	160	14	0	11
king-size w/dark chocolate coating	4-oz bar	220	21	0	17
king-size w/milk chocolate coating	4-oz bar	220	21	0	17
strawberry shortcake	1 bar	220	26	0	18
thin mint	1 bar	250	23	1	19
toasted almond	1 bar	220	27	0	23
vanilla w/milk chocolate coating	1 bar	220	21	0	17
CHIPWICH..Sandwiches					
king-size..single-serve	1 sdw	310	45	<1	19
vanilla	1 sdw	250	37	0	15
vanilla fudge..low-fat	1 sdw	200	36	2	15
SANDWICHES					
Chilly Bears Cookies 'N' Cream	1 sdw	180	24	<1	12
Gingerbread Men	1 sdw	160	26	<1	12
SINGLE-SERVE					
bars					
king-size					
candy center crunch	1 bar	230	21	0	15
chocolate éclair	1 bar	410	31	1	17
premium	1 bar	220	26	0	18
ice cream bar	1 bar	250	23	0	19
giant	1 bar	410	35	2	28
strawberry shortcake	1 bar	250	30	<1	20
toasted almond	1 bar	230	21	0	15
cones..w/chocolate topping & peanuts					
king-size..vanilla w/chocolate	1 cone	250	30	1	19
cups..cookies 'n' cream	1 cup	310	45	1	29
sandwiches					
cookies 'n' cream	1 sdw	230	34	1	18
giant king-size..vanilla	1 sdw	250	36	1	20

Food and Description	Amount	Total Calories	Total Carbs	Fiber	Sugars
■ (Good Humor)					
BARS					
multipacks					
chocolate éclair	1 bar	160	20	<1	12
cookies 'n' cream	1 bar	190	21	<1	15
dark chocolate	1 bar	190	15	<1	12
milk chocolate	1 bar	180	15	0	12
strawberry shortcake	1 bar	170	21	0	12
toasted almond	1 bar	180	22	<1	16
single-serve					
candy center crunch	1 bar	310	24	<1	19
chocolate éclair	1 bar	220	30	<1	16
Number 1 Bar	1 bar	200	21	<1	15
Oreo Cookie	1 bar	250	28	<1	18
Reese's Peanut Butter	1 bar	310	27	<1	23
strawberry shortcake	1 bar	230	30	<1	17
toasted almond	1 bar	230	30	<1	23
CONES & CUPS..Singles					
giant king cone	1 cone	400	44	1	30
king cone	1 cone	250	30	<1	19
premium sundae	1 cone	270	29	<1	18
sundae twist cup	1 cup	160	33	0	29
SANDWICHES..Singles					
premium					
cookie	1 sdw	290	41	1	24
vanilla	1 sdw	160	25	0	12
■ (Häagen-Dazs) multipack bars					
caramel & almond crunch	1 bar	300	28	0	27
chocolate & dark chocolate	1 bar	290	23	2	20
coffee & almond crunch	1 bar	310	23	1	21
dulce de leche caramel	1 bar	300	28	0	27
raspberry cheesecake	1 bar	300	28	0	27
vanilla & almonds	1 bar	320	22	1	20
vanilla & dark chocolate	1 bar	280	22	1	20
vanilla & milk chocolate	1 bar	280	20	0	20
■ (Healthy Choice) low-fat					
BARS					
fudge..6-pack	1 bar	80	13	0	2
mocha fudge..6-pack	1 bar	90	17	1	14
sorbet & cream..6-pack	1 bar	100	20	<1	14
strawberry & cream..6-pack	1 bar	90	17	<1	15
SANDWICHES					
caramel	1 sdw	140	27	<1	17
fudge swirl	1 sdw	140	27	<1	16
vanilla	1 sdw	130	24	<1	14
■ (Hoods)					
BARS					
chocolate-covered ice cream bar					
original	1 bar	160	11	0	11
reduced-fat	1 bar	100	9	0	3

Food and Description	Amount	Total Calories	Total Carbs	Fiber	Sugars
chocolate éclair	1 bar	150	14	0	11
fudge bars					
dipped delights					
chocolate fudge	1 bar	95	21	1	16
java smoothie	1 bar	90	17	0	9
peanut butter chocolate	1 bar	135	14	0	8
orange cream..regular	1 bar	90	18	0	18
Rocket	1 bar	120	23	0	22
sport sundae	1 bar	250	23	0	22
CONES & CUPS					
Nutty Royale	1 cone	220	26	<1	15
Sundae cup swirl w/chocolate &					
strawberry sauce	1 cup	120	19	0	16
SANDWICHES					
Hoodsie					
light	1 sdw	160	29	1	16
low-fat	1 sdw	90	15	0	2
mint	1 sdw	100	15	0	8
original	1 sdw	180	27	1	16
■ (Imagine) nondairy desserts					
DREAM BARS					
chocolate	1 bar	270	32	2	22
chocolate nutty	1 bar	270	23	2	14
vanilla	1 bar	270	33	1	21
vanilla nutty	1 bar	260	23	2	14
DREAM PIES					
chocolate	1 pie	320	39	2	13
mint	1 pie	320	39	2	13
mocha	1 pie	320	40	1	12
vanilla	1 pie	320	40	1	12
■ (Kemp's)					
BARS					
English toffee	1 bar	160	14	0	13
float bar	2 bars	100	20	0	16
fudge bar..6-pack	1 bar	80	17	1	16
Kemp's ice cream bar w/chocolate coating					
2.5 oz	1 bar	160	12	0	11
king	1 bar	240	20	0	17
Kemp's Krunch Bar..12-pack	1 bar	140	12	0	10
Kemp's toffee bar	1 bar	170	14	0	14
Krunch					
junior	2 bars	210	18	0	15
king	1 bar	230	20	0	17
King Malt Ball crunch bar	1 bar	280	22	1	18
Koala bar	1 bar	290	25	0	22
Moo Jr.'s	2 bars	190	20	0	17
orange cream bar					
1.78 oz	1 bar	80	13	0	13
king	1 bar	120	19	0	15
Scooter					

Food and Description	Amount	Total Calories	Total Carbs	Fiber	Sugars
cream	2 bars	90	18	0	18
fudge	2 bars	170	15	0	14
Trios..vanilla	2 bars	210	19	1	18
CONES					
Kemp's sundae cone					
caramel	1 cone	290	33	2	24
combination	1 cone	290	31	2	22
Nutty Royale	1 cone	220	25	1	17
old-fashioned sundae..vanilla	1 cone	290	31	2	22
NO SUGAR ADDED					
fudge bar..12-pack	1 bar	110	22	0	10
ice cream sandwich..vanilla	1 sdw	140	21	0	3
SANDWICHES					
chocolate chip	1 sdw	140	26	0	14
cookies 'n' cream	1 sdw	170	26	0	13
Cow Tracks	1 sdw	190	26	0	15
double chocolate	1 sdw	160	26	0	14
Kemp's king..Neapolitan	1 sdw	280	38	0	23
Kemp's mint chocolate chip	1 sdw	170	24	0	15
Kempwich	1 sdw	340	44	0	33
Pearson's mint patty	1 sdw	180	27	0	15
vanilla					
king	1 sdw	280	38	0	23
mini	1 sdw	100	15	0	8
mini..reduced-fat	1 sdw	90	16	0	8
regular..12-pack	1 sdw	160	25	0	13
■ **(Klondike)**					
BARS					
cappuccino	1 bar	280	24	0	21
caramel crunch	1 bar	270	26	0	24
Chocolate for Chocoholics	1 bar	280	23	<1	21
dark chocolate	1 bar	280	24	<1	20
Heath..single	1 bar	300	26	0	24
Hershey w/almond	1 bar	250	20	<1	17
Krunch..single	1 bar	260	24	0	20
minis snack-size vanilla	1 bar	170	15	0	13
Movie Bites..4.48-oz pkg	1 pkg	310	26	0	23
Neapolitan	1 bar	280	24	<1	21
original vanilla	1 bar	280	24	0	22
Planters caramel & peanut..single	1 bar	300	28	1	24
Slim-a-Bear..no sugar added	1 bar	170	21	4	7
CARB SMART					
ice cream bar					
fudge	1 bar	100	9	1	3
vanilla..w/chocolate coating	1 bar	170	9	2	5
ice cream cone	1 cone	210	14	3	3
ice cream sandwich	1 sdw	80	10	2	3
CONES					
Big Bear Sundae Kone					

Food and Description	Amount	Total Calories	Total Carbs	Fiber	Sugars
sundae..w/caramel center	1 cone	320	35	<1	26
sundae..w/fudge center	1 cone	320	36	<1	26
vanilla	1 cone	300	31	<1	21
chocolate	1 cone	280	29	1	20
vanilla	1 cone	280	29	1	20
caramel	1 cone	300	34	<1	25
fudge	1 cone	300	34	<1	25
Slim-a-Bear 96% fat-free					
chocolate	1 cone	180	36	3	19
vanilla	1 cone	170	35	3	19
SANDWICHES					
Big Bear					
ice cream cookie	1 sdw	270	38	1	23
Neapolitan..single-serve	1 sdw	300	42	<1	25
vanilla..single	1 sdw	300	42	<1	25
giant cookie w/Hershey's chips	1 sdw	470	66	2	38
mini Reese's pieces..4.2 oz	1 pkg	260	37	1	22
Oreo cookie	1 sdw	230	34	2	18
Slim-a-Bear..98% fat-free	1 sdw	130	28	3	14
Slim-a-Bear..no sugar added..vanilla	1 sdw	120	25	3	1
TACOS..Choco Taco..singles	1 bar	290	35	1	24
■ (LeCarb) bars					
chocolate	1 bar	100	6	<1	2
chocolate almond	1 bar	130	6	1	2
lemon	1 bar	100	6	0	3
strawberry	1 bar	100	6	0	3
■ (M&M's Brand)					
CONE	1 cone	230	32	1	22
SANDWICHES					
brownie	1 sdw	220	28	0	20
cookie	1 sdw	220	29	1	19
■ (Nestlé)					
Bon Bons					
dark chocolate	8 pieces	330	29	<1	25
milk chocolate	8 pieces	330	29	<1	26
Butterfinger	1 bar	210	17	0	14
Carnation					
sandwiches					
Neapolitan..singles	1 sdw	240	34	0	24
vanilla..singles	1 sdw	240	34	0	23
sundae cups					
w/chocolate topping	1 cup	200	28	0	23
w/strawberry topping	1 cup	210	28	0	24
Crunch Bar					
caramel	1 bar	210	19	0	16
chocolate & vanilla	1 bar	230	18	0	15
reduced-fat	1 bar	150	17	0	5
vanilla	1 bar	220	18	0	15
drumstick					
caramel	1 cone	360	36	<1	29

Food and Description	Amount	Total Calories	Total Carbs	Fiber	Sugars
chocolate	1 cone	360	33	<1	24
chocolate-dipped	1 cone	340	35	2	20
classic					
fudge sundae	1 cone	340	35	2	20
s'mores	1 cone	310	34	<1	27
strawberry cheesecake	1 cone	340	35	2	20
cookies & cream	1 cone	350	40	<1	31
reduced-fat	1 cone	280	36	<1	27
triple chocolate	1 cone	280	36	<1	27
vanilla	1 cone	340	33	<1	24
caramel	1 cone	340	35	2	20
fudge	1 cone	340	35	2	20
w/chocolate layers	1 cone	280	32	1	19
Husky Bar	1 bar	340	32	0	28
Toll House cookie sandwich					
chocolate chip cookie	1 sdw	520	72	1	4
chocolate chocolate chip cookie	1 sdw	550	67	2	49
■ (Popsicle)					
characters..singles					
Col. Crunch					
chocolate éclair	1 bar	160	20	<1	12
strawberry	1 bar	170	21	0	12
Snoopy ice cream bar	1 bar	150	16	0	13
WWE ice cream bar	1 bar	180	16	0	13
Creamsicle					
CarbSmart pops..1.75 oz..all flavors	1 pop	20	5	1	0
no sugar added/multi-pks/all flavors	1 bar	25	6	0	2
original..single..orange	1 bar	110	20	0	15
pop..1.75 oz..all flavors	1 pop	70	13	0	10
sugar-free..1.65 oz..all flavors	2 pops	45	12	3	0
Fudgsicle					
chocolate..single	1 bar	90	17	<1	14
fat-free	1 bar	60	14	<1	10
mini..1.2 oz	2 pops	80	16	<1	13
no sugar added..1.75 oz	2 pops	90	19	1	3
original..2.5 oz	1 bar	90	16	<1	13
ice cream pops..mini	2 pops	200	18	0	16
ice cream sandwich..mini	2 oz	100	15	0	7
Sprinklers bar..single	1 bar	180	26	0	19
■ (Schwan's)					
BARS					
caramel premium	1 bar	210	20	0	17
chocolate fudge sticks	1 bar	110	22	0	16
chocolate sundae crunch	1 bar	180	22	0	13
English toffee	1 bar	200	28	0	16
Gold'n Nugit	1 bar	250	23	0	19
rainbow stick	1 bar	90	18	0	14
root beer float	1 bar	90	16	0	12
Schwan's ice cream	1 bar	190	17	0	13
Silver Mint	1 bar	150	14	0	12

Food and Description	Amount	Total Calories	Total Carbs	Fiber	Sugars
strawberry crunch	1 bar	170	21	0	14
Trim Creations chocolate fudge stick	1 bar	50	14	0	4
CONES					
banana fudge sundae	1 cone	250	35	<1	21
caramel round top	1 cone	350	41	1	27
chip & mint sundae	1 cone	260	36	1	23
pecan praline sundae	1 cone	260	36	0	23
Race Trax	1 cone	270	35	<1	20
rocky road sundae	1 cone	260	39	2	25
vanilla fudge chocolate sundae	1 cone	260	37	1	23
vanilla sundae	1 cone	210	28	0	15
CUPS					
apple pie à la mode	½ cup	260	35	<1	18
brownie à la mode	½ cup	280	36	1	27
caramel cappuccino	1 cup	300	35	0	28
frozen hot chocolate	½ cup	160	23	<1	13
root beer float	1 cup	140	25	0	23
SANDWICHES					
chocolate chip cookie	1 sdw	260	33	0	21
Glacier Bay Lemon	1 sdw	190	28	1	15
Mississippi Mud	1 sdw	200	29	2	13
■ **(Slim-Fast)**					
chocolate fudge bar	1 bar	110	22	<1	17
ice cream sandwich..all flavors	1 sdw	130	27	<1	14
■ **(Starbucks)**					
FRAPPUCCINO COFFEE BARS					
caffe vanilla	1 bar	110	20	9	5
java fudge	1 bar	130	25	4	16
mocha	1 bar	120	22	3	15
■ **(Tofutti)**					
BARS					
Hooray Hooray	1 bar	150	10	0	0
Marry Me	1 bar	168	22	0	18
Monkey...peanut butter	1 bar	220	22	0	18
SANDWICHES..Cuties					
Blueberry Wave	1 sdw	140	20	0	12
chocolate	1 sdw	130	16	0	9
Chocolate Wave	1 sdw	140	20	0	12
Coffee Break	1 sdw	130	16	0	9
cookies 'n' cream	1 sdw	120	17	0	9
Jazzy	1 sdw	120	17	0	9
mint chocolate chip	1 sdw	120	19	0	11
peanut butter	1 sdw	165	20	0	10
Strawberry Wave	1 sdw	140	20	0	12
Totally Vanilla	1 sdw	120	16	0	9
vanilla..no sugar added	1 sdw	120	17	0	9
SANDWICHES..Too-Too's					
vanilla chocolate chip	1 sdw	230	30	0	18
■ **(Weight Watchers)**					
BARS					

Food and Description	Amount	Total Calories	Total Carbs	Fiber	Sugars
chocolate mousse	1 bar	40	9	1	3
chocolate treat	1 bar	100	20	1	17
English toffee crunch	1 bar	110	12	1	10
fudge treat	1 bar	100	20	1	17
giant...low-fat					
cookies 'n' cream	1 bar	120	24	4	15
fudge	1 bar	80	20	4	15
orange vanilla treat	1 bar	40	10	0	3
CONES					
chocolate sundae	1 cone	130	29	4	12
peanut butter fudge	1 cone	130	29	3	12
vanilla or vanilla fudge	1 cone	130	29	3	12
CUPS...Sundae..Giant					
chocolate chocolate	1 cup	150	39	9	23
peanut butter chocolate	1 cup	150	30	8	24
SANDWICHES..Round					
chocolate	1 sdw	130	27	4	14
mint	1 sdw	130	28	3	15
peanut butter 'n' fudge	1 sdw	130	28	3	15
vanilla	1 sdw	130	28	3	15
ICE CREAM CONES & CUPS					
(Joy Cone)					
cones					
kid's cone	3 cups	15	3	0	0
sugar	1 cone	50	11	0	3
cups..cake					
jumbo	1 cup	30	7	0	0
regular..plain or colored	1 cup	20	3	0	0
sundaes	1 cup	30	6	0	0
waffle					
bowl	1 bowl	80	18	<1	5
cone	1 cone	90	19	<1	5
(Keebler)					
fudge-dipped cup	1 cup	35	6	0	2
ice cream cup/vanilla	1 cup	15	4	0	0
sugar cone	1 cone	50	10	0	4
waffle..bowl or cone	1 bowl or cone	50	10	0	4
(Nabisco)					
Comet..sugar cone	1 cone	60	4	1	1
Oreo..chocolate	1 cone	50	10	1	4
original cup	1 cup	20	4	0	0
rainbow cup	1 cup	20	4	0	1
ICE CREAM SANDWICH (*See* ICE CREAM BARS, CONES & CUPS, SANDWICHES & FROZEN NOVELTIES)					
ICE CREAM TOPPING (*See also* CREAM; DIP; WHIPPED TOPPING)					
BOTTLED, CANNED, or JARRED					
(Hershey's)					
CHOCOLATE SHOPPE TOPPINGS					
double chocolate hot fudge	2 Tbs	120	12	1	18

Food and Description	Amount	Total Calories	Total Carbs	Fiber	Sugars
fat-free	2 Tbs	100	23	1	18
regular	2 Tbs	130	23	<1	17
DESSERT TOPPINGS..Sprinkles					
Reese's peanut butter &					
milk chocolate	2 Tbs	90	12	0	6
triple chocolate	2 Tbs	90	12	<1	7
SHELL TOPPINGS					
chocolate fudge cookie	2 Tbs	190	15	2	12
Heath	2 Tbs	230	17	<1	15
Krackel	2 Tbs	190	14	0	11
milk chocolate	2 Tbs	230	16	1	14
Reese's	2 Tbs	220	17	1	15
SUNDAE SYRUPS					
caramel	2 Tbs	100	25	0	20
double chocolate fudge	1 Tbs	50	13	1	21
SYRUPS..Hershey's					
chocolate					
light	2 Tbs	50	12	0	10
malt..Whoppers	2 Tbs	100	25	0	21
original	2 Tbs	100	24	0	20
strawberry	2 Tbs	100	26	0	26
TOPPING..Hershey's canned					
chocolate fudge	2 Tbs	130	24	<1	17
(Kraft)					
butterscotch	2 Tbs	130	28	0	18
caramel	2 Tbs	120	28	0	20
chocolate-flavored	2 Tbs	110	26	1	20
hot fudge	2 Tbs	140	24	<1	17
pineapple	2 Tbs	110	28	0	19
strawberry	2 Tbs	110	29	0	22
(Smucker's)					
PLATE SCRAPERS DESSERT TOPPINGS					
caramel	2 Tbs	100	25	0	18
chocolate	2 Tbs	100	23	1	11
raspberry	2 Tbs	100	25	0	13
white chocolate	2 Tbs	110	22	0	11
SPECIALTY TOPPINGS					
Dove toppings					
dark chocolate	2 Tbs	140	22	1	15
milk chocolate	2 Tbs	130	21	1	17
dulce de leche (milk caramel)	2 Tbs	110	23	0	19
pecans in syrup	2 Tbs	170	20	<1	13
special recipes					
butterscotch caramel	2 Tbs	130	30	<1	18
hot fudge	2 Tbs	140	22	<1	16
walnuts in syrup	2 Tbs	170	20	1	13
TOPPINGS, OTHER					
3 Musketeers..sundae syrup	2 Tbs	110	23	0	18
butterscotch..sundae syrup	2 Tbs	100	25	0	19
butterscotch & caramel syrup					

Food and Description	Amount	Total Calories	Total Carbs	Fiber	Sugars
regular..spoonable	2 Tbs	130	31	<1	21
sundae	2 Tbs	110	25	0	19
butterscotch & caramel topping					
regular..spoonable	2 Tbs	130	31	<1	21
special recipe	2 Tbs	130	30	<1	28
caramel					
fat-free microwaveable	2 Tbs	130	31	1	21
sundae syrup	2 Tbs	100	25	0	19
chocolate fudge					
microwaveable	2 Tbs	130	28	1	18
regular..spoonable	2 Tbs	130	28	1	18
sundae syrup	2 Tbs	110	26	1	21
chocolate-flavored sundae syrup	2 Tbs	110	26	1	21
chocolate-flavored syrup..sugar-free	2 Tbs	100	24	1	0
dulce de leche (milk caramel)	2 Tbs	140	25	0	22
hot fudge					
light..fat-free	2 Tbs	90	23	2	15
microwaveable..original	2 Tbs	130	24	<1	14
regular..spoonable	2 Tbs	140	24	1	16
special recipe	2 Tbs	140	22	<1	16
sugar-free	2 Tbs	100	24	1	0
Magic Shell toppings					
caramel	2 Tbs	220	14	0	13
chocolate	2 Tbs	220	16	1	15
chocolate fudge	2 Tbs	220	19	1	11
Twix	2 Tbs	210	18	1	15
marshmallow..spoonable	2 Tbs	120	29	0	28
Milky Way..spoonable	2 Tbs	130	24	0	18
pecans in syrup	2 Tbs	170	20	<1	13
pineapple..spoonable	2 Tbs	110	28	0	28
strawberry					
regular..spoonable	2 Tbs	100	26	0	26
sundae syrup	2 Tbs	110	16	0	23

ICE MILK (*See* ICE CREAM & ICE CREAM–LIKE FROZEN DESSERTS)

ICE MILK BAR (*See* ICE CREAM BARS, CONES & CUPS, SANDWICHES & FROZEN NOVELTIES)

ICES (*See* FRUIT ICES, BARS & POPS)

ICING (*See* CAKE FROSTING/ICING)

INDIAN PUDDING (*See* PUDDING & MOUSSE)

J

Food and Description	Amount	Total Calories	Total Carbs	Fiber	Sugars
JACKFRUIT/raw..sliced	1 cup	155	40	3	0
JALAPEÑO (*See* MEXICAN FOOD; PEPPER)					
JAM/JELLY/PRESERVES					
(Bama)					
JAM					
grape	1 Tbs	50	13	0	13
red plum	1 Tbs	50	13	0	13
strawberry	1 Tbs	60	14	0	7
jelly					
all flavors	1 Tbs	50	13	0	13
grape w/peanut butter	1 Tbs	120	17	0	11
preserves					
apricot	1 Tbs	50	13	0	13
blackberry	1 Tbs	50	13	0	13
peach	1 Tbs	30	13	0	13
strawberry	1 Tbs	50	13	0	13
spread..strawberry	1 Tbs	50	13	0	13
(Braswell's) fig preserves	1 Tbs	45	11	0	9
(Cascadian Farm) organic					
fancy fruit spreads..all flavors	1 Tbs	40	10	0	10
(Crosse & Blackwell)					
guava jelly	1 Tbs	60	14	0	13
lemon curd	1 Tbs	50	13	0	10
mint-flavored apple	1 Tbs	60	14	0	13
orange marmalade	1 Tbs	60	16	0	11
red currant jelly	1 Tbs	60	14	0	13
(Empress)					
jam..all flavors	2 tsp	35	9	0	9
jelly..all flavors	2 tsp	35	9	0	9
preserves..all flavors	2 tsp	35	9	0	9
(Fifty/50) fruit spread..all flavors	1 Tbs	10	4	0	1
(Jok'n Al) fruit spread..low-carb					
apricot	1 Tbs	10	2	0	2
black currant	1 Tbs	10	2	0	2
blackberry & apple	1 Tbs	10	2	0	1
orange marmalade	1 Tbs	10	2	0	2
pineapple	1 Tbs	9	2	0	1
raspberry	1 Tbs	10	2	0	1
strawberry	1 Tbs	10	2	0	1

Food and Description	Amount	Total Calories	Total Carbs	Fiber	Sugars
(Knott's Berry Farm)					
jam..all flavors	1 Tbs	35	9	0	6
jelly					
all flavors	½ oz	35	9	0	6
light..all flavors	1 tsp	8	2	0	2
orange marmalade	¾ oz	50	13	0	10
preserves..all flavors	1 Tbs	35	9	0	6
spread..all flavors	½ oz	35	9	0	6
(Maple Grove Farms) jam..all flavors	1 Tbs	50	13	0	9
(Mary Ellen)					
jam..all flavors	1 Tbs	50	13	0	12
jelly..all flavors	1 Tbs	50	13	0	12
(Polaner)					
jam..all flavors	1 Tbs	40	10	0	9
jelly					
mint..real	1 Tbs	60	14	0	8
other flavors..all	1 Tbs	40	10	0	8
preserves					
all flavors	1 Tbs	40	10	0	9
60% less sugar	1 Tbs	20	6	0	5
sugar-free	1 Tbs	10	5	0	0
(Smucker's) fruit spreads..all flavors					
jam	1 Tbs	50	13	0	12
jelly	1 Tbs	50	13	0	12
low-sugar	1 Tbs	25	6	0	5
marmalade..orange	1 Tbs	50	13	0	12
preserves	1 Tbs	50	13	0	12
Simply 100% Fruit spread	1 Tbs	40	10	0	8
sugar-free	1 Tbs	10	5	0	0
(Welch's)					
jam..all flavors	1 Tbs	50	13	0	13
jelly..all flavors	1 Tbs	50	13	0	13
preserves..all flavors	1 Tbs	50	13	0	13
(Wolferman's) fruit spreads..all flavors	1 Tbs	40	10	0	9
JAPANESE FOOD (See ASIAN FOOD)					
JELL-O (See GELATIN)					
JERKY STICKS & STRIPS (See MEAT SNACK)					
JERUSALEM ARTICHOKE..raw..sliced	1 cup	115	26	2	0
JEW'S EAR					
dried	½ cup	35	10	0	0
raw..sliced	½ cup	15	3.5	0	0
JICAMA/YAM BEAN-TUBER/MEXICAN POTATO					
raw..sliced	1 cup	50	11	6	na
JUICE (See individual listings)					
JUJUBE..dried	3 oz	246	63	2.5	na

K

Food and Description	Amount	Total Calories	Total Carbs	Fiber	Sugars
KALE					
CANNED (The Allens) seasoned					
Southern-style	½ cup	35	6	1	2
FROZEN (Best Yet) chopped..cooked	½ cup	30	2	2	1
RAW	½ cup	17	3	1	1
KASHA (*See* BUCKWHEAT GROATS)					
KELP (*See* SEAWEED)					
KETCHUP (*See* CATSUP)					
KIDNEY BEAN					
CANNED					
(The Allens) red frijoles rojos	½ cup	120	22	8	2
(Bush's Best)					
dark red	½ cup	130	21	7	2
light red	½ cup	110	20	7	1
(Eden) 100% organic					
cannellini..white	½ cup	100	17	5	1
red..no salt added	½ cup	100	18	10	0
refried..lightly salted	½ cup	80	15	6	0
(Progresso)					
cannellini/white	½ cup	100	16	5	0
dark red	½ cup	110	20	6	2
(S&W) dark red..all styles	½ cup	100	23	6	7
(Trappey's)					
dark red	½ cup	130	22	8	1
jalapeño	½ cup	120	19	6	2
light red	½ cup	110	22	8	2
New Orleans–style w/bacon	½ cup	110	20	6	3
w/chili gravy	½ cup	110	20	7	3
DRY..bag.. (Springfield) light red	1.35 oz	70	22	14	1
SPROUTED..raw mature seeds	1 cup	55	8	na	0
KIELBASA (*See* SAUSAGE)					
KIWI JUICE/JUICE BLEND (*See also* FRUIT PUNCH; SOFT DRINK MIX; individual listings)					
(After The Fall) Kiwi Bear	8 fl oz	100	24	0	23
(Ocean Spray) Cravin' Less Sugar	8 oz	70	19	0	15
(R. W. Knudsen) kiwi strawberry	8 oz	120	30	0	28
KIWIFRUIT					
fresh/raw	2 medium	100	24	1	16
	1 large	55	13	<1	9
KNOCKWURST (*See* FRANKFURTER; SAUSAGE)					

Food and Description	Amount	Total Calories	Total Carbs	Fiber	Sugars
KOHLRABI..fresh/sliced					
cooked–drained	½ cup	24	6	1	0
raw	1 cup	110	26	6	0
KOOL-AID (*See* SOFT DRINK MIX)					
KRAUT JUICE (*See* SAUERKRAUT JUICE)					
KUMQUAT..fresh/raw	1 medium	12	3	1	0

L

Food and Description	Amount	Total Calories	Total Carbs	Fiber	Sugars
LAMB					

(Note: All serving sizes are cooked portions, unless otherwise stated. "Lean" means lamb trimmed of all separable fat before cooking. In most cases, 4 ounces of raw meat equals 3 ounces of cooked meat.)

Food and Description	Amount	Total Calories	Total Carbs	Fiber	Sugars
domestic..USA					
composite cuts/leg & shoulder					
lean					
braised/cubed	3 oz	190	0	0	0
broiled					
cubed	3 oz	160	0	0	0
ground	3 oz	240	0	0	0
leg/foreshank					
lean					
braised	3 oz	160	0	0	0
broiled/ground	3 oz	240	0	0	0
lean & fat					
braised	3 oz	210	0	0	0
braised/diced	1 cup	340	0	0	0
stewed	3 oz	210	0	0	0
leg/shank					
lean..roasted	3 oz	155	0	0	0
lean & fat..roasted	3 oz	190	0	0	0
leg/sirloin					
lean..roasted	3 oz	175	0	0	0
lean & fat..roasted	3 oz	250	0	0	0
leg/whole					
lean..roasted	3 oz	165	0	0	0
lean & fat..roasted	3 oz	220	0	0	0
loin					

Food and Description	Amount	Total Calories	Total Carbs	Fiber	Sugars
lean..roasted	3 oz	175	0	0	0
lean & fat..roasted	3 oz	265	0	0	0
organs					
brain					
braised	3 oz	125	0	0	0
pan-fried	3 oz	235	0	0	0
heart..braised	3 oz	160	2	0	0
kidney..braised	3 oz	115	1	0	0
liver					
braised	3 oz	190	2	0	0
pan-fried	3 oz	205	3	0	0
tongue/braised	3 oz	235	0	0	0
rib					
lean..roasted	3 oz	200	0	0	0
lean & fat..roasted	3 oz	305	0	0	0
shoulder/arm					
lean					
broiled	3 oz	170	0	0	0
roasted	3 oz	165	0	0	0
shoulder/blade					
lean					
broiled	3 oz	180	0	0	0
roasted	3 oz	180	0	0	0
lean & fat					
broiled	3 oz	235	0	0	0
roasted	3 oz	240	0	0	0
shoulder/whole					
lean					
broiled	3 oz	180	0	0	0
roasted	3 oz	175	0	0	0
lean & fat					
braised/diced	1 cup	485	0	0	0
broiled	3 oz	236	0	0	0
roasted	3 oz	235	0	0	0
LAMB'S QUARTERS					
fresh/cooked..chopped	1 cup	60	9	0	0
LARD (See also FAT; OIL; PORK)	1 Tbs	115	0	0	0
	1 cup	1,850	0	0	0
LASAGNA (See BEEF DISH/ENTRÉE; FROZEN ENTRÉE/DINNER; PASTA ENTRÉE/DINNER)					
LAVER (See SEAWEED)					
LEEK					
freeze-dried	¼ cup	3	1	0	0
fresh					
cooked	¼ cup	8	2	0	0
raw..chopped	¼ cup	14	3	<1	0
whole	1 medium	54	13	2	0
LEMON/fresh	1 medium	17	5	2	0
	1 large	25	12	5	0
LEMON JUICE					

Food and Description	Amount	Total Calories	Total Carbs	Fiber	Sugars
BOTTLED					
(Haggen) from concentrate..natural	2 tsp	0	0	0	0
(Realemon)	1 tsp	0	0	0	0
(Springfield) from concentrate	1 Tbs	3	1	0	0
FRESH	1 Tbs	4	1.5	0	0
	½ cup	30	11	0.5	0
FROZEN (Sunkist)	1 fl oz	7	2	0	0
LEMON PEEL					
candied (S&W)	58 pieces	80	23	2	18
fresh..grated	1 Tbs	3	1	0	0
LEMONADE/LEMONADE-FLAVORED DRINK (*See also* SOFT DRINK; SOFT DRINK MIX; TEA)					
BOTTLED, BOXED, or CANNED					
(Capri Sun) lemonade..pouch	6.75 oz	100	27	0	27
(Crystal Light) all flavors	8 fl oz	5	0	0	0
(Dr. Pepper/Seven Up) Elements Turbulence					
Shredded Lemon Energy	8 fl oz	120	29	0	28
(Minute Maid)					
coolers..pouch	8.45 oz	100	26	0	26
lemonade..box	6.75 oz	90	25	9	24
pink lemonade	8 fl oz	110	30	0	29
regular..all natural	8 fl oz	110	31	0	29
(Newman's Own)					
lemonade..all styles	8 fl oz	110	27	0	27
Lemon-Aided Iced Tea	8 fl oz	110	27	0	27
(Odwalla) lemonade..strawberry	8 fl oz	120	29	0	29
(R. W. Knudsen)					
Recharge..lemon	8 fl oz	70	18	0	17
spritzer..lemon lime	12 fl oz	170	41	0	38
(Santa Cruz Organics) sparkling	12 fl oz	100	26	0	23
(Snapple) all flavors..regular	8 fl oz	110	26	0	24
(Welch's)					
lemonade juice cocktail	10 fl oz	160	41	0	40
	11.5 fl oz	190	47	0	46
single serve	8 fl oz	130	33	0	32
low-cal lemonade drink	8.45 fl oz	15	3	0	2
(Zeigler) chilled..pink or regular	8 fl oz	100	26	0	25
FROZEN					
(Minute Maid) all styles..prepared	8 fl oz	110	30	0	28
frozen concentrate only	2 oz	110	30	0	28
(Old Orchard) all styles..prepared	8 fl oz	110	27	0	26
frozen concentrate only	2 oz	110	27	0	26
MIX...prepared unless otherwise noted					
(Country Time)					
lemonade iced tea					
classic	8 fl oz	90	22	0	22
peach	8 fl oz	90	22	0	22
raspberry	8 fl oz	80	20	0	20
pink					

Food and Description	Amount	Total Calories	Total Carbs	Fiber	Sugars
sugar-free	8 fl oz	5	0	0	0
sweetened	8 fl oz	70	17	0	17
regular					
sugar-free	8 fl oz	5	0	0	0
sweetened	8 fl oz	70	17	0	17
sweetened lemonade drink mix					
cranberry raspberry	8 fl oz	90	22	0	22
raspberry	8 fl oz	80	20	0	20
strawberry	8 fl oz	80	20	0	20
wild berry	8 fl oz	90	22	0	22
(Crystal Light)					
pink or traditional	8 fl oz	5	0	0	0
raspberry peach	8 fl oz	5	1	0	0
(Kool-Aid)					
pink					
regular..prepared w/sugar & water	8 fl oz	100	25	0	25
sugar-free	8 fl oz	5	0	0	0
traditional					
regular..prepared w/sugar & water	8 fl oz	100	25	0	25
sugar-free	8 fl oz	5	0	0	0
LEMON-LIME DRINK (*See* SOFT DRINK; SOFT DRINK MIX)					
LENTIL (*See also* SOUP; VEGETARIAN FOODS)					
CANNED					
(Eden) w/sweet onion & bay leaf	½ cup	90	13	4	0
DRIED					
(Arrowhead Mills) green or red..raw	¾ cup	150	27	9	0
(Goya)	¼ cup	70	19	9	0
MICROWAVEABLE					
(Fantastic Foods)					
country lentil..big cup	½ pkg	180	32	0	2
couscous w/lentil	½ pkg	170	35	5	3
SPROUTED	½ cup	40	8	na	0
LENTIL SOUP (*See* SOUP)					
LETTUCE					
Bibb	med head	21	4	2	0
butterhead	med head	21	4	2	0
cos/shredded	½ cup	4	1	0	0
iceberg	med head	70	11	8	0
loose leaf or Simpson/shredded	½ cup	5	1	0	0
romaine/shredded	½ cup	4	1	0	0
LICHEE NUT/LYCHEE NUT/LITCHI NUT					
dried/shelled	1 oz	80	20	4.5	0
raw	1 medium	6	2	0	0
shelled & seeded	½ cup	65	16	<1	0
LIMA BEAN (*See also* BUTTER BEAN)					
CANNED					
The Allens East Texas Fair) green	½ cup	120	23	8	0
(Aunt Nellie's) Reber butter beans (Bush's Best)	½ cup	140	25	6	4

Food and Description	Amount	Total Calories	Total Carbs	Fiber	Sugars
green					
butter beans	½ cup	110	19	6	0
limas..medium	½ cup	110	17	5	0
speckled butter beans	½ cup	110	19	5	0
(Eden) baby	½ cup	100	17	4	0
(Glory) seasoned					
butter beans	½ cup	120	20	5	0
limas	½ cup	140	24	7	0
(S&W) butter beans	½ cup	80	19	5	2
(Trappey's) baby					
baby green flavored w/slab bacon	½ cup	120	22	6	2
baby white..w/bacon	½ cup	130	21	6	2
large white..w/sausage	½ cup	110	21	6	2
(Veg-All) baby green habas verdes					
tiernas de lima	½ cup	90	17	4	1
DRIED..bag					
(Best Yet)					
baby lima	¼ cup	70	23	15	0
Fordhook	¼ cup	90	17	5	1
large	¼ cup	70	22	12	0
FROZEN					
(Birds Eye)					
baby	½ cup	110	22	5	1
butter	½ cup	100	20	4	1
speckled butter	½ cup	100	20	4	1
(C&W) all styles	½ cup	90	15	5	1
(Green Giant) baby..boil-in-bag	⅔ cup	110	20	4	1
LIME	1 medium	20	7	2	0
LIME JUICE					
BOTTLED					
(Herdez) vegetable juice..spicy lime	11.3 oz	90	19	2	7
(Jero) cocktail mix..sweetened..West India–style					
	1 oz	35	9	0	8
(Major Peters') from concentrate..sweetened..West India–style					
	1 tsp	10	2	0	2
(Realime)	1 fl oz	6	0	0	0
(T. Marzetti) Key Largo lime juice	1 tsp	0	0	0	0
FRESH	⅓ cup	22	7	<1	0
LIME JUICE DRINK (See also SOFT DRINK; SOFT DRINK MIX)					
BOTTLED or CANNED					
(Kern's) from Libby's..limeade	8 fl oz	120	31	0	29
(La Croix) natural lime	12 fl oz	0	0	0	0
(Minute Maid) limeade..cherry	8 fl oz	120	34	0	33
(Odwalla) organic					
Summertime Lime Quencher	8 fl oz	90	24	0	18
(Snapple-a-Day) mango lime..low-carb	11.5 fl oz	90	16	7	7
FROZEN/PREPARED					
(Minute Maid)	8 fl oz	100	26	0	24
(Old Orchard)	8 fl oz	115	27	0	26

Food and Description	Amount	Total Calories	Total Carbs	Fiber	Sugars
LING					
baked or broiled	3 oz	95	0	0	0
LINGCOD					
baked or boiled	3 oz	90	0	0	0
raw	3 oz	75	0	0	0
LINGUINE (*See* FROZEN ENTRÉE/DINNER; PASTA ENTRÉE/DINNER; VEGETARIAN FOODS)					
LIQUEUR (*See also* COCKTAIL; LIQUOR, DISTILLED)					
anisette	¾ fl oz	74	7	0	0
Benedictine	¾ fl oz	69	7	0	0
crème de cacao	1.5 fl oz	150	23	0	na
crème de menthe	1.5 fl oz	186	21	0	na
Curaçao	¾ fl oz	54	6	0	0
Drambuie	1.5 fl oz	157	13	0	na
gin..citrus	1.5 fl oz	114	0	0	0
kirsch	1.5 fl oz	120	9	0	na
Pernod	1.5 fl oz	115	3	0	0
rum..Bacardi Superior	1.5 fl oz	66	0	0	0
sloe gin	1.5 fl oz	130	4	0	0
Southern Comfort	1.5 fl oz	115	5	0	0
triple sec	1.5 fl oz	120	6	0	0
vodka..citrus	1.5 fl oz	100	0	0	0
LIQUOR, DISTILLED					
(NOTE: In all cases, the higher the proof [the % of alcohol], the higher the calories.)					
80-proof	1 fl oz	67	0	0	0
84-proof	1 fl oz	70	0	0	0
86-proof	1 fl oz	72	0	0	0
90-proof	1 fl oz	75	0	0	0
94-proof	1 fl oz	78	0	0	0
97-proof	1 fl oz	81	0	0	0
100-proof	1 fl oz	83	0	0	0
LIVER (*See* BEEF; CHICKEN; GOOSE; LAMB; PÂTÉ; PORK; TURKEY)					
LIVER LOAF (*See* LUNCHEON MEAT)					
LIVERWURST (*See* LUNCHEON MEAT)					
LOBSTER (*See also* SEAFOOD ENTRÉE/DINNER)					
fresh					
northern..cooked–moist heat	3 oz	83	1	0	<1
	1 cup	142	2	0	0
spiny..cooked–moist heat	3 oz	120	3	0	0
spiny..raw	3 oz	95	2	0	0
LOBSTER, IMITATION					
(Louis Kemp) Lobster Delights					
chunk-style	½ cup	80	12	0	5
flake-style	½ cup	80	12	0	4
salad-style	½ cup	80	12	0	4
LOBSTER BISQUE (*See* SOUP)					
LOTUS ROOT					
cooked	½ cup	40	10	2	0
raw..9.5" in length	10 slices	60	14	1.5	0
LOTUS SEED					
dried	1 oz	94	18	na	0

Food and Description	Amount	Total Calories	Total Carbs	Fiber	Sugars
raw	1 oz	25	5	na	0
LOX (See SALMON)					
LUNCHEON LOAF (See LUNCHEON MEAT)					
LUNCHEON MEAT (See also BEEF; CHICKEN; HAM; LUNCHEON MEAT SPREAD; TURKEY; VEGETARIAN FOODS)					
■ **(Alpine Lace)**					
deli meats					
97% fat-free ham					
cooked	2 oz	60	2	0	1
honey	2 oz	60	2	0	1
97% fat-free roast beef	2 oz	70	1	0	0
turkey breast..fat-free	2 oz	50	0	0	0
■ **(Armour)**					
beef..dried..95% fat-free	1 oz	60	2	0	2
bologna..w/chicken & turkey	1 oz	90	2	0	1
Lunch Makers..Cracker Crunchers					
cooked ham	2.6 oz	360	48	1	39
ham	2.6 oz	240	17	2	7
pepperoni pizza	3.3 oz	240	26	1	7
turkey	2.6 oz	360	21	1	5
potted meat	½ oz	130	0	0	0
Treet luncheon loaf					
Light..50% less fat	2 oz	110	4	0	2
original	2 oz	130	3	0	3
Vienna sausage					
barbecue	2.17 oz	150	0	0	0
chicken	1.89 oz	110	1	0	0
hot 'n' spicy	2.17 oz	150	2	0	0
jalapeño	1.89 oz	170	1	0	0
light..50% less fat	1.89 oz	90	1	0	1
original	1.89 oz	150	0	0	0
smoked	1.89 oz	150	0	0	0
■ **(Boar's Head)**					
bologna					
beef	2 oz	150	0	0	0
garlic	2 oz	150	1	0	1
Lebanon	2 oz	100	3	0	3
pork & beef	2 oz	150	<1	0	0
ham..tavern	2 oz	60	2	0	2
Italian delicacies					
abruzzese..hot & sweet	1 oz	100	<1	0	0
capocollo..hot & sweet	1 oz	80	0	0	0
imported porketta	2 oz	70	<1	0	<1
mortadella	2 oz	160	0	0	0
w/pistachio nuts	2 oz	170	2	0	0
pepperoni..sandwich-style	1 oz	130	1	0	0
prosciutto riserva stradolce	1 oz	60	0	0	0
soppressata..hot & sweet	1 oz	100	<1	0	0
liverwurst					
braunschweiger..light	2 oz	120	1	0	0

Food and Description	Amount	Total Calories	Total Carbs	Fiber	Sugars
onion	2 oz	160	1	0	1
smoked	2 oz	170	1	0	1
loaves					
Dutch	2 oz	150	2	0	2
olive	2 oz	130	<1	0	<1
pickle & pepper	2 oz	150	2	0	1
spiced ham	2 oz	120	2	0	1
salami					
Bianco D'Oro..Italian dry	1 oz	110	1	0	0
Genoa	2 oz	180	1	0	0
hard	1 oz	110	<1	0	0
sausages					
hot..smoked	1 link	250	1	0	0
kielbasa	2 oz	120	0	0	0
smoked..natural casing	1 link	360	2	0	0
■ (Butterball)					
turkey breast					
honey-roasted & smoked					
deli-thin..fat-free	2 oz	50	3	0	2
hearty deli-sliced	1 oz	30	1	0	1
oven-roasted					
97% fat-free	1.6 oz	60	1	0	0
premium-carved	1.6 oz	60	1	0	0
■ (Carl Buddig) /sliced					
1.5-oz pkgs..lean smoked					
ham	1 pkg	65	0.5	0	0
ham..honey	1 pkg	70	2	0	0
turkey	1 pkg	65	0.5	0	0
turkey..honey	1 pkg	70	2	0	0
2.5-oz pkgs...lean smoked					
beef	1 pkg	120	1	0	1
chicken	1 pkg	110	1	0	1
corn beef	1 pkg	120	1	0	1
ham	1 pkg	120	1	0	1
ham..honey	1 pkg	120	3	0	3
pastrami	1 pkg	120	1	0	1
turkey	1 pkg	110	1	0	1
honey	1 pkg	120	3	0	3
oven-roasted	1 pkg	110	1	0	1
8-oz pkgs..lean smoked					
beef	¼ pkg	90	1	0	0
chicken	¼ pkg	85	1	0	0
corned beef	¼ pkg	90	1	0	0
ham..honey	¼ pkg	90	2	0	0
turkey..honey	¼ pkg	90	2	0	0
■ (DAK)					
beef..corned beef..can	2 oz	120	1	0	1
ham					
chopped..can	2 oz	170	1	0	1
chunked & ground	2 oz	100	1	0	1

Food and Description	Amount	Total Calories	Total Carbs	Fiber	Sugars
deli-smoked ham..97% fat-free	2 oz	60	1	0	1
imported..98% fat-free	1.6 oz	45	0	0	0
premium					
97% fat-free	1 oz	30	0	0	0
honey..97% fat-free	1 oz	30	0	0	0
imported..97% fat-free	2 oz	50	0	0	0
turkey ham..95% fat-free	1 oz	35	0	0	0
■ (Danola)					
beef					
Angus roast beef	2 oz	60	1	0	0
Cajun-style	2 oz	60	1	0	0
corned beef	2 oz	60	1	0	0
canned	2 oz	120	1	0	1
Italian-style roast beef	2 oz	60	1	0	0
ham					
Black Forest..smoked..97% fat-free	1.6 oz	60	0	0	0
imported..lower sodium..98% fat-free	1.6 oz	40	0	0	0
pepper-smoked..97% fat-free	1.8 oz	50	1	0	1
smoked honey..97% fat-free	1.6 oz	50	2	0	2
supreme					
baked brown sugar	2 oz	60	1	0	1
Black Forest..smoked	2 oz	60	1	0	1
imported w/natural juices	2 oz	50	0	0	0
smoked honey	2 oz	60	1	0	1
smoked maple-flavored honey	2 oz	70	2	0	2
smoked Virginia Brand	2 oz	60	0	0	1
■ (Farmer John)					
bologna..roll..sliced	2 slices	190	0	0	0
bologna..beef..sliced	2 slices	150	0	0	0
cotto salami	2 slices	150	0	0	0
ham					
cooked..sliced	2 slices	60	0	0	0
extra-lean	1 slice	40	0	0	0
steak	2 oz	70	0	0	0
head cheese..sliced	1 slice	110	0	0	0
liverwurst..w/bacon	2 oz	190	0	0	0
mission loaf..sliced	2 slices	80	0	0	0
■ (Galileo)					
coppacola..hot	2 oz	140	1	0	1
cotto salami	2 oz	170	2	0	1
Genoa salami	2 oz	180	0	0	0
hard salami	1 oz	120	0	0	0
mortadella	2 oz	160	2	0	2
salami..Italian dry..thin-sliced	5 slices	110	1	0	1
■ (Healthy Choice)					
COLD CUTS..deli thin-sliced					
chicken breast					
honey-roasted	4 slices	60	3	0	0
honey-roasted & smoked	4 slices	70	4	0	2
oven-roasted	4 slices	60	3	0	0

Food and Description	Amount	Total Calories	Total Carbs	Fiber	Sugars
smoked	4 slices	60	3	0	0
ham					
cooked..baked	4 slices	60	2	0	1
honey	4 slices	60	2	0	2
honey maple	4 slices	60	3	0	2
honey mustard	4 slices	60	2	0	2
Virginia Brand..smoked	4 slices	60	2	0	1
pastrami	4 slices	60	2	0	0
turkey breast					
mesquite-flavor..smoked	4 slices	60	2	0	0
oven-roasted	4 slices	60	2	0	1
rotisserie-seasoned	4 slices	60	2	0	1
COLD CUTS..regular					
bologna	2 slices	80	7	0	2
chicken breast..oven-roasted	1-oz slice	30	2	0	0
ham					
baked cooked	1-oz slice	30	1	0	1
cooked	1-oz slice	30	2	0	1
honey..square	1-oz slice	30	1	0	1
smoked	1-oz slice	30	1	0	1
turkey breast					
honey-roasted & smoked	1-oz slice	35	1	0	1
oven-roasted	1-oz slice	30	0	0	0
smoked	1-oz slice	30	1	0	<1
■ (Hebrew National)					
bologna..beef..lean	1 oz	90	1	0	0
knockwurst..beef	1 link	260	1	0	0
pastrami..deli slices	4 slices	90	1	0	0
salami..beef	3 slices	150	0	0	0
turkey breast					
oven-roasted	5 slices	50	1	0	0
smoked	2 oz	50	1	0	0
■ (Hillshire Farm)					
bologna..deluxe club presliced	1 slice	90	0	0	0
bratwurst	2.5-oz link	250	2	0	2
bratwurst..beer	2.5-oz link	250	2	0	2
Chicken breast..Deli Select..oven-roasted	2 oz	50	1	0	1
ham					
brown sugar.. baked	2 oz	70	3	0	3
brown sugar cured..bone in	3 oz	120	1	0	1
honey-cured..baked	2 oz	60	2	0	2
spiral sliced	3 oz	120	1	0	1
Italian sausage..sweet	2.5 oz	250	2	0	2
pepperoni	1 oz	150	0	0	0
pickle loaf	1 oz	70	1	0	1
Polska kielbasa..turkey	2-oz link	90	2	0	2
Smokeys..Big Red..smoked..skinless	2-oz link	180	2	0	2
Smokeys...Little	2-oz link	170	2	0	2

Food and Description	Amount	Total Calories	Total Carbs	Fiber	Sugars
summer sausage					
beef..Old World	2 oz	180	1	0	1
Yard-O-Beef	2 oz	190	1	0	0
■ (Hormel)					
beef					
dried	10 slices	50	1	0	1
seasoned..roast	2 oz	70	0	0	0
chicken					
breast	2 oz	50	0	0	0
chunk chicken	2 oz	60	0	0	0
lemon	2 oz	50	1	0	0
tomato basil w/garlic	2 oz	50	2	0	2
corned beef..cooked	2 oz	70	0	0	
ham					
Black Label..regular	2 oz	140	3	0	3
Black Forest..97% fat-free	2 oz	60	0	0	0
cooked..97% fat-free	2 oz	60	0	0	0
Cure 81..boneless chunk	3 oz	100	0	0	0
Curemaster	3 oz	80	0	0	0
double-smoked	2 oz	70	0	0	0
honey..sliced	2 oz	70	3	0	3
spiced	2 oz	140	1	0	1
pastrami..cooked	2 oz	70	0	0	0
pepperoni					
Rosa Grande	1 oz	140	0	0	0
turkey	17 slices	80	0	0	0
salami					
Genoa	12 slices	210	0	0	0
hard	1 oz	110	0	0	0
sandwich-style	1 oz	90	0	0	0
Spam..luncheon meat					
BBQ	2 oz	160	4	0	3
w/cheese	2 oz	170	2	0	1
classic single	1 pkg	210	2	0	1
garlic	2 oz	160	1	0	0
hot & spicy	2 oz	180	1	0	0
less salt	2 oz	180	1	0	0
light	2 oz	110	1	0	0
oven-roasted turkey	2 oz	80	1	0	0
regular	2 oz	180	1	0	0
smoked	2 oz	180	2	0	1
turkey single	1 pkg	110	3	0	0
turkey					
breast					
honey-smoked	2 oz	70	3	0	3
roasted	2 oz	50	0	0	0
smoked	2 oz	60	1	0	1
■ (Jennie-O Turkey Store)					
turkey..presliced					
Blue Ribbon breast..deli-shaved	2 oz	50	2	0	0

Food and Description	Amount	Total Calories	Total Carbs	Fiber	Sugars
Grand Champion w/caramel	2 oz	70	0	0	0
Jennie-O	2 oz	50	1	0	0
smoked..deli-shaved	2 oz	50	0	0	0
X-tra Lean					
bologna	2 oz	110	2	0	0
breast..99% fat-free	4 oz	180	5	0	0
hickory-smoked..97% fat-free	2 oz	60	1	0	0
oven-roasted breast	1.5 oz	45	1	0	0
pastrami	2 oz	60	1	0	0
salami	2 oz	70	2	0	0
smoked breast	1.5 oz	40	0	0	0
turkey ham	2 oz	70	1	0	0
■ (Kahn's)					
bologna					
beef	1 slice	90	1	0	0
beef & cheddar	1 slice	90	1	0	0
garlic	1 slice	90	1	0	0
giant..thick-sliced	1 slice	110	1	0	0
thick deluxe	1 slice	140	1	0	0
Dutch loaf	1 slice	80	1	0	0
ham..97% fat-free	1 oz slice	30	1	0	0
honey loaf	1 slice	40	1	0	0
liver loaf	1 slice	170	3	0	0
pickle loaf	1-oz slice	80	2	0	0
salami					
beef..8-oz pkg	1-oz slice	70	1	0	0
cotto salami/regular-sliced	1-oz slice	60	1	0	0
spice loaf					
beef/family pack	1-oz slice	60	1	0	0
regular/family pack	1-oz slice	70	1	0	0
■ (Land O' Frost)					
DELI-SHAVED..12-oz pkg					
chicken	2 oz	100	1	0	0
honey	2 oz	110	3	0	2
ham	2 oz	70	1	0	0
honey	2 oz	80	4	0	3
turkey	2 oz	90	0	0	0
honey	2 oz	100	3	0	2
DELI-STYLE..thin-sliced..2.5-oz pkg					
beef	1 pkg	120	2	0	2
chicken	1 pkg	120	0	0	0
honey	1 pkg	140	6	0	5
corned beef	1 pkg	120	1	0	1
ham	1 pkg	120	2	0	1
honey	1 pkg	100	5	0	3
pastrami	1 pkg	120	1	0	1
turkey	1 pkg	110	0	0	0
honey	1 pkg	120	4	0	1
roasted pepper	1 pkg	120	1	0	1

Food and Description	Amount	Total Calories	Total Carbs	Fiber	Sugars
■ (Libby's) corned beef..canned	2 oz	120	0	0	0
■ (Louis Rich)					
bologna..turkey..lower-fat	1 oz	50	1	0	0
Carving Board					
ham..honey..thin-carved	2.5 oz	70	2	0	2
turkey breast					
oven-roasted..98% fat-free	2.75 oz	70	3	0	0
chicken breast..breast cuts					
honey-roasted	3 oz	130	3	0	3
oven-roasted	3 oz	130	1	0	1
cotto salami..turkey..50% less fat	1 oz	45	3	0	0
ham					
honey-glazed..thin-carved	6 slices	70	2	0	2
turkey ham..50% less fat..all styles	1 oz	35	1	0	0
turkey breast					
hickory-smoked					
98% fat-free	1 oz	30	1	0	0
fat-free	2 oz	50	1	0	0
honey-roasted..fat-free	2 oz	60	3	0	2
oven-roasted..fat-free	2 oz	50	1	0	0
smoked	2 oz	70	3	0	0
smoked..95% fat-free..white	2 oz	35	1	0	0
■ (Oscar Mayer)					
bologna..sliced					
beef	1 oz	90	1	0	1
cheese	1 oz	90	1	0	0
light	1 oz	60	2	0	0
turkey	1 oz	50	1	0	0
chicken breast					
oven-roasted	2.5 oz	70	1	0	1
oven-roasted..deli-style..thin-sliced	2 oz	60	1	0	1
ham					
96% fat-free					
baked..cooked	1 oz	60	4	0	2
boiled	3 oz	60	1	0	1
chopped	1 oz	50	1	0	1
cooked	1 oz	30	0	0	1
honey	2.5 oz	60	2	0	2
honey..chopped	1 oz	60	4	0	2
smoked	2.5 oz	60	0	0	0
deli-style					
brown sugar					
shaved	1.8 oz	60	3	0	3
thin-sliced	1.8 oz	60	3	0	3
honey..shaved	1.8 oz	50	2	0	2
smoked..all styles	1.8 oz	45	0	0	0
loaves & sausages					
braunschweiger..liver sausage	2 oz	290	1	0	1
ham & cheese loaf	1 oz	60	1	0	1
liver cheese	1.3 oz	120	1	0	1

Food and Description	Amount	Total Calories	Total Carbs	Fiber	Sugars
luncheon loaf..spiced	1 oz	60	2	0	1
olive	1 oz	70	2	0	1
pickle & pimento	1 oz	80	2	0	2
Lunchables..individual lunch meat meals					
All Star..burgers..2-count	1 pkg	430	61	1	40
Cracker Stackers..3.8 oz					
bologna/American cheese	1 pkg	530	60	1	44
ham & cheddar	1 pkg	420	37	1	13
turkey & American cheese	1 pkg	430	52	1	36
Deluxe					
turkey & chicken w/cheese	1 pkg	390	25	1	8
turkey & ham w/cheese	1 pkg	370	25	1	7
salami					
beef cotto	1 oz	60	1	0	1
cotto	1 oz	70	1	0	0
hard	1 oz	100	1	0	0
spread..sandwich	2 oz	130	9	0	4
turkey breast					
mesquite-smoked..thin-sliced	2 oz	60	2	0	0
oven-roasted..98% fat-free	1 oz	25	0	0	0
smoked..white..honey..lean	1 oz	35	2	0	1
white..oven-roasted..95% fat-free	1 oz	30	1	0	0
■ (Plumrose)					
ham					
baked..96% fat-free	3 oz	35	0	0	0
brown sugar–baked..97% fat-free	1 oz	30	1	0	1
honey..96% fat-free	1 oz	35	2.5	0	1.5
honey-baked..97% fat-free	1 oz	35	1	1	1
ham steaks..smoked	4.5 oz	150	3	0	2
thin & tasty..97% fat-free					
ham					
baked	2 oz	50	2	0	0
cooked	2 oz	50	2	0	0
smoked	2 oz	50	2	0	0
turkey breast					
fat-free	2 oz	35	0	0	0
honey	2 oz	45	0	0	0
turkey breast					
hickory-smoked..97% fat-free	1 oz	30	0.5	0	0.5
honey..97% fat-free	1 oz	30	0	0	0
turkey ham..95% fat-free	1 oz	35	0	0	0
■ (Sara Lee) Deli Meats					
beef					
corned beef..USDA choice	2 oz	70	0	0	0
corned beef..presliced	2 slices	50	1	0	0
pastrami..USDA choice	2 oz	70	1	0	0
pastrami..presliced	2 slices	60	0	0	0
roast beef					
medium	2 oz	60	1	0	0

Food and Description	Amount	Total Calories	Total Carbs	Fiber	Sugars
peppered	2 oz	70	1	0	0
rare	2 oz	60	1	0	0
chicken breast..oven-roasted	2 oz	45	1	0	1
ham					
Black Forest	2 oz	60	1	0	1
brown sugar	2 oz	70	5	0	4
home-style baked	2 oz	60	2	0	2
honey-cured	2 oz	60	2	0	2
maple honey	2 oz	70	4	0	3
old-fashioned..cooked	2 oz	50	1	0	1
peppered	2 oz	60	2	0	2
smokehouse	2 oz	60	1	0	0
tavern honey	2 oz	60	2	0	2
Virginia-baked..presliced	2 slices	50	2	0	1
sausage..salami					
Genoa	1 oz	110	1	0	0
hard	1 oz	120	0	0	0
sandwich-style pepperoni..sliced	7 slices	140	0	0	0
turkey breast					
golden-roasted	2 oz	50	0	0	0
hardwood-smoked	2 oz	60	1	0	0
honey-roasted	2 oz	60	1	0	1
honey-roasted turkey ham	2 oz	70	2	0	2
mesquite-smoked	2 oz	60	1	0	0
oven-roasted	2 oz	60	0	0	0
oven-roasted rotisserie-flavored	2 oz	70	1	0	0
peppered..cracked	2 oz	50	2	0	1
■ SPAM (*See* (Hormel) in this section)					
■ (Tyson) deli meats..self-serve					
beef bologna	1 slice	80	1	0	1
chicken breast..golden roasted..smoked	3 slices	60	1	0	1
corned beef	2 slices	70	0	0	0
ham					
Black Forest	1 slice	30	0	0	1
brown sugar	1 slice	35	2	0	2
Virginia Brand	1 slice	30	0	0	1
olive loaf	1 slice	70	3	0	2
pastrami	2 slices	70	0	0	0
pepperoni..sandwich	5 slices	130	0	0	0
pickle loaf	1 slice	70	5	0	2
roast beef	2 slices	90	1	0	0
salami..all styles	4 slices	110	1	0	0
turkey breast					
golden-roasted	2 slices	70	2	0	2
hickory-smoked	2 slices	70	1	0	1
honey-flavored	2 slices	70	5	0	2
LUNCHEON MEAT SPREAD (*See also* PÂTÉ)					
(Armour)					
chicken..w/white meat	2.2 oz	110	4	0	1

Food and Description	Amount	Total Calories	Total Carbs	Fiber	Sugars
deviled ham..smoke-flavored	2.2 oz	110	0	0	0
potted meat..all flavors	2.2 oz	80	0	0	0
(Hormel) Spam..meat spread	1.5 oz	140	1	0	1
(Old Wisconsin Sausage) Spreadables..pâté					
braunschweiger..all flavors	2 oz	210	3	0	3
(Oscar Mayer)					
braunschweiger liver sausage	2 oz	190	1	0	1
sandwich spread	2 oz	130	9	0	4
(Underwood)					
chicken..white meat	¼ cup	110	3	0	0
ham..deviled	¼ cup	160	1	0	0
liverwurst	2 oz	170	3	1	1
roast beef	¼ cup	100	2	0	1
LUPIN					
boiled	½ cup	98	8	2.5	0
raw	½ cup	330	35	na	0
LYCHEE					
dried	1 oz	80	20	1	0
fresh	1 fruit	5	1.5	0	0

M

Food and Description	Amount	Total Calories	Total Carbs	Fiber	Sugars
MACADAMIA NUT					
(Diamond of California) chopped	¼ cup	240	4	2	1
(Fisher) Snack 'n' Serve Nut Bowl					
dry-roasted	1 oz	200	14	12	1
halves & pieces	1 oz	210	4	3	1
(Mauna Loa)					
butter candy–glazed	¼ cup	190	10	1	6
chocolate-covered	1 oz	170	19	2	17
dry-roasted..unsalted	¼ cup	200	4	2	1
honey-roasted	1 oz	200	4	2	1
Kona coffee–glazed	¼ cup	210	10	1	6
macadamia mixed nuts	¼ cup	190	8	2	1
macadamia nut butter corn crunch	1 oz	150	18	1	11
macadamia tropical nut & fruit mix	¼ cup	180	23	2	14
Maui onion & garlic	¼ cup	210	4	2	4
mountains milk chocolate–covered	4 pieces	200	21	1	19
MACARONI (See PASTA)					

Food and Description	Amount	Total Calories	Total Carbs	Fiber	Sugars
MACARONI & CHEESE (*See* FROZEN ENTRÉE/DINNER; PASTA ENTRÉE/DINNER; VEGETARIAN FOODS)					
MACE/ground	1 tsp	8	1	0	0
MACKEREL (*See also* SEAFOOD ENTRÉE/DINNER)					
(3 Diamonds) mackerel fillets..box					
in soybean oil	~3 oz	160	0	0	0
water & salt added	~3 oz	70	0	0	0
Atlantic..cooked—dry heat	3 oz	223	0	0	0
jack..canned..drained					
(Geisha) water & salt added	2.5 oz	80	0	0	0
King..cooked—dry heat	3 oz	115	0	0	0
Pacific/mixed species..cooked—dry heat	3 oz	170	0	0	0
smoked..fillets	2 oz	150	0	0	0
Spanish..cooked—dry heat	3 oz	134	0	0	0
MAHI MAHI (*See also* DOLPHIN FISH)					
cooked—dry heat	3 oz	95	0	0	0
Hawaiian-style..frozen..skinless-boneless	4 oz	100	0	0	0
MALT (*See* BARLEY MALT; MILK MIX)					
MALT LIQUOR (*See* BEER, ALE & MALT LIQUOR)					
MAMEY APPLE/MAMMEY APPLE/MAMMEE APPLE					
raw					
peeled..no seeds	3 oz	42	10	3	na
whole	1 medium	435	105	25	na
MANDARIN ORANGE (*See also* TANGERINE)					
CANNED OR JARRED					
(Del Monte) in light syrup..individual					
pull-top can	4 oz	70	17	<1	17
SunFresh..chilled jar	½ cup	80	19	<1	17
(Empress)	½ cup	80	19	<1	17
FRESH					
(Dole)	½ cup	80	19	<1	18
MANGO					
CANNED or JARRED					
(Del Monte) chilled jar					
SunFresh..in extra-light syrup	½ cup	70	19	<1	17
FRESH					
whole	1 medium	135	35	4	30
(Dole)	1 medium	70	17	1	15
FROZEN					
(C&W) chunks	1 cup	90	21	2	13
MANGO JUICE/JUICE BLEND/JUICE DRINK (*See also* FRUIT PUNCH)					
BOTTLED					
(Kern's from Libby's) nectar	5.5 fl oz	100	25	0	21
	8 fl oz	150	36	0	34
	12 fl oz	210	52	0	44
(Knudsen)					
Mango Fandango..spritzer	12 fl oz	190	45	0	45
mango orange	8 fl oz	120	30	0	26
(Libby's) nectar	8 fl oz	100	25	0	21
(Minute Maid) mango tropical..light	12 oz	10	2	0	1
(Snapple) juice drink..Mango Madness					

Food and Description	Amount	Total Calories	Total Carbs	Fiber	Sugars
diet	8 fl oz	15	0	0	0
regular	8 fl oz	110	29	0	29
(Walnut Acres) organic nectar	8 fl oz	120	29	0	28
(Welch's) juice drink..single-serve					
mango passion fruit	10 fl oz	160	39	0	38
	11.5 oz	180	45	0	44

MANICOTTI (*See* FROZEN ENTRÉE/DINNER; PASTA ENTRÉE/DINNER)
MAPLE SYRUP (*See* PANCAKE & WAFFLE SYRUP)
MARGARINE, MARGARINE SPREAD & SPRAY

Food and Description	Amount	Total Calories	Total Carbs	Fiber	Sugars
(Benecol)					
light	1 Tbs	45	0	0	<1
regular	1 Tbs	80	0	0	<1
(Blue Bonnet)					
light					
soft	1 Tbs	40	<1	0	0
stick	1 Tbs	50	<1	0	0
home-style..soft	1 Tbs	60	0	0	0
regular..stick	1 Tbs	80	0	0	0
light	1 Tbs	50	1	0	0
(Breakstone)					
original..unsalted	1 Tbs	100	<1	0	0
whipped..all styles	1 Tbs	60	0	0	<1
(Brummel & Brown) made w/yogurt					
stick	1 Tbs	90	0	0	0
tub	1 Tbs	50	0	0	0
(Fleischmann's) olive oil spread					
original..soft	1 Tbs	80	0	0	0
light	1 Tbs	40	0	0	0
premium blend..squeeze	1 Tbs	70	0	0	0
(Hain) safflower	1 Tbs	100	0	0	0
(Hollywood) safflower	1 Tbs	100	0	0	0
(I Can't Believe It's Not Butter)					
fat-free	1 Tbs	5	0	0	0
light spread..tub	1 Tbs	50	0	0	0
regular	1 Tbs	90	0	0	0
spray	5 sprays	0	0	0	0
squeeze	1 Tbs	80	0	0	0
sweet cream & calcium	1 Tbs	50	0	0	0
sweet cream buttermilk	1 Tbs	90	0	0	0
whipped..squeeze	1 Tbs	60	0	0	0
(Keller's)					
48% vegetable oil..tub	1 Tbs	60	0	0	<1
70% vegetable oil..box	1 Tbs	90	0	0	<1
(Land O' Lakes)					
Country Morning Blend					
stick	1 Tbs	100	0	0	0
light	1 Tbs	50	0	0	0
tub	1 Tbs	100	0	0	0
light	1 Tbs	50	0	0	0

Food and Description	Amount	Total Calories	Total Carbs	Fiber	Sugars
Fresh Buttery Taste					
soft or tub	1 Tbs	80	0	0	0
stick	1 Tbs	90	0	0	0
(Move Over Butter)					
65% vegetable oil..whipped w/sweet					
cream..tub	1 Tbs	60	0	0	0
stick	1 Tbs	90	0	0	0
tub	1 Tbs	90	0	0	0
(Nucoa)					
Heart Beat..corn oil	1 Tbs	25	0	0	0
Smartbeat					
light/unsalted	1 Tbs	25	0	0	0
squeeze/fat-free	1 Tbs	5	0	0	0
super-light/trans-fat-free	1 Tbs	20	0	0	0
soft	1 Tbs	90	0	0	0
stick	1 Tbs	100	0	0	0
(Parkay)					
light..stick or tub	1 Tbs	50	0	0	0
original..60% vegetable oil					
stick	1 Tbs	90	0	0	0
tub	1 Tbs	80	0	0	0
spray					
for cooking	1 spray	0	0	0	0
for topping	5 sprays	0	0	0	0
squeeze	1 Tbs	70	0	0	0
(Promise)					
extra-light	1 Tbs	50	0	0	0
fat-free	1 Tbs	5	0	0	0
regular..stick	1 Tbs	90	0	0	0
sunflower oil	1 Tbs	90	0	0	0
twin tubs	1 Tbs	80	0	0	0
ultra..tub	1 Tbs	35	0	0	0
(Shedd's Spread)					
canola oil blend	1 Tbs	60	0	0	0
churn-style..East Coast					
stick	1 Tbs	80	0	0	0
tub	1 Tbs	60	0	0	0
cinnamon	1 Tbs	70	4	0	4
cooking & topping spray	5 short sprays	0	0	0	0
Country Crock	1 Tbs	70	0	0	0
honey	1 Tbs	70	2	0	2
light	1 Tbs	50	0	0	0
(Weight Watchers)..all styles	1 Tbs	45	0	0	0
MARINADE (See also SEASONINGS)					
BAGGED, BOTTLED, or JARRED					
(A1) Marinade					
Chicago	1 tbs	20	2	0	2
steakhouse..New Orleans Cajun	1 tbs	25	5	0	5
steakhouse..teriyaki	1 Tbs	25	5	0	4
(Andre Prost) hot adobo	1 Tbs	10	2	0	2

Food and Description	Amount	Total Calories	Total Carbs	Fiber	Sugars
(Annie's Naturals)					
Paradise	2 Tbs	50	5	0	4
Smokey Campfire	2 Tbs	60	1	0	1
Spicy Ginger	2 Tbs	35	3	0	2
(Carb Options) (*See* (Lawry's) in this section)					
(Cardini)					
chipotle pepper	1 Tbs	10	2	0	1
fajita mesquite	1 Tbs	10	2	0	1
roasted garlic & herb	1 Tbs	10	2	0	2
spicy Cajun	1 Tbs	10	2	0	2
tangy teriyaki	1 Tbs	20	4	0	3
zesty lemon pepper	1 Tbs	15	4	0	3
(Chef Paul's) Magic Sauce & Marinade					
California sun-dried tomato	1 Tbs	17	6	0	4
Louisiana red pepper	1 Tbs	16	5	0	3
San Francisco teriyaki	1 Tbs	16	5	0	3
Southwest chipotle	1 Tbs	8	2	0	1
(Consorzio) 10-minute marinade					
Baja lime	1 Tbs	60	0	0	0
California teriyaki	1 Tbs	40	5	0	5
Dijon peppercorn	1 Tbs	15	3	0	2
Jamaican Jerk	1 Tbs	10	3	0	2
lemon pepper	1 Tbs	60	1	0	1
roasted garlic & balsamic vinegar	1 Tbs	30	4	0	2
sesame ginger	1 Tbs	25	4	0	4
Southwestern w/smoked chipotles	1 Tbs	30	3	0	1
tropical grill	1 Tbs	40	3	0	3
(Gourmet) marinades					
bold & spicy steakhouse grill	1 Tbs	15	1	0	2
cilantro & lime..Caribbean grill	1 Tbs	10	1	0	1
jalapeño & lime Southwest grill	1 Tbs	10	1	0	1
lemon & pepper citrus grill	1 Tbs	25	4	0	3
pineapple teriyaki..Asian grill	1 Tbs	15	3	0	3
roasted garlic, fine wine & herbs	1 Tbs	10	1	0	1
(KC Masterpiece)					
garlic & herb	1 Tbs	30	5	0	3
ginger & garlic	1 Tbs	30	7	0	7
golden honey Dijon	1 Tbs	40	9	0	8
honey teriyaki	1 Tbs	40	8	0	7
mesquite	1 Tbs	40	7	0	5
spiced Caribbean jerk	1 Tbs	25	6	0	5
zesty lemon pepper	1 Tbs	25	4	0	3
(Kikkoman)					
marinade & sauce					
honey & mustard teriyaki	1 Tbs	30	6	0	5
roasted garlic teriyaki	1 Tbs	25	5	0	3
teriyaki	1 Tbs	15	2	0	2
teriyaki light	1 Tbs	15	3	0	3
Quick & Easy marinade					
gourmet teriyaki	1 Tbs	30	7	0	5

Food and Description	Amount	Total Calories	Total Carbs	Fiber	Sugars
honey & mustard	1 Tbs	30	6	0	5
roasted garlic & herb	1 Tbs	20	4	0	3
toasted sesame teriyaki	1 Tbs	40	8	0	5
stir-fry & marinade					
black bean sauce w/garlic	2 Tbs	50	6	2	4
hoisin sauce	2 Tbs	80	17	0	16
Thai-style chili sauce	2 Tbs	70	15	1	15
(Lawry's)					
Carb Options..Italian garlic	1 Tbs	0	0	0	0
regular marinades					
Caribbean Jerk	1 Tbs	25	6	0	6
citrus grill	1 Tbs	15	3	0	3
Dijon & honey	1 Tbs	20	3	0	3
Havana garlic & lime	1 Tbs	10	2	0	2
Hawaiian	1 Tbs	20	4	0	4
herb & garlic	1 Tbs	10	2	0	2
lemon pepper	1 Tbs	10	2	0	2
Mediterranean w/lime juice	1 Tbs	10	2	0	2
tequila lime	1 Tbs	15	4	0	4
teriyaki..w/pineapple juice	1 Tbs	25	6	0	6
Thai ginger	1 Tbs	10	2	0	2
(McCormick Golden Dip) seafood					
marinade					
Cajun-style	1 Tbs	60	2	0	2
garlic herb	1 Tbs	60	1	0	1
ginger teriyaki	1 Tbs	60	5	1	4
honey mustard	1 Tbs	25	4	0	4
honey soy	1 Tbs	30	7	0	6
lemon herb	1 Tbs	80	0	0	0
lemon pepper	1 Tbs	25	1	0	1
mesquite	1 Tbs	10	1	0	1
white wine	1 Tbs	20	1	0	1
(Patak's) original					
marinade					
golden mango..mild	1 Tbs	30	4	0	4
honey & ginger..mild	1 Tbs	35	5	0	4
sweet & smoky..medium	1 Tbs	35	5	0	4
marinade & grilling sauce					
spicy ginger & garlic..mild	1 Tbs	35	3	1	2
(SeaPak Shrimp) liquid marinade..bag					
Caesar Parmesan	3.3 oz	110	3	0	1
garlic herb	3.3 oz	90	2	1	0
spicy Szechuan	3.3 oz	110	3	0	1
MIX..Mix only					
(Adolph's)					
For The Grill					
fajita	½ tsp	10	2	0	2
hickory barbecue	½ tsp	15	3	0	3
mesquite	½ tsp	10	2	0	2
teriyaki	½ tsp	10	3	0	0

Food and Description	Amount	Total Calories	Total Carbs	Fiber	Sugars
Marinade in Minutes..tenderizing					
original chicken	½ tsp	5	1	0	1
original meat	½ tsp	5	1	0	1
steak sauce	½ tsp	5	1	0	1
(Lawry's)					
beef..tenderizing	½ tsp	0	0	0	0
teriyaki	1 Tbs	25	5	0	5
Weekday Gourmet..liquid mix..beef					
London broil	1 Tbs	10	2	0	2
teriyaki steak	1 Tbs	25	5	0	5
MARINARA SAUCE (*See* SAUCE)					
MARJORAM/dried	1 tsp	2	<1	0	0
MARMALADE (*See* JAM/JELLY/PRESERVES)					
MARSHMALLOW					
(Kraft)					
Funmallows					
large	1.1 oz	100	24	0	19
miniature	~1 oz	100	23	0	16
Jet-Puffed	1 oz	90	23	0	17
miniatures	1 oz	100	24	0	16
toasted coconut	1 oz	100	21	0	16
Jet-Puffed marshmallow cream	2 Tbs	40	10	0	8
(La Nouba) Zero Carb marshmallows	1 piece	15	5	0	0
MATZO (*See* CRACKER; MATZO MEAL & MIX)					
MATZO MEAL & MIX (*See also* CRACKER CRUMBS/MEAL; SOUP)					
MEAL					
(Goodman's) matzo ball..mix only					
50% less salt	2 Tbs	50	11	<1	0
Passover	1 cup	514	109	1	0
regular	2 Tbs	50	11	<1	0
(Manischewitz)	½ cup	243	54	2	0
'Daily'	1 cup	514	109	1	0
Farfel	1 cup	280	60	0	0
MIX					
(Manischewitz) matzo ball..mix only	2 Tbs	50	9	<1	0
MAYONNAISE/MAYONNAISE-TYPE DRESSING (*See also* SALAD DRESSING)					
(Bennett's) real	1 Tbs	110	1	0	0
(Best Foods)					
Dijonnaise Creamy Dijon	1 tsp	5	1	0	0
Just 2 Good!..reduced-fat	1 Tbs	25	2	0	1
light	1 Tbs	50	1	0	0
real	1 Tbs	100	0	0	0
reduced-fat	1 Tbs	40	2	0	1
Squeeze Light..all flavors	1 Tbs	50	1	0	0
Squeeze..low-fat	1 Tbs	25	4	0	3
(Featherweight) soyamaise	1 Tbs	100	0	0	0
(Hain)					
canola					
light..reduced-calorie	1 Tbs	60	0	0	0
regular	1 Tbs	100	0	0	0

Food and Description	Amount	Total Calories	Total Carbs	Fiber	Sugars
eggless	1 Tbs	110	0	0	0
light	1 Tbs	60	0	0	0
safflower	1 Tbs	110	0	0	0
(Hellmann's)					
Dijonaise	1 tsp	5	1	0	0
Bacon & Tomato Twist..light	1 Tbs	50	1	0	0
Garlic Paradise	1 Tbs	50	1	0	0
Herb Sensation..light	1 Tbs	50	1	0	0
Just 2 Good!..reduced-fat	1 Tbs	25	2	0	1
light	1 Tbs	50	1	0	0
real	1 Tbs	100	0	0	0
reduced-fat	1 Tbs	40	2	0	1
(Hollywood) canola	1 Tbs	100	1	0	0
(Kraft)					
mayonnaise					
hot 'n' spicy	1 Tbs	100	0	0	0
Kraft Free..nonfat	1 Tbs	10	2	0	0
light	1 Tbs	50	2	0	1
super-easy squeeze	1 Tbs	45	2	0	1
real	1 Tbs	100	0	0	0
squeeze..easy	1 Tbs	100	0	0	0
Miracle Whip					
hot 'n' spicy	1 Tbs	60	2	0	1
light	1 Tbs	35	2	0	2
nonfat	1 Tbs	15	2	0	2
original	1 Tbs	70	2	0	1
squeeze..super-easy	1 Tbs	60	2	0	1
squeeze..super-easy..light	1 Tbs	35	2	0	2
(La Costena) w/lime juice	1 Tbs	100	0	0	0
(Nasoya) tofu Nayonaise	1 Tbs	40	1	0	0
(Smart Beat) canola or corn oil	1 Tbs	40	1	0	0
(Weight Watchers)					
regular	1 Tbs	50	1	0	0
whipped	1 Tbs	15	3	0	2
MEAL REPLACEMENT (*See* NUTRITIONAL SUPPLEMENT)					
MEAT SEASONING (*See* MARINADE; SEASONINGS)					
MEAT SNACK					
(Armour) dried..sliced beef..jar	~1 oz	60	2	0	2
(Jimmy Dean)					
beef jerky..1-oz pkg					
original	1 pkg	70	4	0	0
teriyaki	1 pkg	80	6	0	6
beef jerky..2-oz..4-oz & 8-oz pkgs					
original	1 oz	70	4	0	0
teriyaki	1 oz	80	6	0	6
giant sticks..beef..1.5 oz	1 pkg	150	2	0	0
kippered steak..1-oz pkg					
original	1 pkg	70	2	0	1

Food and Description	Amount	Total Calories	Total Carbs	Fiber	Sugars
peppered	1 pkg	70	3	0	2
teriyaki	1 pkg	70	5	0	4
sausage..pickled..1 oz	1 pkg	240	3	0	1
(Outpost)					
beef jerky	1 oz	70	4	0	3
beef 'n' cheese	1.5 oz	150	2	0	1
beef sticks	0.25 oz	35	1	0	0
hot sausage	0.875 oz	60	1	0	1
kippered beef steak	0.875 oz	60	4	0	4
kippered beef steak nuggets	1 oz	80	6	0	2
(Pemmican) kippered beef steak					
BBQ	1 oz	60	2	0	1
original	1 oz	60	2	0	2
peppered	1 oz	60	2	0	1
sweet & hot	1 oz	70	6	0	4
teriyaki	1 oz	60	2	0	1
(Penrose) pouch items					
Big Mama	2.4 oz	190	0	2	0
Firecracker	1.2 oz	100	2	1	0
giant	1.7 oz	140	3	1	0
smoked sausage..Big Mama	2 oz	200	2	0	<1
Tijuana Mama	2.4 oz	190	0	2	0
(Slim Jim)					
beef jerky..super jerk	0.31 oz	35	<1	0	0
deli sticks..all flavors	1.8 oz	240	7	0	2
kippered beef steak..all flavors	1.4 oz	110	3	0	0
meat & cheese items					
beef 'n' cheese	1.5 oz	150	3	0	0
chili beef 'n' cheese	1.5 oz	150	3	0	0
pepperoni	1.5 oz	150	2	1	0
Slim Jim items					
big..spicy	0.44 oz	70	<1	0	0
giant					
chili or mild	0.97 oz	150	2	0	0
spicy	0.97 oz	150	1	0	0
mild..super	0.64 oz	100	1	0	0
nacho					
giant	0.97 oz	150	2	0	0
super	0.64 oz	100	1	0	0
sweet & spicy..giant	0.97 oz	140	3	<1	0
Tabasco					
giant	0.97 oz	150	2	0	0
super	0.64 oz	100	<1	0	0
(Tombstone)					
beef jerky	1 stick	35	<1	0	0
beef sticks	1 stick	90	<1	0	0
(Trail's Best)					
beef jerky					
1-oz pkg					
original	1 oz	70	4	0	13
teriyaki	1 oz	80	6	0	6

Food and Description	Amount	Total Calories	Total Carbs	Fiber	Sugars
2-oz pkg					
hot teriyaki	2 oz	150	12	0	12
original	2 oz	140	8	0	7
teriyaki	2 oz	150	12	0	12
giant sticks..1.5-oz pkg					
beef..smoked	1 pkg	150	2	0	0
meat					
hot & spicy	1 pkg	140	6	0	5
pepperoni	1 pkg	150	2	0	<1
teriyaki	1 pkg	140	6	0	5
Happy Trails..meat sticks..1.1-oz pkg	1 pkg	120	3	0	1
kippered..king steak..1.1-oz pkg					
original	1 pkg	80	3	0	1
peppered	1 pkg	80	5	0	5
sweet & hot	1 pkg	80	5	0	5
teriyaki	1 pkg	70	4	0	2
kippered..big steak..1.6-oz pkg					
hot	1 pkg	120	3	0	2
original	1 pkg	110	4	0	2
peppered	1 pkg	110	5	0	3
sweet & hot	1 pkg	120	8	0	7
teriyaki	1 pkg	110	8	0	7
meat & cheese snack..2-oz pkg					
beef	1 pkg	210	3	0	1
ham & cheddar	1 pkg	200	4	0	4
pepperoni & mozzarella	1 pkg	200	2	0	1
spicy beef & jalapeño cheese	1 pkg	200	3	0	<1
sausage..pickled..2-oz pkg					
Blazin' Hot	1 pkg	250	3	0	<1
spicy pickled	1 pkg	240	3	0	<1
w/peppers	1 pkg	250	5	1	1

MEAT SPREAD (*See* LUNCHEON MEAT SPREAD)

MEAT SUBSTITUTE (*See* VEGETARIAN FOODS; individual listings)

MEAT TENDERIZER (*See also* MARINADE; SEASONINGS)

| (Tone's) all styles | 1 tsp | 7 | 1 | 0 | 0 |

MELBA TOAST (*See* CRACKER)

MELON (*See* individual listings)

MEXICAN FOOD (*See also* BEEF DISH/ENTRÉE; BREAKFAST SANDWICH; DIP; FROZEN ENTRÉE/DINNER; PASTA ENTRÉE/DINNER; RICE DISH; SAUCE; SEASONINGS; TOMATO; TOMATO SAUCE; TORTILLA CHIPS; VEGETARIAN FOODS)

■ **BEANS** (*See* Refried Beans in this section)

■ **BURRITO** (*See* Mexican Entrées/Dinners in this section)

■ **CHILI** (*See* BEEF DISH/ENTRÉE; CHILI/CHILI BEANS; SEASONINGS)

■ **CHILI BEANS** (*See* CHILI/CHILI BEANS) and individual bean listings)

■ **CHILI SAUCE** (*See* SAUCE)

■ **CHILIS** (*See* Peppers in this section)

■ **CHURRO**

| frozen (Tio Pepe's) cinnamon..6-oz pkg | 1 piece | 110 | 14 | 2 | na |

■ **ENCHILADA** (*See* Mexican Entrées/Dinners in this section)

Food and Description	Amount	Total Calories	Total Carbs	Fiber	Sugars
■ **GAZPACHO** (*See* SOUP)					
■ **GUACAMOLE** (*See* DIP)					
■ **MENUDO**					
(La Costena) beef tripe & hominy stew	1 cup	180	10	2	1
■ **MEXICAN ENTRÉES/DINNERS**					
FROZEN..MICROWAVEABLE..REFRIGERATED					
(Delimex)					
quesadilla..chicken & cheese	⅙ box	230	25	1	2
rice..chicken fried	6.9 oz	290	47	2	3
rice..grilled chicken teriyaki	1 bowl	450	84	3	14
tacos..rolled..beef & cheddar	⅕ box	410	44	7	0
taquitos					
beef	5 pieces	370	49	8	0
3-cheese	5 pieces	400	50	6	2
(El Monterey)					
APPETIZERS					
fiesta					
family pack/classics	⅓ box	370	33	1	2
taquitos	3 pieces	330	36	1	2
minis					
tacos	4 pieces	260	27	3	1
variety	4.5 oz	370	32	1	2
CARB-FRIENDLY					
chicken & cheese quesadilla	1 quesadilla	210	16	9	0
chipotle, chicken & cheese	1 quesadilla	310	26	14	0
shredded beef steak	1 burrito	320	26	14	1
shredded steak quesadilla	1 quesadilla	260	15	9	1
CRUNCHEROS					
quesadilla					
3-cheese & grilled chicken	4 pieces	450	34	1	3
taquitos					
chicken & cheese	4 pieces	410	52	2	3
shredded steak & cheese	⅙ box	390	38	1	2
Southwest chicken	½ box	400	52	2	2
taco beef & cheese	4 pieces	420	40	2	2
ENCHILADAS					
beef w/sauce	2.5-lb tray	180	18	2	1
cheese w/sauce & garnish	2.5-lb tray	220	16	1	1
chicken w/suiza sauce	1 tray	210	19	1	3
MEXICAN GRILL..charbroiled					
chicken & cheese quesadilla	1 quesadilla	230	20	1	1
chicken breast taquitos	3 taquitos	380	36	1	1
steak burrito	1 burrito	290	39	1	1
MINI FRIED BURRITOS					
cream cheese & jalapeños	3 pieces	370	32	1	2
nacho cheese & beef	3 pieces	330	35	2	1
QUESADILLA..grilled					
chicken & cheese	1 quesadilla	260	20	1	1

Food and Description	Amount	Total Calories	Total Carbs	Fiber	Sugars
QUICK CLASSICS					
beef tamales	1 tamale	300	26	3	1
chicken tamales	1 tamale	260	28	2	1
SOFT TACOS					
beef & cheese	1 taco	440	42	3	0
sausage, egg & cheese	1 taco	370	29	1	0
spicy					
beef & cheese	1 taco	420	40	2	2
chicken & cheese	1 taco	340	44	4	1
TAMALES..shredded beef	1 tamale	200	26	3	1
(Patio)					
BURRITOS..bean & cheese	1 burrito	300	45	4	5
DINNERS..beef enchilada	1 meal	370	53	10	3
(Rosarita) *REFRIGERATED MEALS*					
enchilada..shredded chicken	1 meal	280	24	0	2
fajita..grilled chicken breast	1 meal	160	21	0	1
quesadilla..grilled chicken	1 meal	250	19	0	0
MIXES AND REFRIGERATED DINNER KITS					
(Chi-Chi's)					
fiesta tortilla soup..mix only	⅕ pkg	80	13	1	4
shells & seasonings					
fajita	2 shells	300	54	2	7
soft taco	2 shells	300	54	2	9
white corn	2 shells	200	30	2	3
sweet corn cake..mix only	½ cup	100	22	0	11
(Kraft) refrigerated dinner kits					
fiesta taco dinner bake	⅕ kit	340	28	3	3
Mexican-style lasagna	⅕ kit	310	30	2	3
3-cheese chicken enchilada	⅕ kit	300	29	2	4
(Old El Paso)					
dinner kit..prepared burrito	1 piece	270	27	1	2
cheesy taco pizza	1 taco	350	17	1	3
gordita					
w/ranch sauce	1 gordita	390	34	1	2
w/regular sauce	1 gordita	310	36	1	3
taco					
prepared w/chicken breast	1 taco	260	19	1	2
prepared w/lean ground beef	1 taco	300	19	1	2
(Ortega) dinner kits					
taco..w/shells & seasoning	⅙ box	150	24	3	1
taco kit..soft tortilla w/seasonings	⅕ box	240	47	2	6
(Oscar Mayer) Lunchables					
nachos..cheese dip & salsa	4.4-oz box	380	39	3	3
	4.75-oz box	570	70	4	38
(Taco Bell) dinner kits..Home Originals					
fajita..15.5-oz box	⅕ box	230	38	3	3
soft taco..12.5-oz box	⅕ box	200	32	1	1
soft taco..16.35-oz box	⅕ box	230	38	2	2
taco..1.75-oz box	⅙ box	130	19	2	1

Food and Description	Amount	Total Calories	Total Carbs	Fiber	Sugars
taco..14.25-oz box	⅙ box	230	29	2	2
Ultimate Nachos	¼ box	280	29	4	3
■ **MEXICAN FOOD SEASONINGS** (*See also* SEASONINGS)					
(Chi-Chi's) mix..dry					
fajita	¼ pkg	35	7	0	2
fiesta					
burrito	¼ pkg	35	6	1	2
restaurante	1 Tbs	10	2	0	0
taco	⅕ pkg	25	4	1	1
(Old El Paso) mix..dry					
burrito	2 tsp	15	4	0	0
chili	1 Tbs	15	3	<1	<1
enchilada	2 tsp	10	2	<1	0
fajita	1 tsp	10	3	0	0
taco..all styles	2 tsp	15	4	0	0
(Ortega) mix..dry					
burrito	⅛ pkg	20	3	1	0
fajita	⅛ pkg	15	3	0	1
taco	⅙ pkg	20	4	0	0
(Taco Bell) mix only	2 Tbs	20	3	1	0
■ **MEXICAN POTATO** (*See* JICAMA)					
■ **PEPPERS**					
(Chi-Chi's)					
diced tomatoes & green chilis	¼ cup	20	4	1	3
green chili					
diced	2 Tbs	10	1	0	0
whole	¾ pepper	10	1	0	0
jalapeños					
wheels	19 pieces	10	2	0	0
whole	2-½ peppers	10	2	0	0
(Clemente Jacques)					
chipotle..in adobe sauce	1 oz	25	4	1	2
jalapeños..pickled					
sliced	1 oz	5	1	0	0
whole	1 oz	5	1	0	1
(Embasa)					
jalapeños..all styles	1 oz	5	1	1	0
nopalitos..sliced	~1 oz	5	1	2	0
(La Victoria)					
green					
diced	2 Tbs	0	0	0	0
whole	1 pepper	5	1	0	<1
jalapeño					
marinated	1½ Tbs	10	2	0	<1
sliced	14 pieces	5	<1	0	0
(Old El Paso) jalapeños					
relish	1 Tbs	5	1	0	0
whole..pickled	2 medium	5	1	0	0
(Ortega)					
green chili..all styles	1 oz	10	2	0	1

Food and Description	Amount	Total Calories	Total Carbs	Fiber	Sugars
jalapeños					
sliced..hot	1 oz	10	2	0	1
whole	1 oz	10	2	0	1
(Ro*Tel)					
green chilis..blended in spicy tomato sauce					
chunky	½ cup	20	4	1	3
diced in sauce	½ cup	40	8	<1	7
extra-hot	½ cup	20	4	1	3
Mexican festival	½ cup	30	6	1	3
milder	½ cup	20	4	1	3
original	½ cup	20	4	1	3
(Vlasic)					
jalapeños..Mexican hot	1 oz	8	2	0	0
Mexican..tiny hot	1 oz	6	2	0	0
pepperoncini..mild	1 oz	5	1	0	0
■ REFRIED BEANS					
(Amy's) organic					
traditional vegetarian	½ cup	140	21	6	1
vegetarian black beans	½ cup	140	20	6	1
w/green chilis	½ cup	130	20	6	1
(Comida Sabrosa)	½ cup	140	23	9	2
(Eden) refried					
black beans	½ cup	110	18	7	0
black beans..spicy	½ cup	110	18	7	0
black soy & black beans	½ cup	90	13	6	1
kidney beans	½ cup	80	15	6	0
pinto beans	½ cup	90	19	7	0
pinto beans..spicy	½ cup	90	18	7	0
(La Costena)					
black beans					
refried	½ cup	180	20	7	1
whole	½ cup	70	15	6	1
pinto..refried	½ cup	160	20	9	1
(Old El Paso)					
beans & cheese	½ cup	120	15	6	2
beans & green chilis	½ cup	100	18	6	1
beans & sausage	½ cup	200	14	4	1
fat-free	½ cup	100	18	6	1
traditional	½ cup	100	17	6	1
vegetarian	½ cup	100	17	6	2
(Rosarita)					
authentic home-style	½ cup	140	15	3	0
traditional..98% fat-free	½ cup	110	19	5	1
traditional..no fat	½ cup	100	19	5	1
(Taco Bell) Home Originals					
original..fat-free	½ cup	110	21	6	1
vegetarian blend	½ cup	140	23	7	1
■ SALSA/SAUCE (See also SAUCE)					
(Chi-Chi's)					
picante..all styles	2 Tbs	10	2	0	2

Food and Description	Amount	Total Calories	Total Carbs	Fiber	Sugars
salsa					
con queso	2 Tbs	45	3	0	1
fiesta..hot	2 Tbs	10	2	0	2
garden	2 Tbs	15	3	0	1
hot	2 Tbs	10	2	0	2
medium	2 Tbs	10	2	0	2
mild	2 Tbs	10	2	0	2
original..all styles	2 Tbs	10	2	0	1
roasted tomato	2 Tbs	10	2	0	1
taco..thick & chunky	1 Tbs	10	1	0	1
(Embasa)					
Mexicana..original recipe..all styles	2 Tbs	5	1	1	1
(Hain) salsa/green chili..all styles	¼ cup	20	4	0	0
(Herdez)					
Salsa Casera..all styles	1 oz	10	1	0	0
Salsa Ranchera	1 oz	15	1	0	0
Salsa Taquera					
medium	1 oz	10	2	0	0
Mexicana picante	1 oz	25	6	0	2
(La Costena)					
Mexican hot sauce..all styles	~1 oz	10	2	0	0
Mexican sauce..all styles	~1 oz	10	2	0	0
tomato sauce..fried..seasoned	2 oz	40	6	1	1
(La Victoria)					
chili..red	2 oz	15	2	0	1
enchilada					
hot picante	¼ cup	25	2	0	0
mild green chili	¼ cup	15	3	0	1
red	¼ cup	20	2	0	0
salsa..all styles and flavors	2 Tbs	10	2	0	1
(Muir Glen) organic fat-free					
hot..habañero	2 Tbs	10	2	0	1
medium..black bean & corn	2 Tbs	15	2	0	1
medium..other flavors..all	2 Tbs	10	2	0	1
(Newman's Own) Bandito salsa					
all "heat" styles	2 Tbs	10	1	0	1
peach	2 Tbs	25	6	1	5
pineapple	2 Tbs	15	3	1	3
roasted garlic	2 Tbs	10	2	1	1
(Old El Paso)					
enchilada..all flavors	¼ cup	30	1	0	0
picante..all flavors	2 Tbs	10	2	0	1
salsa					
garden pepper..all flavors	2 Tbs	10	2	<1	1
Make Mine Medium	2 Tbs	10	2	<1	1
Wild for Mild	2 Tbs	10	2	<1	1
thick 'n' chunky..all flavors	2 Tbs	10	2	0	1
taco..all flavors	1 Tbs	5	1	0	0
(Ortega) salsa					
garden-style					

Food and Description	Amount	Total Calories	Total Carbs	Fiber	Sugars
medium	2 Tbs	10	2	1	1
mild	2 Tbs	10	2	0	1
home-style..all styles	2 Tbs	10	2	0	1
Mexican-style..mild	2 Tbs	15	3	1	1
roasted garlic..medium	2 Tbs	10	2	0	1
(Pace)					
enchilada sauce	¼ cup	25	5	1	4
Mexican Creations Sauce					
cilantro & lime	1 cup	25	6	0	5
roasted ranchero	1 cup	35	6	1	4
sweet roasted onion & garlic	¼ cup	30	7	0	5
taco					
classic	2 Tbs	20	4	1	3
mild	2 Tbs	15	4	1	3
verde w/tomatillos & jalapeños	1 cup	20	5	0	2
salsa					
chunky	2 Tbs	10	2	<1	2
chipotle	2 Tbs	10	3	<1	2
cilantro	2 Tbs	10	2	>1	2
fire-roasted tomato	2 Tbs	10	2	<1	2
grande garlic	2 Tbs	10	3	<1	2
roasted pepper & garlic	2 Tbs	10	3	<1	2
con queso	2 Tbs	45	4	<1	1
(Ro*Tel) diced tomatoes & green chilis					
salsa..all styles	½ cup	20	4	1	3
(Taco Bell) Home Originals					
hot sauce	1 tsp	0	0	0	0
picante..Smooth'n Zesty..mild	2 Tbs	15	3	1	2
salsa					
con queso					
medium	2 Tbs	40	2	0	0
mild	2 Tbs	40	3	0	1
thick & chunky					
medium	2 Tbs	15	2	1	2
mild	2 Tbs	15	3	1	2
taco sauce					
medium	2 Tbs	10	2	1	1
mild	2 Tbs	15	3	1	1
(Tostitos) salsa					
con queso..restaurant-style	2 Tbs	40	5	<1	<1
fire-roasted tomato	2 Tbs	15	2	1	1
hot, medium, or mild	2 Tbs	15	3	1	2
restaurant-style	2 Tbs	15	2	<1	1
roasted garlic	2 Tbs	15	3	1	2
■ SHELLS					
TACO					
(Chi-Chi's) white or yellow	2 shells	170	22	2	0
(Mission) jumbo	1 shell	90	11	1	0
(Old El Paso)					
mini..fun-size	7 shells	150	19	1	0

Food and Description	Amount	Total Calories	Total Carbs	Fiber	Sugars
salad	1 shell	110	14	<1	0
super stuffer	2 shells	180	23	2	0
yellow or white corn	3 shells	150	20	1	0
TOSTADA..corn					
(Old El Paso)	3 shells	150	20	1	0
(Rosarita)	1 shell	60	8	<1	0

■ **TACO** (*See* BREAKFAST SANDWICH; and *see* Mexican Entrées/Dinners; Mexican Food Seasonings in this section)
■ **TACO SEASONING** (*See* Mexican Food Seasonings in this section)
■ **TACO SHELL** (*See* Shells in this section)
■ **TAMALE** (*See also* Mexican Entrées/Dinners in this section)

CANNED					
(Derby)	2 tamales	160	15	1	na
(Hormel)					
beef					
hot-spicy	2 tamales	140	15	2	2
regular	7.6 oz	200	22	3	2
chicken	2 tamales	130	15	1	2
(Wolf)	2 tamales	210	23	4	0

■ **TOMATILLO**

CANNED					
(La Costena)	4 medium	40	4	4	0

■ **TORTILLA** (*See also* Shells in this section)

(Abuelita)					
tortilla..6"					
yellow corn	4 tortillas	160	34	2	0
white corn/table	2 tortillas	150	32	4	0
tortilla..8" lower carbs	1 tortilla	80	10	5	0
tortilla..9"..whole wheat	1 tortilla	110	20	1	<1
tortilla..12"					
cheese	1 tortilla	217	29	1	1
chili	1 tortilla	238	33	1.5	1
pesto	1 tortilla	216	30	1	1
tomato	1 tortilla	237	33	2	1
whole wheat	1 tortilla	178	25	1.5	0
tortilla..12"..hand-stretched..original	1 tortilla	110	20	1	<1
tortilla..12"..pressed	1 tortilla	270	44	0	1
(Adios Carbs)					
tortilla..10-count					
garlic & herb	1 tortilla	87	8	0	2
green onion	1 tortilla	87	8	0	2
jalapeño pepper	1 tortilla	87	8	0	2
regular	1 tortilla	87	8	0	2
tortilla..chocolate dessert..8-count	1 tortilla	87	8	0	2
tortilla..red chili pepper..10-count	1 tortilla	87	8	0	2
(Cruz)					
corn..stone-ground	2 tortillas	110	21	2	0
flour					
burrito-size	1 tortilla	130	22	1	0
chimichanga	1 tortilla	130	22	1	0
97% fat-free	1 tortilla	120	24	1	1
restaurant-style	1 tortilla	300	52	1	1

Food and Description	Amount	Total Calories	Total Carbs	Fiber	Sugars
whole wheat..8-count	1 tortilla	130	15	10	1
(Guerrero)					
corn..50-count	2 tortillas	120	25	2	0
estilo ranchero..50-count	2 tortillas	120	23	2	0
flour					
fajita..20-count	1 tortilla	110	0	0	0
fresqui ricas..10-count	1 tortilla	140	19	1	0
riquisimas..12-count	1 tortilla	320	44	2	1
riquisimas..30-count	1 tortilla	140	20	1	1
triguenas..whole wheat	1 tortilla	140	20	1	1
(Labrada)					
tortilla wraps..all flavors	1 wrap	60	5	3	0
(Mission)					
corn					
como hechas en casa	1 tortilla	70	13	1	0
Estilo Casero..regular-size	1 tortilla	70	13	1	0
super-size	1 tortilla	80	14	1	0
white corn..12-count	2 tortillas	80	15	1	0
flour					
burrito-size					
98% fat-free	1 tortilla	160	33	3	1
regular-size	1 tortilla	220	36	2	2
Estilo Casero sabrositas					
burrito-size	1 tortilla	220	36	2	2
burrito-size..98% fat-free	1 tortilla	160	33	3	1
regular-size	1 tortilla	140	24	1	2
fajita-size	1 tortilla	120	19	1	1
grande	1 tortilla	130	22	1	2
restaurant-style	1 tortilla	100	17	1	1
low-carb					
fajita-size	1 tortilla	80	12	7	0
soft taco-size	1 tortilla	110	18	11	0
whole wheat..burrito	1 tortilla	200	31	21	0
whole wheat..fajita	1 tortilla	80	12	8	0
soft taco–size..regular-size..20-count	1 tortilla	150	25	1	2
(Reser's) Baja Café..flour tortillas					
burrito-size..10-count	1 tortilla	180	29	1	0
home-style..10-count	1 tortilla	130	22	1	0
soft taco–size..12-count	1 tortilla	130	21	1	0
(Taco Bell) flour..soft for tacos..12-count	1 tortilla	200	32	1	1

■ **TORTILLA CHIPS** (*See* TORTILLA CHIPS)

■ **TORTILLA MIX**

(Quaker) mix only					
harina, preparada para tortillas	⅓ cup	160	27	1	1
masa harina	¼ cup	110	24	3	0
(White Wings) tortilla mix flour	¼ cup	220	40	1	0

■ **TOSTADA** (*See* Mexican Entrées/Dinners in this section)

■ **TOSTADA SHELL** (*See* Shells in this section)

Food and Description	Amount	Total Calories	Total Carbs	Fiber	Sugars
MILK (*See also* MILK SUBSTITUTE; RICE DRINK; SOY MILK)					
BUFFALO	1 cup	236	13	0	0
COW..CANNED					
condensed..sweetened					
(Borden) Eagle Brand					
fat-free	1.4 oz	110	24	0	24
low-fat	1.4 oz	120	23	0	23
original	1.4 oz	130	23	0	23
(Carnation)	2 Tbs	130	22	0	22
(Magnolia)	1.4 oz	130	23	0	23
COW..EVAPORATED					
(Carnation)					
fat-free	2 Tbs	25	4	0	4
low-fat	2 Tbs	25	3	0	3
whole..regular	2 Tbs	40	3	0	3
(Milnot)					
fat-free	2 Tbs	25	4	0	4
whole	2 Tbs	40	3	0	3
COW..FRESH					
(Blue Bunny)					
1% low-fat	1 cup	100	12	0	12
2% reduced-fat					
chocolate	1 cup	180	25	0	24
regular	1 cup	120	11	0	11
fat-free	1 cup	90	12	0	12
vitamin D	1 cup	150	11	0	11
(Borden)					
2% reduced-fat	1 cup	120	11	0	11
chocolate-flavored					
Dutch..2% reduced-fat	1 cup	170	23	<1	22
skim	1 cup	80	22	<1	11
whole	1 cup	150	11	0	11
(Darigold)					
1% fat..light	1 cup	110	13	0	12
2% fat..reduced-fat	1 cup	130	13	0	12
acidophilus bifidus..fat-free	1 cup	100	1	0	1
acidophilus..low-fat	1 cup	110	13	0	12
buttermilk..low-fat	1 cup	110	13	0	12
extra calcium	1 cup	110	13	0	12
fat-free	1 cup	90	13	0	12
fat-free..Trim Deluxe	1 cup	100	14	0	13
flavored milk					
chocolate..reduced-fat	1 cup	210	33	<1	32
eggnog..classic	1 cup	200	26	0	23
extra chocolate	1 cup	240	33	<1	31
strawberry..reduced-fat	1 cup	210	33	0	32
vanilla	1 cup	210	33	0	32
homogenized	1 cup	150	12	0	12

Food and Description	Amount	Total Calories	Total Carbs	Fiber	Sugars
(Hersheys)					
chocolate					
fat-free	1 cup	150	29	<1	26
reduced-fat	1 cup	200	31	1	28
shake					
cookies & cream	7 fl oz	200	1	1	28
creamy chocolate	7 fl oz	200	1	1	28
mint chocolate	7 fl oz	300	53	1	51
strawberry	7 fl oz	280	44	0	44
vanilla cream	7 fl oz	320	55	0	44
(Hood)					
Carb Countdown..dairy beverage					
2% reduced-fat	1 cup	100	3	0	3
chocolate	1 cup	100	3	0	3
fat-free	1 cup	70	3	0	3
homogenized	1 cup	130	3	0	3
regular milk products					
buttermilk	1 cup	90	13	0	12
chocolate...1%	1 cup	170	28	<1	26
chocolate...whole	1 cup	230	31	<1	29
coffee..1%	1 cup	170	28	0	26
LightBlock					
fat-free	1 cup	80	13	0	12
whole	1 cup	150	12	0	12
Simply Smart..1%	1 cup	120	13	0	12
Simply Smart..fat-free	1 cup	90	13	0	12
whole w/vitamin D	1 cup	150	12	0	12
(Horizon) Organic					
1% low-fat	8 oz	100	12	0	11
2% reduced-fat	8 oz	120	12	0	11
chocolate..reduced-fat	8 oz	160	26	1	24
fat-free	8 oz	80	12	0	11
whole	8 oz	150	11	0	11
(Kemp's) Flavored					
café mocha..reduced-fat	12 oz	200	29	0	27
chocolate	1 cup	220	29	0	25
French vanilla	12 oz	210	25	0	25
(Nestlé USA) Nesquik..ready-to-drink					
Buncha Banana	1 cup	200	30	0	29
chocolate					
fat-free	1 cup	160	32	<1	30
whole	1 cup	230	31	<1	29
double chocolate	1 cup	230	30	<1	17
Very Vanilla	1 cup	220	29	0	28
(Umpqua)					
1% low-fat	8 oz	100	11	0	11
2% reduced-fat	8 oz	120	11	0	11
buttermilk..low-fat	8 oz	110	13	0	12
chocolate..Dutch-style	8 oz	190	26	1	25

Food and Description	Amount	Total Calories	Total Carbs	Fiber	Sugars
fat-free white milk	8 oz	80	11	0	11
homogenized w/vitamin D	8 oz	150	11	0	11
COW..LACTOSE-REDUCED (See MILK SUBSTITUTE)					
DRY..POWDERED					
(Alba) nonfat..prepared	1 cup	80	12	0	12
(Carnation) mix only..nonfat	⅓ cup	80	12	0	12
(Nestlé USA) Nido..dry mix..whole	⅓ cup	150	12	0	12
(Saco)					
buttermilk..prepared	1 cup	80	13	0	12
nonfat milk..prepared	1 cup	80	12	0	12
GOAT					
canned..evaporated (Meyenberg)	8 oz	145	10	0	10
carton					
powder mixed w/water	1 cup	145	11	0	11
REFRIGERATED					
1% low-fat	1 cup	90	9	0	9
whole	1 cup	145	10	0	10
FRESH	1 cup	168	11	0	11
HUMAN	1 cup	170	17	0	0
SHEEP	8 fl oz	264	13	0	0
MILK MIX (*See also* BREAKFAST DRINK; COCOA; MILK SHAKE)					
(Carnation) mix only..malted milk					
chocolate	2 Tbs	90	18	1	14
original	2 Tbs	90	15	1	10
(Choco Milk) mix only..all flavors	2 Tbs	90	21	0	21
(Ghirardelli) cocoa					
double chocolate..hot	3 Tbs	100	24	2	20
sweet ground chocolate & cocoa	3 Tbs	100	24	2	20
unsweetened	1 Tbs	20	4	2	0
(Hersheys)					
chocolate milk mix	3 Tbs	90	23	<1	21
Hot Cocoa Collection					
Dutch chocolate	1 envelope	140	29	1	25
French vanilla	1 envelope	140	28	0	25
syrups					
chocolate	2 Tbs	100	24	0	20
light	2 Tbs	50	12	0	10
strawberry	2 Tbs	100	26	0	26
Whoppers chocolate malt	2 Tbs	100	25	0	21
(Land O' Lakes) Cappuccino Classics					
Amaretto Italia	1 pkt	130	23	0	22
French vanilla	1 pkt	130	23	0	22
mocha	1 pkt	130	23	0	22
Suisse Mocha	1 pkt	140	25	1	22
suprema	1 pkt	130	23	0	22
(Nestlé)					
Nesquik..flavored syrup					
chocolate	2 Tbs	100	24	1	23
strawberry	2 Tbs	110	27	0	26

Food and Description	Amount	Total Calories	Total Carbs	Fiber	Sugars
Nesquik..mix only					
chocolate	2 Tbs	90	19	1	18
double chocolate	2 Tbs	90	17	1	17
strawberry	2 Tbs	90	21	0	21
(Swiss Miss) mix only					
Chocolate Sensations	1 pkt	150	27	2	23
cocoa					
fat-free..regular	1 pkt	50	9	1	7
light	1 pkt	70	17	2	16
no sugar added..regular	1 pkt	50	9	1	7
double-rich	1 pkt	110	22	0	0
French vanilla..fat-free	1 pkt	120	22	1	13
Marshmallow Lovers					
fat-free	1 pkt	60	13	1	12
regular	1 pkt	140	27	2	21
milk chocolate					
regular					
cannister	¼ cup	140	27	2	21
	1 pkt	120	22	1	17
w/marshmallows	1 pkt	120	22	1	18
MILK SHAKE (See MILK; individual FAST FOOD listings)					
MILK SUBSTITUTE (See also RICE DRINK; SOY MILK; YOGURT DRINK)					
(Dairy Ease) 100% lactose-free					
fat-free	1 cup	80	12	0	11
reduced-fat	1 cup	130	12	0	12
whole	1 cup	160	11	0	11
(EdenSoy) soy milk					
carob	8 fl oz	170	27	0	13
original	8 fl oz	130	13	0	7
vanilla..original	8 fl oz	150	23	0	15
(Full Circle) organic..enriched					
lactose-free					
chocolate	8 fl oz	100	11	2	7
original	8 fl oz	170	26	2	19
(Kikkoman Pearl) organic					
creamy vanilla	8 oz	110	11	0	10
green tea	8 oz	110	13	1	10
original	8 oz	110	12	1	9
tropical delight w/7 juices	8 oz	110	14	0	13
(Lactaid) 100% lactose-free					
chocolate..2% reduced-fat	1 cup	150	24	1	23
regular					
fat-free	1 cup	80	13	0	12
low-fat	1 cup	110	13	0	12
reduced-fat	1 cup	130	13	0	12
whole	1 cup	150	12	9	12
fat-free	1 cup	80	13	0	12
(Le Carb) less lactose..fewer carbs					
chocolate	1 cup	130	6	1	3

Food and Description	Amount	Total Calories	Total Carbs	Fiber	Sugars
white					
2% low-fat	1 cup	110	4.5	0	4
homogenized	1 cup	140	4	0	4
(Sno*E) tofu-based milk mix					
low-fat	3 Tbs	70	10	1	7
regular	3 Tbs	80	20	0	27
(Vitasoy) soy milk					
classic original	8 oz	120	11	1	15
rich chocolate	8 oz	100	9	2	5
smooth vanilla	8 oz	110	11	2	7
unsweetened original	8 oz	80	5	0	1
vanilla delight	8 oz	120	13	1	8
MILKFISH					
cooked—dry heat	3 oz	165	0	0	0
raw	3 oz	125	0	0	0
MILLET (See also CEREAL; FLOUR)					
(Arrowhead Mills) hulled	¼ cup	150	34	3	0
MINCEMEAT (See PIE FILLING)					
MINERAL WATER (See WATER)					
MINESTRONE (See SOUP)					
MISO (See also SOUP)					
(Eden)					
genmai..brown rice	1 Tbs	25	3	1	1
hacho..soybean	1 Tbs	35	2	1	0
mugi..soybean & barley	1 Tbs	25	3	1	1
shiro..soybean..sweet	1 Tbs	35	5	1	3
(Westbrae) pasteurized					
miso bags					
barley	1 tsp	10	2	0	0
brown rice	1 tsp	10	<1	0	0
soybean	1 tsp	10	0	0	0
miso soups..instant..all types	1 pkt	35	3	0	0
miso tubs..mellow					
barley	1 tsp	10	1	<1	<1
brown rice	1 tsp	10	2	<1	<1
red	1 tsp	10	2	<1	<1
white	1 tsp	10	2	<1	<1
MOLASSES					
(Brer Rabbit)					
blackstrap	1 Tbs	60	13	0	12
full flavor	1 Tbs	60	15	0	11
mild	1 Tbs	60	16	0	13
unsulphured	1 Tbs	60	13	0	12
(Mott's) Grandma's..all styles	1 Tbs	50	12	0	12
MONKFISH..cooked—dry heat	3 oz	85	0	0	0
MOOSE..boneless..roasted	3 oz	115	0	0	0
MORTADELLA (See SAUSAGE)					
MOTH BEAN..boiled	½ cup	105	18	0	0
MOUNTAIN YAM					
Hawaiian..steamed	½ cup	60	14	0	na

Food and Description	Amount	Total Calories	Total Carbs	Fiber	Sugars
MOUSSE (*See* PUDDING & MOUSSE)					
MUFFIN (*See also* BREAKFAST SANDWICH; PASTRY, TOASTER)					
■ **FROZEN**					
(Sara Lee) Thaw & Serve..FOOD SERVICE					
LARGE..4.25 oz					
apple cranberry nut	1 muffin	440	53	2	30
banana nut	1 muffin	440	73	1	29
blueberry	1 muffin	430	64	2	41
reduced-fat	1 muffin	270	43	1	21
bran	1 muffin	440	54	2	22
carrot nut	1 muffin	440	60	2	46
cheese streusel	1 muffin	440	53	2	34
cinnamon pecan coffee cake	1 muffin	490	59	2	40
corn	1 muffin	490	58	1	44
double chocolate chunk	1 muffin	440	63	3	43
lemon poppyseed	1 muffin	460	60	3	34
orange streusel	1 muffin	450	63	1	31
triple berry	1 muffin	370	56	2	40
SMALL..2.125 oz					
apple cranberry nut	1 muffin	220	26	1	15
blueberry	1 muffin	210	32	<1	21
bran	1 muffin	200	28	1	21
cheese streusel	1 muffin	220	27	1	16
corn	1 muffin	250	32	1	17
double chocolate chunk	1 muffin	230	29	1	19
(Weight Watchers)					
chocolate chocolate chip	1 muffin	190	39	2	21
■ **MIX**					
(Betty Crocker) mix..prepared					
ORIGINAL BOX MIX					
apple streusel	1 muffin	210	33	0	18
banana nut	1 muffin	170	27	1	12
cranberry orange	1 muffin	150	25	0	13
double chocolate	1 muffin	200	30	0	20
lemon poppyseed	1 muffin	190	29	0	14
Twice the Blueberry	1 muffin	140	25	1	12
wild blueberry	1 muffin	170	28	<1	14
POUCH..MADE W/WATER..PREPARED					
apple cinnamon	1 muffin	130	21	0	10
banana nut	1 muffin	130	21	0	11
chocolate chip	1 muffin	130	21	0	11
lemon poppyseed	1 muffin	130	22	0	11
triple berry	1 muffin	120	23	0	12
(Duncan Hines) box mix					
BAKERY-STYLE..PREPARED					
blueberry streusel	1 muffin	170	31	1	17
chocolate chip	1 muffin	180	31	1	16
cinnamon swirl	1 muffin	190	34	1	20
wild Maine blueberry	1 muffin	140	25	1	12

Food and Description	Amount	Total Calories	Total Carbs	Fiber	Sugars
(Jiffy) dry mix only					
apple cinnamon	¼ cup	170	28	1	13
banana nut	¼ cup	160	25	2	11
blueberry	¼ cup	160	28	1	13
bran w/dates	¼ cup	150	26	3	12
corn	¼ cup	160	28	1	8
raspberry	¼ cup	170	26	1	12
(Krusteaz)..prepared					
FAT-FREE					
banana	1 muffin	140	33	2	19
blueberry	1 muffin	130	30	2	15
cinnamon apple	1 muffin	130	31	2	20
corn..honey corn bread & muffin	1 muffin	120	27	1	8
cranberry orange	1 muffin	140	32	2	18
LOW-FAT					
apple oat bran	1 muffin	170	33	4	12
ORIGINAL					
almond poppyseed	1 muffin	180	30	1	17
apple cinnamon	1 muffin	170	31	1	16
blueberry	1 muffin	180	30	2	15
honey bran	1 muffin	180	29	3	15
lemon poppyseed	1 muffin	170	30	<1	16
oat bran	1 muffin	180	32	2	15
wild blueberry	1 muffin	150	26	<1	14
(Martha White) prepared					
apple cinnamon	1 muffin	160	28	0	16
banana nut	1 muffin	150	24	1	12
blackberry	1 muffin	160	28	0	16
blueberry	1 muffin	160	28	0	16
blueberry cheese	1 muffin	170	26	0	15
carrot cake	1 muffin	160	30	1	18
chocolate chip	1 muffin	160	28	1	16
cinnamon	1 muffin	180	33	1	17
lemon poppyseed	1 muffin	150	25	1	11
(Pillsbury) mix only					
QUICK BREAD & MUFFIN MIX					
apple cinnamon	1/14 pkg	130	26	1	16
banana	1/12 pkg	130	26	1	14
blueberry	1/12 pkg	140	24	1	13
cranberry	1/14 pkg	110	30	1	16
lemon poppyseed	1/12 pkg	150	28	1	14
pumpkin	1/12 pkg	130	27	1	14
MUFFIN MIX					
blueberry	1/6 pkg	170	30	0	17
chocolate chip	1/6 pkg	180	30	1	16
(White Lily) mix only					
apple cinnamon	1/5 pkg	190	32	1	18
banana nut	1/5 pkg	180	30	1	13
blackberry	1/5 pkg	190	32	1	17
blueberry	1/5 pkg	190	32	1	18

Food and Description	Amount	Total Calories	Total Carbs	Fiber	Sugars
chocolate chip..real milk chocolate	⅕ pkg	180	30	1	13
cinnamon raisin	⅕ pkg	180	30	1	13
corn	⅕ pkg	190	33	1	10
wild berry	⅕ pkg	200	32	1	18
■ READY-TO-SERVE					
(Awrey's)					
MUFFINS..1.5 oz					
apple	1 muffin	140	18	0	8
banana nut	1 muffin	170	20	0	10
blueberry	1 muffin	140	18	0	8
raisin bran	1 muffin	160	21	2	11
MUFFINS..GRANDE..4 oz					
banana nut	1 muffin	410	46	1	23
blueberry	1 muffin	360	45	1	23
cheese streusel	1 muffin	400	51	1	28
chocolate chip	1 muffin	370	41	1	24
(Bay's) English muffins					
original	1 muffin	140	27	1	2
sourdough	1 muffin	130	26	2	2
(Earth Grains) English muffins					
cinnamon raisin	1 muffin	150	31	2	2
sourdough..premium	1 muffin	130	26	1	2
(Entenmann's)					
CARB COUNTING..blueberry breakfast	1 muffin	170	22	4	2
LITTLE BITES..pouches					
blueberry	1 pouch	190	26	1	15
chocolate chip	1 pouch	210	26	1	15
(Hostess)					
LARGER MUFFINS..hearty					
banana nut	1 muffin	620	78	2	39
blueberry	1 muffin	590	78	1	41
chocolate chip	1 muffin	620	78	2	41
cranberry orange	1 muffin	590	79	1	41
cream cheese	1 muffin	620	73	1	41
oat bran	1 muffin	160	21	1	9
MINI MUFFINS..0.5 oz					
banana walnut	3 muffins	160	16	0	8
blueberry	3 muffins	150	18	0	8
chocolate chip	3 muffins	150	17	1	10
cinnamon apple	3 muffins	160	16	0	8
MUFFIN LOAF					
apple spice	1 loaf	430	61	1	41
banana nut	1 loaf	460	63	0	29
blueberry	1 loaf	440	62	2	34
chocolate chip cookie	1 loaf	400	58	2	32
raspberry	1 loaf	440	62	2	34
(Otis Spunkmeyer)					
LOW-FAT..2.25 oz					
apple cinnamon	1 muffin	210	42	<1	28
banana nut	1 muffin	200	40	<1	25

Food and Description	Amount	Total Calories	Total Carbs	Fiber	Sugars
chocolate chocolate chip	1 muffin	210	41	1	26
wild blueberry	1 muffin	200	38	<1	24
REGULAR..1.8 oz					
apple	1 muffin	180	22	<1	11
banana	1 muffin	190	23	<1	12
blueberry	1 muffin	180	22	<1	11
chocolate	1 muffin	180	25	2	11
REGULAR..2.25 oz					
apple cinnamon	1 muffin	240	30	<1	18
banana nut	1 muffin	270	33	<1	20
chocolate chocolate chip	1 muffin	260	33	1	22
corn	1 muffin	250	30	<1	15
harvest bran	1 muffin	230	33	3	19
wild blueberry	1 muffin	230	27	1	20
REGULAR..4 oz					
almond poppyseed	½ muffin	210	23	<1	17
apple cinnamon	½ muffin	220	27	<1	16
banana nut	½ muffin	240	30	<1	18
blueberry	½ muffin	210	27	2	13
cheese streusel	½ muffin	220	30	<1	18
chocolate chip	½ muffin	240	28	>1	18
chocolate chocolate chip	½ muffin	230	29	<1	19
corn	½ muffin	230	26	0	14
cranberry orange	½ muffin	210	25	0	14
harvest bran	½ muffin	200	29	2	17
lemon	½ muffin	230	27	1	15
orange	½ muffin	230	27	<1	16
pumpkin walnut	½ muffin	220	25	<1	14
raspberry chese streusel	½ muffin	190	28	1	14
REGULAR..6.5 oz					
banana	½ muffin	370	47	2	27
blueberry	½ muffin	340	39	<1	22
cheese streusel	½ muffin	340	51	2	27
chocolate chocolate chip	½ muffin	350	43	2	25
corn	½ muffin	360	43	1	21
SPECIAL CAFÉ COLLECTION..6.5 oz					
banana walnut	½ muffin	380	46	2	26
chocolate chocolate chip	½ muffin	360	46	2	20
wild blueberry	½ muffin	330	43	2	23
(Pepperidge Farm) English muffins					
cinnamon raisin	1 muffin	140	28	2	8
sourdough	1 muffin	130	27	2	<1
(Sara Lee)					
INDIVIDUALLY WRAPPED..2.0 oz					
banana nut	1 muffin	190	30	<1	19
blueberry	1 muffin	170	26	<1	16
bran	1 muffin	190	24	1	11
cheese streusel	1 muffin	220	28	1	16
INDIVIDUALLY WRAPPED..4.75 oz					
banana nut	1 muffin	480	73	2	45

Food and Description	Amount	Total Calories	Total Carbs	Fiber	Sugars
blueberry	1 muffin	440	69	2	32
bran	1 muffin	470	62	3	27
carrot nut	1 muffin	480	63	3	32
cheese streusel	1 muffin	500	61	2	34
chocolate chip cookie	1 muffin	550	75	3	47
chocolate chunk	1 muffin	470	69	4	41
cinnamon pecan coffee cake	1 muffin	560	72	2	42
corn	1 muffin	510	67	2	32
(Thomas') English muffins					
CARB CONSIDER..original	1 muffin	100	23	9	0
REGULAR					
hearty grains					
honey wheat	1 muffin	130	27	2	4
oat bran	1 muffin	130	27	2	2
whole wheat..100%	1 muffin	120	22	3	2
multigrain..light	1 muffin	200	2	8	0
oatbran	1 muffin	130	27	2	2
sourdough	1 muffin	120	25	1	0
Toast R Cakes..corn	1 muffin	110	18	1	8
(Wolferman's)					
CAKE MUFFINS..5 oz					
almond poppyseed	1 muffin	590	67	<1	37
apple cinnamon	1 muffin	570	68	<1	39
cherry cream cheese	1 muffin	570	68	<1	39
chocolate caramel pecan	1 muffin	570	64	1	38
ENGLISH MUFFINS..Miniature					
1910 original recipe	2 muffins	130	24	2	1
cinnamon raisin	2 muffins	125	28	2	6
cranberry citrus	2 muffins	140	30	2	6
San Francisco sourdough	2 muffins	110	23	<1	0
SIGNATURE SELECTIONS..English muffins					
1910 original recipe	1 muffin	230	48	2	2
apple orchard	1 muffin	260	49	2	10
cinnamon & raisin	1 muffin	260	55	3	14
cranberry citrus	1 muffin	250	53	3	9
honey & oats	1 muffin	260	50	3	7
mixed berry	1 muffin	250	51	2	11
multigrain & honey	1 muffin	240	49	4	7
natural cheese	1 muffin	250	45	2	3
pumpkin spice	1 muffin	250	51	2	7
San Francisco sourdough	1 muffin	230	48	2	2
smoked onion & garlic	1 muffin	220	45	2	2
wild Maine blueberry	1 muffin	250	51	2	8
MULBERRY/fresh	1 cup	60	14	2	na
MULLET/striped..cooked—dry heat	3 oz	127	0	0	0
MUNG BEAN					
dried/generic					
boiled	½ cup	106	20	7.5	na
raw	½ cup	361	65	7.5	na

Food and Description	Amount	Total Calories	Total Carbs	Fiber	Sugars
sprouted					
canned	½ cup	8	1	1	na
raw	½ cup	16	3	1	na
stir-fried	½ cup	31	6.5	1	na
MUNGO BEAN					
boiled	½ cup	95	17	6	na
raw	½ cup	355	61	19	na
MUSHROOM					
CANNED or JARRED					
(3 Diamonds) stems & pieces..4 oz	1 can	28	4	2	1
(BinB) broiled in butter					
sliced	1 can	40	4	1	<1
sliced w/garlic	1 can	40	5	1	1
whole	1 can	40	4	1	<1
(Geisha) pieces & stems..4 oz	1 can	30	4	2	1
(Green Giant) white					
mushrooms & garlic	½ cup	25	4	1	<1
pieces & stems	½ cup	30	4	2	1
sliced or whole	1 can	40	4	1	1
whole	1 can	40	4	1	<1
DRIED					
(Frieda's)					
chanterelle	2 pieces	15	2	1	0
morel	3 pieces	15	2	0	0
oyster	3 pieces	15	2	0	0
paddy straw	6 pieces	15	2	0	0
porcini	5 pieces	15	2	1	0
shiitake	¼ cup	10	3	0	0
wood ear	3 pieces	15	2	0	0
FRESH					
(Frieda's)					
enoki..raw	~1 oz	10	2	1	1
oyster..raw	3 oz	20	4	1	0
shiitake..cooked	4 oz	40	10	1.5	0
FROZEN (Nancy's) mushroom turnovers	12 pieces	490	45	4	9
MUSHROOM DISH (*See* FROZEN ENTRÉE/DINNER; VEGETABLES, MIXED; individual FAST FOOD listings)					
MUSKMELON (*See* CANTALOUPE)					
MUSKRAT..roasted..meat only	3 oz	200	0	0	0
MUSSEL					
CANNED (Reese's) in red sauce	4 oz	120	4	0	na
FRESH..blue					
cooked—moist heat	3 oz	147	6	0	0
raw	3 oz	73	3	0	0
SMOKED (Ducktrap River)	¼ cup	140	3	0	0
MUSTARD					
DRY (Spice Islands) ground	1 tsp	10	0	0	0
PREPARED					
(Annie's Naturals) organic					
Dijon	1 tsp	0	0	0	0

Food and Description	Amount	Total Calories	Total Carbs	Fiber	Sugars
honey	1 tsp	0	0	0	0
horseradish	1 tsp	5	1	0	<1
raspberry	1 tsp	5	1	0	1
(Best Foods/Hellmann's)					
Dijonnaise	1 tsp	10	1	0	0
(Grey Poupon)					
country Dijon	1 tsp	5	1	0	0
Dijon	1 tsp	5	1	0	0
Parisian	1 tsp	5	0	0	0
(Gulden's)					
spicy brown	1 tsp	5	0	0	0
zesty honey	1 tsp	10	2	0	2
(Hebrew National) deli mustard	1 tsp	0	0	0	0
(Heinz) spicy brown	1 Tbs	14	1	0	0
(Jack Daniel's) all styles	1 tsp	5	0	0	0
(Kraft) all styles	1 tsp	0	0	0	0
(Plochman's) Celebrations					
cranberry orange	1 tsp	5	1	0	0
Definitely Dill	1 tsp	5	1	0	0
Lager Bier	1 tsp	5	1	0	0
Lemon Really?	1 tsp	5	1	0	0
Raspberry Rhapsody	1 tsp	5	1	0	0
sun-dried tomato & oregano	1 tsp	5	1	0	0
Sweet Hot Jazz	1 tsp	10	2	0	1
(Westbrae)					
Asian-style	1 tsp	5	1	0	0
Dijon-style	1 tsp	0	0	0	0
organic					
honey	1 tsp	5	1	0	0
yellow	1 tsp	0	0	0	0
stoneground	1 tsp	0	0	0	0
(Zatarain's) Creole	1 tsp	0	0	0	0
MUSTARD GREENS					
CANNED					
(The Allens)					
seasoned Southern-style	½ cup	45	6	1	2
w/turnips..Southern-style	½ cup	45	6	1	2
(Glory Foods) seasoned	½ cup	50	7	3	3
FRESH (Glory) raw..bag	2 cups	20	4	3	<1
MUSTARD SAUCE (*See* SAUCE)					
MUSTARD SEED..yellow..whole	1 tsp	15	1	0	0

N

Food and Description	Amount	Total Calories	Total Carbs	Fiber	Sugars
NACHOS (*See* MEXICAN FOOD)					
NAPOLEON (*See* PASTRY)					
NATAL PLUM (*See* CARISSA)					
NAVY BEAN					
CANNED					
(Bush's Best)	½ cup	110	19	6	0
(Eden Foods) organic	½ cup	110	20	7	0
(Trappey's) seasoned					
w/slab bacon	½ cup	110	17	7	3
w/slab bacon & jalapeños	½ cup	110	16	6	3
DRIED (Haggen)	½ cup	80	23	12	1
NECTARINE..fresh					
whole..~5 oz	1 medium	70	16	2	12
NEUFCHÂTEL CHEESE (*See* CHEESE; CHEESE SPREAD)					
NEWBURG SAUCE (*See* SAUCE)					
NONDAIRY FROZEN DESSERT (*See* ICE CREAM & ICE CREAM-LIKE FROZEN DESSERT; ICE CREAM BARS, CONES & CUPS, SANDWICHES & FROZEN NOVELTIES; RICE FROZEN DESSERT; SHERBET; TOFU FROZEN DESSERT)					
NOODLE (*See* ASIAN FOOD; PASTA)					
NORI (*See* SEAWEED)					
NUTMEG..ground	1 tsp	11	1	0	0
NUTRITION BAR (*See* GRANOLA/GRANOLA-TYPE BAR)					
NUTRITIONAL LIQUID SUPPLEMENT (*See also* BREAKFAST/CEREAL BAR; BREAKFAST DRINK; GRANOLA/GRANOLA-TYPE BAR)					
(Atkins) Advantage shakes					
café au lait	11 fl oz	170	5	3	1
chocolate delight	11 fl oz	170	5	4	1
chocolate royale	11 fl oz	170	6	4	1
creamy vanilla	11 fl oz	170	4	3	1
strawberry supreme	11 fl oz	170	5	3	1
(Boost)					
Boost Plus..all flavors	8 fl oz	360	45	0	22
Breeze..all flavors	8 fl oz	160	31	0	31
high-protein drink					
chocolate	8 fl oz	240	33	0	25
strawberry	8 fl oz	240	33	0	18
vanilla	8 fl oz	240	33	0	16
regular-protein drink					
butter pecan	8 fl oz	240	41	0	23

Food and Description	Amount	Total Calories	Total Carbs	Fiber	Sugars
chocolate	8 fl oz	240	41	0	27
chocolate malt	8 fl oz	240	41	0	27
chocolate mocha	8 fl oz	240	41	0	23
strawberry	8 fl oz	240	41	0	23
vanilla	8 fl oz	240	41	0	23
(Carb Solutions) high-protein drink					
creamy vanilla	11 fl oz	100	4	2	1
rich chocolate	11 fl oz	110	5	3	1
(Celebrity) Hollywood Diet					
two-day juice fast..all flavors	4 fl oz	100	26	0	26
(ChoiceDM) nutrition drink					
chocolate	8 fl oz	220	24	3	10
chocolate fudge	11 fl oz	125	11	9	0
French vanilla	11 fl oz	100	7	6	0
strawberries 'n' cream	11 fl oz	100	7	6	0
vanilla	8 fl oz	220	24	3	10
(Ensure)					
Enlive! clear liquid nutrition..					
all flavors	8 fl oz	300	65	0	15
Ensure					
balanced nutrition..lactose-free					
all flavors	8 fl oz	250	40	0	18
fiber w/FOS..all flavors	8 fl oz	250	42	3	12
high calcium..all flavors	8 fl oz	225	31	0	19
high protein..all flavors	8 fl oz	230	31	0	19
light..all flavors	8 fl oz	200	33	0	18
plus..all flavors	8 fl oz	360	50	0	16
(Odwalla)					
Future Shakes					
Dutch Chocolate	8 fl oz	160	27	2	19
Vanilla Al'mondo	8 fl oz	190	24	3	16
Nutritionals..juices					
Citrus C Monster	8 fl oz	150	33	2	30
Mo' Beta	8 fl oz	140	34	1	26
Strawberry C Monster	8 fl oz	150	34	<1	27
Super Protein 2001/02	8 fl oz	170	33	2	28
Superfood	8 fl oz	140	32	2	26
Wellness	8 fl oz	150	33	1	24
(Ross) (*See* (Ensure) in this section)					
(Slim-Fast)					
HEALTHY..ready-to-drink meal					
apple cranberry raspberry	11 fl oz	220	46	5	39
banana cream	11 fl oz	220	40	5	35
cappuccino delight	11 fl oz	220	42	8	35
chocolate..rich royale	11 fl oz	220	40	5	35
chocolate soy..lactose-free	11 fl oz	220	39	5	31
creamy chocolate	11 fl oz	220	40	5	34
dark chocolate fudge	11 fl oz	220	42	5	33
French vanilla	11 fl oz	220	40	5	35

Food and Description	Amount	Total Calories	Total Carbs	Fiber	Sugars
milk chocolate	11 fl oz	220	40	5	34
orange cream	11 fl oz	220	35	5	29
orange pineapple w/soy protein	11 fl oz	220	46	5	39
orange strawberry banana					
w/soy protein	11 fl oz	220	46	5	39
strawberries 'n' cream	11 fl oz	220	40	5	35
vanilla w/soy lactose-free	11 fl oz	220	38	5	31
LOW-CARB..ready-to-drink meal					
café latte	11 fl oz	190	4	2	2
chocolate royale	11 fl oz	190	6	4	1
creamy chocolate	11 fl oz	190	6	4	1
strawberries & cream	11 fl oz	190	6	4	1
vanilla cream	11 fl oz	180	4	2	1
SLIM-FAST OPTIMA..ready-to-drink meal					
all flavors	11 fl oz	180	24	5	17
NUTS, MIXED (*See also* ICE CREAM TOPPING; individual nut listings)					
(Ann's House of Nuts)					
Cajun	⅓ cup	170	16	2	1
California	¼ cup	130	21	2	16
cranberry fruit & nut	3 Tbs	110	15	2	12
deluxe..mixed	¼ cup	220	7	3	2
honey nut crunch	3 Tbs	150	14	2	13
nut 'n' fruit	3 Tbs	120	16	2	13
nuts..Swiss	3 Tbs	130	17	1	14
(Fisher)					
Fisher Chef's Naturals..nut topping	1 oz	170	6	2	2
Fisher Deluxe..mixed..no peanuts	1 oz	170	6	2	1
glazed nut mix & cashews					
praline	1 oz	170	11	0	8
toffee	1 oz	160	11	2	7
Gourmet Select..imperial mixed nuts	1 oz	180	6	2	1
Nuts & Crunches					
Bayou blend..spicy sweet	1 oz	150	13	2	4
golden crisp	1 oz	140	14	1	3
honey crunch	1 oz	140	17	1	5
Nuts & Fruits snack mix					
California-style	1 oz	140	15	2	8
raisin cranberry	1 oz	150	13	2	9
trail-style	1 oz	150	11	2	8
Snack 'n' Serve nut bowl					
mixed deluxe w/o peanuts	1 oz	180	5	2	2
(Kettle) Roaster Fresh mixed nuts					
camping mix	1 oz	140	11	2	7
chocolate lover's					
natural	1 oz	120	15	2	11
regular	1 oz	130	16	2	13
deluxe nut	1 oz	170	6	2	1
honey cranberry	1 oz	120	16	2	12
honey roast					
harvest	1 oz	130	15	2	8

Food and Description	Amount	Total Calories	Total Carbs	Fiber	Sugars
nuts & fruit	1 oz	120	16	2	13
plain	1 oz	160	8	2	1
Organic Sunrise..soy & mango	1 oz	120	13	3	9
Raw Hikers	1 oz	120	15	2	12
Southwest BBQ	1 oz	150	11	2	1
Truffle Trail	1 oz	120	17	2	14
X-Treme Trail	1 oz	150	9	2	5
(Planters) mixed					
cashew almond pecan	1 oz	170	7	2	<1
deluxe	1 oz	170	6	2	<1
macadamia cashew mix w/almonds	23 pieces	180	6	2	0

Food and Description	Amount	Total Calories	Total Carbs	Fiber	Sugars
OAT BRAN (See BRAN; CEREAL)					
OATS (See also CEREAL; FLOUR)					
(Arrowhead Mills)					
groats	¼ cup	160	29	4	0
rolled flakes	⅓ cup	130	23	4	0
steel-cut	¼ cup	170	29	5	0
whole grain	1 oz	110	19	5	0
OCEAN PERCH (See also FROZEN ENTRÉE/DINNER; SEAFOOD ENTRÉE/DINNER)					
Atlantic..cooked-dry heat	3 oz	103	0	0	0
OCTOPUS (See also SEAFOOD ENTRÉE/DINNER; SQUID)					
CANNED					
(Goya) spiced	¼ cup	140	3	0	na
(Reese's)	¼ cup	120	4	0	na
cooked—moist heat	3 oz	140	4	0	0
raw	3 oz	70	2	0	9
OIL (See also ASIAN FOOD/SAUCES & SEASONINGS; COOKING SPRAY)					
FLAVORED					
(House of Tsang)					
all flavors	1 tsp	45	0	0	0
wok	1 Tbs	130	0	0	0
PLAIN					
all 100% vegetable & fish oils	1 tsp	45	0	0	0
	1 Tbs	120	0	0	0

Food and Description	Amount	Total Calories	Total Carbs	Fiber	Sugars
(Smucker's) Baking Healthy Oil & Shortening oil-replacement for baking	1 Tbs	30	7	0	4
OKRA (See also VEGETABLES, MIXED)					
CANNED or JARRED					
(Best Maid) pickled..all styles	1 oz	10	2	0	1
(Mt. Olive) pickled..all styles	1.5 oz	15	2	0	0
(Trappey's)					
Creole gumbo	½ cup	35	6	3	1
cut	½ cup	25	6	3	1
w/tomatoes & corn	½ cup	30	6	4	1
FRESH..baked..no seasonings	½ cup	25	6	2	0
FROZEN					
(Best Yet) breaded	3.2 oz	80	16	1	4
(McKenzie's)					
breaded	2.66 oz	90	19	3	2
cut	3.2 oz	25	5	3	1
OLIVE					
(Black Pearls) ripe					
chopped	½ oz	25	1	0	0
colossal..pitted	½ oz	20	1	0	0
jalapeño..sliced	½ oz	25	1	0	0
jumbo..pitted	½ oz	20	1	0	0
jumbo..whole	½ oz	25	1	0	0
large..pitted	½ oz	25	1	0	0
medium..pitted	½ oz	15	1	0	0
Spanish salad olives	½ oz	25	1	0	0
(Burgundy Pearls) pitted					
Caesar Parmesan	½ oz	25	2	1	0
classic Italian	½ oz	25	2	1	0
roasted pepper	½ oz	25	2	1	0
(Green Pearls)					
jumbo..whole..Sicilian-style	½ oz	20	1	0	0
Manzanilla pimento..sliced	½ oz	25	1	0	0
Manzanilla pimento..stuffed	½ oz	25	1	0	0
queen pimento..stuffed	½ oz	20	1	0	0
queen..whole	½ oz	20	1	0	0
super colossal..Sicilian-style	½ oz	20	1	0	0
zesty..sliced..Sicilian-style	½ oz	20	1	0	0
(Mediterranean Pearls)					
garlic..stuffed queen	½ oz	20	1	0	0
jalapeño..stuffed queen	½ oz	20	1	0	0
Kalamata..whole	½ oz	35	1	0	0
(Peloponnese) naturally brine-cured					
Amfissa	½ oz	40	1	0	0
cracked	½ oz	20	1	0	0
Ionian	½ oz	25	1	0	0
Kalamata	½ oz	40	1	0	0
gourmet black olives	½ oz	40	1	0	0
mixed	½ oz	40	1	0	0

Food and Description	Amount	Total Calories	Total Carbs	Fiber	Sugars
(Star) Spanish olives					
Manzanillas	½ oz	15	1	0	0
queens	½ oz	15	1	0	0
OLIVE LOAF (*See* LUNCHEON MEAT)					
OLIVE OIL (*See* OIL)					
OMELET (*See* EGG DISH/MEAL)					
ONION (*See also* SCALLION; VEGETABLES, MIXED)					
CANNED or JARRED					
(Aunt Nellie's) whole..Holland-style	½ cup	40	6	2	5
(Best Yet) French fried..crispy	¼ oz	43	3	0	0
(Crosse & Blackwell) cocktail	1 Tbs	5	1	0	0
(Vlasic) cocktail..all styles	1 oz	4	1	0	0
DRIED					
flakes	1 Tbs	16	4	0.5	0
powder..ground	1 tsp	7	1.5	<1	0
FRESH..all types..mature					
(Dole)..whole	1 medium	60	14	3	9
(Frieda's) baby Hawaiian	⅓ cup	10	3	1	0
raw..chopped	½ oz	18	1	0	0
FROZEN					
(Birds Eye) Southern vegetables..diced	⅔ cup	30	6	<1	3
(C&W) petite..whole	⅔ cup	30	7	1	4
(McKenzie's) onion rounds	⅓ pkg	220	28	2	3
ONION, GREEN or **SPRING** (*See* SCALLION)					
ONION DISH (*See also* FROZEN ENTRÉE/DINNER; VEGETABLES, MIXED; VEGETARIAN FOODS)					
FROZEN					
(Birds Eye) vegetables w/sauce					
pearl onions in real cream sauce	½ cup	60	9	1	6
(Mrs. Paul's) onion rings	7 rings	190	22	1	3
(Ore-Ida)					
gourmet onion rings	4 pieces	210	28	1	2
Onion Ringers	6 rings	220	25	3	5
ONION POWDER	1 tsp	10	2	0	0
ONION RINGS (*See* ONION DISH; individual FAST FOOD listings)					
ONION SOUP (*See* SOUP)					
OPOSSUM..braised or roasted	3 oz	190	0	0	0
ORANGE (*See also* MANDARIN ORANGE)					
FRESH					
California navel					
peeled sections	1 cup	75	19	4	12
whole	1 medium	65	16	1	14
(Dole)	1 medium	70	21	7	14
Florida					
peeled sections	1 cup	85	21	4	14
whole	1 medium	70	17	4	14
(SunKist) all types	1 medium	80	21	7	14

Food and Description	Amount	Total Calories	Total Carbs	Fiber	Sugars
ORANGE JUICE/JUICE BLEND/JUICE DRINK (*See also* FRUIT PUNCH; SOFT DRINK; SOFT DRINK MIX; TEA)					
BOTTLED, BOXED, or CANNED					
(Dole)					
orange juice..all styles	8 fl oz	120	27	0	23
orange juice blends					
peach mango	8 fl oz	120	28	0	23
tropical fruit	8 fl oz	120	27	0	25
(Minute Maid)					
orange juice..premium					
all juice styles	8 fl oz	110	27	0	20
original..100% pure	12 fl oz	170	40	0	36
pulp-free	8 fl oz	110	27	0	24
(Ocean Spray) orange citrus spritzer	11.75 fl oz	160	40	0	40
(Odwalla) Essentials..organic					
carrot orange apple blend	8 fl oz	100	23	1	21
(R. W. Knudsen) orange mango juice	8 fl oz	120	30	0	26
(Snapple) juice drinks					
orange carrot..diet	8 fl oz	10	3	0	1
orangeade	8 fl oz	120	29	0	29
(Sunny D) fruit juice drink					
orange	8 fl oz	130	43	0	40
smooth California-style w/calcium	8 fl oz	140	35	0	31
(Tropicana)					
orange juice					
Essentials..Light 'N Healthy	10 fl oz	140	33	0	28
Grovestand	8 fl oz	110	26	0	22
Healthy Heart	8 fl oz	110	26	0	22
Home-style	14 fl oz	190	43	0	39
Immunity Defense..orange plus	8 fl oz	110	26	0	22
plus calcium	14 fl oz	190	43	0	39
Pure Premium	6 fl oz	80	20	0	17
orange..plus calcium	8 fl oz	110	26	0	22
Sweet Valencia..w/ or w/o pulp	8 fl oz	110	26	0	22
Orange Twisters					
Orange Cranberry Clash	10 fl oz	160	37	9	36
Orange Strawberry Banana Burst	11.5 oz	180	45	0	40
(V8 Splash)					
juice drink..orange pineapple	8 fl oz	110	27	0	25
smoothie..orange cream	8 fl oz	130	29	1	25
(Welch's)					
orange juice	11.5 oz	170	43	0	41
orange pineapple					
juice cocktail	11.5 fl oz	180	45	0	44
juice drink	10 fl oz	140	36	0	35
FROZEN					
(Old Orchard) prepared..unless noted otherwise					
orange juice	8 fl oz	120	27	0	24
pineapple orange banana	8 fl oz	120	29	0	26

Food and Description	Amount	Total Calories	Total Carbs	Fiber	Sugars
(Welch's) orange pineapple apple juice cocktail..prepared	8 fl oz	140	35	0	34
MIX					
(Tang) breakfast drink..prepared					
natural orange flavor	8 fl oz	90	24	0	24
orange..naranja..cannister	8 fl oz	90	24	0	24
orange pineapple	8 fl oz	100	24	0	24
ORANGE PEEL					
CANDIED					
(Seneca)	2 Tbs	70	18	1	11
(S&W)	58 pieces	80	23	2	18
FRESH..grated	1 Tbs	5	2	1	0
ORANGE ROUGHY (*See also* SEAFOOD ENTRÉE/DINNER)					
cooked—dry heat	3 oz	80	0	0	0
raw	3 oz	60	0	0	0
OREGANO..ground	1 tsp	5	1	0	0
ORIENTAL FOOD (*See* ASIAN FOOD; FROZEN ENTRÉE/DINNER; PASTA ENTRÉE/DINNER; RICE DISH; VEGETARIAN FOODS; individual listings)					
OSTRICH..(New West)..ostrich steak	4 oz	130	0	0	0
OYSTER (*See also* SEAFOOD ENTRÉE/DINNER)					
CANNED					
(3 Diamonds) whole in salted water	2 oz	60	2	0	0
(Bumble Bee) Fancy					
smoked	2 oz	120	6	0	0
whole	2 oz	70	3	0	0
(Chicken of the Sea)					
smoked	2.3 oz	140	8	0	0
in oil	3.75 oz	140	8	0	0
teriyaki	3.75 oz	120	12	1	6
in water	3.75 oz	120	10	0	0
whole	2 oz	80	6	0	0
(Crown Prince) smoked in oil	¼ cup	60	0	0	0
(Orleans) fancy smoked	2 oz	120	6	0	0
FRESH					
Eastern					
breaded & fried	6 medium	175	10	na	0
	3 oz	165	10	na	0
steamed	6 medium	60	3	0	9
	3 oz	115	7	0	0
Pacific/Western					
raw	1 medium	40	2	0	0
steamed	1 medium	40	2	0	0
	3 oz	140	8	0	0

P

Food and Description	Amount	Total Calories	Total Carbs	Fiber	Sugars
PANCAKE					
FROZEN or REFRIGERATED					
(Aunt Jemima)					
blueberry	3 pancakes	210	40	2	8
buttermilk	3 pancakes	200	37	2	9
home-style	3 pancakes	200	37	<1	8
low-fat	3 pancakes	190	35	2	7
mini	3 pancakes	240	46	2	8
original	3 pancakes	210	40	2	8
Syrup Dunkers	~½ box	520	114	2	53
(Pillsbury)					
blueberry	3 pancakes	260	50	1	15
buttermilk	3 pancakes	260	51	1	14
mini	3 pancakes	260	44	<1	12
original	3 pancakes	260	51	1	13
MIX (NOTE: Unless otherwise stated, data are for dry mix only.)					
(Arrowhead Mills)					
blue corn	⅓ cup	160	28	5	0
buckwheat	⅓ cup	170	29	5	0
gluten-free	¼ cup	150	36	0	1
kamut	¼ cup	140	24	4	0
oat bran	¼ cup	120	21	6	1
whole grain	¼ cup	120	24	4	4
wild rice	¼ cup	130	28	2	0
(Aunt Jemima) pancake & waffle..mix only					
buckwheat	¼ cup	100	23	3	3
buttermilk	¼ cup	110	23	1	4
buttermilk..complete	⅓ cup	160	31	1	6
buttermilk..reduced-calorie..complete	⅓ cup	130	28	5	6
complete	⅓ cup	160	32	1	7
original	⅓ cup	150	33	1	7
whole wheat	¼ cup	120	26	3	4
(Betty Crocker) mix..prepared w/water					
box					
buttermilk	3 pancakes	200	39	1	7
original	3 pancakes	200	39	1	9

Food and Description	Amount	Total Calories	Total Carbs	Fiber	Sugars
pouch					
complete..mix w/water..					
buttermilk	3 pancakes	210	37	1	8
original	3 pancakes	250	39	1	6
(Bisquick) Shake 'N Pour..pancake & waffle mix..prepared					
blueberry	3 pancakes	210	40	1	8
buttermilk	3 pancakes	200	38	1	6
original	3 pancakes	210	39	<1	9
(Hodgson Mill)					
buckwheat	⅓ cup	190	40	3	1
multigrain buttermilk					
w/milled flax seed & soy	⅓ cup	150	31	5	2
(Hungry Jack) pancake & waffle..mix only					
blueberry..4-count	⅛ pkg	200	40	1	12
buttermilk	⅓ cup	150	31	1	7
(Jiffy) buttermilk complete..prepared	3 pancakes	160	32	<1	4
(Krusteaz) prepared					
apple spice	3 pancakes	210	40	3	11
blueberry	3 pancakes	240	47	2	11
buttermilk					
fat-free	3 pancakes	200	46	6	8
original	3 pancakes	210	40	1	7
chocolate chip	3 pancakes	220	41	1	11
home-style	3 pancakes	230	39	1	8
oat bran					
light	3 pancakes	140	34	8	6
low-fat	3 pancakes	230	45	4	10
wheat & honey	3 pancakes	220	42	4	6
(Maple Grove Farms) pancake & waffle..mix only					
buckwheat w/honey..24-oz box	¹⁄₁₉ box	130	28	4	3
buttermilk w/honey..24-oz box	¹⁄₁₉ box	130	28	3	4
(Shawnee Mills)					
pancake..mix only					
buttermilk..complete..low-fat	1.5 oz	150	29	1	3
pancake & waffle..mix only					
buttermilk	¼ pkg	180	31	2	4
buttermilk..low-fat	1.5 oz	160	29	1	2
whole wheat	⅓ pkg	170	30	5	3
PANCAKE & WAFFLE MIX (*See* PANCAKE, Mix entry)					
PANCAKE & WAFFLE SYRUP (*See also* ICE CREAM TOPPING; SYRUP)					
(Aunt Jemima)					
butter light	¼ cup	100	26	1	25
butter rich	¼ cup	210	52	0	29
country rich..all flavors	¼ cup	210	53	0	30
light	¼ cup	100	26	1	25
original	¼ cup	210	52	0	32
(Bob White)					
butter maple	¼ cup	220	55	0	29
crystal white fancy	2 Tbs	130	32	0	29

Food and Description	Amount	Total Calories	Total Carbs	Fiber	Sugars
(Golden Griddle)					
cinnamon	¼ cup	240	60	0	27
light	¼ cup	90	24	0	19
original	¼ cup	220	60	0	30
(Karo) pancake					
dark	2 Tbs	120	31	0	11
golden	2 Tbs	130	33	0	17
light	2 Tbs	130	33	0	17
original..dark corn syrup	¼ cup	240	63	0	25
(Maple Grove Farms)					
apricot	¼ cup	210	54	1	52
blueberry	¼ cup	210	52	0	49
boysenberry	¼ cup	210	43	0	52
maple					
pure					
100%	¼ cup	200	53	0	53
dark amber	¼ cup	200	53	0	53
medium amber	¼ cup	200	53	0	53
red raspberry	¼ cup	210	53	0	42
strawberry swirl	¼ cup	210	53	0	52
(Roddenbery's) Northwoods					
butter maple	¼ cup	230	58	0	29
light	¼ cup	100	24	0	19
original	¼ cup	230	57	0	28
sugar-free	¼ cup	100	24	0	19
(Smucker's)					
breakfast..sugar-free..squeeze	¼ cup	30	8	0	0
fruit syrups..all flavors	¼ cup	210	52	0	52
PAPAYA					
CANNED or JARRED					
(Del Monte) Sun Fresh..refrigerated					
in extra-light syrup	½ cup	70	17	1	16
DRIED					
(Sun-Maid) Tropical Trio					
pineapple papaya mango	1.4 oz	130	34	1	27
FRESH					
cubed..peeled	1 cup	60	14	3	8
(Dole)	½ medium	70	19	2	9
PAPAYA JUICE/NECTAR (*See also* FRUIT PUNCH)					
BOTTLED, BOXED, or CANNED					
(After The Fall) Pele papaya	8 fl oz	120	25	0	22
(Knudsen) nectar	8 fl oz	140	35	0	31
(Libby's)	11.5 fl oz	210	51	0	47
PAPRIKA (Durkee) ground	1 tsp	8	0	0	0
PARFAIT (*See* CANDY; ICE CREAM BARS, CUPS & CONES, SANDWICHES & FROZEN NOVELTIES; PUDDING & MOUSSE)					
PARSLEY					
dried	1 tsp	1	0	0	0
freeze-dried	any amount	0	0	0	0
fresh	10 sprigs	3	1	0	0

Food and Description	Amount	Total Calories	Total Carbs	Fiber	Sugars
PARSNIP..fresh					
cooked	½ cup	65	15	3	0
raw/sliced	½ cup	50	12	3.5	0
PASSION FRUIT/GRANADILLA					
fresh	1 medium	18	4	2	0
(Frieda's)	5 oz	140	33	15	16
PASSION FRUIT JUICE/JUICE BLEND (*See also* FRUIT PUNCH)					
generic..fresh					
purple	1 cup	126	34	0.5	na
yellow	1 cup	149	36	0.5	na
(Knudsen) orange passion fruit spritzer	12 fl oz	160	40	0	38
(Welch's) passion fruit juice cocktail	8 fl oz	150	38	0	37
PASTA (*See also* COUSCOUS)					
(Adrienne's) Gourmet/wheat-free & gluten-free Papadini Hi-Protein Pure Lentil Bean Pasta					
all styles	2 oz	190	33	5	1
(American Beauty) dry					
angel hair	2 oz	210	42	2	2
capellini	2 oz	210	42	2	2
curly roni	2 oz	210	42	2	2
egg noodles					
bow ties	2 oz	210	39	1	2
crinkly	2 oz	210	40	2	2
extra-wide	2 oz	210	40	2	2
fine	2 oz	210	40	2	2
wide	2 oz	210	40	2	2
elbow roni	2 oz	210	40	2	2
fettuccini..egg	2 oz	210	42	2	2
fettuccini..Florentine	2 oz	210	42	2	2
lasagna	2 oz	210	42	2	2
manicotti	2 oz	210	42	2	2
mostaccioli	2 oz	210	40	2	2
penne rigate	2 oz	210	42	2	2
rainbow shells	2 oz	210	42	2	2
rigatoni..enriched	2 oz	210	42	2	2
roni mac	2 oz	210	42	2	2
rotini..enriched	2 oz	210	42	2	2
sea shells	2 oz	210	42	2	2
shell roni..all sizes	2 oz	210	42	2	2
shells..medium	2 oz	210	40	2	2
Soups 'n' Sides..all styles	2 oz	210	42	2	2
spaghetti..all styles	2 oz	210	40	2	2
trio Italiano..rotini mostaccioli	2 oz	210	42	2	2
vermicelli	2 oz	210	44	1	2
vermicelli fideo..enriched	2 oz	200	44	1	2
(Amish Kitchens) egg noodle..all styles	2 oz	220	38	1	2
(Azumaya) cooked					
pasta..soy					
large square wrappers	8 wraps	160	31	1	1
round	10 wraps	160	31	1	1

Food and Description	Amount	Total Calories	Total Carbs	Fiber	Sugars
pasta wrappers..egg rolls	7 wraps	170	35	1	1
spinach pasta	1 cup	210	42	2	1
thin-cut noodles	1 cup	210	43	2	1
(Barilla)					
angel hair	2 oz	200	42	2	1
egg	2 oz	210	40	2	1
campanelle	2 oz	200	42	2	1
cellentani	2 oz	200	42	2	1
ditalini	2 oz	200	42	2	1
egg noodles..all styles	2 oz	210	40	2	1
elbows	2 oz	200	40	2	1
farfalle	2 oz	200	42	2	1
fettuccini	2 oz	200	42	2	1
gemelli	2 oz	200	42	2	1
linguine	2 oz	200	42	2	1
manicotti	~2 oz	180	37	2	2
orzo	2 oz	200	42	2	1
penne	2 oz	200	42	2	1
rigitoni	2 oz	200	42	2	1
rotini..all styles	2 oz	200	42	2	1
shells					
jumbo	2 oz	180	38	2	2
large	2 oz	200	42	2	1
medium	2 oz	200	42	2	1
spaghetti..all styles	2 oz	200	42	2	1
ziti	2 oz	200	42	2	1
(Buitoni) refrigerated cut pasta					
FAMILY-SIZE					
cheese					
ravioli	1¼ cups	330	40	3	3
tortellini	1 cup	320	50	3	4
herb chicken & tortellini	1 cup	340	52	2	3
mixed-cheese tortellini	1 cup	320	50	3	3
mozzarella					
& herb grande ravioli	1½ cups	340	43	3	3
& pepperoni tortelloni	1 cup	330	45	2	3
REGULAR-SIZE					
angel hair	1¼ cups	230	43	2	1
beef ravioletti	1 cup	300	46	2	3
cheese & roasted garlic tortelloni	1 cup	270	37	2	2
chicken					
& herb tortellini	1 cup	340	52	2	3
Parmesan ravioli	1¼ cups	310	45	7	3
& prosciutto tortelloni	1 cup	330	47	2	2
roasted w/garlic ravioli	1¼ cups	340	47	2	3
classic beef ravioli	1¼ cups	340	48	2	4
fettuccini	1¼ cups	240	45	2	1
4-cheese ravioli	1¼ cups	330	40	3	3
4-cheese ravioli..light	1¼ cups	230	37	2	3

Food and Description	Amount	Total Calories	Total Carbs	Fiber	Sugars
garden vegetable ravioli	1 cup	250	39	2	4
linguine	1¼ cups	240	45	2	1
mozzarella					
& herb tortelloni	1 cup	330	46	2	3
& pepperoni tortelloni	1 cup	330	45	2	3
portobello mushroom & cheese					
tortelloni	1 cup	270	46	3	2
spinach fettuccini	1¼ cups	220	45	2	1
sun-dried tomato tortelloni	1 cup	310	46	3	4
sweet Italian sausage tortelloni	1 cup	330	48	3	5
3-cheese					
ravioletti	1 cup	270	43	2	3
tortellini	1 cup	320	50	3	4
(Creamette) dry					
egg noodles					
extra-wide	2 oz	210	38	1	2
no egg yolk..all styles	2 oz	210	42	2	3
regular..all styles	2 oz	210	42	2	3
enriched pasta..all styles	2 oz	210	42	2	3
Healthy Harvest..all styles	2 oz	210	41	3	2
Kid's Club..all shapes	2 oz	210	42	2	3
other dry pasta..all styles & shapes	2 oz	210	42	2	3
(Da Vinci) organic..all styles & shapes	2 oz	200	41	1	3
(Di Giorno) refrigerated					
low-fat..cholesterol-free					
fettuccini					
red bell pepper	3 oz	200	38	2	1
regular	3 oz	200	38	2	1
spinach	3 oz	190	38	2	1
tortelloni..3-cheese	3 oz	250	37	2	2
(Eden) dry					
artichoke ribbons	2 oz	210	40	2	1
bell pepper	2 oz	210	40	2	1
creste dei gallo..parsley garlic	2 oz	210	41	4	2
extra-fine pasta	2 oz	210	40	3	1
mung bean..Harusame	2 oz	190	47	0	0
pesto gemelli	2 oz	210	41	4	2
quinoa..organic	~1.5 oz	180	29	11	2
ribbons durum..golden amber..organic					
parsley garlic	2 oz	210	40	3	1
pesto	2 oz	210	40	3	1
saffron	2 oz	210	49	3	1
wheat pesto					
80% whole grain	2 oz	200	41	5	1
100% whole grain	2 oz	210	41	5	1
rice pasta..bifun	2 oz	200	44	0	0
rigatoni..endless tubes	2 oz	210	41	4	2
soba					
40% buckwheat	2 oz	190	43	3	2

Food and Description	Amount	Total Calories	Total Carbs	Fiber	Sugars
100% buckwheat	2 oz	200	43	3	2
Japanese	2 oz	190	37	3	2
lotus root	2 oz	190	37	4	2
mugwort	2 oz	190	37	2	2
wild yam jinenjo	2 oz	190	37	2	2
spaghetti..organic					
kamut	2 oz	190	38	6	2
parsley garlic	2 oz	210	41	4	2
spirals..organic					
flax rice..60% whole grain	2 oz	200	40	4	0
kamut	2 oz	190	40	6	3
mixed grain	2 oz	210	41	7	3
rye	2 oz	200	44	8	1
sesame rice	2 oz	200	36	4	1
udon					
brown rice..organic	2 oz	200	38	3	1
Japanese	2 oz	190	37	3	5
Japanese brown	2 oz	190	38	2	2
vegetable shells..small	2 oz	210	49	4	1
ziti rigati..parsley garlic	2 oz	210	41	5	2
(Goodman's) dry					
alphabets	2 oz	210	42	2	3
bows..large	2 oz	220	40	1	2
egg flakes	2 oz	220	40	1	2
egg noodles..all sizes	2 oz	210	39	1	2
yolk-free ribbons	2 oz	210	42	2	3
(Hodgson Mill) dry					
organic whole wheat w/milled flaxseed & soy					
fettuccini	2 oz	200	40	6	0
penne	2 oz	200	40	6	0
spaghetti	2 oz	200	40	6	0
spirals	2 oz	200	40	6	0
veggie...all types & sizes	2 oz	200	41	1	0
whole wheat					
angel hair	2 oz	190	34	6	0
couscous	⅓ cup	210	47	5	1
couscous w/milled flaxseed & soy	⅓ cup	230	48	5	1
couscous..garlic & basil w/milled flaxseed & soy	⅓ cup	235	50	6	1
couscous..Parmesan cheese w/milled flaxseed & soy	⅓ cup	240	50	6	3
egg noodles	2 oz	190	34	4	0
spinach	2 oz	190	32	5	0
fettuccini w/flaxseed	2 oz	190	40	6	0
yokeless pasta ribbons	2 oz	190	34	5	0
(Lundberg Family Farms) brown rice pasta					
all styles & shapes	2 oz	210	44	3	3
(Monterey) refrigerated pasta..cooked					
Carb-Smart	3 oz	200	27	5	1

Food and Description	Amount	Total Calories	Total Carbs	Fiber	Sugars
fettuccini..classic egg	3 oz	200	27	5	1
ravioli	3.6 oz	260	17	5	1
4-cheese & chives	3.6 oz	220	18	5	1
seafood w/lobster & crab	3.6 oz	240	18	5	1
spinach ricotta	3.6 oz	230	21	6	1
other pasta	3 oz	270	36	1	1
grandi	3 oz	230	30	0	0
ravioli..low-fat	3 oz	240	36	2	1
ravioli..snow crab	3 oz	240	35	1	1
spinach ricotta	3 oz	300	40	1	1
tortellini	3 oz	340	36	0	0
classic Italian cheese	3 oz	280	51	0	0
rainbow..5-cheese	3 oz	250	37	1	1
(Mrs. Weiss') dry					
egg noodles	2 oz	210	39	2	2
egg farvel	2 oz	210	39	1	2
egg flakes	2 oz	210	39	1	2
extra-fine	2 oz	210	39	1	2
ha-lush-ka	2 oz	210	39	2	2
kluski	2 oz	210	39	2	2
kluski..enriched	2 oz	210	39	1	2
medium	2 oz	210	39	1	2
wide	2 oz	180	35	2.5	3
(Reames) frozen					
egg noodles	½ cup	210	39	1	1
golden ribbons	½ cup	170	32	1	1
home-style	½ cup	240	42	2	3
quick cook	1 cup	230	42	2	3
hearty home-style chicken noodle	3 oz	130	21	1	2
home-style	½ cup	190	35	2	1
flat dumplings	½ cup	160	32	1	1
free..no yolk	½ cup	160	32	1	1
(Ronzoni) dry					
acini pepe-44	2 oz	210	42	2	2
angel hair..lemon pepper	2 oz	210	41	2	2
egg pastina	2 oz	210	40	2	2
macarrones	2 oz	210	40	2	2
campanelle-73	2 oz	210	42	2	2
capellini-11	2 oz	210	42	2	2
farfalle-66	2 oz	210	42	2	2
spaghetti	2 oz	210	42	2	2
spinach ricotta	2 oz	210	42	2	2
(Strom Products)					
No Yolks..all shapes	2 oz	210	41	3	0
Wacky Mac..all styles and shapes	2 oz	200	41	1	0
(VitaSpelt) pasta..dry					
white spelt..all shapes and types	2 oz	210	42	2	9
whole grain..all shapes and types	2 oz	190	40	5	4
(Westbrae Natural) dry					
angel hair..corn	2 oz	210	46	0	0

Food and Description	Amount	Total Calories	Total Carbs	Fiber	Sugars
lasagna..whole wheat..no egg					
plain	2 oz	200	39	9	1
spinach	2 oz	180	35	8	1
spaghetti..whole wheat..no egg					
plain	2 oz	200	39	9	1
spinach	2 oz	180	38	8	1

PASTA ENTRÉE/DINNER (*See also* ASIAN FOOD; FROZEN ENTRÉE/DINNER; VEGETARIAN FOODS; individual listings)

CANNED

Food and Description	Amount	Total Calories	Total Carbs	Fiber	Sugars
(Annie's) homegrown organic					
All-Stars	1 cup	150	31	<1	11
Arthur Loops	1 cup	150	32	1	11
cheesy ravioli	1 cup	190	31	3	9
P'Sghetti Loops w/soy meatballs	1 cup	190	29	2	9
(Chef Boyardee)					
Beefaroni					
big w/beef in tomato sauce	1 cup	270	35	5	7
macaroni w/beef in sauce	1 cup	260	37	5	9
Chili Mac	1 cup	270	30	1	5
lasagna..beef & tomato sauce	10.5 oz	300	42	3	9
macaroni..cheesy burger	1 cup	220	32	0	4
pasta shells & meatballs..mini bites	1 cup	300	36	3	7
Pepperoni Pizzazaroli	1 cup	320	46	3	11
ravioli					
beef in tomato & meat sauce	1 cup	230	35	3	6
cheesy burger	1 cup	300	48	0	13
mini beef in tomato & meat sauce	1 cup	300	36	3	7
mini bites..beef & meatballs	1 cup	280	31	2	8
overstuffed w/tomato meat sauce	1 cup	280	48	4	12
spaghetti & meatballs	7.5 oz	270	34	1	8
jumbo	1 cup	280	30	3	8
mini bites w/meatballs	7.5 oz	280	31	1	8
X-Men..in tomato & cheese sauce	7.5 oz	200	43	2	12
X-Men..w/meatballs..in tomato sauce	7.5 oz	290	39	2	9
(Franco-American)					
beef ravioli..in meat sauce	1 cup	260	39	5	13
beef ravioliOs..in meat sauce	1 cup	290	39	3	11
Fun Shapes SpaghettiOs					
Smilers	1 cup	180	36	3	15
w/meatball Smilers	1 cup	260	33	3	12
Knights & castles SpaghettiOs	1 cup	190	37	2	12
w/meatballs	1 cup	260	33	3	9
spaghetti..in tomato & cheese sauce	1 cup	210	40	2	14
SpaghettiOs	1 cup	180	37	3	14
A to Zs	1 cup	180	36	3	15
w/meatballs	1 cup	260	33	3	12
w/sliced franks	1 cup	230	33	2	12
w/meatballs	1 cup	240	32	3	11
w/sliced franks	1 cup	230	27	5	9

Food and Description	Amount	Total Calories	Total Carbs	Fiber	Sugars
FRESH					
(Reser's) pasta salads..ready-to-serve					
elbow macaroni	¾ cup	320	28	2	8
California pasta	¾ cup	160	29	2	10
gourmet macaroni & cheese	¾ cup	280	29	2	8
Italian	½ cup	160	18	3	3
Thai noodle	⅔ cup	230	26	3	10
traditional macaroni	¾ cup	320	28	2	8
FROZEN					
(Birds Eye) Pasta Secrets..prepared					
Italian pesto	1 cup	240	32	2	6
primavera	1 cup	230	26	3	4
radiatore pasta & vegetables	1 cup	200	27	1	5
ranch	1 cup	300	29	2	8
3-cheese	1 cup	230	31	2	8
white cheddar	1 cup	200	27	1	5
zesty garlic	1 cup	240	31	2	6
(Cascadian Farm) bowls..veggie					
Japanese noodles & vegetables	1 bowl	180	29	4	7
pasta marinara	1 bowl	180	30	3	7
pasta primavera	1 bowl	270	37	2	7
(Green Giant)					
Complete Skillet Meal..as packaged					
chicken Alfredo	¼ pkg	270	35	2	5
chicken cheesy pasta	¼ pkg	270	37	3	7
creamy chix noodle	¼ pkg	290	42	3	11
garlic chicken pasta	¼ pkg	260	31	2	5
Create A Meal..as packaged					
beefy noodle	1¾ cups	170	31	3	4
cheesy pasta & vegetable	1¾ cups	210	27	2	7
chicken Alfredo	2 cups	230	33	3	6
garlic herb chicken	1⅓ cups	230	30	3	3
Parmesan herb chix	1¾ cups	160	29	5	3
skillet lasagna	1¾ cups	150	31	3	10
Pasta Accents..as packaged					
Alfredo	2 cups	200	27	3	4
creamy cheddar	2⅓ cups	250	36	3	5
garden herb seasoning	2 cups	230	32	7	4
garlic seasoning	2 cups	260	36	3	6
3-cheese	2 cups	350	42	4	7
white cheddar sauce	1¾ cups	290	37	3	7
(Uncle Ben's) Noodle & Pasta Bowls					
3-cheese ravioli	1 bowl	380	55	6	12
4-cheese lasagna w/meat sauce	1 bowl	330	41	7	8
chicken fettuccini Alfredo	1 bowl	350	47	2	10
garlic & herb chicken	1 bowl	380	55	4	10
honey ginger chicken	1 bowl	430	69	3	23
orange-glazed beef	1 bowl	440	70	4	26
Parmesan shrimp penne	1 bowl	380	58	2	19
spicy peanut chicken	1 bowl	420	58	5	15

Food and Description	Amount	Total Calories	Total Carbs	Fiber	Sugars
Thai-style chicken	1 bowl	400	60	6	13
tomato sausage rotini	1 bowl	420	67	6	12
■ MICROWAVE CONTAINER					
(Betty Crocker) Bowl Appétit!					
home-style chicken pasta	1 bowl	260	42	2	3
macaroni & cheese	1 bowl	370	56	1	8
pasta Alfredo	1 bowl	360	42	1	8
3-cheese rotini	1 bowl	360	56	2	12
tomato Parmesan penne	1 bowl	350	59	2	8
(Dinty Moore) American Classics					
beef ravioli	1 bowl	300	34	3	8
chicken & noodles	1 bowl	260	28	2	3
lasagna	1 bowl	340	28	3	6
macaroni & cheese w/Cure 81 ham	1 bowl	330	29	1	2
spaghetti..w/meatballs	1 bowl	290	44	3	17
(Hormel) shelf-staple entrées					
Kid's Kitchen					
beefy macaroni	1 cup	180	24	2	4
cheesy mac & beef	1 cup	260	32	1	3
mini ravioli	1 cup	240	35	1	6
noodle rings & chicken	1 cup	140	18	1	2
spaghetti & meatballs	1 cup	230	26	2	11
spaghetti rings & franks	1 cup	240	32	1	11
spaghetti rings & meatballs	1 cup	230	31	1	12
(Kraft) It's Pasta Anytime					
fettuccini w/classic Alfredo sauce	1 meal	580	74	4	7
spaghetti w/tomato sauce	1 meal	550	103	8	18
■ MIX					
(Annie's) prepared					
Deluxe Mac & Cheese					
elbows & 4-cheese sauce	1 cup	320	45	2	3
real aged Wisconsin cheddar	1 cup	320	44	2	5
rotini w/white cheddar	1 cup	300	44	2	4
macaroni & cheese					
Alfredo shells & cheddar	1 cup	370	47	1	2
family-size shells & white cheddar	1 cup	370	48	1	2
mild Mexican shells & cheddar	1 cup	280	49	1	21
peace & pasta Parmesan	1 cup	280	49	1	2
shells & real aged Wisconsin cheddar	1 cup	370	49	1	2
shells & white cheddar	1 cup	370	48	1	2
whole wheat shells & cheddar	1 cup	360	47	5	2
Totally Natural Pasta Meals made w/organic pasta					
curly fettuccini w/white cheddar & broccoli sauce	1 cup	350	51	1	2
penne pasta w/Alfredo cheese sauce	1 cup	360	49	1	2
radiatore pasta w/sun-dried tomato & basil sauce	1 cup	350	52	1	2
rotini pasta w/4-cheese sauce	1 cup	350	51	1	2

Food and Description	Amount	Total Calories	Total Carbs	Fiber	Sugars
(Atkins) Quick Quisine					
elbows & cheese	½ pkg	250	17	9	0
pesto cream	½ pkg	240	17	10	1
(Bean Cuisine)..mix only					
Mediterranean black beans & fusili	¼ pkg	210	30	4	2
pasta & Barcelona red beans w/radiatore	¼ pkg	210	29	4	2
(Betty Crocker) Suddenly Salad..prepared					
Caesar	1 cup	250	34	1	4
classic	1 cup	240	37	2	5
creamy Parmesan	1 cup	360	30	1	4
ranch & bacon	¾ cup	330	31	1	3
roasted garlic..Parmesan	¾ cup	340	34	1	4
(Carapelli) pasta & sauce..box mix					
4-cheese w/cavatappi pasta	½ box	240	47	4	5
creamy Alfredo w/penne pasta	½ box	240	47	4	6
creamy tomato w/spirals	½ box	240	49	4	8
(Fantastic Foods)					
Carb'tastic..Fast Naturals..ready meals					
penne Alfredo	1 pkg	280	25	21	3
penne w/meat sauce	1 pkg	240	22	14	7
vegetarian pesto primavera	1 pkg	270	22	14	6
Ramen noodle cups					
big cup..vegetable curry	½ pkg	110	29	2	2
small cup					
vegetable miso	1 cup	130	25	2	2
vegetarian..chicken-free	1 cup	140	26	4	4
vegetable miso	½ pkg	100	19	1	3
vegetarian..chicken-free	½ pkg	100	19	2	1
(Golden Grain) Pasta Roni..prepared as directed					
angel hair					
w/herbs	1 cup	320	42	2	7
w/lemon & butter	1 cup	360	48	2	4
w/Parmesan cheese	1 cup	320	40	2	7
broccoli					
au gratin	1 cup	280	41	2	7
regular	1 cup	330	42	2	6
chicken					
& garlic..low-fat	1 cup	300	40	2	4
regular	1 cup	310	41	2	5
corkscrew pasta					
w/creamy garlic sauce	1 cup	420	350	40	8
w/4-cheese sauce	1 cup	390	49	2	9
fettuccini					
w/Alfredo sauce					
original	1 cup	460	58	2	7
reduced-fat	1 cup	310	49	2	7
w/broccoli au gratin	1 cup	280	41	2	7
w/Romanoff sauce	1 cup	400	48	2	9

Food and Description	Amount	Total Calories	Total Carbs	Fiber	Sugars
w/Stroganoff sauce	1 cup	370	49	2	9
garlic Alfredo	1 cup	360	49	2	8
herb w/butter rigatoni	1 cup	350	42	2	6
home-style chicken	1 cup	230	39	3	4
linguine					
w/chicken & broccoli	1 cup	380	49	2	4
w/creamy chicken Parmesan	1 cup	410	51	3	7
parmesano	1 cup	390	50	2	7
rigatoni w/white cheddar &					
broccoli sauce	1 cup	320	40	2	7
Romanoff	1 cup	400	48	2	9
shells w/white cheddar sauce	1 cup	310	40	2	7
Stroganoff	1 cup	370	49	2	9
vermicelli w/roasted garlic & olive oil	1 cup	360	49	2	2
(Knorr)					
bow tie & beans	½ pkg	260	47	6	6
fettuccini w/classic Alfredo sauce	½ pkg	280	43	2	3
penne w/sun-dried tomato					
Parmesan sauce	½ pkg	270	50	3	4
rotini w/delicate mushroom sauce	½ pkg	260	50	1	7
(Kraft)					
macaroni & cheese..mix only, unless noted otherwise					
Blue's Clues	2.75 oz	260	47	1	7
Crazy Noodles..Green Wigglers	2.75 oz	260	48	2	8
deluxe					
4-cheese blend	3.5 oz	320	44	1	4
half the fat	3.5 oz	290	49	2	7
original	3.5 oz	320	44	2	4
sharp cheddar	2.8 oz	270	38	1	4
premium					
cheesy Alfredo	2.4 oz	260	44	2	7
mild white cheddar	2.4 oz	260	48	2	7
3-cheese	2.4 oz	260	48	2	7
Spirals	2.75 oz	260	47	1	7
SpongeBob Square Pants	2.75 oz	260	48	1	7
pasta salads					
classic ranch w/bacon	¼ pkg	130	26	2	2
creamy Caesar	¼ pkg	190	35	2	6
garlic Parmesan	¼ pkg	180	33	2	3
Italian	¼ pkg	160	30	2	3
ranch w/tuna..prepared	¼ pkg	300	27	1	2
side dishes..deluxe rotini & white					
cheddar sauce w/broccoli	½ box	400	48	2	6
spaghetti dinner/meat sauce..					
prepared	5.5 oz	330	45	3	8
Velveeta..prepared					
radiatore & cheese..herb & garlic	1 cup	360	46	2	6
shells & cheese					
bacon	1 cup	400	47	2	5
light	1 cup	320	51	2	8

Food and Description	Amount	Total Calories	Total Carbs	Fiber	Sugars
original	1 cup	360	46	2	6
salsa	1 cup	380	47	2	5
(Lipton)					
Asian Side Dishes					
beef lo mein	½ pkg	230	42	2	2
sweet & sour	½ pkg	260	50	2	8
teriyaki	½ pkg	250	46	2	5
Thai sesame	½ pkg	230	42	2	2
Fiesta Sides					
jalapeño jack	½ pkg	230	44	2	4
nacho	½ pkg	230	44	1	2
Pasta & Sauce..mix only					
Alfredo	½ pkg	240	39	1	3
Alfredo broccoli	½ pkg	250	40	1	3
butter	½ pkg	240	43	1	4
butter & herb	½ pkg	240	42	1	4
cheddar broccoli	½ pkg	250	48	2	4
cheesy cheddar	½ pkg	220	41	2	3
chicken	½ pkg	220	43	1	1
chicken broccoli	½ pkg	220	41	2	1
creamy chicken flavor	½ pkg	230	40	1	2
Parmesan	½ pkg	230	39	1	2
Stroganoff	½ pkg	210	39	1	2
Pasta & Sauce..Italian sides					
creamy garlic	½ pkg	270	47	1	4
4-cheese bowtie	½ pkg	220	38	1	2
tomato Parmesan	½ pkg	240	41	2	4
(Near East) prepared as directed					
couscous					
broccoli	1 cup	210	42	3	3
herbed chicken	1 cup	220	42	3	2
Mediterranean curry	1 cup	220	42	3	3
Moroccan pasta	1¼ cups	260	46	2	3
Parmesan	1 cup	220	41	2	3
roasted garlic & olive oil	1 cup	230	41	2	1
toasted pine nuts	1 cup	230	40	2	2
tomato lentil	1 cup	220	42	3	3
wild mushroom..herb	1 cup	230	42	3	2
Creative Grains					
chicken & herbs	1 cup	270	51	6	2
creamy Parmesan	1 cup	280	48	3	2
roasted garlic	1 cup	220	41	5	1
roasted pecan & garlic	1 cup	240	37	4	1
pastas w/delicate sauce					
angel hair..spicy tomato	1 cup	240	41	3	3
fusilli..Parmesan & Romano	1 cup	300	50	3	3
gemelli..tomato Parmesan	1 cup	330	52	4	3
radiatore..basil & herb	1 cup	260	41	3	2
vermicelli..garlic & olive oil	1 cup	260	39	2	3

Food and Description	Amount	Total Calories	Total Carbs	Fiber	Sugars
(Ragu) Ragu Express Pasta Dinners					
classic meat flavor	⅙ box	200	36	2	6
sweet tomato & garlic	⅙ box	500	39	3	8
traditional tomato	⅙ box	190	36	2	6
(Velveeta) (*See* (Kraft) in this section)					
PASTA SAUCE (*See* SAUCE)					
PASTRAMI (*See* LUNCHEON MEAT)					
PASTRY (*See also* CAKE; DONUT; PASTRY, TOASTER; PASTRY DOUGH; PIE CRUST)					
■ **FROZEN OR REFRIGERATED**					
(Alouette) pastry kit..baked Brie in pastry w/raspberries & almonds	⅑ kit	220	15	1	5
(Athens) baklava pastry..bite-size	2 pieces	230	28	<1	17
(Nancy's) pecan tartlets	6 tartlets	470	53	2	27
(Pepperidge Farm) turnovers					
apple	1 turnover	290	36	2	13
blueberry	1 turnover	280	33	1	14
peach	1 turnover	290	35	1	16
raspberry	1 turnover	290	35	1	16
(Pillsbury)					
sweet roll..Home-baked Classics					
cinnamon roll w/icing	1 roll	330	53	1	21
sweet rolls..dulce de leche caramel	1 roll	160	22	0	9
turnover					
apple	1 turnover	170	23	<1	11
cherry	1 turnover	170	23	0	12
(Rhodes)					
Bake-N-Serv Rolls..prepared					
apple cinnamon w/sweet topping	1 roll	190	28	<1	10
cinnamon w/rich vanilla icing	1 roll	195	28	<1	9
orange rolls w/cream cheese icing	1 roll	285	49	1	15.5
raspberry w/rich vanilla icing	1 roll	180	29	<1	6
strawberry w/rich vanilla icing	1 roll	180	29	<1	6
Rolls Anytime!					
cinnamon w/cream cheese icing	1 roll	240	42	1	14
orange w/cream cheese icing	1 roll	300	51	1	21
(Rich's) Temptations Éclairs					
Bavarian cream	1 éclair	220	25	0	10
Bavarian cream..mini	4 éclairs	250	29	1	21
cappuccino	1 éclair	220	25	0	19
(Sara Lee)					
cinnamon roll..deluxe w/icing	1 roll	320	41	1	21
coffee cakes					
butter streusel	⅙ cake	190	25	1	10
crumb	⅛ cake	190	30	1	18
pecan	⅙ cake	140	23	1	9
■ **READY-TO-SERVE**					
(Athens) filo pastries					
spanakopita..spinach & cheese 0.5 oz	10 pieces	390	34	2	3

Food and Description	Amount	Total Calories	Total Carbs	Fiber	Sugars
1.0 oz	5 pieces	390	34	2	3
2.0 oz	2½ pieces	390	34	2	3
tiropita..3-cheese					
0.5 oz	10 pieces	450	25	1	4
1.0 oz	5 pieces	450	25	1	4
2.0 oz	2½ pieces	390	34	2	3
(Awrey's)					
almond tea bites	1 tea bite	430	49	2	20
apple-filled pastries..petite	1 pastry	180	23	<1	9
bear claws..gourmet	1 pastry	430	48	2	29
cinnamon rolls w/cream-cheese icing	1 roll	650	94	3	35
cinnamon swirl pastries	1 pastry	430	56	2	23
Danish cinnamon swirl..6-pack	1 Danish	320	42	1	19
Long John coffee cake	1 slice	200	24	<1	10
raspberry cheese swirl pastries	1 pastry	400	53	1	21
sweet roll..8-pack Danish	1 Danish	300	39	<1	17
(Dunkin' Donuts) (*See* DONUT in this section; *see also* individual FAST FOOD listing)					
(Entenmann's)					
cinnamon buns..light	1 bun	170	33	2	18
cinnamon swirl buns	1 bun	310	43	1	20
coffee cake..crumb	1/10 cake	250	33	1	13
crumb cake					
crumb delight..light	1/9 cake	210	37	1	20
Little Bites	1 pouch	280	36	1	19
Ultimate for Crumb Lovers	1/10 cake	250	33	1	17
lemon twist..fat-free	1/8 twist	130	30	1	16
pecan Danish ring	2-oz piece	250	25	1	12
raspberry twist					
fat-free	1/8 twist	140	32	2	19
original	1/8 twist	220	28	1	15
walnut Danish ring	2-oz slice	240	25	1	12
(Hostess)					
honey buns					
glazed	1 bun	320	34	1	26
iced..frosted	1 bun	410	42	1	31
sweet rolls					
cherry	1 roll	220	35	0	21
cinnamon	1 roll	210	34	0	14
(Lance) snack					
cinnamon roll	4-oz roll	370	70	2	34
honey bun	3-oz bun	320	47	4	13
(Little Debbie) snack					
boxed					
honey bun..1.78 oz	1 pkg	230	24	<1	13
iced..2 oz	1 pkg	250	31	1	17
pecan spinwheel	1 pkg	100	16	0	7
individual packages					
honey bun..3.98 oz	1 bun	460	57	1	32
honey bun..pecan	1 pkg	220	26	1	13
pecan spinwheel..2 oz	1 pkg	210	32	<1	15

Food and Description	Amount	Total Calories	Total Carbs	Fiber	Sugars
(Otis Spunkmeyer)					
Café Collection cinnamon rolls..4 oz	½ roll	190	31	1	12
Café Collection Coffee Cakes					
apple cinnamon	1 cake	370	50	2	30
cheese	1 cake	340	46	2	24
Danish					
bear claw	2 oz	250	27	1	16
breakfast claw	2 oz	240	30	<1	18
buttercrumb	2 oz	250	31	<1	18
cinnamon					
Danish	2 oz	250	31	<1	18
roll	2.75 oz	340	43	2	24
twist	1.8 oz	230	25	1	10
fruit	2 oz	240	30	<1	17
(Sara Lee)					
breakfast cakes..crumb					
blueberry	1 cake	180	30	<1	9
French crumb	1 cake	180	33	0	20
breakfast cakes..home-style					
blueberry yogurt	1 slice	300	47	1	32
lemon poppyseed	1 slice	300	45	2	28
cinnamon rolls					
cinnamon supreme..2.125 oz	1 roll	240	33	2	17
cinnamon supreme..4.25 oz	1 roll	470	65	3	29
Nutti-Sticky bun..4.0 oz	1 bun	480	52	2	29
original Cinnaswirl..5.75 oz	1 roll	600	92	5	45
Danish					
large..Pastries Elite					
apple twist..4 oz	1 Danish	420	53	2	12
cheese butterfly..4 oz	1 Danish	450	49	4	18
cinnamon almond bear					
claw..3.5 oz	1 Danish	410	50	2	13
small..demi-Danish..1.25 oz					
apple	1 Danish	120	17	1	8
cheese	1 Danish	130	16	<1	7
cinnnamon raisin	1 Danish	140	19	<1	8
pecan	1 Danish	150	16	<1	6
individually wrapped					
cinnamon rolls					
ultimate cinnamon roll..4.25 oz	1 roll	570	79	4	44
single-serve..microwave					
cinnamon roll..4.75 oz	1 roll	540	68	2	34
Danish..3.25 oz					
apple orchard	1 Danish	340	45	1	21
cinnamon raisin	1 Danish	370	47	3	22
creamy cheese	1 Danish	230	27	2	17
red raspberry	1 Danish	250	50	2	26
sweet cheese	1 Danish	330	39	2	17
(TastyKake) snack					
apple fritter..Oxford	1 fritter	170	21	1	7

Food and Description	Amount	Total Calories	Total Carbs	Fiber	Sugars
honey bun					
glazed	1 bun	390	45	1	20
iced	1 bun	400	46	1	22
maple..iced	1 bun	390	46	1	21
Koffee Kake..cream-filled					
2 oz	1 cake	270	35	0	22
3 oz	1 cake	390	51	<1	33
raspberry..low-fat	1 cake	170	35	0	21
(Wolferman's)					
baklava	1 piece	337	44	2	29
povitica					
cream cheese	1 slice	150	19	0	11
English walnut	1 slice	180	20	1	11
rugelach	1 slice	150	14	0	7
PASTRY, TOASTER					
(Kellogg's) Pop Tarts					
low-fat..frosted..all flavors	1 pastry	190	39	1	20
Pastry Swirls					
apple cinnamon	1 pastry	250	37	<1	14
cheese	1 pastry	260	36	0	15
cheese & cherry	1 pastry	250	37	<1	16
regular..frosted					
blueberry	2 pastries	400	75	2	36
brown sugar cinnamon	1 pastry	210	34	1	17
cherry	1 pastry	200	38	1	19
chocolate fudge	1 pastry	200	37	1	19
hot fudge sundae	1 pastry	200	37	1	20
raspberry	1 pastry	210	37	1	19
s'mores	1 pastry	200	36	1	18
strawberry	1 pastry	200	38	1	19
wild berry	1 pastry	210	39	1	21
regular..unfrosted					
apple cinnamon	1 pastry	210	37	<1	17
blueberry	1 pastry	210	35	1	14
brown sugar cinnamon	1 pastry	210	37	<1	17
chocolate chip	1 pastry	220	35	<1	18
French toast	1 pastry	220	34	<1	15
Snack-Stix..frosted					
caramel chocolate	1 pastry	200	36	<1	19
double chocolate	1 pastry	200	37	<1	20
Yogurt Blasts..all flavors	1 pastry	210	37	<1	18
(Pillsbury) Toaster Strudel					
apple	1 pastry	190	26	<1	10
blueberry	1 pastry	190	26	<1	10
brown sugar cinnamon	1 pastry	190	26	<1	11
caramel apple	1 pastry	200	28	0	11
chocolate	1 pastry	190	25	<1	11
cream cheese	1 pastry	200	23	<1	8
cream cheese & cherry	1 pastry	200	24	<1	9
cream cheese & raspberry	1 pastry	200	24	0	9

Food and Description	Amount	Total Calories	Total Carbs	Fiber	Sugars
cream cheese & strawberry	1 pastry	200	24	<1	9
Danish-style cream cheese	1 pastry	200	23	<1	8
raspberry	1 pastry	190	26	0	10
strawberry	1 pastry	190	26	<1	10
wild berry	1 pastry	190	25	<1	10
(Quaker) Breakfast Squares..toastable					
apple cinnamon brown sugar					
iced	1 pastry	190	36	0	19
un-iced	1 pastry	190	35	1	17
blueberry..iced	1 pastry	190	36	0	19
cherry cobbler..un-iced	1 pastry	190	36	0	17
strawberry					
iced	1 pastry	190	36	0	19
un-iced	1 pastry	190	36	0	17
PASTRY DOUGH (See also PIE CRUST)					
(Apollo) filo dough	3 sheets	180	35	1	1
(Athens/Apollo Foods)..ready-to-go					
baklava dough					
rectangles	2 pieces	310	39	1	23
triangles	2 pieces	540	67	2	38
chocolate					
almond blossoms	2 pieces	590	61	3	33
almond rolls	4 pieces	580	64	3	28
swirls	1 swirl	230	34	2	22
triangles	2 pieces	550	67	2	36
large shells..traditional	1 shell	160	13	0	0
pastry sheets..filo					
12" x 17"	3 sheets	160	30	<1	1
14" x 18"	2½ sheets	180	37	1	1
pecan blossoms	2 pieces	590	60	1	26
pecan tarts	9 pieces	600	60	2	35
shredded dough..kataifi	⅛ pkg	180	35	4	1
(Pepperidge Farm)					
pastry shell	1 shell	190	16	<1	1
puff pastry dough sheet	⅙ sheet	170	14	<1	1
PÂTÉ (See also LUNCHEON MEAT; LUNCHEON MEAT SPREAD; VEGETARIAN FOODS)					
(Boar's Head) liverwurst..smoked	2 oz	170	1	0	1
(Old Wisconsin Sausage)					
braunschweiger..all styles	2 oz	210	3	0	3
(Sell's) liver	2.25 oz	190	3	0	1
(Tofutti)					
mackerel..smoked	3.5 oz	230	2	0	0
salmon	3.5 oz	145	2	0	0
PEA (See also BLACK-EYED PEA; PIGEON PEA; PURPLE HULL PEA; SNOW PEA; VEGETABLES, MIXED)					
CANNED					
(The Allens..East Texas Fair)					
lady cream peas	½ cup	100	17	5	0
peas 'n' pork	½ cup	110	17	5	0

Food and Description	Amount	Total Calories	Total Carbs	Fiber	Sugars
pepper peas w/jalapeños	½ cup	120	22	6	0
purple hull	½ cup	120	21	6	1
white acre	½ cup	100	17	5	0
(Blue Boy) sweet peas	½ cup	70	12	4	5
(Bush's Best) purple hull peas	½ cup	110	8	5	0
(Del Monte) sweet					
regular	½ cup	60	13	4	6
very young small	½ cup	60	13	4	5
(Green Giant)					
sweet peas	½ cup	60	11	3	3
less sodium	½ cup	60	11	3	2
w/tiny pearl onions	½ cup	60	11	3	3
(S&W)					
petit pois..early June	½ cup	70	12	4	4
sweet..young & tender..medium	½ cup	70	12	4	4
w/tiny pearl onions	½ cup	40	11	3	1
(Trappey's) field peas					
w/bacon	½ cup	90	15	5	0
w/snaps & bacon	½ cup	110	19	<1	0
DRIED					
(Arrowhead Mills) green split	2 oz	200	35	8	na
(Frieda's)	⅓ cup	130	22	9	1
(Hurst) green split w/ham	3 Tbs	120	22	11	1
FRESH					
green..raw (Frieda's)	⅓ cup	130	22	9	0
snow..raw (Frieda's)	1 cup	35	6	2	3
sugar snap					
(Dole)	½ cup	40	5	2	3
(Frieda's)	⅔ cup	35	6	2	3
FROZEN					
(Birds Eye)					
garden	⅔ cup	70	12	4	4
purple hull	½ cup	110	21	4	1
sugar snap	⅔ cup	40	7	2	2
sweet peas..w/pearl onions	⅔ cup	60	12	3	5
(C&W)					
baby pea pods	⅔ cup	40	7	3	2
petite..all types	⅔ cup	70	12	4	6
sugar snap	⅔ cup	35	6	2	2
(Cascadian Farm)					
peas & pearl onions	¾ cup	60	11	4	5
sugar snap peas	¾ cup	35	6	2	3
(Green Giant)..boil-in-bag					
baby sweet peas	⅔ cup	80	16	3	1
baby sweet peas & butter	¾ cup	90	14	4	7
sugar snap peas	⅔ cup	50	10	3	5
sweet peas & pearl onions	½ cup	50	10	3	5

PEA, BLACK-EYED (*See* BLACK-EYED PEA)
PEA, PIGEON (*See* PIGEON PEA)

Food and Description	Amount	Total Calories	Total Carbs	Fiber	Sugars
PEA, PURPLE HULL (*See* PURPLE HULL PEA)					
PEA, SNOW (*See* SNOW PEA)					
PEACH					
CAN OR CUP					
(Del Monte)					
cups..plastic..all styles	1 bowl	70	17	<1	16
freestone					
halves..in heavy syrup	½ cup	100	24	1	23
light	½ cup	60	15	1	14
slices..in heavy syrup	½ cup	100	24	1	23
light	½ cup	60	14	1	13
harvest spice..sliced	½ cup	80	21	<1	20
pull-top cans..4 oz					
diced..in light syrup	1 can	80	20	<1	19
in 100% juice	1 can	60	13	<1	12
light	1 can	50	13	<1	12
sliced..light	1 can	60	15	1	14
sliced					
in 100% juice	½ cup	60	15	1	14
in raspberry-flavored syrup	½ cup	80	20	<1	19
spiced..whole	½ cup	100	24	<1	23
yellow cling..Fruit Natural..chunks	½ cup	70	17	<1	16
(Dole) fruit bowls					
diced	4 oz cup	70	18	1	17
in strawberry gel	4.3 oz cup	80	21	1	19
yellow cling..sliced..in light syrup	3.5 oz	80	19	1	18
(Libby's) light..in juice..all styles	½ cup	50	13	1	12
(S&W)					
slices					
in heavy syrup	½ cup	100	24	1	23
in light syrup	½ cup	70	17	1	16
natural-style	½ cup	80	19	1	18
Snow peaches..in light syrup	½ cup	80	20	1	19
Sweet Memory..w/cinnamon	½ cup	80	19	1	19
whole..spiced..in heavy syrup	1 peach	100	24	1	23
DRIED					
(Del Monte) sun-dried	⅓ cup	90	28	5	21
(Sonoma) 4 pieces	1.4 oz	130	31	3	23
(Sun-Maid)	¼ cup	100	25	3	16
FRESH					
peeled..sliced	½ cup	37	10	2	9
whole..(Dole)	1 medium	40	10	2	9
FROZEN					
(Big Valley) freestone	⅔ cup	50	13	1	9
(C&W) sliced	⅔ cup	50	13	2	9
PEACH JUICE/JUICE BLEND/JUICE DRINK (*See also* FRUIT PUNCH; SOFT DRINK; SOFT DRINK MIX)					
BOTTLED, BOXED, or CANNED					
(Goya) nectar	6 fl oz	110	27	0	24

Food and Description	Amount	Total Calories	Total Carbs	Fiber	Sugars
(Kern's) nectar	11.5 oz	200	46	0	42
	8 fl oz	150	36	0	33
(Libby's) Juicy Juice	8 fl oz	130	32	0	29
(R. W. Knudsen)					
After The Fall..Georgia peach	8 fl oz	100	27	0	25
nectar	8 fl oz	120	30	0	28
peach spritzer	12 fl oz	160	37	0	26
(Snapple) juice drinks					
peach tea..diet	8 fl oz	0	0	0	0
raspberry peach	8 fl oz	120	29	0	27
(V8 Splash)					
juice drink..peach lemonade	8 fl oz	110	27	0	25
smoothie..peach mango	8 fl oz	120	27	0	27
(Walnut Acres) peach juice	8 fl oz	120	32	0	29
PEANUT					
(Ballpark)	1 oz	180	5	1	0
(Barcelona) Virginia..blanched..all styles	¼ cup	200	8	3	1
(Beer Nuts)					
kettle-cooked..simply salted	1 oz	185	6	2	0
original	1 oz	170	7	2	2
(Fisher)					
dry..honey-roasted	1 oz	170	7	2	4
dry..roasted	1 oz	170	6	2	2
Holiday Selections					
butter toffee..honey-roasted	1 oz	170	7	2	4
peanut carousel	1 oz	160	8	1	2
peanut trio	1 oz	160	8	1	2
honey-roasted	1 oz	170	7	1	4
raw..Chef's Naturals	1 oz	160	8	3	1
salted in shell..dry-roasted	1 oz	160	7	2	1
Snack Nuts & Seeds					
butter toffee	1 oz	130	17	1	15
honey-roasted	1 oz	170	7	2	4
honey-roasted..dry-roasted	1 oz	170	7	1	4
party	1 oz	160	5	2	1
Spanish..redskin..12-oz can	1 oz	180	6	2	2
(Kettle) hand-crafted nuts					
honey-roasted peanuts	1 oz	160	8	2	1
Spanish..jumbo..salted or no salt	1 oz	160	5	2	1
Spanish..raw	1 oz	160	4	3	1
(Lance)					
honey-roasted..1.375-oz	1 pkg	220	13	3	5
hot 'n' spicy..1.75-oz	1 pkg	290	13	2	2
salted..original..1.75-oz	1 pkg	200	6	4	0
(Mojave) peanuts					
w/mild chili	1 oz	160	5	2	0
w/spicy chili	1 oz	160	5	2	0
(Planters)					
cocktail					
honey-roasted..sweet 'n' crunchy	1 oz	170	6	2	1

Food and Description	Amount	Total Calories	Total Carbs	Fiber	Sugars
lightly salted	1 oz	170	5	2	1
party pack..unsalted	1 oz	170	6	2	1
dry-roasted	1 oz	160	6	2	1
lightly salted	1 oz	170	5	3	1
unsalted	1 oz	160	6	2	1
honey..dry-roasted	1 oz	160	8	2	4
Nut Poppers					
cheddar	1 oz	140	15	1	1
nutty original	1 oz	140	15	1	3
oil-roasted cocktail					
lightly salted	1 oz	170	6	2	1
unsalted	1 oz	170	6	0	2
redskin	1 oz	180	5	2	<1
Spanish..raw	1 oz	150	6	3	1
Sweet 'n' Crunchy	1 oz	140	16	2	13
(Weight Watchers) honey-roasted	0.7 oz	100	7	2	3
PEANUT BUTTER					
(Adams)					
100% natural	2 Tbs	200	4	1	1
no-stir..no sugar added..creamy	2 Tbs	210	7	2	2
(Arrowhead Mills) 100% Valencia					
sodium-free..all styles	2 Tbs	200	6	1	1
(Bama)					
original..all styles	2 Tbs	200	8	2	4
swirl w/jam or jelly..all styles	2 Tbs	120	17	0	11
(Jif)					
Chocolate Silk Sensations	2 Tbs	190	14	1	12
original..all styles	2 Tbs	190	7	2	3
reduced-fat..all styles	2 Tbs	190	15	2	4
Simply Jif					
creamy	2 Tbs	190	6	2	2
crunchy	2 Tbs	190	7	2	2
(Peter Pan)					
creamy					
regular	2 Tbs	190	7	2	3
very low-sodium	2 Tbs	200	7	2	3
crunchy					
regular	2 Tbs	190	6	2	3
very low-sodium	2 Tbs	200	6	2	3
Peter Pan Plus..creamy	2 Tbs	190	6	2	3
(Roaster Fresh) organic	2 Tbs	170	5	0	0
(Skippy)					
Doubly Delicious					
w/Nestlé Crunch pieces	2 Tbs	210	11	2	7
w/Nestlé Toll House pieces	2 Tbs	210	11	2	8
reduced-fat					
creamy	2 Tbs	190	15	2	5
super chunk	2 Tbs	180	13	2	4
roasted honey nut..creamy..all styles	2 Tbs	190	7	2	3

Food and Description	Amount	Total Calories	Total Carbs	Fiber	Sugars
(Smucker's)					
Chocolate Silk Smooth Sensation	2 Tbs	190	14	1	12
Goober PB&J					
grape	3 Tbs	230	24	2	21
strawberry	3 Tbs	230	24	2	21
old-fashioned natural					
chunky	2 Tbs	200	7	2	2
creamy	2 Tbs	200	7	2	2
honey	2 Tbs	200	9	2	4
reduced-fat					
creamy or crunchy	2 Tbs	190	15	2	4
natural	2 Tbs	200	12	2	2
PEANUT BUTTER–FLAVORED BAKING CHIPS (*See* BAKING BITS, BARS, CHIPS, CHUNKS & PIECES)					
PEANUT FLOUR (*See* FLOUR)					
PEAR					
CANNED or JARRED					
(Del Monte)					
halves					
in extra-light syrup..light	½ cup	60	15	1	14
in heavy syrup	½ cup	100	24	1	23
in light syrup..cinnamon-flavored	½ cup	80	21	1	19
in pear juice..Fruit Naturals	½ cup	60	15	1	14
Orchard Select sliced Bartlett	½ cup	80	20	2	19
individual pull-top cans..4.5 oz					
halves in heavy syrup	1 can	100	24	1	23
light	1 can	60	15	1	14
sliced..in heavy syrup	1 can	100	24	1	23
(Libby's) light..all styles	½ cup	60	15	1	14
(S&W)					
Bartlett halves..in heavy syrup	½ cup	90	22	2	18
California Sun..in light syrup	½ cup	80	20	<1	15
natural..Bartlett..halves or slices	½ cup	80	21	2	17
quartered..in heavy syrup	½ cup	90	23	1	22
sliced..in pear juice	½ cup	80	21	2	17
DRIED (Sonoma Organic) 4 pieces	1.4 oz	140	32	7	na
FRESH (Dole) Bartlett	1 medium	100	25	4	17
PEAR JUICE/NECTAR					
CANNED or JARRED					
(Goya) nectar	6 fl oz	120	29	1	na
(Kern's) nectar	8 fl oz	150	37	3	24
	12 fl oz	220	54	4	35
(Libby's) nectar	5.5 fl oz	100	25	0	21
(R. W. Knudsen) organic	6 fl oz	120	30	0	23
PECAN					
(Azar) all styles	1 oz	210	22	3	1
(Diamond of California) all styles	¼ cup	220	5	3	1
(Fisher)					
Dulects..pecan clusters	1.2 oz	150	15	1	14

Food and Description	Amount	Total Calories	Total Carbs	Fiber	Sugars
chopped	1 oz	200	4	2	1
ground	1 oz	200	3	3	0
halves	1 oz	200	4	2	1
salad toppings..pecan pieces	1 oz	190	4	3	1
(Planters)					
chips	2 oz	390	9	7	2
halves					
Gold Measure	2 oz	390	9	7	2
regular	1 oz	170	4	3	1
pieces	1 oz	390	9	7	2
(Smucker's) topping..pecans in syrup	1.25 oz	170	20	<1	13
PEPPER (*See also* MEXICAN FOOD; PEPPER, GROUND; SEASONINGS)					
CANNED or JARRED					
(Arnold's) Chilito's Encurtidos	1 oz	10	1	0	0
(B&G)					
hot jalapeños..slices	1 oz	0	0	0	0
roasted	1 oz	0	0	0	0
w/garlic	1 oz	15	2	0	1
w/imported balsamic vinegar	1 oz	10	3	0	2
sandwich toppers..peppers					
hot..chopped	1 oz	0	0	0	0
sweet	1 oz	20	5	0	3
sweet bell	1 oz	20	5	0	3
sweet	1 oz	10	3	0	2
sweet red	2 oz	20	5	0	3
(Hebrew National)					
filet peppers	1 oz	9	2	0	0
hot cherry	1 oz	11	2	0	0
red filet peppers	1 oz	9	2	0	0
(Heinz)					
banana..hot	1 pepper	6	1	0	0
hot rings..slices	1 pepper	4	1	0	0
Sweet Pepper Momentos	1 oz	6	1	0	0
(Mt. Olive)					
banana peppers..hot	1 oz	10	2	0	0
cherry rings..hot	1 oz	10	2	0	0
chow-chow..all styles	1 oz	15	1	0	0
jalapeño slices	2 oz	5	1	0	0
pepper rings..banana..all styles	1 oz	10	2	0	0
pepperoncini..imported	1 oz	10	2	0	0
sweet 'n' hot peppers..salad	1 oz	40	9	7	0
(Progresso) drained					
cherry	2 Tbs	30	2	1	1
whole..hot	1 medium	10	3	1	0
diced..drained	2 Tbs	30	2	1	1
diced..fried	2 tbs	60	3	1	2
pepper salad	2 Tbs	15	1	1	0
roasted	2 peppers	10	2	<1	1
Tuscan	3 peppers	10	3	1	0

Food and Description	Amount	Total Calories	Total Carbs	Fiber	Sugars
(Trappey's)					
banana					
slices	21 slices	6	1	0	1
whole	3 peppers	6	1	0	1
cherry..all styles	1 oz	10	3	1	0
jalapeño..hot					
sliced	1 oz	5	1	0	1
whole	1 oz	10	3	1	0
serrano..hot	1 oz	10	3	1	0
tempero..Greek pepperoncini..mild	1 pepper	10	3	1	0
torrido..Santa Fe Grande..hot	1 pepper	10	3	1	0
(Vlasic)					
banana..hot	1 oz	4	1	0	0
cherry					
hot	1 oz	10	2	0	0
mild	1 oz	8	2	0	0
Greek pepperoncini salad					
hot	1 oz	10	2	0	0
mild	1 oz	5	1	0	0
Mexican..hot	1 oz	8	2	0	0
Mexican..tiny hot	1 oz	6	2	0	0
DRIED red or green	1 Tbs	1	0	0	0
FREEZE-DRIED sweet red or green	1 Tbs	1	0	0	0
FRESH					
green chili..hot					
chopped	½ cup	16	3	1	0
whole	1 medium	15	4	1	0
jalapeño					
chopped	½ cup	17	2	<1	0
whole	2 medium	14	1	0	0
red chili..hot					
chopped	½ cup	14	3	1	0
whole	1 medium	15	4	1	0
red or green..sweet					
chopped	½ cup	20	5	1.5	0
whole..2.5" diameter	1 medium	30	8	2	0
yellow..sweet					
chopped	10 strips	14	3	1	0
whole..3" diameter	1 medium	50	12	2	0
FROZEN					
(Birds Eye) green & red..stir-fry	3 oz	25	5	2	3
(C&W) green & red..strips	3 oz	25	4	2	1
PEPPER, GROUND (*See also* PEPPER; SEASONINGS)					
(Durkee)					
black	1 tsp	8	0	0	0
red/cayenne	1 tsp	9	1	1	0
white	1 tsp	8	2	0	0
(Lawry's) lemon	1 tsp	6	1.5	<1	0
PEPPERONI (*See* SAUSAGE)					

Food and Description	Amount	Total Calories	Total Carbs	Fiber	Sugars
PERCH (*See* OCEAN PERCH; SEAFOOD ENTRÉE/DINNER)					
PERSIMMON					
Japanese/kaki..~2.5" diameter					
dried	1 medium	93	25	5	17
fresh	1 medium	118	31	6	na
PESTO SAUCE (*See* SAUCE)					
PHEASANT..raw					
breast..meat only	5 oz	189	0	0	0
leg meat..meat only	3 oz	114	0	0	0
PICANTE SAUCE (*See* MEXICAN FOOD; SAUCE)					
PICCALILLI (*See* PICKLE RELISH)					
PICKLE (*See also* PICKLE RELISH)					
(Arnold's)					
dill..all types	1 oz	0	0	0	0
garden mix..so hot	1 oz	0	0	0	0
hamburger slices	1 oz	0	0	0	0
(Claussen's)					
bread 'n' butter					
chips	4 slices	20	5	0	3
sandwich slices	2 slices	20	5	0	3
half sours..New York–deli-style	½ pickle	5	1	0	0
hamburger dills					
chips	10 chips	5	1	0	0
slices	10 slices	5	1	0	0
hearty garlic..deli-style..all styles	1 oz	5	1	0	0
kosher dills					
burger slices	4 slices	5	1	0	0
halves	½ pickle	5	1	0	0
mini	1 pickle	5	1	0	0
sandwich slices	2 slices	5	1	0	0
slices	4 slices	5	1	0	0
spears	1 spear	5	1	0	0
whole	½ pickle	5	1	0	0
sweet gherkins	1 oz	30	7	0	6
sweet pickle relish	1 Tbs	15	2	0	1
(Del Monte)					
pickle relish					
hamburger-style	1 Tbs	20	5	<1	5
hot dog–style	1 Tbs	15	4	<1	3
sweet					
gherkins	1 oz	40	10	1	10
midget	2 oz	40	10	1	10
pickle	2 oz	40	10	1	10
pickles					
dill..all types	1 oz	5	1	1	0
sweet					
dill chips	1 oz	40	10	1	10
gherkins	1 oz	40	10	1	10

Food and Description	Amount	Total Calories	Total Carbs	Fiber	Sugars
midget	1 oz	40	10	1	10
whole	1 oz	40	10	1	10
(Hebrew National)					
barrel-cured dill	1 pouch	23	4	0	0
kosher..all types	1 oz	4	1	0	0
(Heinz)					
dill..kosher..all types	1 oz	4	1	0	0
sweet					
gherkins..midget or regular	1 oz	35	8	0	8
pickles	1 oz	35	8	0	8
salad cubes	1 oz	30	7	0	7
sweet cucumber					
slices	1 oz	20	5	0	5
sticks	1 oz	25	6	0	6
(Mrs. Klein's) fancy imported					
pepperoncini	1 oz	5	1	0	0
Southern hot mix	1 oz	0	0	0	0
(Mt. Olive)					
bread & butter	1 oz	25	6	0	5
no sugar added	1 oz	0	0	0	0
old-fashioned sweet	1 oz	25	6	0	5
old-fashioned sweet..strips	1 oz	25	6	0	5
zesty..chips	1 oz	25	6	0	5
cocktail midgets	1 oz	5	1	0	0
dill..all types	1 oz	0	0	0	0
hot..mixed	1 oz	0	0	0	0
salad...sweet cubes..green or red	1 Tbs	20	4	0	2
sweet	1 oz	35	8	0	7
cucumber strips	1 oz	20	4	0	2
gherkins..no sugar added	1 oz	0	0	0	0
midgets	1 oz	35	8	0	7
super-sweet dill strips	1 oz	40	10	0	8
(Peter Piper's)					
bread & butter..all styles	1 oz	30	7	0	7
kosher dills..all types	1 oz	0	0	0	0
sweet					
gherkins	1 oz	35	8	0	8
midgets	1 oz	40	10	0	10
salad cubes	1 Tbs	20	4	0	4
(Schorr's)					
kosher..all types	1 oz	4	1	0	0
sour					
garlic whole	1 oz	3	1	0	0
half spears	1 oz	4	1	0	0
halves	1 oz	4	1	0	0
(Steinfeld's)					
crunchy..all types	1 oz	5	1	0	0
Greek pepperoncini	1 oz	5	1	0	0
kosher dills..all types	1 oz	5	1	0	0
Polish dills	1 oz	5	1	0	0

Food and Description	Amount	Total Calories	Total Carbs	Fiber	Sugars
sandwich builders					
kosher dills..all styles	1 oz	5	1	0	0
Polish dills	1 oz	0	0	0	0
zesty dills	1 oz	0	0	0	0
sweet..all types	1 oz	30	8	0	7
(Vlasic)					
Half-The-Salt					
hamburger dill chips	1 oz	10	3	0	2
sweet butter chips	1 oz	30	7	0	7
kosher dills..all types	1 oz	4	1	0	1
refrigerated deli bread & butter	1 oz	35	9	0	9
regular					
bread & butter chunks	1 oz	25	6	0	6
original dills					
Polish snack chunks	1 oz	4	1	0	1
sweet butter chips	1 oz	30	7	0	7
sweet butter stix	1 oz	18	5	0	5
zesty crunchy dills	1 oz	4	1	0	1
zesty dill snack chunks or spears	1 oz	4	1	0	1
sweet gherkins	1 oz	35	9	0	9
PICKLE RELISH (*See also* PICKLE)					
(Arnold's) sweet	1 Tbs	15	3	0	2
(Cascadian Farm)					
dill	1 Tbs	5	0	0	0
sweet	1 Tbs	20	5	0	5
(Crosse & Blackwell) chow-chow	1 Tbs	10	1	0	<1
(Heinz)					
piccalilli	1 Tbs	15	4	0	4
relish					
hamburger	1 Tbs	15	3	0	2
hot dog	1 Tbs	15	3	0	2
sweet	1 Tbs	20	5	0	5
(Mt. Olive)					
dill	1 Tbs	0	0	0	0
hot dog	1 Tbs	20	5	0	3
India	1 Tbs	20	4	0	2
jalapeño..mild	1 Tbs	20	4	0	2
sweet	1 Tbs	20	5	0	3
(Vlasic) sweet	½ oz	15	4	0	4
PIE & COBBLER (*See also* PIE CRUST; PIE FILLING)					
FROZEN or REFRIGERATED					
(Bistro Gourmet) thaw & serve					
DESSERT PIES					
Apple Cherry Orchard	1 slice	420	68	3	54
Bourbon Street Pecan	1 slice	550	56	3	36
chocolate caramel peanut	1 slice	550	56	3	36
Chocolate Oblivion w/crushed Oreos	1 slice	540	52	2	37
Fudgy Peanut Butter Clutter	1 slice	580	48	3	36
Islander's Key Lime	1 slice	420	58	3	41

Food and Description	Amount	Total Calories	Total Carbs	Fiber	Sugars
malted chocolate caramel	1 slice	710	70	6	47
Plantation Pecan	1 slice	520	59	3	41
GOURMET TARTS..individual					
pecan	1 tart	860	120	11	62
rustic apple	1 tart	540	71	7	23
(Chef Pierre)					
COBBLERS..5-pound					
apple	1/18 cobbler	230	34	1	19
blackberry	1/18 cobbler	260	42	2	28
blueberry	1/18 cobbler	260	39	2	25
cherry	1/18 cobbler	260	42	2	28
peach	1/18 cobbler	240	37	2	20
strawberry	1/18 cobbler	240	35	2	19
CREAM PIES..10"					
apples, cinnamon & cream..					
fruit de la cream	1/8 pie	430	48	1	38
banana..crème de la cream	1/10 pie	360	28	1	16
chocolate cream layer	1/8 pie	520	49	2	32
chocolate..crème de la cream	1/9 pie	470	43	2	27
coconut..crème de la cream	1/8 pie	350	39	2	35
cookies & cream..crème de la cream	1/8 pie	410	35	2	24
crème de la cream..variety pack	1/10 pie	300	39	2	35
double chocolate..crème de la cream	1/10 pie	360	44	2	32
gourmet					
chocolate peanut butter silk	1/8 pie	500	41	3	26
French silk	1/8 pie	570	48	3	32
peanut butter cream	1/8 pie	460	43	2	23
pumpkin cream layer	1/8 pie	380	42	1	33
strawberries & cream					
Fruit de la Crème	1/8 pie	400	45	1	38
toffee crunch cream de la crème	1/9 pie	430	38	2	31
LATTICE-TOP PIES..prebaked					
apple	1/8 pie	320	50	2	28
cherry	1/8 pie	310	48	3	29
peach	1/8 pie	300	45	3	26
MERINGUE PIES..traditional					
chocolate..traditional	1/8 pie	370	54	2	24
chocolate icebox..condensed	1/9 pie	340	49	2	20
coconut..traditional	1/8 pie	340	49	3	37
coconut icebox..condensed	1/9 pie	330	50	2	37
key lime	1/8 pie	440	70	4	53
Key West lime icebox..condensed	1/8 pie	460	69	4	54
lemon..traditional	1/8 pie	290	52	2	34
lemon icebox..condensed	1/8 pie	380	65	3	52
lime icebox..condensed	1/8 pie	360	63	3	54
OPEN-FACED SPECIALTY..10" pies					
French coconut	1/8 pie	490	68	4	37
pumpkin	1/10 pie	320	51	3	34

Food and Description	Amount	Total Calories	Total Carbs	Fiber	Sugars
Southern pecan	1/10 pie	570	80	3	40
sweet potato	1/9 pie	400	53	2	32
TRADITIONAL..10" pies					
banana cream	1/8 pie	400	49	3	33
Boston cream	1/6 pie	220	36	2	27
chocolate cream	1/6 pie	410	49	2	24
coconut cream	1/8 pie	430	49	3	25
lemon cream	1/6 pie	420	50	3	25
strawberry cream	1/6 pie	420	52	2	30
(Edward's)					
Chocolate butter pecan..limited	1/8 pie	560	63	2	36
FAMILY RECIPE..ready-to-serve					
lemon meringue..34 oz	1/8 pie	350	62	1	57
GOURMET..ready-to-serve..36 oz					
key lime	1/8 pie	440	57	2	46
Mocha Mudslide	1/8 pie	410	52	1	37
pecan cheesecake	1/8 pie	530	59	1	32
turtle	1/8 pie	390	46	1	34
SUNDAE CREATIONS..ready-to-serve..25.5 oz					
caramel	1/6 pie	440	50	9	37
chocolate	1/6 pie	480	44	1	30
cookie dough	1/6 pie	450	54	1	36
strawberry	1/6 pie	410	48	0	34
(Marie Callender's)					
COBBLERS					
apple	1/4 cobbler	370	45	2	31
berry..16 oz	1/4 cobbler	370	41	1	29
cherry	1/4 cobbler	380	50	0	32
peach..16 oz	1/4 cobbler	360	47	0	24
(Mrs. Smith's)					
COBBLERS					
apple	1/8 cobbler	270	43	2	20
w/toasted oatmeal topping	1/8 cobbler	280	44	2	24
blackberry	1/8 cobbler	260	43	2	20
cherry	1/8 cobbler	280	46	1	24
w/almond crumb topping	1/8 cobbler	290	45	1	23
peach..2-lb cobbler	1/8 cobbler	320	49	2	16
strawberry w/toasted crumb top	1/6 cobbler	330	52	1	26
PIES..CREAM					
Boston cream	1/10 pie	210	31	0	23
Caramel Caribou..2-count	1 pie	350	37	1	25
chocolate..restaurant classics					
French silk	1/8 pie	490	47	2	30
chocolate..Soda Shoppe	1/8 pie	340	42	1	23
coconut cream..Soda Shoppe	1/8 pie	360	42	1	23
coconut custard	1/8 pie	250	30	1	16
moose tracks..2-count	1 pie	370	37	1	25
PIES..FRUIT					
apple					
caramel..flip-it cakes	1/2 pkg	480	90	2	58

Food and Description	Amount	Total Calories	Total Carbs	Fiber	Sugars
crumb..deep-dish	1/10 pie	320	49	2	25
deep-dish	1/12 pie	330	45	2	24
Dutch apple crumb	1/8 pie	360	52	2	24
no sugar added	1/8 pie	350	42	3	7
old-fashioned	1/8 pie	350	46	2	21
blueberry	1/8 pie	330	43	3	16
cherry	1/8 pie	340	45	1	21
deep-dish crumb	1/10 pie	300	48	1	23
festival of berries..deep-dish	1/10 pie	300	44	2	24
peach					
deep-dish	1/10 pie	270	36	2	20
traditional	1/8 pie	320	40	2	16
strawberry w/toasted oatmeal crumb top	1/6 pie	330	52	1	26
strawberry delight..flip-it cakes	1/2 pkg	380	73	1	47
PIES..OTHER					
key lime..restaurant classics	1/8 pie	410	59	1	46
lemon meringue	1/8 pie	290	47	1	31
mince	1/8 pie	380	53	2	26
pecan..Southern..special recipe	1/8 pie	550	75	2	44
pumpkin					
custard	1/8 pie	240	36	2	20
hearty	1/8 pie	260	38	3	18
Special Recipe..homemade	1/10 pie	280	40	2	23
red raspberry	1/8 pie	340	45	1	19
sweet potato	1/8 pie	330	45	2	25
(Pet-Ritz)					
COBBLERS..home-style					
apple cinnamon	1/6 cobbler	280	40	0	26
blackberry	1/6 cobbler	260	12	1	22
cherry	1/6 cobbler	300	57	1	22
peach	1/6 cobbler	240	37	1	19
PIES..home-style					
apple	1/4 pie	380	53	2	22
berry banana cream	1/4 pie	320	38	1	23
cherry	1/4 pie	400	57	1	22
chocolate drizzle cream	1/4 pie	330	39	1	25
coconut cream..toasted	1/4 pie	330	37	1	23
lemon raspberry	1/4 pie	320	39	1	23
(Sara Lee's)					
COBBLER ANYTIME..2-count box					
apple	1 cobbler	350	46	2	10
blackberry	1 cobbler	350	47	2	20
peach	1 cobbler	340	43	1	15
PIES					
French silk..24 oz	1/5 pie	340	34	2	31
lemon meringue..tangy..30 oz	1/6 pie	220	41	1	37
PIES..OVEN-FRESH..37 oz					
apple	1/8 pie	340	46	1	26
blueberry	1/8 pie	360	53	2	22

Food and Description	Amount	Total Calories	Total Carbs	Fiber	Sugars
cherry	⅛ pie	320	44	0	16
Dutch apple	⅛ pie	350	53	2	30
mince	⅛ pie	370	55	2	26
peach	⅛ pie	330	50	2	30
pumpkin	⅛ pie	260	37	2	18
raspberry	⅛ pie	360	50	3	18
Southern sweet potato	⅛ pie	280	45	2	26
SIGNATURE SELECTIONS					
apple orchard deep-dish	⅒ pie	400	43	3	39
caramel applenut	⅑ pie	370	45	2	26
cherry..deep-dish gourmet	⅒ pie	380	59	3	32
cinnamon French apple	⅒ pie	360	48	2	31
dulce de leche caramel swirl	⅛ pie	400	37	2	20
fruits of the forest	⅑ pie	340	41	9	22
golden peach..deep-dish	⅒ pie	340	46	2	29
Key West lime	⅛ pie	400	41	2	30
pumpkin..traditional	⅒ pie	250	34	2	17
Southern pecan	⅛ pie	520	70	3	28
strawberries & cream	⅛ pie	400	33	2	20
(Schwan's)					
Andes mint cream	1 piece	500	59	1	41
pecan caramel cream slices	1 slice	280	35	1	26
(Weight Watchers) Smart Ones					
key lime	1 piece	200	34	0	24
peanut butter	1 piece	210	27	1	14
READY-TO-SERVE					
(Entenmann's) pie					
original					
apple..home-style	1 serving	370	55	3	25
reduced-fat	⅙ pie	280	56	3	30
single deluxe cream pie	1 pie	430	55	1	28
single lemon pie	1 pie	450	62	1	31
(Hostess) snack					
apple	1 pie	480	67	2	36
blackberry	1 pie	520	79	2	29
blueberry	1 pie	480	70	2	31
cherry	1 pie	470	65	1	35
French apple	1 pie	480	67	2	36
lemon	1 pie	500	66	0	46
peach	1 pie	480	68	1	30
pineapple	1 pie	460	62	1	29
strawberry fruit	1 pie	510	71	2	35
(Lance) snack..pecan	3 oz	350	46	3	35
(TastyKake) snack					
apple	1 pie	260	41	1	20
banana	1 pie	370	53	<1	30
blueberry	1 pie	290	48	1	24
cherry	1 pie	290	47	1	26
coconut cream	1 pie	370	42	1	21

Food and Description	Amount	Total Calories	Total Carbs	Fiber	Sugars
French apple	1 pie	330	55	1	32
lemon	1 pie	300	44	<1	22
peach	1 pie	270	41	1	20
pineapple	1 pie	290	46	1	25
pumpkin	1 pie	320	45	1	21
strawberry	1 pie	330	55	1	33
Tasty-Klair	1 pie	390	49	0	26
PIE CRUST (*See also* PASTRY)					
FROZEN					
(Chef Pierre) food service..unbaked					
deep dish..9" crust	1/9 crust	130	13	0	0
regular..10" crust	1/9 crust	110	11	0	1
vegetable shortening					
9" deep dish crust	1/8 crust	130	12	0	1
10" crust	1/9 crust	120	11	0	0
(Mrs. Smith's)					
flaky home-style..9" deep-dish	1/10 crust	120	14	0	2
home-style shortbread..9" deep-dish	1/16 crust	130	14	0	4
(Oronoque)					
6" crust	1/4 crust	110	9	0	0
9" deep-dish crust	1/8 crust	100	8	0	0
9" regular	1/8 crust	80	7	0	0
(Pet-Ritz) ready-to-bake					
deep-dish					
9" all-vegetable shortening	1/8 crust	110	12	0	0
9" crust	1/8 crust	90	11	0	0
regular					
9" all-vegetable shortening	1/8 crust	80	10	0	0
9" crust	1/8 crust	80	9	0	0
MIX					
(Betty Crocker) 9" crust..prepared	1/8 crust	110	9	0	<1
(Flako) mix only	1/4 cup	130	13	1	0
(Jiffy) mix only	1/4 cup	160	19	<1	0
(Krusteaz) mix...prepared..9" crust	1/8 crust	90	10	<1	1
(Nabisco) mix..prepared..9" crust					
Honey Maid..graham	1/8 crust	140	18	1	8
Nilla..cookie crumb	1/8 crust	140	18	1	10
Oreo..cookie crumb	1/8 crust	140	18	1	9
READY-TO-USE					
(Keebler) Ready Crust					
chocolate					
9" pie	1/8 crust	110	12	<1	6
single-serve	1 tart	110	15	<1	6
graham cracker					
9" pie	0.75 oz	110	14	0	6
	0.92 oz	130	17	0	7
reduced-fat	1/8 crust	90	14	0	6
shortbread	1/8 crust	110	14	0	6
single-serve tarts	1 tart	120	15	<1	6

Food and Description	Amount	Total Calories	Total Carbs	Fiber	Sugars
(Nabisco) Oreo	1 oz	140	18	1	9
(Pillsbury) refrigerated	⅛ crust	120	13	0	<1
PIE FILLING (*See also* PUDDING & MOUSSE)					
CANNED or JARRED					
(Borden) None Such mincemeat					
original..classic..condensed					
w/apples & raisins	½ cup	150	36	1	31
ready-to-use					
original..classic	½ cup	190	45	0	39
w/brandy & rum	½ cup	200	47	0	44
(Comstock)					
apple					
cinnamon 'n' spice	⅓ cup	100	25	2	22
French	⅓ cup	100	25	2	22
MoreFruit	⅓ cup	80	20	1	18
original..country	⅓ cup	90	23	0	18
blueberry..MoreFruit	⅓ cup	80	21	1	15
cherry					
dark sweet..MoreFruit	⅓ cup	100	25	2	22
light	⅓ cup	60	15	1	14
regular	⅓ cup	90	23	0	18
original					
light	⅓ cup	60	15	1	14
red ruby	⅓ cup	90	23	0	18
lemon	⅓ cup	130	28	0	20
mincemeat	⅓ cup	170	43	1	31
peach..MoreFruit	⅓ cup	80	19	1	17
pumpkin pie mix	⅓ cup	90	23	0	18
raspberry	⅓ cup	100	25	2	17
strawberry	⅓ cup	100	23	1	15
(Crosse & Blackwell)					
mincemeat	¼ cup	180	43	1	31
w/rum and brandy	¼ cup	180	43	1	31
(Libby's) pumpkin pie mix	⅓ cup	90	20	2	17
(None Such) Mincemeat (*See* (Borden) in this section)					
(Thank You)					
apple					
cinnamon 'n' spice	⅓ cup	100	25	2	22
French	⅓ cup	100	25	2	22
MoreFruit	⅓ cup	80	20	1	18
original..country	⅓ cup	90	23	0	18
blueberry..MoreFruit	⅓ cup	80	21	1	15
cherry					
dark sweet..MoreFruit	⅓ cup	100	25	2	22
light	⅓ cup	60	15	1	14
regular	⅓ cup	90	23	0	18
original					
light	⅓ cup	60	15	1	14
red ruby	⅓ cup	90	23	0	18
lemon	⅓ cup	130	28	0	20

Food and Description	Amount	Total Calories	Total Carbs	Fiber	Sugars
mincemeat	⅓ cup	170	43	1	31
peach..MoreFruit	⅓ cup	80	19	1	17
pumpkin pie mix	⅓ cup	90	23	0	18
raspberry	⅓ cup	100	25	2	17
strawberry	⅓ cup	100	23	1	15
MIX (NOTE: Unless stated otherwise, 1 serving of mix = the amount in ½ cup prepared.)					
(Banquet) Dessert Bakes					
apple crisp	⅙ box	220	41	1	23
cherry cobbler	⅕ cobbler	250	48	4	24
peach cobbler	⅙ cobbler	220	41	4	16
(Calhoun Bend Mill) mix only					
apple cinnamon crisp topping	3 Tbs	140	33	1	20
cherry oatmeal crunch topping	3 Tbs	120	28	1	16
cinnamon crisp topping	¼ cup	140	34	1	23
fruit cobbler	¼ cup	140	33	0	22
oatmeal crunch topping	¼ cup	140	31	1	18
peach cobbler	3 Tbs	95	21	2	10
pecan pie	⅛ cup	110	27	0	18
(Jell-O) pudding & pie filling..dry mix only					
cook & serve					
fat-free					
chocolate	¼ pkg	130	29	0	21
vanilla	¼ pkg	140	20	0	16
original					
banana cream	¼ pkg	80	20	0	15
butterscotch	¼ pkg	100	24	1	19
chocolate	¼ pkg	90	22	1	15
chocolate fudge	¼ pkg	90	22	1	15
coconut cream	¼ pkg	90	18	1	14
lemon	⅙ pkg	50	12	0	6
milk chocolate	¼ pkg	90	22	0	16
vanilla	⅙ pkg	80	20	0	16
sugar-free..reduced-calorie					
chocolate	¼ pkg	30	7	<1	0
vanilla	⅙ pkg	20	5	0	0
instant					
regular					
banana cream	⅙ pkg	90	23	0	18
butterscotch	¼ pkg	90	23	0	18
cheesecake	¼ pkg	100	24	0	20
chocolate	¼ pkg	100	25	1	10
chocolate cherry	¼ pkg	100	25	1	19
chocolate fudge	¼ pkg	100	25	1	17
coconut cream	⅙ pkg	100	21	1	16
devil's food	¼ pkg	140	25	1	19
French vanilla	¼ pkg	90	23	0	18
lemon	¼ pkg	90	24	0	19
Oreo cookies 'n' cream	¼ pkg	120	28	0	21
vanilla	¼ pkg	90	23	0	19
white chocolate	¼ pkg	90	23	0	19

Food and Description	Amount	Total Calories	Total Carbs	Fiber	Sugars
sugar-free..banana cream	¼ pkg	25	6	0	0
sugar-free..fat-free					
banana cream	¼ pkg	25	6	0	0
butterscotch	¼ pkg	25	6	0	0
chocolate fudge	¼ pkg	35	8	1	0
pistachio	¼ pkg	30	6	0	0
vanilla	¼ pkg	25	6	0	0
white chocolate	¼ pkg	25	6	0	0
PIEROGI/POTATO DUMPLING (See PASTA; FROZEN ENTRÉE/DINNER)					
PIGEON (See SQUAB/PIGEON)					
PIGEON PEA					
CANNED (Goya) green	8 oz	10	26	8	0
FRESH					
cooked—drained	½ cup	90	15	2.5	1
raw	½ cup	105	18.5	3	3
SEEDS..immature					
boiled—drained	½ cup	85	2	0	0
raw	20 seeds	10	2	0	0
PIGNOLIA (See PINE NUT)					
PIG'S FEET (See PORK; PORK ENTRÉE/DINNER)					
PIKE					
northern..cooked—dry heat	3 oz	95	0	0	0
walleye..cooked—dry heat	3 oz	100	0	0	0
PILAF (See PASTA ENTRÉE/DINNER; RICE DISH)					
PIMIENTO					
CANNED					
(Dromedary)	1 oz	10	2	0	0
(Goya) fancy	½ oz	4	1	0	0
PIÑA COLADA (See COCKTAIL)					
PINE NUT					
CANNED (Diamond of California)	1 oz	180	5	2	0
DRIED					
(Frieda's)	¼ cup	150	4	1	0
pignolia	1 oz	146	4	1	0
pinyon	1 oz	161	4	1	0
JARRED (Progresso) pignolia nuts	1 oz	170	2	0	0
PINEAPPLE					
BOWL, CAN, CUP, or JAR					
(Del Monte)					
chunks					
in heavy syrup	½ cup	90	24	1	22
in juice	½ cup	70	17	1	15
crushed					
in heavy syrup	½ cup	90	24	1	22
in juice	½ cup	70	17	1	15
Fruit Naturals	½ cup	70	18	<1	15
individual 4.3-oz pull-top cans					
tidbits..100% juice	1 can	50	15	<1	13
wedges..100% juice	1 can	70	17	1	15

Food and Description	Amount	Total Calories	Total Carbs	Fiber	Sugars
sliced					
in heavy syrup	2 slices	90	23	1	21
in juice	2 slices	60	16	1	14
SunFresh..slightly sweetened	½ cup	70	18	1	15
tidbits..in juice..bowl..100% juice	1 bowl	70	18	1	15
(Dole)					
chunks-					
in clarified juice	½ cup	60	15	1	13
in heavy syrup	½ cup	90	24	1	22
coarse-cut crushed..in juice	½ cup	70	17	1	13
crushed					
in heavy syrup	½ cup	90	23	1	21
in juice	½ cup	70	17	1	13
Dole fruit bowls	1 bowl	60	15	1	13
pieces..in light syrup	½ cup	80	20	1	18
tidbits					
in clarified juice	½ cup	60	15	1	13
in heavy syrup	½ cup	90	24	1	22
in light syrup	½ cup	80	20	1	18
CANDIED					
(S&W) glacé					
slices..all types	1 piece	180	46	0	43
wedges..all types	5 pieces	80	21	0	20
DRIED					
(Ann's House of Nuts)	10 pieces	140	35	2	30
(Sun-Maid) Tropical Trio					
w/ pineapple, papaya & mango	1.4 oz	130	34	1	27
FRESH					
(Dole) slices..¾" thick	2 slices	60	16	1	13
PINEAPPLE JUICE/JUICE BLEND/JUICE DRINK (*See also* FRUIT PUNCH)					
BOTTLED, BOXED, or CANNED					
(Del Monte) from concentrate	6 fl oz	80	20	0	17
(Dole)					
CANNED					
pineapple..from concentrate	8 fl oz	120	29	9	25
pineapple grapefruit	6 fl oz	100	25	0	na
pineapple orange banana	6 fl oz	100	24	0	na
REFRIGERATED					
pineapple	8 fl oz	130	30	0	26
pineapple mango	8 fl oz	120	30	1	29
pineapple orange	8 fl oz	120	29	0	25
pineapple orange berry	8 fl oz	130	30	0	26
pineapple orange guava	8 fl oz	120	29	0	25
pineapple passion banana	8 fl oz	120	29	0	25
(Kern's) nectar..pineapple mango	8 fl oz	150	36	0	33
(Orlando Sun)					
pineapple orange banana	8 fl oz	100	25	0	25
pineapple orange cherry	8 fl oz	100	25	0	25

Food and Description	Amount	Total Calories	Total Carbs	Fiber	Sugars
(R. W. Knudsen)					
pineapple coconut	8 fl oz	130	31	0	26
pineapple nectar	8 fl oz	140	34	0	28
(Welch's)					
pineapple banana..juice blended	8 fl oz	130	33	0	32
pineapple orange..juice cocktail	11.5 fl oz	150	37	0	36
(Whipper Snapple) pineapple orange	10 fl oz	160	41	0	39
FROZEN					
(Dole) prepared					
100% pineapple juice	8 fl oz	130	29	0	25
pineapple grapefruit	8 fl oz	130	29	0	25
pineapple orange	8 fl oz	120	29	0	25
pineapple orange banana	8 fl oz	130	29	0	25
pineapple orange guava	8 fl oz	120	29	0	25
pineapple orange strawberry	8 fl oz	130	29	0	25
pineapple passion banana	8 fl oz	120	29	0	25
pineapple strawberry	8 fl oz	130	29	0	25
PINK BEAN					
CANNED					
(Goya) habichuelas rosadas					
Spanish-style	½ cup	80	32	10	0
DRIED					
boiled	½ cup	125	24	4.5	0
raw	½ cup	360	68	13.5	0
PIÑON/PINYON (*See* PINE NUT)					
PINTO BEAN					
CANNED					
(Bush's)					
w/bacon	½ cup	110	19	6	0
w/bacon & jalapeños	½ cup	110	19	6	0
w/pork	½ cup	120	17	6	0
(Eden) organic					
original	½ cup	100	18	6	0
refried..all flavors	½ cup	90	19	7	0
(Goya) Spanish-style	7.5 oz	140	31	10	0
(Hain)	½ cup	110	18	8	0
(Luck's) seasoned w/pork					
regular	½ cup	140	19	6	0
w/onions	½ cup	150	24	6	0
(Trappey's) w/bacon					
jalapinto	½ cup	120	22	8	0
original	½ cup	120	20	7	0
(Westbrae) organic	½ cup	100	19	7	2
DRIED..(Arrowhead Mills)..raw	¼ cup	150	27	8	0
PINYON (*See* PINE NUT)					
PISTACHIO					
(Alma) extra-jumbo..all styles	1 oz	160	6	<1	<1
(Ann's House of Nuts) natural	¼ cup	190	9	3	3
(Blue Diamond) raw	1 oz	200	10	3	0
(Dole) dry-roasted					

Food and Description	Amount	Total Calories	Total Carbs	Fiber	Sugars
shelled	1 oz	160	7	0	0
unshelled	1 oz	90	3	0	0
(Fisher) natural..in shell	1 oz	170	7	0	0
(Lance) roasted in shell..1.125-oz pkg	1 pkg	90	4	2	0
(Planters) dry-roasted					
shelled					
Munch 'N Go	2 oz	330	14	6	4
regular	1 oz	170	7	3	2
unshelled..all styles	1 oz	160	7	3	2
(Sunkist)					
California dry-roasted	1 oz	170	9	3	2
& salted in shell	1 oz	180	9	3	3
PITA BREAD (*See* BREAD)					
PITANGA/BRAZILIAN CHERRY/SURINAM CHERRY					
fresh..raw	1 medium	2	0.5	<1	0
	1 cup	57	13	<1	0
PIZZA (*See also* FROZEN ENTRÉE/DINNER; VEGETARIAN FOODS; individual FAST FOOD listings)					
■ **(Atkins)**					
Quick Quisine					
pepperoni	1 pkg	440	22	11	3
smokehouse	1 pkg	420	22	11	3
supreme	1 pkg	360	22	11	3
■ **(Banquet)** French Bread Pizza					
cheese	1 pizza	330	43	4	5
deluxe	1 pizza	330	42	3	6
pepperoni	1 pizza	380	44	4	6
■ **(California Pizza Kitchen)**					
3-piece pizza					
BBQ chicken recipe	⅓ pizza	280	33	1	9
5-cheese & tomato	⅓ pizza	320	35	2	7
Jamaican Jerk	⅓ pizza	270	33	2	8
Thai chicken recipe	⅓ pizza	290	33	3	9
6-piece pizza					
BBQ recipe chicken	⅙ pizza	310	38	2	10
5-cheese & tomato	⅙ pizza	350	35	2	7
Thai chicken recipe	⅓ pizza	310	38	3	10
■ **(Celeste)**					
Pizza for One					
cheese	1 pizza	420	43	4	5
deluxe	1 pizza	470	46	5	6
4-cheese					
original	1 pizza	470	41	4	5
zesty	1 pizza	470	43	4	5
pepperoni	1 pizza	470	43	4	5
sausage	1 pizza	480	45	4	5
sausage & pepperoni	1 pizza	560	43	4	5
suprema	1 pizza	530	48	6	6
vegetable	1 pizza	430	45	5	5
zesty chicken supreme	1 pizza	380	38	5	6

Food and Description	Amount	Total Calories	Total Carbs	Fiber	Sugars
Pizza/Large					
cheese	¼ pizza	300	33	3	4
deluxe	¼ pizza	340	34	5	6
pepperoni	¼ pizza	350	38	3	4
Pizza..Rising Crust..fresh-baked					
4-cheese	⅙ pizza	320	42	4	6
pepperoni	⅙ pizza	330	42	4	8
supreme	⅙ pizza	360	41	6	6
3-meat	⅙ pizza	340	42	6	9
■ (Di Giorno)					
Deep Dish					
pepperoni	⅛ pizza	390	33	2	5
supreme	⅛ pizza	310	25	2	4
Rising Crust					
12-inch					
cheese-stuffed	⅙ pizza	390	37	3	6
4-cheese	⅙ pizza	310	40	3	8
sausage & pepperoni	⅙ pizza	360	40	2	8
Rising Crust					
4-cheese	⅙ pizza	310	40	3	8
pepperoni	⅙ pizza	360	40	2	8
supreme	⅓ pizza	320	35	3	7
Rising Crust..Half & Half					
pepperoni & cheese	⅙ pizza	390	40	3	8
supreme	⅙ pizza	370	41	3	8
Rising Crust..Microwave					
4-cheese	½ pizza	370	44	3	7
pepperoni	½ pizza	390	43	3	7
supreme	½ pizza	410	44	3	7
Thin Crispy Crust					
4-cheese	⅕ pizza	300	34	3	6
4-meat	⅕ pizza	320	37	2	6
grilled chicken, tomato & spinach	⅕ pizza	260	33	2	5
pepperoni	⅕ pizza	310	34	2	5
■ (Dining In)					
3-piece..Self-Rising Crust					
pepperoni..6-cheese	⅓ pizza	290	42	2	2
portobello mushroom & 5 cheeses	⅓ pizza	250	33	1	2
supreme..6-cheese	⅓ pizza	310	34	2	2
3-meat..6-cheese	⅓ pizza	280	33	1	2
tomato w/basil & 6 cheeses	⅓ pizza	250	33	1	2
6-piece..Self-Rising Crust..6 cheese					
cheese	⅙ pizza	290	42	2	2
pepperoni	⅙ pizza	340	43	2	2
supreme	⅙ pizza	350	43	2	2
3-meat	⅙ pizza	340	42	2	2
Half & Half					
pepperoni..6-cheese	⅓ pizza	370	43	2	2

Food and Description	Amount	Total Calories	Total Carbs	Fiber	Sugars
Other					
BBQ-recipe chicken	⅓ pizza	300	38	1	7
roasted vegetable & 5-cheese	⅓ pizza	240	33	3	3
■ **(Freschetta)**					
8-inch					
4-cheese	½ pizza	410	48	2	5
mozzarella & basil margherita	½ pizza	370	46	2	4
pepperoni	½ pizza	450	48	2	5
roasted-garlic chicken	½ pizza	370	49	3	4
Southwest-style	½ pizza	360	48	2	6
supreme	½ pizza	460	50	3	6
12-inch					
4-meat	⅙ pizza	350	40	2	4
4-cheese	⅕ pizza	390	47	2	5
pepperoni	⅙ pizza	360	30	2	4
sausage	⅙ pizza	360	40	2	5
sausage & pepperoni	⅙ pizza	360	40	2	4
special deluxe	⅙ pizza	350	40	2	5
supreme	⅙ pizza	360	41	2	5
Brick Oven..fire-baked crust					
cheese & bacon	¼ pizza	320	35	1	2
classic supreme	¼ pizza	370	38	2	3
5-Italian cheese	¼ pizza	330	36	1	3
Italian-style pepperoni	¼ pizza	410	37	2	3
portobello mushroom & spinach	¼ pizza	290	38	2	3
Southwest-style chicken	¼ pizza	340	39	2	3
Stuffed Crust					
4-cheese	⅕ pizza	340	43	2	6
pepperoni	⅕ pizza	370	42	2	6
sausage & pepperoni..25-oz pkg	⅕ pizza	370	42	2	6
supreme w/grilled vegetables	⅙ pizza	310	38	2	5
vegetable medley	⅕ pizza	310	44	2	6
■ **(Jack's)**					
Pizza Bursts..7-oz box					
combination sausage & pepperoni	½ pkg	250	25	1	2
pepperoni	½ pkg	260	25	1	3
sausage	½ pkg	250	25	1	3
SuperCheese	½ pkg	250	25	1	3
supreme	½ pkg	260	25	1	2
■ **(Jenos)**					
Crisp 'n' Tasty Pizza					
Canadian-style bacon	1 pizza	440	51	2	6
cheese	1 pizza	460	51	2	5
combination	1 pizza	500	50	2	5
hamburger	1 pizza	500	51	2	5
pepperoni	1 pizza	510	50	2	5
sausage	1 pizza	480	51	2	5
supreme	1 pizza	500	50	2	5
3-meat	1 pizza	490	49	2	5

Food and Description	Amount	Total Calories	Total Carbs	Fiber	Sugars
■ (Lean Cuisine)					
deluxe	1 pizza	370	55	3	7
4-cheese	1 pizza	380	55	3	7
pepperoni	1 pizza	380	60	3	8
roasted vegetable	1 pizza	330	57	3	7
■ (Lunchables)					
Fun Pack					
extra cheesy..3-count					
4.5 oz	1 pack	300	28	2	4
4.8 oz	1 pack	450	62	2	35
Pizza Dunks..5.1 oz	1 pack	490	84	3	41
Pizza Swirls..4.6 oz	1 pack	480	73	2	46
Mega Pack					
extra cheese..deep dish	1 pizza	700	104	4	61
pepperoni..deep dish	1 pizza	760	105	4	65
■ OSCAR MAYER (*See* (Lunchables) in this section)					
■ (Red Baron)					
Deep Dish Mini..8-count pkg					
cheese	½ pkg	380	44	2	4
pepperoni	½ pkg	400	41	2	4
sausage & pepperoni	½ pkg	310	31	1	3
supreme	½ pkg	320	32	1	3
Deep Dish Pan–style					
4-cheese	⅓ pizza	370	39	2	3
meat trio	⅓ pizza	390	38	2	3
pepperoni	⅓ pizza	400	41	2	4
supreme	⅓ pizza	410	40	2	3
Deep Dish Singles					
4-cheese	1 pizza	440	41	2	3
cheese	1 pizza	420	41	2	4
meat trio	1 pizza	420	42	2	4
pepperoni	1 pizza	460	41	2	3
sausage	1 pizza	480	41	2	3
special deluxe	1 pizza	430	40	2	3
supreme	1 pizza	470	40	2	3
vegetable supreme	1 pizza	400	42	2	4
Original..Classic					
Canadian bacon	¼ pizza	380	36	1	3
4-cheese	¼ pizza	420	36	1	3
hamburger	⅕ pizza	330	29	1	2
Mexican-style	⅕ pizza	360	29	2	2
pepperoni	¼ pizza	440	36	1	3
sausage	⅕ pizza	330	33	1	3
sausage & pepperoni	⅕ pizza	360	29	1	3
special deluxe	⅕ pizza	340	30	2	3
supreme	⅕ pizza	350	30	2	3
Pizzeria-style					
4-cheese	⅙ pizza	360	43	2	5
meat trio	⅙ pizza	370	43	2	5
pepperoni	⅙ pizza	370	43	2	5

Food and Description	Amount	Total Calories	Total Carbs	Fiber	Sugars
sausage	⅙ pizza	370	43	2	5
special deluxe	⅙ pizza	390	44	2	5
supreme	⅙ pizza	360	44	2	5
Stuffed Pizza Slices..2-count pkg					
Italian sausage	½ pkg	340	36	2	6
Italian sausage & pepperoni	½ pkg	360	36	1	6
pepperoni	½ pkg	370	36	1	6
roasted garlic chicken	½ pkg	290	35	1	6
supreme	½ pkg	340	37	2	6
■ **(San Francisco Foods)**					
Stuffed Pizza					
5-cheese	¼ pizza	420	53	3	5
meat combo	¼ pizza	430	50	3	4
pepperoni	¼ pizza	410	48	2	3
spinach & feta	¼ pizza	400	50	3	2
supreme	¼ pizza	400	46	3	4
western chicken	¼ pizza	310	39	2	5
■ **(Schwan's)**					
Deep Dish..single-serve					
4-cheese	1 pizza	450	46	2	4
pepperoni	1 pizza	480	46	2	4
sausage	1 pizza	460	44	2	4
supreme	1 pizza	450	43	2	3
Self-Rising					
4-cheese	⅙ pizza	410	46	2	5
pepperoni	⅙ pizza	380	39	2	4
supreme	⅙ pizza	380	39	2	4
special recipe					
4-cheese	⅓ pizza	400	33	1	3
pepperoni	⅓ pizza	460	34	1	3
sausage	¼ pizza	370	26	1	2
sausage & pepperoni	¼ pizza	380	26	1	2
supreme	¼ pizza	360	26	1	2
Stuffed Pizza Slices					
pepperoni	1 slice	370	36	1	6
supreme	1 slice	340	37	2	6
■ **(Tombstone)**					
Deep Dish					
cheese	1 pizza	460	51	3	9
pepperoni & cheese supreme	1 pizza	500	51	3	9
supreme	1 pizza	470	52	3	9
Half & Half					
cheese & pepperoni					
cheese portion	¼ pizza	340	37	4	6
pepperoni portion	¼ pizza	430	38	4	6
Mexican-style					
chicken fajita	¼ pizza	300	29	2	4
nacho grande	¼ pizza	380	37	3	5
taco supreme	¼ pizza	360	37	3	5

Food and Description	Amount	Total Calories	Total Carbs	Fiber	Sugars
Original					
cheese & pepperoni	¼ pizza	400	37	4	6
extra cheese	¼ pizza	340	36	4	6
supreme	⅕ pizza	310	30	3	5
Oven-Rising Crust					
pepperoni	⅙ pizza	380	33	3	7
3-cheese	⅙ pizza	300	36	2	9
Stuffed Crust..cheese	⅕ pizza	390	40	1	8
Tombstone for One					
pepperoni	1 pizza	550	41	3	8
veggie	1 pizza	350	46	4	8
■ **(Tony's)**					
Deep Dish					
cheese..5.5 oz	1 pizza	410	40	2	2
pepperoni..6.27 oz	1 pizza	510	43	2	3
sausage..6.33 oz	1 pizza	490	42	2	3
supreme..6.5 oz	1 pizza	470	43	2	4
Mini Pizza for One					
Canadian bacon	1 pizza	510	49	2	5
cheese	1 pizza	550	53	2	5
pepperoni	1 pizza	620	54	2	5
sausage	1 pizza	620	55	3	6
sausage & pepperoni	1 pizza	620	55	2	5
supreme	1 pizza	640	56	3	6
Original w/Italian-style pastry crust					
Canadian bacon	⅓ pizza	390	33	1	3
cheese	⅓ pizza	390	33	1	3
4-cheese	⅓ pizza	390	33	1	3
hamburger	⅓ pizza	420	33	2	3
meat trio	¼ pizza	350	26	1	2
Mexican..fiesta-style	¼ pizza	340	25	2	2
pepperoni	⅓ pizza	440	33	1	3
sausage	⅓ pizza	440	34	2	3
sausage & mushroom	½ pizza	340	26	2	2
sausage & pepperoni	⅓ pizza	450	34	2	3
supreme	¼ pizza	310	29	1	2
vegetable	⅓ pizza	400	34	2	4
Super Rise					
4-cheese	¼ pizza	340	49	2	4
meat trio	¼ pizza	380	41	2	4
pepperoni	¼ pizza	410	42	2	4
sausage	¼ pizza	390	41	2	4
supreme	⅕ pizza	330	34	2	3
Thin Crust					
cheese	⅓ pizza	310	31	1	3
hamburger	⅓ pizza	330	32	1	3
pepperoni	⅓ pizza	330	33	1	4
sausage	⅓ pizza	340	32	2	3
sausage & pepperoni	⅓ pizza	350	33	2	4
supreme	⅓ pizza	350	33	2	3

Food and Description	Amount	Total Calories	Total Carbs	Fiber	Sugars
■ (Totino's)					
Family-size					
cheese	⅓ pizza	370	39	2	4
combination	¼ pizza	310	29	1	3
pepperoni	⅓ pizza	420	38	2	4
sausage	¼ pizza	300	29	1	3
Party Pizza..crisp crust					
bacon burger	½ pizza	390	35	2	4
Canadian-style bacon	½ pizza	330	34	1	3
cheese	½ pizza	320	34	2	4
combination	½ pizza	390	35	2	3
hamburger	½ pizza	370	34	2	3
Mexican-style	½ pizza	320	31	2	2
pepperoni	½ pizza	380	34	1	3
sausage	½ pizza	360	35	2	3
sausage & mushroom	½ pizza	360	34	2	4
sausage & sliced pepperoni	½ pizza	380	35	2	4
sliced pepperoni	½ pizza	380	35	1	4
supreme	½ pizza	380	35	2	3
3-cheese	½ pizza	330	33	1	3
3-meat	½ pizza	360	34	2	3
zesty Italiano	½ pizza	390	36	2	4
Pizza Rolls					
cheese	6 rolls	200	26	1	3
cheesy taco	6 rolls	210	23	1	2
combination	6 rolls	230	23	1	2
hamburger	6 rolls	210	24	1	3
pepperoni	6 rolls	230	24	1	2
pepperoni supreme	6 rolls	220	24	1	3
sausage	6 rolls	230	24	1	3
spicy pepperoni	6 rolls	230	24	1	2
supreme	6 rolls	220	24	1	3
3-meat	6 rolls	220	24	1	3
■ (Weight Watchers) Bistro Selections					
BBQ-style chicken	1 pizza	380	61	3	6
4-cheese	1 pizza	400	61	3	3
pepperoni	1 pizza	400	61	3	3
spicy sausage	1 pizza	390	53	3	3
veggie..ultimate crust	1 pizza	400	69	5	2
■ (Wolfgang Puck)					
Rising Crust					
cheeseless	⅓ pizza	150	31	2	2
4-cheese	½ pizza	270	29	2	3
mushroom & spinach	⅓ pizza	230	29	2	3
pepperoni & mushrooms	⅓ pizza	310	32	2	3
sausage & herb	⅓ pizza	350	27	2	3
spicy chicken	⅓ pizza	270	28	2	3
Sourdough Crust					
pepperoni..8"	½ pizza	390	43	3	4
vegetable..12"	¼ pizza	360	40	5	5

Food and Description	Amount	Total Calories	Total Carbs	Fiber	Sugars
Whole Wheat Crust					
artichoke..8"	½ pizza	320	34	3	4
4-cheese	½ pizza	360	40	5	5
PIZZA CRUST					
(Better Pizza Crusts) ready-to-eat	½ crust	80	9	0	0
(Betty Crocker) pouch mix.. prepared..9"	¼ crust	160	33	1	1
(Boboli) Italian bread shell..prebaked					
Italian..8-oz pkg	¼ shell	150	24	1	1
Italian original..14-oz pkg	⅛ shell	140	23	1	1
Italian personal-size..10-oz pkg	¼ shell	200	31	1	1
Italian thin..10-oz pkg	⅕ shell	170	28	1	1
(Carbsense) mix..prepared..garlic & herb	¹⁄₁₂ pizza	105	7	4	0
(Flax O Meal) mix..prepared.. Italian herb	¹⁄₁₆ slice	130	7	4	1
(Jiffy) mix only..equal ¼ crust	⅓ cup	160	31	2	2
(Mama Mary's) fresh-baked gourmet					
7" dia	⅛ slice	200	32	3	2
12" dia	¹⁄₁₂ slice	200	32	2	2
(Martha White) mix..crust only					
crispy crust	1 slice	160	32	1	2
deep pan	1 slice	140	28	1	1
(Pillsbury) refrigerated..prebaked	⅕ crust	150	27	<1	4
PIZZA SAUCE (See SAUCE)					
PLANTAIN/BAKING BANANA/COOKING BANANA					
cooked..sliced	1 cup	180	48	4	na
raw					
sliced	½ cup	90	23	1.5	na
whole	1 medium	220	57	4	na
PLUM					
CANNED					
(Giant) whole..in heavy syrup	½ cup	100	25	2	19
(S&W) whole..peeled..in heavy syrup	½ cup	130	33	2	26
DRIED					
(Sunsweet) California..pitted	~1 oz	110	26	2	13
FRESH (Dole)..raw	2 medium	80	19	2	10
POI	½ cup	135	32	0.5	0
POKEBERRY/fresh					
cooked	½ cup	16	2.5	1	0
raw	½ cup	20	3	1.5	0
POLENTA					
chilled (Frieda's) traditional flavor..½"	2 slices	70	15	1	1
mix (Fantastic Foods) mix only	¼ cup	260	46	4	3
POLISH SAUSAGE (See SAUSAGE)					
POLLACK/POLLOCK (See also SEAFOOD ENTRÉE/DINNER)					
Alaskan/walleye..cooked—dry heat	3 oz	100	0	0	0
Atlantic..cooked—dry heat	3 oz	100	0	0	0
POMEGRANATE-fresh					
(Dole)	1 medium	104	26	1	14
(Frieda's)	5 oz	100	24	1	12

Food and Description	Amount	Total Calories	Total Carbs	Fiber	Sugars
POMEGRANATE JUICE					
(R. W. Knudsen)	8 fl oz	150	37	0	34
POMPANO/Florida					
cooked—dry heat	3 oz	180	0	0	0
POP TART (See PASTRY, TOASTER)					
POPCORN (See also POPCORN CAKES)					
(NOTE: Unless stated otherwise, data are for popped corn.)					
(ACT II) microwave					
butter	⅓ pkg	160	18	3	0
light	½ pkg	110	19	3	0
mini bags	⅙ pkg	210	23	4	0
classic white	⅓ pkg	180	15	3	0
kettle corn					
94% fat-free	⅓ pkg	130	28	5	0
buttery	⅓ pkg	170	17	3	0
original	⅓ pkg	170	16	3	0
movie theater..butter	⅓ pkg	170	16	3	0
sweet corn on the cob	⅓ pkg	180	15	3	0
extreme butter	⅓ pkg	180	16	3	0
(ASAP) microwave..butter					
baseball/basketballs	⅑ pkg	170	18	4	0
Bugs Bunny	⅑ pkg	160	18	4	0
Happy Birthday	⅑ pkg	170	18	4	0
low-fat	⅙ pkg	110	27	4	0
Powerpuff Girls	⅑ pkg	160	18	4	0
Scooby-Doo	⅑ pkg	160	18	4	0
sunflowers..natural	⅑ pkg	160	19	4	0
(Bearitos) ready-to-eat					
buttery	2½ cups	170	14	1	0
buttery..light	3½ cups	140	13	3	0
caramel..fat-free	1 cup	120	27	1	14
cheddar..white	2⅓ cups	170	14	1	0
no oil	5 cups	110	23	4	0
no oil..no salt	5 cups	120	24	1	0
(Betty Crocker) Pop Secret..popped					
94% fat-free..butter	1 cup	20	26	4	4
butter					
extra	1 cup	40	17	3	0
Jumbo Pop	1 cup	40	18	3	0
light	1 cup	20	20	4	0
Movie Theater	1 cup	40	17	3	0
toffee butter	1 cup	35	15	3	0
home-style	1 cup	35	17	3	0
honey butter	1 cup	35	15	3	0
kettle corn	1 cup	35	15	3	0
(Cape Cod)					
cheese-flavored	3 cups	200	17	3	0
old-fashioned butter	3 cups	170	16	2	0
(Chester's) prepopped					
butter	3 cups	170	16	3	<1

Food and Description	Amount	Total Calories	Total Carbs	Fiber	Sugars
cheddar cheese	3 cups	200	17	2	2
Flamin' Hot	2½ cups	170	14	3	1
(Cracker Jack)					
butter toffee	½ cup	140	22	1	12
caramel	½ cup	120	23	1	15
Nothing But Nuts..unpopped					
butter toffee	4 Tbs	200	9	2	6
original	3 Tbs	170	9	2	0
(Crunch & Munch) buttery popcorn					
almond supreme	1 oz	140	22	1	14
caramel	1 oz	160	23	1	11
toffee					
buttery	1 oz	150	22	1	13
fat-free	1 oz	110	26	1	15
(Fiddle Faddle) ready-to-eat					
butter toffee	⅔ cup	120	22	<1	16
caramel w/Planters peanuts	⅔ cup	120	23	<1	16
honey nut	½ cup	130	24	1<1	15
w/Heath toffee bits	½ cup	100	23	0	15
(Jolly Time) microwaveable					
Big Cheez Ultimate cheddar cheese	⅓ pkg	140	17	6	1
butter					
American's best					
butter..94% fat-free	1 oz	90	23	9	1
Blast 'O Butter Theatre-Style	1.16 oz	150	19	9	0
Crispy 'N White..natural					
light	3 cups	120	20	7	0
regular	3 cups	150	16	6	1
Healthy Pop..94% fat-free butter	3 cups	90	23	9	1
(Michael Season's) ready-to-eat					
caramel	1 cup	110	25	1	15
old-fashioned	2 cups	120	25	2	14
(Newman's Own) Old-style Picture Show Microwave					
butter					
Butter Boom	3½ cups	170	15	3	0
fat-free..94%	3½ cups	110	22	2	0
light	3½ cups	110	20	3	0
regular	3½ cups	170	16	3	0
natural					
light	3½ cups	110	20	3	0
original	3½ cups	170	16	3	0
white cheddar..genius food	3½ cups	190	19	3	0
(Orville Redenbacher's) unpopped, unless otherwise specified					
bag..original..popped	1 cup	120	29	6	0
Clusters..ready-to-eat..bag					
butter toffee	½ cup	130	20	1	11
caramel nut	½ cup	130	22	1	12
Drizzlers..ready-to-eat					
milk chocolate	⅔ cup	150	23	1	16
white fudge	⅔ cup	150	24	<1	15

Food and Description	Amount	Total Calories	Total Carbs	Fiber	Sugars
microwaveable					
butter					
light	3-oz pkg	110	19	4	0
movie theater					
butter	⅓ pkg	170	16	4	0
mini bags	1.5-oz bag	210	20	3	0
old-fashioned	⅓ pack	160	17	4	0
Pour Over Movie Theater	½ pack	170	14	3	0
Smart Pop..94% fat-free	⅓ pack	110	26	6	0
mini bags	¼ pack	110	24	4	0
Sweet'n buttery	⅓ pack	180	15	3	0
Ultimate Butter	⅓ pkg	160	15	4	0
Cinnabon	⅓ pkg	180	15	2	3
honey butter	⅓ pack	180	16	3	0
kettle corn..original	⅓ pack	180	16	3	0
kettle corn..Smart Pop	⅓ pack	120	27	6	0
movie theater					
light..popped	1 cup	20	19	5	0
Smart Pop..94% fat-free	1 pkg	120	28	7	0
regular popcorn kernels..unpopped					
white or yellow	3 Tbs	120	29	6	0
(Pop Secret) (See (Betty Crocker) in this section)					
(Poppycock) ready-to-eat					
cashew lovers	½ cup	140	21	<1	12
chocolate lovers	½ cup	160	22	<1	13
low-carb..original	½ cup	120	15	1	3
just the nuts..deluxe	¼ cup	150	20	0	12
just the nuts..fancy cashews	¼ cup	190	15	2	10
original	½ cup	160	20	1	13
pecan delight	½ cup	150	20	0	12
(Vic's) Corn Popper..ready-to-eat					
caramel					
light	1 cup	90	15	0	15
regular	1 cup	165	30	0	30
cheese..white or yellow					
light	1 cup	60	6	0	0
regular	1 cup	135	6	0	0
white					
light	1 cup	35	6	0	0
regular..original	1 cup	60	6	0	0
(Weight Watchers)					
microwaveable	1 pouch	100	22	1	0
ready-to-eat					
butter	0.66 oz	90	13	0	0
butter toffee	0.9 oz	110	21	1	11
caramel	0.9 oz	100	22	1	11
white cheddar	0.66 oz	100	20	0	0
(Wise) ready-to-eat					
buttery cheddar	1 oz	160	13	2	1
hot cheese–flavored	1 oz	150	15	2	2

Food and Description	Amount	Total Calories	Total Carbs	Fiber	Sugars
light butter	1 oz	140	22	3	0
original butter	1 oz	150	14	2	0
POPCORN CAKES (*See also* POPCORN; RICE CAKES)					
(Hain)					
butter					
mini	7 cakes	50	10	<1	0
regular	1 cake	50	10	<1	0
caramel..mini	6 cakes	50	12	<1	4
mild cheddar..mini	6 cakes	50	10	<1	1
plain..regular	1 cake	35	8	1	0
white cheddar..regular	6 cakes	50	10	<1	0
(Mother's) butter	1 cake	35	7	<1	0
(Orville Redenbacher's)					
butter					
mini	8 cakes	60	12	1	0
regular	2 cakes	60	14	2	0
caramel					
mini	6 cakes	60	13	1	4
regular	1 cake	40	10	1	3
chocolate peanut crunch					
mini	6 cakes	60	12	2	4
regular	1 cake	45	10	1	4
peanut caramel crunch..mini	6 cakes	60	12	1	4
sour cream & onion..mini	8 cakes	60	12	2	0
white cheddar..regular	2 cakes	60	13	2	0
(Quaker)					
butter					
mini	6 cakes	50	11	2	0
regular	1 cake	35	7	<1	0
caramel					
mini	5 cakes	50	12	1	4
regular	1 cake	50	12	1	4
cheddar cheese..mini	6 cakes	50	11	1	1
strawberry crunch	1 cake	50	11	1	1
POPCORN OIL (*See* OIL)					
POPPYSEED	1 tsp	15	1	0	0
	1 Tbs	50	2	1	0

POPSICLE (*See* FRUIT ICES, BARS & POPS; ICE CREAM BARS, CONES & CUPS, SANDWICHES & FROZEN NOVELTIES)

PORK (*See also* BACON; HAM; LUNCHEON MEAT; PORK ENTRÉE/DINNER; SAUSAGE)
(NOTE: The information listed under Today's Leaner Pork was provided by the National Pork, Livestock, and Meat Board. Following this is nutritional information provided by the United States Department of Agriculture. "Lean" means pork trimmed of separable fat before cooking, "Lean & Fat" means untrimmed and cooked or eaten as purchased. In most cases, 4 ounces of raw pork yields approximately 3 ounces cooked. Serving amounts do not include bone.)

■ **TODAY'S LEANER PORK**
(NOTE: Unless otherwise stated, meat has been trimmed of all separable fat and roasted.)

Food and Description	Amount	Total Calories	Total Carbs	Fiber	Sugars
blade steak	3 oz	193	0	0	0
center loin chop	3 oz	165	0	0	0
center rib chop	3 oz	179	0	0	0
loin chop	3 oz	173	0	0	0
loin roast	3 oz	165	0	0	0
rib chop	3 oz	186	0	0	0
rib roast	3 oz	182	0	0	0
ribs (country-style)	3 oz	210	0	0	0
sirloin chop	3 oz	164	0	0	0
sirloin roast	3 oz	184	0	0	0
tenderloin	3 oz	139	0	0	0
top loin chop	3 oz	165	0	0	0
■ PORK CUTS/FRESH					
backfat/raw	1 oz	230	0	0	0
	3.5 oz	805	0	0	0
backribs/lean & fat/roasted	3 oz	315	0	0	0
belly/raw	1 oz	150	0	0	0
center loin/bone-in					
chop					
lean					
broiled	3 oz	170	0	0	0
pan-fried	3 oz	200	0	0	0
lean & fat					
broiled	3 oz	205	0	0	0
pan-fried	3 oz	235	0	0	0
roast/roasted					
lean	3 oz	170	0	0	0
lean & fat	3 oz	200	0	0	0
ground..broiled or grilled	3 oz	250	0	0	0
leg					
rump half					
lean					
roasted	3 oz	175	0	0	0
roasted/chopped or diced	1 cup	280	0	0	0
lean & fat					
roasted	3 oz	215	0	0	0
roasted/chopped or diced	1 cup	340	0	0	0
shank half					
lean					
roasted	3 oz	185	0	0	0
roasted/chopped or diced	1 cup	290	0	0	0
lean & fat					
roasted	3 oz	245	0	0	0
roasted/chopped or diced	1 cup	390	0	0	0
whole					
lean					
roasted	3 oz	180	0	0	0
roasted/chopped or diced	1 cup	285	0	0	0

Food and Description	Amount	Total Calories	Total Carbs	Fiber	Sugars
lean & fat					
roasted	3 oz	230	0	0	0
roasted/chopped or diced	1 cup	370	0	0	0
loin					
blade/bone-in/chop					
lean					
broiled	3 oz	200	0	0	0
roasted	3 oz	210	0	0	0
lean & fat					
broiled	3 oz	275	0	0	0
roasted	3 oz	275	0	0	0
center rib					
chop/bone-in					
lean..broiled	3 oz	190	0	0	0
lean & fat..broiled	3 oz	225	0	0	0
chop/boneless..lean..broiled	3 oz	185	0	0	0
ribs/country-style					
lean..roasted	3 oz	210	0	0	0
lean & fat..roasted	3 oz	280	0	0	0
whole					
lean					
broiled	3 oz	180	0	0	0
roasted	3 oz	180	0	0	0
lean & fat					
broiled	3 oz	210	0	0	0
roasted	3 oz	210	0	0	0
shoulder					
arm picnic					
lean..roasted	3 oz	195	0	0	0
lean & fat..roasted	3 oz	250	0	0	0
Boston blade					
roast					
lean..roasted	3 oz	200	0	0	0
lean & fat..roasted	3 oz	230	0	0	0
steak					
lean..broiled	3 oz	195	0	0	0
lean & fat..broiled	3 oz	220	0	0	0
whole					
lean..roasted	3 oz	200	0	0	0
lean & fat..roasted	3 oz	250	0	0	0
sirloin					
chop/bone-in					
lean..broiled	3 oz	180	0	0	0
lean & fat..broiled	3 oz	220	0	0	0
chop/boneless					
lean..broiled	3 oz	165	0	0	0
lean & fat..broiled	3 oz	180	0	0	0
roast/bone-in					
lean..roasted	3 oz	185	0	0	0

Food and Description	Amount	Total Calories	Total Carbs	Fiber	Sugars
lean & fat..roasted	3 oz	225	0	0	0
roast/boneless					
lean..roasted	3 oz	170	0	0	0
lean & fat..roasted	3 oz	175	0	0	0
spareribs..lean & fat..braised	3 oz	337	0	0	0
tenderloin					
lean					
broiled	3 oz	160	0	0	0
roasted	3 oz	140	0	0	0
lean & fat					
broiled	3 oz	170	0	0	0
roasted	3 oz	150	0	0	0
top loin					
chop/boneless					
lean..broiled	3 oz	175	0	0	0
lean & fat..broiled	3 oz	195	0	0	0
roast/boneless					
lean..roasted	3 oz	165	0	0	0
lean & fat..roasted	3 oz	195	0	0	0
■ **PORK CUTS, ORGANS & OTHER/FRESH**					
brain..braised	3 oz	120	0	0	0
chitterlings/chitlins..simmered	3 oz	260	0	0	0
ear..simmered	1 ear	185	0	0	0
feet..simmered	3 oz	165	0	0	0
heart					
braised	1 heart	190	1	0	0
braised..chopped or diced	1 cup	215	0	0	0
jowl..raw	4 oz	740	0	0	0
kidney..braised	3 oz	130	0	0	0
liver..braised	3 oz	140	3	0	0
lung..braised	3 oz	85	0	0	0
pancreas..braised	3 oz	190	0	0	0
spleen..braised	3 oz	130	0	0	0
tail..simmered	3 oz	340	0	0	0
tongue..braised	3 oz	230	0	0	0
■ **PORK CUTS/FRESH..BY BRAND**					
(Hormel)					
Always Tender					
seasoned					
garlic pork tenderloin	4 oz	130	1	0	0
honey mustard pork loin fillet	4 oz	140	4	0	4
mesquite pork tenderloin	4 oz	130	2	0	0
mojo pork loin fillet	4 oz	140	3	0	2
onion garlic pork shoulder roast	4 oz	180	2	0	0
peppercorn pork tenderloin	4 oz	140	2	0	0
teriyaki tenderloin	4 oz	140	5	0	4
unseasoned					
baby back ribs	4 oz	240	0	0	0

Food and Description	Amount	Total Calories	Total Carbs	Fiber	Sugars
boneless					
pork loin..center cut	4 oz	160	0	0	0
pork tenderloin	4 oz	120	0	0	0
sirloin roast	4 oz	130	0	0	0
crown roast	4 oz	190	0	0	0
picnic cut	4 oz	230	0	0	0
pork butts	4 oz	250	0	0	0
pork roast	4 oz	170	0	0	0
shoulder roast	4 oz	180	0	0	0
spareribs	4 oz	280	0	0	0
PORK & BEANS (*See* BEANS, BAKED & VARIETY)					
PORK ENTRÉE/DINNER (*See also* ASIAN FOOD; FROZEN ENTRÉE/DINNER)					
(Betty Crocker) Pork Helper Mix..prepared					
breaded pork chops					
& mashed potatoes	⅙ box	340	28	1	3
pork chops & stuffing	⅕ pkg	320	23	1	3
pork fried rice	⅕ pkg	340	24	<1	1
(Bryan) frozen..precooked					
baby back ribs	3 oz	310	0	0	0
Boston butt	3 oz	110	0	0	0
St. Louis–style ribs	3 oz	240	0	0	0
(Castleberry's) BBQ pork..smoked sauce	2.2 oz	160	2	1	1
(Delores) pig's feet	2 oz	90	6	0	0
(Hillshire Farm) frozen..cooked					
BBQ ribs..St. Louis–style w/sauce	5 oz	350	9	0	9
boneless cooked pork roast	3 oz	170	<1	0	1
(Hormel)					
fully cooked entrées					
pork chops w/gravy	5 oz	160	3	0	2
pork roast	5 oz	180	0	0	0
pulled BBQ pork	2 oz	90	10	0	10
sliced BBQ pork	5 oz	200	23	0	23
Southwestern pork carnitas	2 oz	60	2	0	2
pickled					
pig's feet	2 oz	80	0	0	0
pork hocks	2 oz	110	0	0	0
(KC Masterpiece) BBQ pork..shredded	2 oz	130	11	0	10
(Plumrose) ready-to-eat					
baby back ribs w/smoky BBQ sauce	5 oz	280	28	0	25
(Sara Lee) frozen					
Carver's Collection..pork roast	4 oz	120	1	0	0
PORK FAT (*See* LARD)					
PORK RIND (*See* PORK ENTRÉE/DINNER; SNACKS)					
PORK SAUSAGE (*See* SAUSAGE)					
POT PIE (*See* BEEF DISH/ENTRÉE; CHICKEN ENTRÉE/DINNER; FROZEN ENTRÉE/DINNER; TURKEY ENTRÉE/DINNER; VEGETARIAN FOODS)					
POTATO (*See also* POTATO DISH/ENTRÉE; SWEET POTATO; YAM)					
CANNED					
(The Allens Butterfield) new					
diced	6 oz	100	22	3	0

Food and Description	Amount	Total Calories	Total Carbs	Fiber	Sugars
sliced	6 oz	100	22	4	0
whole	6 oz	90	20	2	0
(Bush's Best) all styles	½ cup	40	8	0	0
(Del Monte)					
new					
diced	½ cup	45	11	<1	0
sliced	⅔ cup	60	13	2	0
whole..w/liquid	~2 medium	60	13	2	0
Savory Sides..potatoes au gratin	½ cup	80	13	1	1
(S&W) new..small..whole	½ cup	60	14	1	0
FLAKES or GRANULES					
(Betty Crocker) Potato Buds					
original..mix only	⅓ cup	80	18	1	0
(Idahoan) mashed..dehydrated..mix only					
complete	⅛ box	110	20	2	0
real..premium	⅒ box	80	17	1	1
FRESH					
baked					
in microwave..w/skin	1 medium	212	49	5	9
in oven..w/skin	1 medium	220	50	5	9
boiled					
w/skin	½ cup	68	16	1.5	na
w/o skin	½ cup	67	15.5	1.5	na
raw w/skin	1 medium	100	26	3	3
FROZEN or REFRIGERATED					
(Bob Evans)					
hash browns..original	1 serving	80	17	2	1
home fries..restaurant recipe	1 serving	80	17	2	0
mashed					
garlic	1 serving	150	19	2	0
original	1 serving	160	20	2	0
(Inland Valley)					
Crinkle Cuts..French fried–style	8 oz	150	25	2	<1
Crispy Classics..French fries	3 oz	180	28	3	1
Curley QQQ's	1⅓ cups	180	25	2	<1
French fries	3 oz	180	21	2	<1
hash browns					
O'Brien	1 cup	60	14	2	<1
Simply Shreds	1 cup	70	15	2	1
mashed..home-style	⅔ cup	160	22	3	2
potato pancakes	1 pancake	120	12	2	<1
seasoned & coated					
CrissCut fries	3 oz	160	22	2	<1
fajita fries	3 oz	170	22	2	1
Santa Fe corn fries	8 oz	180	25	2	<1
Tasty QQQ's	1⅓ cups	190	25	2	<1
Tater Babies	3 oz	130	19	2	<1
shredded..seasoned potato patties	1 patty	130	15	2	<1
skins..twice-baked					
gourmet..5 oz	1 skin	280	28	2	8

Food and Description	Amount	Total Calories	Total Carbs	Fiber	Sugars
sour cream, bacon & cheddar	1 skin	240	86	0	2
triple cheese..5.1 oz	1 skin	250	33	3	3
triple cheese..stuffed shell	8 oz	400	51	5	6
steak fries	3 oz	110	18	2	<1
Stuffed Spudz	8 oz	210	23	2	<1
Tater Puffs	3 oz	160	20	2	<1
(Lamb Weston)					
Colossal Crinkles	4.5 oz	170	25	3	<1
crinkle cuts					
slim	4 oz	170	25	3	<1
wedge-cut..skin on	5 oz	160	24	3	<1
Munchers					
cheddar..bite-size rounds	4 oz	180	18	3	1
natural	4 oz	120	19	2	<1
Southwest cheddar					
bite-size rounds	4 oz	180	20	2	2
regular cuts..skin on	4.5 oz	160	25	2	<1
regular cuts..thin..skin on	4 oz	170	27	2	<1
shoestrings	4 oz	190	26	3	<1
steak house fries..skin on	5 oz	140	20	3	<1
(Michael Foods) Simply Potatoes					
diced w/onion	⅙ pkg	80	18	2	0
hash browns					
shredded	½ pkg	70	16	1	0
Southwest-style	½ pkg	70	14	2	1
sliced home fries	⅙ pkg	90	20	1	0
wedges	½ pkg	50	10	2	2
(Ore-Ida)					
baked..topped w/broccoli & cheese	10.25 oz	310	47	5	8
Crispers! Texas	3 oz	150	20	2	1
Crispy Crowns	3 oz	170	21	2	1
French fries					
country-style	3 oz	120	18	2	1
fast-food..extra crispy	3 oz	180	21	1	1
golden fries	3 oz	120	20	2	1
pixie crinkles	3 oz	130	21	2	1
shoestrings	3 oz	150	22	1	1
steak					
country-style	3 oz	110	19	2	1
seasoned w/skins	3 oz	110	18	2	1
thick-cut	3 oz	120	17	2	1
waffle	3 oz	150	21	2	1
golden twirls	3 oz	160	22	2	1
hash browns					
country-style..shredded	1¼ cups	80	17	2	1
Southern-style	⅔ cup	70	16	1	1
toaster	3.5 oz	220	25	2	1
Hot Bites!					
deep-dish minis					
3-cheese	2 bites	240	26	1	6

Food and Description	Amount	Total Calories	Total Carbs	Fiber	Sugars
cheese, sausage & pepperoni	2 bites	260	28	1	6
pepperoni & cheese	2 bites	280	26	1	6
nacho dippers	5 bites	260	30	2	2
tater dogs	4 bites	280	18	1	2
mashed potatoes	½ cup	90	16	1	1
Potatoes O'Brien	⅓ pkg	60	14	1	1
sweet potatoes..candied w/sauce	5 oz	180	41	2	31
Tater Tots					
seasoned	¹⁄₁₁ pkg	150	20	2	1
w/onion	9 pieces	170	21	2	1
twice-baked..butter flavor					
w/cheese	5 oz	160	24	3	2
wedges w/skin on					
country-style	3 oz	110	18	1	1
regular	3 oz	110	10	2	1
Zesties!	3 oz	150	20	1	1
POTATO CHIPS & SNACKS (See also SNACKS)					
(Aunt Lisa's) Classic Selects..hearty thick					
all-natural	1 oz	150	14	1	0
no salt added	1 oz	150	14	1	0
smokehouse BBQ	1 oz	150	14	1	2
(Borden)					
all natural..all styles	1 oz	150	15	1	0
regular					
BBQ	1 oz	160	15	1	1
cheddar & sour cream	1 oz	160	15	2	1
honey BBQ	1 oz	150	15	1	2
hot	1 oz	160	14	0	0
New York deli jalapeño	1 oz	140	16	1	0
onion garlic	1 oz	150	14	1	1
plain	1 oz	150	14	1	0
salt & vinegar	1 oz	150	14	1	0
Smoky Mountain BBQ	1 oz	150	15	1	2
sour cream & onion	1 oz	150	14	1	1
Ridgies					
BBQ	1 oz	150	15	1	1
cheddar & sour cream	1 oz	160	15	1	2
original	1 oz	150	14	1	0
sour cream & onion	1 oz	150	14	1	1
rippled	1 oz	150	14	1	0
(Frito-Lay)					
Lay's baked potato crisps					
BBQ..KB Masterpiece	1 oz	120	22	2	2
original	1 oz	110	23	2	2
sour cream & onion	1 oz	120	21	2	3
Lay's Bistro & Gourmet					
applewood BBQ & smoked cheddar	1 oz	150	14	1	1
peppercorn ranch	1 oz	150	15	1	1
roasted garlic & herb	1 oz	150	15	1	<1
sharp cheddar & jalapeño	1 oz	150	14	1	<1

Food and Description	Amount	Total Calories	Total Carbs	Fiber	Sugars
Lay's Kettle Cooked					
classic potato	1 oz	150	16	1	0
jalapeño..extra-crunchy	1 oz	140	16	1	0
mesquite BBQ	1 oz	140	16	<1	1
Lay's original potato chips					
classic	1 oz	150	15	1	0
country BBQ..thick cut	1 oz	160	15	1	<1
Cracker Barrel..sharp cheddar	1 oz	150	16	1	2
deli-style original	1 oz	150	16	1	0
KC Masterpiece BBQ	1 oz	150	15	1	2
salt & vinegar	1 oz	150	15	1	1
Santa Fe ranch	1 oz	150	15	1	<1
sea salt & vinegar	1 oz	160	16	1	<1
sour cream & onion	1 oz	160	12	1	<1
Taste of America..all flavors	1 oz	160	14	1	<1
Ruffles baked potato chips					
cheddar & sour cream	1 oz	120	21	2	2
regular	1 oz	120	22	2	2
Ruffles original potato chips					
3 D's					
BBQ	1 oz	140	18	1	2
maximum cheddar	1 oz	140	17	1	1
Bull's Eye..BBQ	1 oz	150	14	1	1
cheddar & sour cream	1 oz	160	14	1	0
Flavor Rush					
big BBQ & cheddar	1 oz	160	15	1	1
Buffalo Wild Wings & ranch	1 oz	150	15	1	2
KC Masterpiece BBQ	1 oz	150	15	1	1
reduced-fat..all styles	1 oz	140	19	1	0
Wow! fat-free potato chips					
Ruffles					
cheddar & sour cream	1 oz	75	16	1	<1
original	1 oz	75	17	1	0
(Kettle Chips) Natural Gourmet					
crinkle-cut					
dill & sour cream	1 oz	140	15	1	1
salsa w/mesquite	1 oz	140	15	1	0
salt & fresh ground pepper	1 oz	150	15	1	0
Krisps..low-fat..baked..all flavors	1 oz	110	22	2	1
original					
habañero chili w/ginger	1 oz	140	15	<1	0
honey Dijon	1 oz	150	16	1	1
lightly salted..crinkle-cut or regular	1 oz	150	15	1	0
New York cheddar w/herbs	1 oz	150	15	1	1
Parmesan & black pepper	1 oz	150	16	1	0
salsa w/mesquite..crinkle-cut	1 oz	140	15	1	0
sea salt & vinegar	1 oz	150	15	1	0
yogurt & green onion	1 oz	150	15	1	1
(Lance)					
BBQ Originals	1 oz	160	15	1	1

Food and Description	Amount	Total Calories	Total Carbs	Fiber	Sugars
Boomin' Barbecue Rumble	22 chips	140	16	<1	2
Classic Originals	1 oz	160	15	1	0
Howlin' Hot & Spicy Rumble	22 chips	140	15	1	<1
Rumble					
buffalo wings & blue cheese	22 chips	150	16	<1	<1
original	23 chips	160	15	1	0
Wild Sour Cream & Onion	22 chips	150	15	<1	<1
Stormy Salt & Vinegar Rumble	22 chips	150	16	<1	<1
(Louise's) potato chips					
Maui onion..fat-free	1 oz	110	24	2	0
mesquite BBQ					
fat-free	1 oz	110	23	2	1
"1g"	1 oz	110	24	2	0
70% less fat	1 oz	110	21	2	0
original					
fat-free	1 oz	110	23	2	0
"1g"	1 oz	110	24	2	0
70% less fat	1 oz	110	21	2	0
(Michael Season's)					
kettle-cooked					
jalapeño & cheese	1 oz	150	17	1	1
lightly salted	1 oz	140	17	1	1
mesquite barbecue	1 oz	140	17	1	1
reduced-fat					
honey barbecue	1 oz	150	20	1	1
ranch	1 oz	140	18	1	0
unsalted	1 oz	140	17	1	0
yogurt & green onion	1 oz	140	17	1	0
(Pringles) potato crisps					
BBQ..sweet mesquite					
fat-free	1 oz	70	15	2	0
regular	1 oz	160	15	1	0
Right Crisp	1 oz	140	19	1	0
Cheez-ums..regular	1 oz	160	15	1	0
Pizza-Licious..regular	1 oz	160	15	1	0
ranch					
fat-free	1 oz	70	15	2	0
Right Crisp	1 oz	140	19	1	0
salt & vinegar	1 oz	160	15	1	0
sour cream 'n' onion	1 oz	160	15	1	0
(Route 11)					
classic chips					
lightly salted	1 oz	150	16	1	0
salt 'n' vinegar	1 oz	150	16	1	0
classic chips..all other flavors	1 oz	150	16	1	1
specialty chips					
Hayman	1 oz	150	16	1	1
Mama Zuma's Revenge					
green chile enchilada	1 oz	150	16	<1	1
Mama Zuma's Revenge Habañero	1 oz	150	16	<1	1

Food and Description	Amount	Total Calories	Total Carbs	Fiber	Sugars
Route 11					
mixed vegetable	1 oz	150	16	1	1
sweet potato chips	1 oz	150	16	1	1
Tabard Farm Yukon Golds	1 oz	150	16	1	1
taro	1 oz	150	16	<1	1
(Snyder's of Hanover) regular chips					
BBQ	1 oz	150	21	2	0
BBQ rib	1 oz	140	17	4	1
buffalo wing..hot	1 oz	150	20	4	0
Coney Island	1 oz	150	20	3	0
jalapeño	1 oz	150	20	4	1
kosher dill	1 oz	140	20	3	1
original	1 oz	140	19	3	0
salt & vinegar	1 oz	140	19	2	0
sour cream & onion	1 oz	150	19	2	0
taco fiesta	1 oz	150	20	2	0
(Terra) chips					
blues	1 oz	140	17	1	1
frites					
Américaine	1 oz	150	18	3	7
malt vinegar	1 oz	150	18	3	7
seasoned salt	1 oz	150	18	3	7
original	1 oz	140	18	3	1
potpourri	1 oz	140	17	4	2
red bliss					
olive oil fine herbs	1 oz	140	18	3	1
roasted garlic & Parmesan	1 oz	140	16	2	2
sun-dried tomatoes					
w/balsamic vinegar	1 oz	140	18	3	1
30% less fat	1 oz	140	18	2	0
sweet potato					
jalapeño or spiced	1 oz	140	18	1	4
original..no salt	1 oz	140	18	1	2
spiced sweet	1 oz	140	16	3	3
Terra					
Mediterranean	1 oz	140	18	4	3
original	1 oz	140	18	3	1
spiced taro chips	1 oz	130	20	2	2
zesty tomato	1 oz	140	18	4	3
Yukon Gold..50% less fat					
barbecue	1 oz	130	18	2	1
onion & garlic	1 oz	130	19	2	1
original	1 oz	130	19	0	0
salt & vinegar	1 oz	130	20	2	1
yogurt & green onion	1 oz	130	19	1	1
(Wise)					
all-natural..all styles	1 oz	150	15	1	0
Krunchers					
jalapeño	1 oz	140	16	1	2

Food and Description	Amount	Total Calories	Total Carbs	Fiber	Sugars
mesquite	1 oz	140	16	1	2
regular					
BBQ	1 oz	160	15	1	1
cheddar & sour cream	1 oz	160	15	2	1
honey BBQ	1 oz	150	15	1	2
hot	1 oz	160	14	0	0
New York–deli jalapeño	1 oz	140	16	1	0
onion garlic	1 oz	150	14	1	1
Smoky Mountain BBQ	1 oz	150	15	1	2
sour cream & onion	1 oz	150	14	1	1
POTATO DISH/ENTRÉE (*See also* FROZEN ENTRÉE/DINNER; POTATO; SEASONINGS; VEGETARIAN FOODS)					
CANNED, FRESH, or MICROWAVEABLE					
(Fantastic) microwaveable..creamy mashed					
Potato Big Cups					
broccoli & cheddar	½ cup	110	20	2	3
garlic & herbs	½ cup	110	21	2	2
sour cream & chives	½ cup	110	21	2	3
white cheddar cheese	½ cup	110	20	2	3
(Purely Idaho) potatoes..heat & serve					
au gratin	¼ pkg	185	26	2	2
cheddar crusted	¼ pkg	120	26	2	1
garlic Parmesan	¼ pkg	120	26	2	1
hash browns	¼ pkg	100	22	2	1
herb-roasted	¼ pkg	110	26	2	1
home-style..mashed	¼ pkg	170	25	2	3
roasted garlic..mashed	⅕ pkg	150	21	1	1
Southwest-style..scalloped	¼ pkg	170	26	2	2
(Read) canned potato salad..German	½ cup	120	22	2	8
(Reser's) fresh					
Potato Express					
mashed					
caramelized	½ cup	160	21	2	1
country	½ cup	130	22	3	0
creamy deluxe	½ cup	160	19	2	1
garlic	½ cup	150	19	2	0
low-sodium	½ cup	130	21	3	1
premium	½ cup	130	22	3	1
red skin	½ cup	140	22	2	1
sweet potato	½ cup	140	22	3	8
potato salad					
deviled egg	½ cup	230	23	2	8
farm-style	½ cup	190	24	3	5
mustard	½ cup	180	25	3	5
red potato	½ cup	270	22	3	1
regular	½ cup	230	28	3	8
FROZEN or REFRIGERATED					
(Larry's) stuffed potatoes					
bacon & cheese	1 potato	200	24	1	8
bacon, onion & tomato	1 potato	190	24	1	8

Food and Description	Amount	Total Calories	Total Carbs	Fiber	Sugars
broccoli & cheese	1 potato	190	23	1	8
cheddar cheese	1 potato	200	24	1	9
creamy ranch	1 potato	170	22	1	5
old-fashioned butter	1 potato	190	25	1	9
Parmesan & garlic	1 potato	170	22	1	4
Parmesan & herb w/potato skins	1 potato	170	21	1	4
roasted garlic	1 potato	200	24	1	9
sour cream & chives	1 potato	190	24	1	9
toasted onion & cheddar	1 potato	170	22	1	4
w/classic beef gravy	1 potato	160	21	1	4
w/classic chicken gravy	1 potato	170	21	1	4
(Mrs. T's) pierogies					
potato					
& cheddar	¼ pkg	180	34	1	1
mini	¼ pkg	130	25	1	1
& cheese blend	¼ pkg	160	27	1	1
& onion	¼ pkg	180	33	1	1
& roasted garlic	4 oz	190	36	2	2
American cheese	4 oz	180	32	1	1
broccoli & cheddar	4 oz	200	33	2	2
cheddar & bacon..mini	¼ pkg	140	25	1	1
cheddar & jalapeño	¼ pkg	180	34	1	2
4-cheese blend	4 oz	220	36	1	2
mini	¼ pkg	130	25	0	2
sour cream & chive	4 oz	200	34	1	2
(Schwan's)					
baked potato..topped					
w/broccoli & cheese	2 halves	370	50	4	7
w/ham & cheese	2 halves	400	49	4	6
pierogies	3 pieces	200	37	2	1
potato croquettes	1 piece	150	18	2	2
red-skinned w/garlic..mashed	⅔ cup	120	20	2	1
stuffed potato					
plain	1 potato	180	24	2	3
supreme-baked	1 potato	240	23	2	3
(T.G.I. Friday's) stuffed potatoes					
broccoli & cheddar	⅓ pkg	140	16	4	1
cheddar & bacon	⅓ pkg	170	16	3	1
4-cheese & pepperoni	⅓ pkg	160	16	3	1
MIX					
(Betty Crocker) specialty potatoes..prepared by regular recipe					
au gratin	½ cup	150	22	1	3
broccoli au gratin	½ cup	120	20	2	<1
butter & herb..mashed	½ cup	160	20	1	3
cheddar & bacon	½ cup	130	21	1	2
cheddar & bacon..mashed	½ cup	150	19	1	1
cheesy scalloped..home-style	½ cup	150	21	2	2
chicken & herb	½ cup	150	21	1	3
creamy butter..mashed	½ cup	160	21	1	2
deluxe cheesy cheddar					

Food and Description	Amount	Total Calories	Total Carbs	Fiber	Sugars
au gratin	½ cup	180	22	1	3
4-cheese..mashed	½ cup	160	20	1	3
hash browns	½ cup	160	26	2	0
julienne	⅔ cup	110	19	2	2
mashed					
w/gravy & hearty beef	½ cup	170	24	2	2
w/gravy & roast chicken	¾ cup	170	25	1	2
roasted garlic	½ cup	160	20	1	1
roasted garlic & cheddar	½ cup	160	20	3	1
sour cream 'n' chives	½ cup	150	21	3	1
ranch	⅔ cup	130	25	1	2
roasted garlic	½ cup	120	20	1	1
scalloped	½ cup	130	22	3	1
sour cream 'n' chives	⅔ cup	120	21	3	1
3-cheese	⅔ cup	130	21	1	2
twice-baked..cheddar & bacon	¾ cup	180	21	1	3
(Hungry Jack) mix only					
Easy Mash'd..all styles & flavors	¼ box	90	18	2	1
other					
au gratin	⅕ box	100	22	1	1
cheesy scalloped	⅕ box	160	21	1	2
creamy scalloped	⅕ box	110	21	2	1
4-cheese	⅕ box	110	20	1	1
mashed	1 serving	80	18	1	0
sour cream & chives	⅕ box	110	20	2	1
(Idahoan) mix only					
au gratin	⅕ box	110	20	2	2
hash brown..skillet	⅕ box	90	18	1	0
mashed					
butter & herb	¼ box	110	20	1	2
buttery home-style	¼ box	110	20	1	2
complete	⅛ box	110	20	2	0
4-cheese	¼ box	100	19	1	2
loaded..baked-flavor	¼ box	110	10	2	2
original	¼ box	80	18	2	0
roasted garlic	¼ box	110	20	1	3
scalloped	⅕ box	100	21	1	2
Southwestern	¼ pkg	110	20	2	2
(Manischewitz)					
potato pancake..mix only	3 Tbs	80	18	2	na
(Mrs. Manischewitz) Latka..mix only	2 Tbs	80	18	2	na
(Panni) mix only					
Bavarian potato dumpling	⅐ pkg	80	10	2	0
Bavarian potato pancake	1/12 pkg	50	12	1	0
POTATO PANCAKE (*See* POTATO DISH/ENTRÉE)					
POTATO SNACKS (*See* POTATO CHIPS & SNACKS)					
POTATO STARCH					
(Manischewitz)	1 Tbs	30	8	0	0
	½ cup	285	70	0	0

Food and Description	Amount	Total Calories	Total Carbs	Fiber	Sugars
POTTED MEAT (*See* LUNCHEON MEAT; LUNCHEON MEAT SPREAD)					
POULTRY SEASONING (*See* SEASONINGS)					
POUT, OCEAN..cooked—dry heat	3 oz	87	0	0	0
PRETZEL					
(Ann's House of Nuts)					
chocolate	8 pieces	190	27	1	15
yogurt	6 pieces	150	18	0	18
(Auntie Anne's) soft-baked..large w/butter					
almond	1 pretzel	400	72	2	15
w/cinnamon sugar	1 pretzel	450	83	3	26
cinnamon sugar	1 pretzel	450	83	3	26
garlic	1 pretzel	350	68	2	9
Glazin' Raisin	1 pretzel	510	107	4	38
jalapeño	1 pretzel	310	59	2	9
maple crumb	1 pretzel	550	112	3	42
original	1 pretzel	370	72	3	10
Parmesan herb	1 pretzel	440	72	9	10
sesame	1 pretzel	410	64	7	9
Smart Bites	1 bite	10	2	1	0
	15 bites	150	30	15	0
sour cream & onion	1 pretzel	340	66	2	10
sticks					
cinnamon sugar	1 stick	300	55	2	17
original	1 stick	247	48	2	7
whole wheat	1 stick	370	72	7	10
(Combos)					
cheddar cheese..single bag	1.8 oz	240	35	1	8
nacho cheese..single bag	1.8 oz	240	34	1	8
pizzeria..single bag	1.8 oz	230	35	1	7
(Michael Season's) sweet organic					
cinnamon twists	1 cup	130	21	0	7
(Mrs. Manischewitz) bagel pretzel					
all styles & flavors	4 pretzels	110	22	1	<1
(Newman's Own) organic					
Bavarian sourdough	1 pretzel	90	19	1	1
high-protein	1 oz	120	22	4	1
nuggets or rods	1 oz	120	25	2	1
rounds					
regular or unsalted	1 oz	110	24	<1	1
salt & pepper	1 oz	100	24	1	1
spelt	1 oz	120	23	4	0
thins					
regular or unsalted	1 oz	110	24	<1	1
salt & pepper	1 oz	120	24	1	1
sticks	1 oz	110	24	1	1
(Rold Gold)					
Cracker Barrel..sharp cheddar	1 oz	110	22	1	<1
fat-free..tiny twists	1 oz	100	23	1	<1
regular					
classic					

Food and Description	Amount	Total Calories	Total Carbs	Fiber	Sugars
cheddar cheese..tiny twists	1 oz	110	23	1	<1
honey mustard					
nuggets	1 oz	130	20	1	2
tiny twists	1 oz	110	23	1	<1
sticks	1 oz	120	22	1	<1
thin twists	1 oz	120	22	1	<1
tiny twists	1 oz	110	23	1	<1
hard sourdough	1 oz	100	21	1	<1
honey mustard	1 oz	130	22	1	1
Parmesan herb	1 oz	130	18	1	1
rods	1 oz	110	22	1	1
snack mix					
Colossal Cheddar	¾ cup	160	19	1	2
Munchies	¾ cup	140	17	1	1
original	¾ cup	160	18	1	2
(Snyder's of Hanover)					
organic pretzels					
classic..mini	1 oz	110	25	1	1
honey wheat sticks	1 oz	130	24	1	4
oat bran sticks	1 oz	120	25	2	3
pumpernickel & onion sticks	1 oz	120	24	1	0
pretzels					
butter snaps	1 oz	120	25	1	1
hard..all styles	1 oz	100	22	1	0
hearth-baked sourdough	1 oz	110	23	1	0
honey wheat w/sesame seeds	1 oz	120	24	2	4
mini	1 oz	110	25	1	1
oat bran	1 oz	110	25	2	3
old-fashioned dipping sticks	1 oz	100	24	1	1
Olde Tyme	1 oz	120	24	1	1
real milk chocolate–dipped	1 oz	130	19	1	10
rod	1 oz	120	24	1	1
snaps	1 oz	120	25	1	1
soft-baked..6-count	1 pretzel	180	36	2	1
specials	1 oz	120	23	1	0
sticks	1 oz	110	23	1	1
sticks..honey wheat	1 oz	120	24	2	4
thin	1 oz	110	23	1	1
tiny butter sticks	1 oz	120	25	1	1
snack mix	1 oz	150	16	1	2
(SuperPretzel) soft-baked..frozen					
pretzels					
bites	5 bites	140	29	1	1
original..6-count box	1 pretzel	180	36	2	1
PretzelFils					
onion veggie	2 sticks	140	22	1	1
pepper jack	2 sticks	140	22	1	1
pizza	2 sticks	140	23	1	1
Softstix..cheddar	2 sticks	140	23	1	1
PRICKLY PEAR	1 medium	42	10	4	0

Food and Description	Amount	Total Calories	Total Carbs	Fiber	Sugars
PROSCIUTTO (*See* SAUSAGE)					
PRUNE					
CANNED					
(Best Yet) all styles	1.33 oz	110	26	2	13
(Oregon Fruit Products) pitted Italian..whole in heavy syrup	4.25 oz	130	28	7	23
DRIED					
(Del Monte) uncooked					
pitted	¼ cup	120	29	3	14
unpitted	⅓ cup	110	12	1	13
(Dole) pitted	¼ cup	110	26	2	13
(Sun-Maid) California pitted plums	1 oz	110	26	2	13
PRUNE JUICE..BOTTLED or CANNED					
(Del Monte) unsweetened	8 fl oz	170	43	1	27
(Langer's)	8 fl oz	180	41	1	23
(Sunsweet) prune pulp	8 fl oz	170	43	3	27
PUDDING & MOUSSE (*See also* CUSTARD; PIE FILLING)					
MIX (NOTE: Unless stated otherwise, 1 serving of mix = the amount in ½ cup prepared.)					
(Crosse & Blackwell) plum pudding	⅓ pkg	460	87	5	58
(Jell-O) pudding & pie filling..dry mix only					
Americana pudding & custard					
rice pudding	¼ pkg	90	23	0	13
tapioca pudding..prepared	¼ pkg	90	22	0	15
cook & serve					
fat-free					
chocolate	¼ pkg	130	29	0	21
vanilla	¼ pkg	140	20	0	16
original					
banana cream	¼ pkg	80	20	0	15
butterscotch	¼ pkg	100	24	1	19
chocolate fudge	¼ pkg	90	22	1	15
coconut cream	¼ pkg	90	18	1	14
lemon	⅙ pkg	50	12	0	6
milk chocolate	¼ pkg	90	22	0	16
vanilla	⅙ pkg	80	20	0	16
sugar-free..reduced-calorie					
chocolate	¼ pkg	30	7	<1	0
vanilla	⅙ pkg	20	5	0	0
instant					
regular					
banana cream	⅙ pkg	90	23	0	18
butterscotch	¼ pkg	90	23	0	18
cheesecake	¼ pkg	100	24	0	20
chocolate	¼ pkg	100	25	1	10
chocolate fudge	¼ pkg	100	25	1	17
coconut cream	⅙ pkg	100	21	1	16
devil's food	¼ pkg	140	25	1	19
French vanilla	¼ pkg	90	23	0	18
lemon	¼ pkg	90	24	0	19

Food and Description	Amount	Total Calories	Total Carbs	Fiber	Sugars
Oreo cookies 'n' cream	¼ pkg	120	28	0	21
white chocolate	¼ pkg	90	23	0	19
sugar-free..banana cream	¼ pkg	25	6	0	0
sugar-free..fat-free					
banana cream	¼ pkg	25	6	0	0
butterscotch	¼ pkg	25	6	0	0
chocolate fudge	¼ pkg	35	8	1	0
pistachio	¼ pkg	30	6	0	0
vanilla	¼ pkg	25	6	0	0
white chocolate	¼ pkg	25	6	0	0
(Kraft) Kraft Minute..pudding mix..rice	¼ pkg	90	23	0	13
(Uncle Ben's) dry mix					
cinnamon & raisin rice pudding	⅓ pkg	160	37	0	15
French vanilla rice pudding	⅓ pkg	120	28	1	10
READY-TO-SERVE					
(Hunt's)					
Snack Pack					
banana cream pie	1 snack	140	23	0	17
butterscotch	1 snack	130	21	0	15
chocolate	1 snack	140	22	0	17
chocolate brownie	1 snack	140	23	0	17
chocolate fudge	1 snack	150	23	0	16
chocolate marshmallow	1 snack	130	21	0	16
chocolate peanut butter pie	1 snack	140	23	0	17
chocolate vanilla	1 snack	130	21	0	18
dulce de leche	1 snack	140	23	0	17
lemon meringue pie	1 snack	140	23	0	17
S'mores Swirl	1 snack	140	21	0	17
tapioca	1 snack	130	21	0	13
vanilla	1 snack	130	21	0	17
Snack Pack..fat-free					
chocolate	1 snack	90	21	0	15
vanilla or tapioca	1 snack	80	18	0	13
(Jell-O)					
Kraft..Handi-Snacks					
chocolate					
fat-free	1 snack	90	21	0	16
mega-cup	1 snack	170	31	1	23
regular	1 snack	120	22	0	16
chocolate chip cookie	1 snack	120	22	1	16
chocolate vanilla	1 snack	110	21	1	15
rice	1 snack	140	19	0	11
tapioca	1 snack	130	25	0	19
vanilla	1 snack	130	24	0	19
Pudding Snacks					
chocolate	1 snack	140	27	1	21
chocolate fudge sundaes	1 snack	140	25	0	20
Oreo	1 snack	140	27	1	21
tapioca	1 snack	130	25	0	19
vanilla	1 snack	130	24	0	19

Food and Description	Amount	Total Calories	Total Carbs	Fiber	Sugars
X-treme chocolate	1 snack	80	16	1	12
Pudding Snacks..Cream Savers					
chocolate & caramel creme-swirled	1 snack	160	28	0	23
chocolate vanilla swirls	1 snack	140	26	1	20
strawberry & creme-swirled	1 snack	130	25	0	20
Pudding Snacks..fat-free					
chocolate	1 snack	100	21	0	16
chocolate vanilla swirls	1 snack	100	23	1	17
tapioca	1 snack	100	23	0	17
vanilla & chocolate	1 snack	100	24	0	17
vanilla caramel sundaes	1 snack	100	23	0	16
(Kozy Shack) cups					
banana	4 oz	130	22	0	17
chocolate	4 oz	140	24	<1	19
rice	4 oz	140	22	1	16
tapioca	4 oz	130	23	0	20
vanilla	4 oz	130	22	0	17
(Swiss Miss) Pudding Snacks					
apple pie à la mode	1 snack	170	26	0	20
banana cream pie	1 snack	140	20	0	14
butterscotch	1 snack	130	21	0	15
caramel cream	1 snack	140	23	0	22
chocolate					
fat-free	1 snack	90	20	0	15
light	1 snack	140	27	0	19
regular	1 snack	140	22	0	16
chocolate brownie	1 snack	180	27	0	23
chocolate cookie dough	1 snack	140	22	0	16
Chocolate Dare Devil	1 snack	140	23	0	19
chocolate fudge	1 snack	150	23	0	16
chocolate marshmallow	1 snack	130	21	0	16
chocolate mud pie	1 snack	140	24	0	22
chocolate vanilla	1 snack	130	21	0	16
German chocolate cake	1 snack	160	30	0	24
lemon	1 snack	120	23	0	20
lemon meringue pie	1 snack	130	26	0	21
milk chocolate	1 snack	140	23	0	17
tapioca					
fat-free	1 snack	80	19	0	13
regular	1 snack	130	20	0	14
vanilla					
fat-free	1 snack	80	18	0	13
regular	1 snack	130	31	0	17
PUMMELO/POMELO					
FRESH					
sections	1 cup	70	18	2	0
whole	1 medium	230	59	6	0
PUMPKIN					
CANNED					

Food and Description	Amount	Total Calories	Total Carbs	Fiber	Sugars
(Comstock)	½ cup	50	10	4	4
(Libby's) pure pumpkin	½ cup	40	9	5	4
FRESH boiled..mashed	1 cup	48	12	3	na
PUMPKIN CUBES					
(Knorr) pumpkin cubes	1 cube	5	0	0	0
PUMPKIN PIE SPICE (*See* SEASONINGS)					
PUMPKIN SEEDS					
(David) dried..kernels..roasted	¼ cup	160	3	1	0
single bag	2.25 oz	280	6	2	1
PUNCH (*See* FRUIT PUNCH; SOFT DRINK; SOFT DRINK MIX)					
PURPLE HULL PEA					
CANNED (Allens Fresh)	½ cup	100	16	0	–
FROZEN					
(Birds Eye) Southern	½ cup	110	21	4	1
(Frosty Acres)	3.3 oz	130	23	0	–
PURSLANE					
boiled	½ cup	10	1	0	0
raw	1 cup	7	1	0	0

Food and Description	Amount	Total Calories	Total Carbs	Fiber	Sugars
QUAIL/raw					
breast meat only	~2 oz	69	0	0	0
meat & skin	~4 oz	210	0	0	0
meat only	~4 oz	135	0	0	0
QUICHE (*See* EGG DISH/MEAL)					
QUINCE/fresh	1 medium	53	14	0	0
QUINOA (*See also* FLOUR; PASTA; QUINOA SEED)					
whole grain/dry					
(Eden)	¼ cup	180	29	11	2
(Quinoa Corporation)	¼ cup	166	30	3	1
QUINOA SEED (Arrowhead Mills)	¼ cup	140	25	4	0

R

Food and Description	Amount	Total Calories	Total Carbs	Fiber	Sugars
RABBIT					
domesticated/meat only					
roasted	4 oz	225	0	0	0
stewed	4 oz	235	0	0	0
wild/meat only..stewed	4 oz	200	0	0	0
RACCOON/meat only..roasted	3 oz	220	0	0	0
RADICCHIO/raw..shredded	½ cup	5	1	0	0
RADISH					
dried..Chinese	½ cup	155	37	5	–
fresh					
black	1 oz	5	1	0	0
Chinese					
cooked-drained..sliced	½ cup	15	2.5	1	0
raw..whole	1 medium	60	14	5.5	0
daikon					
cooked-drained..sliced	½ cup	15	1	0	0
raw..whole	1 medium	60	14	5.5	0
red/raw (Dole) whole	7 medium	20	3	0	0
white icicle/raw	1 medium	2	0.5	<1	0
RADISH SPROUTS	½ cup	8	1	0	0
RAISIN (*See also* SNACK MIX)					
(Del Monte)					
golden or natural	¼ cup	130	31	2	29
	1 oz box	90	22	2	20
yogurt raisin snack bag..all flavors	0.9 oz	110	20	<1	17
(Dole) all styles	¼ cup	130	31	2	29
(Sun-Maid)					
baking	¼ cup	120	28	2	26
golden	1.3 oz	130	31	2	29
& cherries	1.5 oz	130	31	2	27
yogurt raisins					
chocolate	1 oz	123	22	1	19
vanilla	1 oz	130	20	1	19
RASPBERRY					
FRESH (Dole)	1 cup	50	17	8	12
FROZEN					
(Birds Eye) red..in light syrup	4.5 oz	90	22	5	22
(C&W) red..sweetened	¾ cup	130	29	2	6
(Cascadian Farms)	1 cup	60	15	7	2

Food and Description	Amount	Total Calories	Total Carbs	Fiber	Sugars

RASPBERRY JUICE/JUICE BLEND/JUICE DRINK (*See also* FRUIT PUNCH; LEMONADE; SOFT DRINK; SOFT DRINK MIX)
BOTTLED, BOXED, or CANNED

Food and Description	Amount	Total Calories	Total Carbs	Fiber	Sugars
(After The Fall) raspberry spritzer	12 fl oz	170	42	0	38
(Dole) raspberry kiwi	8 fl oz	120	30	0	26
(Knudsen) red raspberry spritzer	12 fl oz	170	38	0	32
(Smucker's) juice	8 fl oz	120	30	0	29
(Walnut Acres) raspberry juice	8 fl oz	130	32	0	28
(Welch's) wild raspberry	8 fl oz	140	35	0	34

FROZEN (Dole) prepared

Food and Description	Amount	Total Calories	Total Carbs	Fiber	Sugars
country raspberry 100% juice blend	8 fl oz	140	34	0	33

RAVIOLI (*See* BEEF DISH/ENTRÉE; FROZEN ENTRÉE/DINNER; PASTA ENTRÉE/DINNER; VEGETARIAN FOODS)
RED BEAN (*See also* BEANS, BAKED & VARIETY; RICE DISH)
CANNED

Food and Description	Amount	Total Calories	Total Carbs	Fiber	Sugars
(Bush's Best)	½ cup	110	10	6	0
(Eden) small red	½ cup	100	17	5	1
(Knorr) refried	½ cup	120	22	5	0
(S&W) Louisiana-style w/tomato, onions & Cajun sauce	½ cup	80	20	5	2

RED BEAN SOUP (*See* SOUP)
REFRIED BEANS (*See* MEXICAN FOOD)
RELISH (*See* CHUTNEY; CORN DISH; PICKLE RELISH)
RHUBARB
FRESH

Food and Description	Amount	Total Calories	Total Carbs	Fiber	Sugars
cooked..sweetened	1 cup	280	75	5	na
raw..diced	½ cup	13	3	0	0

RICE (*See also* ASIAN FOOD; RICE DISH)
(NOTE: Unless otherwise stated, data are for dry mix only.)
(Arrowhead Mills) brown

Food and Description	Amount	Total Calories	Total Carbs	Fiber	Sugars
long-grain	¼ cup	150	33	2	0
medium-grain	¼ cup	160	34	1	0
short-grain	¼ cup	170	36	2	0
(Fantastic Foods)					
Elegant Grains..all styles	¼ cup	160	36	<1	0
Organic					
couscous	¼ cup	190	43	2	1
whole wheat couscous	¼ cup	210	45	7	0
(Gourmet House) wild..blends					
brown & wild	¼ cup	160	34	1	1
cultivated..Minnesota	¼ cup	170	35	2	0
other..Minnesota cultivated..cracked	¼ cup	170	35	2	0
quick-cooking	¼ cup	170	25	2	0
(Kraft)					
boil-in-bag..long-grain white..enriched	1.5 oz	180	42	1	0
instant					
long-grain..white..all styles	1.5 oz	160	36	1	0
whole-grain..brown	1.5 oz	170	34	2	0
(Lundberg Family Farms)					

Food and Description	Amount	Total Calories	Total Carbs	Fiber	Sugars
Christmas red	¼ cup	170	37	<1	0
Jubilee..gourmet brown-rice blend	¼ cup	170	39	3	0
Lundberg Wehani..brown	1.5 oz	170	38	3	0
Lundberg Wild Blend..wild & brown	1.5 oz	150	35	3	0
organic black japonica..black & mahogany	1.5 oz	170	39	3	1
(Mahatma)					
basmati..Indian fragrance	1.5 oz	160	36	0	0
brown	1.5 oz	160	36	<1	0
instant	1.5 oz	160	36	2	0
Valencia..short-grain	1.5 oz	160	36	1	0
white..long-grain	1.5 oz	150	35	0	0
(Patak's original)					
basmati	1 pouch	430	87	2	1
coconut	1 pouch	500	87	4	5
garlic & cilantro	1 pouch	420	86	3	2
yellow rice	1 pkg	440	89	2	6
(Riceland)					
brown..natural..extra-long-grain	1.67 oz	150	32	1	0
enriched					
extra-long-grain	1.67 oz	160	35	0	0
long-grain..gold..parboiled	1.67 oz	170	37	0	0
medium-grain plump & tender	1.67 oz	170	37	0	0
(S&W)					
brown..natural..all styles	¼ cup	150	32	1	0
Indian basmati	¼ cup	160	36	0	0
Italian arborio	¼ cup	150	35	1	0
organic..brown..natural	¼ cup	150	35	0	0
Thai jasmine	¼ cup	160	36	2	6
white..long-grain					
premium	¼ cup	150	35	0	0
& wild	¼ cup	140	32	<1	0
(Success) as packaged					
brown					
boil-in-bag..prepared	½ cup	150	33	2	0
10-minute..prepared	½ cup	190	43	<1	0
brown & wild	½ cup	190	41	3	1
white..natural long-grain..precooked	½ cup	190	43	<1	0
(A Taste of Thai)					
rice..soft jasmine	¼ cup	160	36	0	0
rice noodles..all styles	2 oz	200	46	2	0
(Tony Chachere's) Creole..dirty rice dinner	⅕ box	160	34	2	2
(Uncle Ben's)					
brown					
instant	½ cup	190	42	2	0
original	¼ cup	170	35	0	0
white					
boil-in-bag	⅓ cup	190	44	1	0
converted	¼ cup	170	38	0	0

Food and Description	Amount	Total Calories	Total Carbs	Fiber	Sugars
Rice-in-an-Instant	½ cup	190	43	1	0
wild/combinations/fast-cooking	1 serving	120	36	2	1
RICE BRAN (*See also* CEREAL)					
crude	½ cup	130	59	25	0
RICE BRAN OIL					
(Hain)	1 Tbs	120	0	0	0
(Hollywood)	1 Tbs	120	0	0	0
RICE CAKES (*See also* POPCORN CAKES)					
(Hain)					
mini					
apple cinnamon	6 cakes	60	13	0	0
honey nut	6 cakes	60	13	0	0
plain	6 cakes	60	12	0	0
ranch	6 cakes	70	9	0	0
regular					
apple cinnamon	1 cake	50	11	0	0
honey nut	1 cake	50	11	0	0
plain	1 cake	40	8	0	0
(Lundberg Family Farms)					
classic cakes					
nutra-farmed					
brown rice					
regular	1 cake	70	15	0	0
salt-free	1 cake	70	16	0	0
organic					
brown rice					
regular	1 cake	70	15	0	0
salt-free	1 cake	70	16	0	0
mochi sweet	1 cake	70	15	0	0
wild rice	1 cake	70	15	0	0
savory cakes					
nutra-farmed					
sesame tamari	1 cake	70	16	2	0
toasted sesame	1 cake	70	15	1	0
koku					
seaweed	1 cake	80	17	1	1
sesame	1 cake	80	17	2	1
organic					
sesame tamari	1 cake	70	15	0	0
tamari seaweed	1 cake	70	16	2	14
sweet cakes..nutra-farmed..					
all flavors	1 cake	80	18	1	2
(Quaker)					
mini rice snacks					
apple cinnamon	8 cakes	60	15	0	6
BBQ	10 cakes	70	12	0	2
caramel corn	7 cakes	60	13	0	6
cheddar cheese	9 cakes	70	11	0	0
chocolate crunch	7 cakes	60	13	0	5

Food and Description	Amount	Total Calories	Total Carbs	Fiber	Sugars
nacho	9 cakes	70	11	0	0
sour cream & onion	10 cakes	70	12	0	1
Quaker rice snacks					
apple cinnamon	8 pieces	60	15	0	6
BBQ	10 pieces	70	12	0	2
caramel corn	7 pieces	60	13	0	6
cheddar cheese	9 pieces	70	11	0	0
chocolate crunch	7 pieces	60	13	0	5
creamy ranch	10 pieces	70	12	0	0
nacho	9 pieces	70	11	0	0
sour cream & onion	10 pieces	70	12	0	1
regular..large rice cakes					
apple cinnamon	1 cake	50	11	0	4
banana nut crunch	1 cake	50	11	0	5
buttered popcorn	1 cake	35	7	0	0
caramel apple	1 cake	60	11	0	4
caramel chocolate chip	1 cake	60	13	0	5
caramel corn	1 cake	50	11	0	4
chocolate crunch	1 cake	60	12	0	4
cinnamon streusel	1 cake	60	12	0	4
peanut butter	1 cake	60	12	0	5
plain	1 cake	35	7	0	0
strawberry crunch	1 cake	50	11	0	4
white cheddar corn	1 cake	45	8	0	0
(Westbrae Natural)					
rice cakes..all flavors	2 cakes	50	10	0	1
rice wafers..all flavors	7 wafers	50	11	0	0
RICE DISH (*See also* ASIAN FOOD; FROZEN ENTRÉE/DINNER; MEXICAN FOOD)					
CANNED					
(Old El Paso) Spanish rice	1 cup	140	39	1	2
FROZEN					
(Green Giant) Rice & Vegetable Combinations					
cheesy rice & broccoli	1 pkg	300	56	2	7
rice medley	1 pkg	280	52	4	4
rice pilaf	1 pkg	230	44	3	5
(Uncle Ben's) rice bowls					
Cajun-style..chicken & sausage	1 bowl	350	56	3	8
chicken fried rice	1 bowl	410	65	3	8
chicken stir-fry	1 bowl	360	58	3	17
chicken vegetable	1 bowl	360	56	3	8
chili w/beans & rice	1 bowl	360	48	6	7
honey Dijon chicken	1 bowl	400	73	3	20
Mexican-style..beef fajita	1 bowl	300	45	3	5
spicy beef & broccoli	1 bowl	370	62	1	13
sweet & sour chicken	1 bowl	360	65	2	20
turkey w/wild rice & cranberries	1 bowl	360	61	3	13
MIX					
(Casbah) pilaf..prepared					
nutted	1 cup	220	49	1	0
original	1 cup	200	44	1	0

Food and Description	Amount	Total Calories	Total Carbs	Fiber	Sugars
Spanish	1 cup	200	44	1	0
(Fantastic Foods)					
Carb'Tastic..ready meals					
ginger shiitake w/rice noodles	1 meal	340	58	4	3
pad Thai w/rice noodles	1 meal	400	59	5	7
Spanish paella	1 meal	280	55	4	2
Thai lemongrass	1 meal	340	48	5	4
Tuscan mushroom risotto	1 meal	310	50	2	1
pilaf..dry mix only					
basmati	¼ cup	150	34	<1	1
4-grain	½ cup	160	34	2	1
Hacienda Spanish	¼ cup	150	33	1	1
organic	¼ cup	160	34	<1	0
vegetarian chicken	¼ cup	180	34	<1	0
rice & beans..dry mix only					
Bombay curry	½ pkg	190	39	4	6
Cajun/cup	½ pkg	180	35	6	4
risotto..dry mix only					
classico	¼ cup	160	32	<1	3
Tuscan mushroom	¼ cup	130	24	<1	1
(Golden Grain) prepared according to pkg directions					
Rice-A-Roni					
beef & mushroom	1 cup	290	50	2	4
beef flavor	1 cup	310	51	2	3
broccoli	1 cup	280	41	1	1
broccoli au gratin	1 cup	270	40	2	5
chicken & broccoli	1 cup	230	41	2	2
chicken..Cajun	1 cup	250	41	2	2
chicken & garlic	1 cup	260	42	1	2
chicken & mushroom	1 cup	360	52	2	4
chicken & vegetables	1 cup	290	51	2	3
chicken flavor..original	1 cup	310	52	2	2
chicken					
4-cheese	1 cup	280	37	1	4
fried rice	1 cup	320	50	2	5
garden vegetable	1 cup	240	41	2	3
herb & butter	1 cup	320	53	1	2
herb roasted chicken	1 cup	260	41	1	3
long grain & wild rice..original	1 cup	240	42	2	2
Mexican-style	1 cup	250	41	2	3
Oriental stir-fry	1 cup	290	54	2	2
rice pilaf	1 cup	310	52	1	1
savory chicken..vegetable..low-fat	1 cup	210	41	2	3
Spanish rice	1 cup	300	51	3	6
Stroganoff	1 cup	360	49	1	5
white cheddar & herbs	1 cup	340	49	1	4
(Health Valley) rice cups..low-fat					
Cantonese	½ cup	140	27	2	2
chicken-flavored	½ cup	140	26	3	2

Food and Description	Amount	Total Calories	Total Carbs	Fiber	Sugars
rice primavera	½ cup	140	26	2	2
shiitake	½ cup	140	26	2	2
Thai	½ cup	140	27	2	3
(Kashi) 7 whole grain & sesame..cooked	½ cup	170	30	6	0
(Knorr) dry mix only					
Italian risotto Milanese arborio-style	2.55 oz	260	59	1	2
lemon herb pilaf	2.55 oz	260	55	1	3
Mexican-style	1.95 oz	200	44	0	0
Spanish-style	¼ box	200	44	1	0
yellow	2.28 oz	230	51	1	2
(Lipton) mix only					
Asian side dishes					
chicken fried rice	½ cup	240	49	1	1
teriyaki rice	½ cup	240	50	1	4
rice & sauce..Cajun-style					
dirty rice	½ cup	250	50	2	1
garlic butter	½ cup	260	49	1	1
New Orleans–style chicken	½ cup	240	51	2	2
w/rice and beans	½ cup	290	62	4	1
fiesta sides					
Mexican rice	½ cup	250	5	2	1
smoked chipotle	½ cup	260	55	2	5
Spanish	½ cup	240	51	2	3
rice sides					
beef	½ cup	240	48	1	1
cheddar broccoli	½ cup	260	50	2	2
chicken					
broccoli	½ cup	240	48	1	1
creamy	½ cup	270	59	1	2
flavored	½ cup	250	48	1	<1
& Parmesan risotto	½ cup	220	43	1	0
herb & butter	½ cup	250	46	1	0
medley	½ cup	230	46	1	1
(Luzianne) dinner kit..mix only					
"dirty" rice	⅕ box	160	35	0	0
étouffée	¼ box	200	42	1	2
gumbo	⅕ box	160	33	1	3
jambalaya	⅕ box	200	43	1	0
shrimp Creole	⅕ box	150	34	1	1
(Mahatma) dry mix only					
black bean	⅓ pkg	200	39	5	0
broccoli & cheese	⅓ pkg	200	39	1	2
chicken & rice	½ pkg	190	42	<1	0
jambalaya	⅙ pkg	190	42	1	1
nacho cheese	¼ pkg	250	49	<1	5
pilaf..classic	½ pkg	190	43	1	0
Spanish..authentic	½ pkg	180	42	2	1
yellow					
saffron	⅓ pkg	190	43	<1	1
spicy	¼ pkg	180	41	<1	2

Food and Description	Amount	Total Calories	Total Carbs	Fiber	Sugars
(Near East)					
Creative Grains..mixes..prepared					
chicken & herb	1 cup	270	51	6	2
creamy Parmesan	1 cup	280	48	3	2
roasted garlic	1 cup	220	41	5	1
roasted pecan & garlic	1 cup	240	37	4	1
rice pilaf..prepared					
brown rice	1 cup	210	41	3	1
chicken-flavor	1 cup	220	43	2	1
curry	1 cup	220	44	2	0
garlic & herb	1 cup	220	44	1	0
lentil	1 cup	200	36	8	3
long grain & wild rice	1 cup	220	43	2	0
Mediterranean chicken w/wild rice	1 cup	210	44	2	na
rice	1 cup	220	44	1	0
roasted chicken & garlic	1 cup	220	43	2	1
Spanish rice	1 cup	310	54	2	2
toasted almond	1 cup	230	40	2	1
wheat	1 cup	220	40	9	2
wild mushroom & herb	1 cup	220	44	2	1
(Old El Paso) mix only..all styles & flavors	⅓ pkg	250	55	2	2
Rice-A-Roni (See (Golden Grain) in this section)					
(Spice Hunter) risotto cups					
spinach & garlic	1 cup	230	48	>1	1
3-cheese	1 cup	240	47	>1	1
wild mushroom	1 cup	220	47	<1	1
(Success) as packaged..boil-in-bag					
beef	1 serving	190	43	2	2
broccoli & cheese	1 serving	210	40	1	4
brown & wild	1 serving	190	41	3	1
cheesy rice	1 serving	220	39	1	2
chicken..classic	1 serving	220	32	1	0
grilled chicken & broccoli	1 serving	190	42	1	1
long-grain & wild	1 serving	190	42	1	2
pilaf	1 serving	200	44	2	3
red beans & rice	1 serving	240	51	8	1
Spanish	1 serving	190	43	1	2
yellow	1 serving	150	33	<1	0
(A Taste of Thai) prepared					
coconut ginger	¾ cup	190	42	2	1.5
garlic basil	¾ cup	160	35	0	2
golden	¾ cup	180	38	0	2
(Uncle Ben's) prepared					
Brown & Wild Rice..mushroom recipe	1 cup	190	40	2	1
Country Inn					
broccoli rice au gratin	1 cup	200	43	1	1
chicken					
& broccoli	1 cup	190	43	1	0
& vegetable	1 cup	190	42	1	0

Food and Description	Amount	Total Calories	Total Carbs	Fiber	Sugars
& wild rice	1 cup	200	43	1	0
Mexican fiesta	1 cup	200	43	1	1
Oriental..fried	1 cup	200	43	1	1
3-cheese	1 cup	200	41	1	4
Flavorful Rice					
chicken herb	1 cup	200	42	1	0
garlic & butter	1 cup	200	43	1	0
lemon & herb	1 cup	190	43	<1	1
Parmesan & butter	1 cup	200	43	0	0
Spanish	1 cup	200	43	0	2
tomato & herb	1 cup	190	43	1	0
Long-Grain & Wild Rice..prepared					
butter & herb	1 cup	190	40	1	1
original recipe	1 cup	190	41	1	1
roasted garlic	1 cup	190	41	1	0
vegetable & herb	1 cup	210	43	1	2
Ready Rice					
long-grain & wild	4.4 oz	180	36	2	1
original long-grain	4.4 oz	190	40	2	0
roasted chicken	4.4 oz	190	37	2	1
Spanish-style	4.4 oz	190	36	2	2
whole grain..brown	4.4 oz	190	36	2	1
(Zatarain's) prepared					
New Orleans jambalaya	1 cup	130	29	0	0
red beans & rice..New Orleans–style	1 cup	90	20	2	0
RICE DRINK					
(Lundberg Family Farms) lactose-free					
drink..rice..all styles	8 fl oz	120	44	3	3
(Rice Dream)					
regular					
carob	8 fl oz	150	32	0	24
chocolate	8 fl oz	170	36	0	25
enriched					
chocolate	8 fl oz	170	36	0	25
original	8 fl oz	120	25	0	11
vanilla	8 fl oz	130	28	0	12
Heartwise					
original	8 fl oz	130	27	3	9
vanilla	8 fl oz	140	30	3	10
(Westbrae)					
plain	1 cup	100	18	0	14
vanilla	1 cup	120	22	0	17
RICE FROZEN DESSERT					
(Rice Dream)					
Dream Bar					
chocolate chocolate	1 bar	270	32	2	22
chocolate nutty	1 bar	270	23	2	14
vanilla	1 bar	270	33	1	21
vanilla nutty	1 bar	260	23	2	14
nondairy frozen dessert					
cappuccino	½ cup	150	23	1	17

Food and Description	Amount	Total Calories	Total Carbs	Fiber	Sugars
carob	½ cup	150	24	2	17
carob almond	½ cup	170	24	2	17
cocoa marble fudge	½ cup	150	25	2	15
Cookies 'N' Dream	½ cup	170	26	1	17
mint carob chip	½ cup	170	26	1	18
mint chocolate chip	½ cup	170	26	1	19
Neapolitan	½ cup	150	24	2	18
orange vanilla swirl	½ cup	150	24	1	18
strawberry	½ cup	140	24	1	19
vanilla	½ cup	150	23	1	17
vanilla Swiss almond	½ cup	180	25	1	18
Rice Dream nondairy pies					
chocolate	1 pie	320	39	2	13
mint	1 pie	320	39	2	13
mocha	1 pie	320	40	1	12
vanilla	1 pie	320	40	1	12
Rice Dream Supreme..Pralines 'n' Dream	½ cup	180	24	1	16
RICE NOODLE (*See* ASIAN FOOD)					
RICE SYRUP (*See also* PANCAKE & WAFFLE SYRUP)					
(Lundberg Family Farms) Sweet Dreams	1.5 oz	110	31	0	25
ROAST BEEF (*See* BEEF; LUNCHEON MEAT)					
ROAST BEEF HASH (*See* BEEF; BEEF DISH/ENTRÉE)					
ROAST BEEF SPREAD (*See* LUNCHEON MEAT SPREAD)					
ROLL (*See also* CROISSANT; PASTRY; SCONE)					
BROWN & SERVE					
(Bread du Jour)					
honey wheat	1 roll	90	18	0	3
Italian rolls	1 roll	90	16	0	2
petite dinner	1 roll	230	45	2	4
(Francisco International)					
Bolillos dinner rolls	1 roll	130	23	1	1
French rolls..6-count	1 roll	210	39	1	2
(Pepperidge Farm)					
bakery..French	½ roll	180	36	1	2
crusty	1 roll	170	15	1	2
European Bake Shoppe..club	1 roll	130	24	1	2
garlic	1 roll	160	25	1	2
(San Francisco) French..sweet..6-pack	1 roll	140	29	1	1
(Wonder) Rolls du Jour					
crusty Italian	1 roll	90	16	0	2
w/buttermilk	1 roll	80	13	1	1
FROZEN					
(Rhodes) bread dough..baked					
cinnamon roll	1 roll	240	42	1	10
cracked wheat	1 roll	140	24	3	3
fat-free	1 roll	85	17	1	1
Rhodes Anytime!..crusty..heat & serve	1 roll	100	20	1	1
sweet dough	1 slice	145	24	1	3
Texas dinner					

Food and Description	Amount	Total Calories	Total Carbs	Fiber	Sugars
wheat	1 roll	140	24	2	2
white	1 roll	150	27	1	3
white dinner	1 roll	95	17	0	2
(Sara Lee) Food Service..soft					
cloverleaf	1 roll	90	14	<1	1
Parker House	3 rolls	170	26	1	3
wheat bakery	1 roll	200	38	3	6
MIX					
(Pillsbury) Specialty Mix..hot roll..					
mix only	¼ cup	110	21	1	2
READY-YO-SERVE					
(Arnold)					
Bran'ola hot dog buns	1 bun	110	22	3	3
Bran'ola buns w/bran	1 bun	140	27	3	4
dinner rolls..enriched	1 roll	130	22	1	4
Francisco French	1 roll	190	35	2	2
hamburger buns..original..8-count	1 bun	140	24	1	4
hot dog buns..8-count					
original	1 bun	120	7	1	3
potato buns..Dutch-style	1 bun	130	24	1	4
sandwich rolls					
country wheat	1 roll	200	37	5	6
country white	1 roll	200	36	2	7
potato rolls..Dutch-style..8-count	1 roll	180	30	1	5
potato rolls..Dutch-style..sesame..					
8-count	1 roll	180	30	1	5
sesame..8-count	1 roll	140	24	1	4
(Awrey's)					
dinner..cracked wheat	2 rolls	120	22	2	4
hoagie	1 roll	230	46	1	3
kaiser	1 roll	190	37	1	4
(Brownberry)					
Bran'ola hot dog buns	1 bun	110	22	3	3
Bran'ola buns w/bran	1 bun	140	27	3	4
dinner rolls..enriched	1 roll	130	22	1	4
Francisco French	1 roll	190	35	2	2
hamburger buns..original..8-count	1 bun	140	24	1	4
hot dog buns..8-count					
original	1 bun	120	7	1	3
potato buns..Dutch-style	1 bun	130	24	1	4
sandwich rolls					
country wheat	1 roll	200	37	5	6
country white	1 roll	200	36	2	7
potato rolls..Dutch-style..8-count	1 roll	180	30	1	5
potato rolls..Dutch-style..sesame..					
8-count	1 roll	180	30	1	5
sesame..8-count	1 roll	140	24	1	4
(Ciabatta)					
dinner	1 roll	90	18	0	1
sandwich	1 roll	180	36	1	1

Food and Description	Amount	Total Calories	Total Carbs	Fiber	Sugars
(Earth Grains)					
French	1 roll	220	43	2	2
hoagies	1 roll	190	35	2	4
kaiser..cornmeal premium	1 roll	180	36	1	5
(King's Hawaiian)					
honey wheat	1 roll	90	15	0	4
multigrain	1 roll	100	15	1	4
regular	1 roll	90	15	0	4
(Panera) breads					
Asiago cheese..demi loaf	2-oz roll	140	21	<1	1
baguette loaf..roll	2.5 oz	160	32	1	1
French roll	2-oz roll	120	25	1	1
sourdough roll	2.5 oz	160	32	1	1
(Pepperidge Farm) bakery					
country-style..dinner	1 roll	90	15	<1	2
Farmhouse					
country wheat	1 roll	210	36	1	5
golden potato classic	1 roll	220	36	<1	6
hearty white	1 roll	210	35	<1	5
sesame white	1 roll	230	36	5	5
frankfurter..sliced	1 roll	140	24	<1	4
hamburger..sliced	1 roll	120	21	1	3
hoagie..soft	1 roll	200	33	2	3
Hot & Crusty					
French	1 roll	100	20	1	1
7-grain	1 roll	80	19	2	3
sourdough	1 roll	100	19	1	1
onion sandwich buns					
w/poppy seeds	1 roll	150	25	1	3
Parker House	1 roll	80	13	<1	2
(San Francisco)					
49'ers sourdough rolls	1 roll	100	20	1	1
French rolls..6 pack	1 roll	170	33	1	1
hamburger buns	1 roll	230	45	1	2
hoagie rolls	1 roll	190	36	1	2
sourdough					
dinner..8 pack	1 roll	110	21	0	1
sandwich..4 pack	1 roll	240	47	3	1
sliced..6 pack	1 roll	170	37	1	1
sweet French rolls..6 pack	1 roll	200	18	0	1
(Sara Lee)					
classic					
hamburger buns..white	1 bun	200	37	1	5
wheat baker buns	1 bun	200	36	3	6
deli rolls..center-split premium	1 roll	200	38	2	5
gourmet hot dog buns	1 bun	120	23	1	4
(SunBeam) potato..all styles					
(Wenner)					
onion swirl buns	1 bun	150	29	1	4
salt stick crescent rolls	1 roll	160	31	1	2

Food and Description	Amount	Total Calories	Total Carbs	Fiber	Sugars
(Wonder)					
hamburger or hot dog..light	1 roll	80	18	4	<1
hamburger or hot dog..original	1 bun	120	22	1	5
REFRIGERATED					
(Pillsbury)					
crescent					
Grands!	1 roll	270	22	<1	5
original	1 roll	110	11	0	2
reduced-fat	1 roll	100	12	0	2
dinner..home-baked..crusty French	1 roll	110	19	0	2
traditional..wheat or white	1 roll	110	18	<1	3
ROSELLE..raw	½ cup	15	3	<1	0
ROSEMARY..dried	1 tsp	4	1	1	0
ROTINI (*See* PASTA; PASTA ENTRÉE/DINNER)					
ROUGHY (*See* ORANGE ROUGHY; SEAFOOD ENTRÉE/DINNER)					
RUM (*See* LIQUOR, DISTILLED)					
RUTABAGA..fresh					
boiled-drained..mashed	½ cup	40	10	2	0
raw..cubed	½ cup	25	5.5	2	0
RYE (*See also* CEREAL; FLOUR; LIQUOR, DISTILLED)					
(Arrowhead Mills)					
flakes..rolled	⅓ cup	110	24	4	0
whole grain	¼ cup	160	34	6	0

S

Food and Description	Amount	Total Calories	Total Carbs	Fiber	Sugars
SABLEFISH					
cooked—dry heat	3 oz	213	0	0	0
raw	3 oz	165	0	0	0
smoked	3 oz	220	0	0	0
SAFFLOWER MARGARINE/SPREAD (*See* MARGARINE, MARGARINE SPREAD & SPRAY)					
SAFFLOWER OIL (*See* OIL)					
SAFFLOWER SEED..kernels..dried	1 oz	150	10	1	0
SAFFRON..dried	1 tsp	2	<1	0	0
SAGE..ground	1 tsp	4	<1	0	0
SALAD, CANNED/DELI/PACKAGED					
(Bumble Bee) *PACKAGED..WITH CRACKERS*					
chicken	3.5 oz	140	10	0	6
seafood w/crab	3.3 oz	200	10	0	4

Food and Description	Amount	Total Calories	Total Carbs	Fiber	Sugars
tuna					
fat-free	3.5 oz	70	10	0	5
regular	3.5 oz	190	6	1	3
(Read's) *CANNED*					
4-bean	½ cup	110	23	2	15
German potato	½ cup	120	22	2	8
3-bean	½ cup	100	23	3	15
SALAD DRESSING (*See also* MAYONNAISE/MAYONNAISE-TYPE DRESSING)					
MIX (NOTE: Unless otherwise stated, mixes prepared as directed on package.)					
(Good Seasons) mix only (makes 2 Tbs..prepared)					
cheese garlic	⅛ pkt	5	1	0	1
garlic & herb	⅛ pkt	5	1	0	1
Italian					
fat-free	⅛ pkt	10	2	0	2
mild	⅛ pkt	10	2	0	2
regular	⅛ pkt	5	1	0	1
zesty	⅛ pkt	5	1	0	1
Oriental sesame	⅛ pkt	15	3	0	2
roasted garlic	⅛ pkt	10	2	0	2
(Lawry's) mix only					
Caesar	1 pkg	75	9	0	na
Italian					
regular	1 pkg	45	9	0	na
w/cheese	1 pkg	75	12	0	na
(A Taste of Thai) spicy peanut	2 Tbs	40	7	1	5
(Weight Watchers) mix only					
(NOTE: 1 serving of mix = the amount in 2 Tbs prepared.)					
blue cheese	1 serving	8	1	0	0
French	1 serving	4	1	0	0
Italian					
creamy	1 serving	5	1	0	0
regular	1 serving	4	1	0	0
Russian	1 serving	4	1	0	0
Thousand Island	1 serving	4	1	0	0
READY-TO-USE					
(Annie's) wild herbal organics					
Asian sesame	2 Tbs	140	4	0	3
balsamic	2 Tbs	100	3	0	3
Caesar	2 Tbs	120	1	0	1
cilantro & lime	2 Tbs	100	2	1	2
Cowgirl Ranch	2 Tbs	120	3	0	2
garden-style	2 Tbs	120	2	0	<1
Gingerly	2 Tbs	100	4	0	3
Goddess	2 Tbs	130	2	0	<1
green garlic	2 Tbs	90	2	0	1
Green Goddess	2 Tbs	130	2	0	<1
papaya poppyseed	2 Tbs	120	4	0	3
Pizza Pie	2 Tbs	110	1	0	1
Thousand Island	2 Tbs	90	5	0	4
Tutti Frutti..85% organic	2 Tbs	80	3	0	2

Food and Description	Amount	Total Calories	Total Carbs	Fiber	Sugars
vinaigrettes					
balsamic	2 Tbs	100	3	0	3
basil & garlic	2 Tbs	130	1	0	0
Gingerly..low-fat	2 Tbs	40	4	0	3
honey mustard..low-fat	2 Tbs	45	6	0	6
raspberry..low-fat	2 Tbs	35	5	0	4
red wine & olive oil	2 Tbs	160	1	0	1
roasted red pepper	2 Tbs	70	3	0	2
sea veggie & sesame	2 Tbs	110	4	0	3
sesame ginger	2 Tbs	100	1	0	1
shiitake & sesame	2 Tbs	120	1	0	1
Tuscan Italian	2 Tbs	80	5	0	4
Zoom	2 Tbs	150	4	0	3
(Bernstein's)					
fat-free..cheese & garlic Italian	2 Tbs	10	2	0	1
Light Fantastic					
Cheese Fantastico	2 Tbs	25	3	0	1
Classico Italian	2 Tbs	25	3	0	2
Italian w/cheese	2 Tbs	25	2	1	0
Oriental	2 Tbs	60	10	0	6
Parmesan garlic ranch	2 Tbs	50	6	0	2
restaurant ranch	2 Tbs	45	5	0	2
roasted garlic balsamic	2 Tbs	45	3	0	2
regular					
balsamic Italian	2 Tbs	110	2	0	1
Caesar..creamy	2 Tbs	120	1	0	0
Cheese Fantastico	2 Tbs	100	3	0	1
cheese & garlic Italian	2 Tbs	110	2	0	1
chunky blue cheese	2 Tbs	120	2	0	1
creamy roasted garlic	2 Tbs	150	3	0	4
herb & garlic Italian	2 Tbs	130	3	0	2
herb garden French	2 Tbs	130	8	0	7
Italian dressing & marinade	2 Tbs	110	1	0	1
olive oil vinaigrette	2 Tbs	90	3	0	2
Parmesan garlic ranch	2 Tbs	140	2	0	1
red wine & garlic Italian	2 Tbs	110	2	0	1
restaurant-recipe Italian	2 Tbs	120	1	0	0
sweet herb Italian	2 Tbs	130	8	0	5
(Cardini's)					
aged Parmesan ranch	2 Tbs	150	2	0	1
balsamic vinaigrette	2 Tbs	150	2	0	2
Caesar					
fat-free	2 Tbs	40	9	0	3
light	2 Tbs	80	5	0	2
regular	2 Tbs	160	1	0	0
honey mustard	2 Tbs	150	5	0	4
Italian w/blue cheese crumbles	2 Tbs	130	2	0	1
Kalamata olive & Romano cheese	2 Tbs	120	2	0	1
poppyseed w/shallots	2 Tbs	160	8	0	7

Food and Description	Amount	Total Calories	Total Carbs	Fiber	Sugars
roasted Asian sesame	2 Tbs	120	7	0	6
roasted garlic	2 Tbs	130	1	0	0
Southwest Caesar	2 Tbs	140	3	0	2
white wine	2 Tbs	110	1	0	1
(Dorothy Lynch)					
fat-free	2 Tbs	30	14	0	14
home-style	2 Tbs	55	12	0	12
(Emeril's)					
Caesar	2 Tbs	130	2	0	1
honey mustard	2 Tbs	100	3	0	2
house herb vinaigrette	2 Tbs	100	1	0	1
Kicked-Up French	2 Tbs	80	8	0	7
(Girard's)					
balsamic vinaigrette					
fat-free	2 Tbs	25	6	0	4
regular	2 Tbs	90	3	0	2
blue cheese vinaigrette	2 Tbs	100	3	0	3
Caesar					
light	2 Tbs	80	5	0	1
regular	2 Tbs	150	1	0	1
champagne					
light	2 Tbs	60	2	0	1
regular	2 Tbs	150	2	0	1
French..original	2 Tbs	120	0	0	0
Greek feta vinaigrette	2 Tbs	100	1	0	0
honey Dijon peppercorn	2 Tbs	140	7	1	7
Italian					
Olde Venice	2 Tbs	130	2	0	1
Romano cheese	2 Tbs	130	2	0	1
Oriental	2 Tbs	120	6	0	5
Parmesan peppercorn	2 Tbs	160	1	0	1
raspberry					
fat-free	2 Tbs	50	13	0	11
regular	2 Tbs	120	9	0	9
red wine vinaigrette					
fat-free	2 Tbs	20	5	0	5
shiitake & chardonnay vinaigrette	2 Tbs	100	4	0	3
spinach	2 Tbs	80	14	0	12
(Henri's)					
bacon & tomato	2 Tbs	130	10	0	7
balsamic..fat-free	2 Tbs	15	4	0	3
Caesar ranch..classic	2 Tbs	140	2	0	2
cucumber..creamy	2 Tbs	90	9	0	2
French					
fat-free	2 Tbs	40	11	0	6
light..low-fat	2 Tbs	70	13	0	7
original..classic	2 Tbs	120	6	0	4
honey mustard..classic..fat-free	2 Tbs	50	12	0	10
Italian..fat-free	2 Tbs	15	4	0	2

Food and Description	Amount	Total Calories	Total Carbs	Fiber	Sugars
mustard vinaigrette	2 Tbs	90	5	0	3
ranch chef's recipe..light	2 Tbs	60	12	0	10
raspberry vinaigrette..fat-free	2 Tbs	35	10	0	7
red wine vinaigrette..fat-free	2 Tbs	15	5	0	0
slaw..fat-free	2 Tbs	50	13	0	na
sweet & sour	2 Tbs	110	8	0	na
Thousand Island..classic	2 Tbs	100	5	0	4
tomato-roasted vinaigrette	2 Tbs	90	3	0	2
(Hollywood)					
buttermilk..old-fashioned	1 Tbs	75	1	0	0
Dijon vinaigrette	1 Tbs	60	2	0	0
French..creamy	1 Tbs	70	2	0	0
Italian	1 Tbs	90	1	0	0
poppyseed ranchers	1 Tbs	75	1	0	0
(Knott's Berry Farm)					
California fruit	2 Tbs	70	8	0	6
honey poppyseed	2 Tbs	120	10	0	9
Oriental chicken salad	2 Tbs	130	5	0	4
raspberry vinaigrette..low-fat	2 Tbs	50	8	0	7
sun-dried tomato vinaigrette	2 Tbs	100	3	0	3
tropical vinaigrette..low-fat	2 Tbs	45	9	0	8
(Kraft)					
CarbWell					
classic Caesar	2 Tbs	110	0	0	0
Italian	2 Tbs	70	0	0	0
ranch	2 Tbs	100	0	0	0
Roka blue cheese	2 Tbs	120	0	0	0
fat-free					
Catalina	2 Tbs	35	8	1	7
honey Dijon	2 Tbs	50	10	1	4
Italian	2 Tbs	15	4	0	2
ranch	2 Tbs	50	11	1	2
Thousand Island	2 Tbs	40	9	1	5
Light Done Right					
blue cheese..Roka	2 Tbs	70	3	0	1
Catalina	2 Tbs	60	12	0	9
Caesar..classic	2 Tbs	60	3	0	<1
Caesar..golden	2 Tbs	70	2	0	2
creamy French	2 Tbs	80	9	0	6
Italian	2 Tbs	70	3	0	2
house	2 Tbs	40	3	0	2
regular	2 Tbs	40	3	0	2
zesty	2 Tbs	25	2	0	2
ranch	2 Tbs	80	3	0	1
buttermilk					
cucumber	2 Tbs	45	3	0	2
regular	2 Tbs	70	7	0	1
3-cheese	2 Tbs	70	2	0	1
raspberry vinaigrette	2 Tbs	60	5	0	5

Food and Description	Amount	Total Calories	Total Carbs	Fiber	Sugars
red wine vinaigrette	2 Tbs	45	3	0	2
Thousand Island	2 Tbs	60	10	0	7
Regular Dressings					
blue cheese..Roka	2 Tbs	130	2	1	1
Caesar	2 Tbs	140	1	0	0
creamy French	2 Tbs	160	5	0	5
honey Dijon	2 Tbs	110	6	0	4
Italian					
creamy	2 Tbs	110	2	0	2
3-cheese	2 Tbs	130	1	0	1
zesty	2 Tbs	110	2	0	2
ranch..original	2 Tbs	170	2	0	1
Thousand Island					
regular	2 Tbs	120	5	0	4
w/bacon	2 Tbs	130	5	0	5
Special Collection					
balsamic vinaigrette	2 Tbs	90	4	0	3
Caesar Italian w/oregano	2 Tbs	100	2	0	1
Caesar vinaigrette w/Parmesan	2 Tbs	60	1	0	1
classic Italian vinaigrette	2 Tbs	50	4	0	2
Greek	2 Tbs	110	2	0	1
Italian					
Parmesan w/basil	2 Tbs	90	2	0	2
pesto	2 Tbs	70	5	0	2
roasted garlic vinaigrette	2 Tbs	50	3	0	2
Parmesan Romano	2 Tbs	140	1	0	1
poppyseed..creamy	2 Tbs	130	8	0	8
sweet honey Catalina	2 Tbs	130	8	0	7
tangy tomato bacon	2 Tbs	130	8	0	7
(Litehouse)					
fat-free					
Caesar	2 Tbs	15	2	0	1
honey bacon	2 Tbs	50	11	0	6
honey Dijon	2 Tbs	35	8	0	5
ranch	2 Tbs	10	3	0	2
raspberry vinaigrette	2 Tbs	15	4	0	0
sesame ginger dressing & sauce	1 Tbs	18	4	0	0
vinaigrette	2 Tbs	5	2	0	1
Naturals					
balsamic vinaigrette	2 Tbs	80	4	0	3
bleu cheese vinaigrette	2 Tbs	130	3	0	2
chipotle ranch	2 Tbs	60	1	0	0
cranberry vinaigrette..fat-free	2 Tbs	25	6	0	5
creamy garlic Caesar	2 Tbs	80	<1	0	0
other..jars					
bleu cheese					
Big Bleu	2 Tbs	160	1	0	1
light	2 Tbs	70	2	0	1
original	2 Tbs	150	1	0	1

Food and Description	Amount	Total Calories	Total Carbs	Fiber	Sugars
Caesar	2 Tbs	140	1	0	0
coleslaw	2 Tbs	90	7	0	5
country ranch	2 Tbs	120	1	0	1
poppyseed	2 Tbs	130	6	0	5
ranch					
light	2 Tbs	60	2	0	1
peppercorn	2 Tbs	100	2	0	1
regular	2 Tbs	120	2	0	2
Roquefort	2 Tbs	130	1	0	1
sweet red French	2 Tbs	110	11	0	8
Thousand Island	2 Tbs	120	3	0	2
(Luna Rossa)					
key lime Caesar	2 Tbs	116	0.5	0	0
lemon garlic caper	2 Tbs	152	1	0	1
tomato Italiano	2 Tbs	152	1	0	1
Vidalia onion vinaigrette	2 Tbs	110	6	0	6
wild raspberry vinaigrette	2 Tbs	27	6	<1	3
(Maple Grove Farms)					
fat-free					
balsamic vinaigrette	2 Tbs	10	2	0	2
cranberry balsamic vinaigrette	2 Tbs	30	7	0	6
honey Dijon	2 Tbs	45	10	0	1
lime basil vinaigrette	2 Tbs	25	6	0	5
raspberry vinaigrette	2 Tbs	35	9	0	8
other dressings					
Caesar..light	2 Tbs	70	5	0	4
honey mustard..light	2 Tbs	80	9	0	9
Romano..light	2 Tbs	40	1	0	1
Vermont honey mustard	2 Tbs	120	9	0	9
(Marie's)					
blue cheese					
chunky	2 Tbs	180	3	0	0
light	2 Tbs	100	7	1	3
Caesar..creamy	2 Tbs	180	3	1	1
coleslaw	2 Tbs	150	6	0	6
feta cheese & herb	2 Tbs	170	2	1	1
honey Dijon	2 Tbs	150	6	0	6
Italian cheese blend	2 Tbs	80	3	0	2
Italian garlic..creamy	2 Tbs	180	1	0	0
jalapeño ranch	2 Tbs	160	1	0	1
Parmesan ranch	2 Tbs	180	1	0	1
peppercorn ranch	2 Tbs	130	3	0	1
poppyseed	2 Tbs	150	8	0	7
ranch..creamy	2 Tbs	190	3	0	1
raspberry vinaigrette..fat-free	2 Tbs	35	8	0	5
red wine vinaigrette	2 Tbs	60	5	0	5
Marzetti (*See* (T. Marzetti) in this section)					
(Nasoya) vegi dressings					
dill..creamy	2 Tbs	70	2	0	2
Italian..creamy	2 Tbs	60	2	0	2

Food and Description	Amount	Total Calories	Total Carbs	Fiber	Sugars
sesame garlic	2 Tbs	60	2	0	2
Thousand Island	2 Tbs	70	3	0	3
(Naturally Fresh)					
fat-free					
balsamic vinaigrette	2 Tbs	5	2	0	1
balsamic vinaigrette II	2 Tbs	80	3	0	2
honey ranch	2 Tbs	25	7	0	6
ranch	2 Tbs	20	4	0	2
raspberry vinaigrette	2 Tbs	25	7	0	6
other dressings					
bleu cheese					
classic	2 Tbs	130	1	0	0
light	2 Tbs	100	1	0	1
regular	2 Tbs	170	0	0	0
Caesar					
classic	2 Tbs	170	1	0	0
grilled	2 Tbs	140	1	0	0
classic Oriental	2 Tbs	100	9	0	8
cranberry orange	2 Tbs	45	13	<1	10
cranberry walnut	2 Tbs	110	6	0	5
French..honey	2 Tbs	120	5	0	5
ginger	2 Tbs	70	1	0	0
honey mustard					
bacon	2 Tbs	70	7	0	4
Dijon	2 Tbs	110	8	0	8
light	2 Tbs	80	6	<1	5
Italian					
fat-free	2 Tbs	5	2	0	1
4-cheese	2 Tbs	110	3	0	3
herb vinaigrette	2 Tbs	110	0	0	0
light	2 Tbs	5	2	0	1
poppyseed	2 Tbs	140	6	0	5
ranch					
classic	2 Tbs	150	1	0	1
fat-free	2 Tbs	20	4	0	2
light	2 Tbs	80	2	0	1
pesto	2 Tbs	70	2	0	1
slaw	2 Tbs	120	6	0	6
Thousand Island	2 Tbs	120	4	0	3
wine & cheese	2 Tbs	140	3	0	2
(Newman's Own)					
balsamic vinaigrette					
light	2 Tbs	45	2	0	1
regular	2 Tbs	90	3	0	1
Caesar					
creamy	2 Tbs	150	1	0	1
original	2 Tbs	150	1	1	1
family recipe					
Italian..light	2 Tbs	60	0	0	0
Italian..original	2 Tbs	150	1	0	1

Food and Description	Amount	Total Calories	Total Carbs	Fiber	Sugars
olive oil & vinegar	2 Tbs	150	1	0	1
Parmesan roasted garlic	2 Tbs	110	2	0	1
parmesano Italiano	2 Tbs	140	2	0	1
ranch	2 Tbs	140	2	0	2
raspberry walnut..light	2 Tbs	70	5	1	5
red wine vinegar & olive oil	2 Tbs	110	3	0	3
Two Thousand Island	2 Tbs	140	4	0	3
(Pfeiffer)					
balsamic vinaigrette	2 Tbs	100	4	0	4
blue cheese	2 Tbs	170	1	0	1
Caesar..original	2 Tbs	120	1	0	1
coleslaw	2 Tbs	170	6	0	6
French..California					
fat-free	2 Tbs	40	9	0	9
original	2 Tbs	150	7	0	7
honey Dijon	2 Tbs	140	6	0	6
Italian					
creamy	2 Tbs	160	1	0	1
original					
fat-free	2 Tbs	20	4	0	3
light	2 Tbs	50	3	0	2
regular	2 Tbs	100	3	0	2
Tuscan	2 Tbs	110	1	0	1
zesty garlic	2 Tbs	100	3	0	2
peppercorn..regular	2 Tbs	180	2	0	1
ranch					
garden	2 Tbs	160	1	0	1
original	2 Tbs	150	1	0	1
red wine vinaigrette	2 Tbs	90	3	0	3
roasted garlic vinaigrette	2 Tbs	130	8	0	8
Russian	2 Tbs	140	4	0	4
sweet & sour	2 Tbs	160	10	0	10
Thousand Island					
fat-free	2 Tbs	45	0	0	0
light	2 Tbs	70	6	0	5
regular	2 Tbs	140	4	0	4
(S&W) Vintage Lites..fat-free					
Italian balsamic	2 Tbs	35	8	0	8
raspberry blush	2 Tbs	40	10	0	10
red wine & herb	2 Tbs	40	10	0	10
white wine & herb	2 Tbs	40	10	0	10
(Seven Seas)					
blue cheese..chunky	2 Tbs	130	2	<1	<1
Caesar..classic	2 Tbs	100	2	0	1
Green Goddess	2 Tbs	130	1	0	1
herbs & spices	2 Tbs	90	1	0	1
Italian					
creamy					
reduced-fat	2 Tbs	45	2	0	1
regular	2 Tbs	110	2	0	2

Food and Description	Amount	Total Calories	Total Carbs	Fiber	Sugars
Viva					
fat-free	2 Tbs	15	2	0	2
reduced-fat	2 Tbs	45	2	0	1
regular	2 Tbs	90	2	0	1
robust	2 Tbs	90	2	1	1
w/olive oil	2 Tbs	50	2	0	2
ranch					
fat-free	2 Tbs	45	11	1	2
reduced-calorie	2 Tbs	100	5	0	2
regular	2 Tbs	160	2	0	1
raspberry vinaigrette	2 Tbs	30	7	0	7
red wine vinegar..fat-free	2 Tbs	15	3	0	3
red wine vinegar & oil					
reduced-fat	2 Tbs	45	3	0	2
regular	2 Tbs	90	2	0	2
(Simply Delicious) organic					
curry peanut	2 Tbs	80	1	0	0
ginger plum	2 Tbs	70	1	0	0
herb garlic	2 Tbs	90	1	0	0
honey mustard	2 Tbs	90	4	0	3
lemon tahini	2 Tbs	110	1	0	0
miso sesame	2 Tbs	70	1	0	0
shiitake sesame	2 Tbs	80	1	0	0
tofu poppyseed	2 Tbs	90	1	0	0
(T. Marzetti)					
balsamic vinaigrette					
light	2 Tbs	50	4	0	4
Marzetti	2 Tbs	100	4	0	4
Marzetti organic	2 Tbs	150	1	0	0
organic	2 Tbs	90	3	0	3
regular	2 Tbs	100	4	0	4
blue cheese					
chunky	2 Tbs	150	2	0	1
Italian vinaigrette	2 Tbs	100	3	0	3
light	2 Tbs	90	6	1	2
organic	2 Tbs	130	1	0	1
sour cream	2 Tbs	170	1	0	0
Caesar					
creamy	2 Tbs	150	1	0	1
light	2 Tbs	70	2	0	2
Marzetti creamy	2 Tbs	160	1	0	0
organic	2 Tbs	150	1	0	0
original	2 Tbs	120	1	0	1
French					
blue cheese	2 Tbs	160	11	0	10
California					
fat-free	2 Tbs	40	10	0	8
light	2 Tbs	90	8	0	7
regular	2 Tbs	160	11	0	11
country..pourable	2 Tbs	160	7	0	6

Food and Description	Amount	Total Calories	Total Carbs	Fiber	Sugars
honey	2 Tbs	80	12	0	12
honey..produce	2 Tbs	170	10	0	10
garlic vinaigrette..Marzetti	2 Tbs	90	4	0	4
Greek vinaigrette	2 Tbs	80	1	0	1
honey Dijon					
fat-free	2 Tbs	50	12	0	11
regular	2 Tbs	140	6	0	6
Italian					
creamy	2 Tbs	160	1	0	1
fat-free	2 Tbs	20	4	0	3
garlic	2 Tbs	100	3	0	2
light	2 Tbs	60	3	0	2
original	2 Tbs	100	3	0	2
roasted garlic vinaigrette	2 Tbs	120	2	0	1
Romano..pourable	2 Tbs	150	1	0	1
Tuscan..Marzetti	2 Tbs	110	1	0	1
Parmesan..organic	2 Tbs	140	2	0	1
peppercorn Parmesan	2 Tbs	160	1	0	1
poppyseed					
fat-free	2 Tbs	60	14	0	9
pourable..Marzetti	2 Tbs	160	11	0	10
regular	2 Tbs	140	10	0	10
ranch					
buttermilk					
light	2 Tbs	90	3	0	1
regular	2 Tbs	160	2	0	1
original					
fat-free	2 Tbs	25	7	1	3
light	2 Tbs	80	5	1	2
regular	2 Tbs	150	1	0	1
Parmesan	2 Tbs	140	2	0	1
peppercorn	2 Tbs	180	2	0	1
raspberry vinaigrette	2 Tbs	100	6	0	6
red wine vinaigrette	2 Tbs	90	3	0	3
roasted garlic dressing	2 Tbs	150	2	0	1
roasted garlic vinaigrette	2 Tbs	130	8	0	8
sesame Oriental..Marzetti	2 Tbs	110	8	0	8
slaw					
light	2 Tbs	100	10	0	8
low-fat	2 Tbs	60	11	0	9
regular	2 Tbs	170	6	0	6
Southern recipe	2 Tbs	150	14	0	14
spinach	2 Tbs	80	14	0	12
sun-dried tomato vinaigrette	2 Tbs	130	6	0	6
sweet & sour	2 Tbs	160	10	0	10
sweet Italian..produce	2 Tbs	150	7	0	7
Thousand Island					
fat-free	2 Tbs	45	11	0	7
light	2 Tbs	70	6	0	5
original	2 Tbs	140	4	0	4

Food and Description	Amount	Total Calories	Total Carbs	Fiber	Sugars
(Walden Farms)					
carb-free..sugar-free					
balsamic vinegar	2 Tbs	40	0	0	0
hot bacon	2 Tbs	40	0	0	0
Italian	2 Tbs	20	2	0	0
ranch	2 Tbs	40	0	0	0
Thousand Island	2 Tbs	40	0	0	0
fat-free..calorie-free..carb & sugar-free..					
all styles & flavors	2 Tbs	0	0	0	0
organic dressings					
balsamic vinaigrette	2 Tbs	80	5	0	4
bleu cheese	2 Tbs	110	2	0	2
Caesar	2 Tbs	120	2	0	1
honey Dijon	2 Tbs	100	6	0	5
ranch	2 Tbs	110	4	0	4
(Weight Watchers)					
Salad Celebrations..fat-free					
French	2 Tbs	40	9	0	6
honey Dijon	2 Tbs	45	11	0	5
Italian					
creamy	2 Tbs	30	7	0	2
regular	2 Tbs	10	2	0	1
ranch	2 Tbs	35	7	0	3
(Western)					
blue cheese	2 Tbs	140	12	0	11
French					
creamy	2 Tbs	140	11	0	9
fat-free	2 Tbs	45	11	0	10
Just 2 Good!					
low-fat	2 Tbs	70	13	0	12
regular	2 Tbs	70	12	0	11
The Original	2 Tbs	160	12	0	11
w/bacon flavor	2 Tbs	140	10	0	8
(Wish-Bone)					
balsamic vinaigrette	2 Tbs	60	3	0	3
Italian	2 Tbs	70	5	0	4
berry vinaigrette	2 Tbs	50	2	0	2
blue cheese					
chunky					
fat-free	2 Tbs	35	7	<1	3
regular	2 Tbs	160	2	0	1
Just 2 Good!	2 Tbs	45	6	0	2
Caesar					
creamy	2 Tbs	170	1	0	<1
low-fat	2 Tbs	40	7	0	2
Just 2 Good!..classic	2 Tbs	45	5	0	2
citrus splash vinaigrette	2 Tbs	90	7	0	4
creamy roasted garlic..fat-free	2 Tbs	40	9	0	3
French					
Just 2 Good!					

Food and Description	Amount	Total Calories	Total Carbs	Fiber	Sugars
deluxe	2 Tbs	50	8	<1	6
sweet 'n' spicy	2 Tbs	50	9	0	5
sweet 'n' spicy	2 Tbs	130	6	0	5
honey Dijon					
Just 2 Good!..low-fat	2 Tbs	50	8	0	5
vinaigrette	2 Tbs	80	6	0	4
Italian					
creamy..fat-free	2 Tbs	10	2	0	1
5-cheese	2 Tbs	120	6	0	2
house	2 Tbs	100	3	0	2
Just 2 Good!					
country	2 Tbs	30	3	0	2
low-fat	2 Tbs	35	5	0	4
Parmesan basil..low-fat	2 Tbs	45	6	0	2
regular	2 Tbs	35	5	0	4
original					
fat-free	2 Tbs	10	2	0	1
regular	2 Tbs	80	3	0	2
robusto	2 Tbs	90	4	0	3
lemon garlic & herb vinaigrette	2 Tbs	70	5	0	3
olive oil vinaigrette	2 Tbs	60	4	0	3
Parmesan & onion	2 Tbs	110	5	0	1
ranch					
classic	2 Tbs	140	2	0	1
fat-free	2 Tbs	40	9	1	2
garlic	2 Tbs	150	2	0	1
Just 2 Good! low-fat	2 Tbs	40	5	0	2
original	2 Tbs	160	1	0	1
peppercorn..low-fat	2 Tbs	45	6	1	0
spring onion	2 Tbs	140	2	0	1
zesty	2 Tbs	140	2	0	2
red wine vinaigrette					
fat-free	2 Tbs	30	7	0	6
regular	2 Tbs	90	9	0	8
roasted garlic vinaigrette	2 Tbs	70	3	0	3
Russian	2 Tbs	110	14	0	6
Thousand Island					
Just 2 Good!	2 Tbs	60	9	0	5
regular	2 Tbs	130	6	0	6
zesty	2 Tbs	140	2	0	2
SALAD TOPPINGS & MIXES (*See also* BACON BITS, CHIPS & PIECES; CROUTONS; SEASONINGS)					
(Fresh Gourmet)					
Almond Toppers					
country ranch	1 Tbs	40	1	1	0
roasted garlic	1 Tbs	40	1	1	0
robust Parmesan	1 Tbs	40	1	1	0
spicy Szechuan	1 Tbs	40	1	1	0
sun-dried tomato basil	1 Tbs	45	1	1	0
(Hidden Valley)					

Food and Description	Amount	Total Calories	Total Carbs	Fiber	Sugars
Salad Crispins					
bacon & onion	1 Tbs	35	4	0	2
cheddar & onion	1 Tbs	35	4	0	2
Italian Parmesan	1 Tbs	35	4	0	2
ranch	1 Tbs	35	4	0	2
sour cream & herb	1 Tbs	35	4	0	2
(McCormick/Schilling)					
Salad Toppins					
garden vegetable	1⅓ Tbs	30	2	0	2
original	1⅓ Tbs	35	2	0	2
SALAMI (See LUNCHEON MEAT; SAUSAGE)					
SALMON (See also SALMON SPREAD; SEAFOOD ENTRÉE/DINNER)					
CANNED					
(Black Top) chum..Alaska	2.10 oz	90	0	0	0
pink	2.25 oz	90	0	0	0
Alaska	2.10 oz	90	0	0	0
chunk-style..skinless..boneless	2.4 oz	60	0	0	0
red..sockeye					
fancy	2.25 oz	110	0	0	0
fancy Alaska	2.10 oz	110	0	0	0
(Bumble Bee)					
blueback..Alaska..fancy	2.14 oz	110	0	0	0
keta..Alaska	2.11 oz	90	0	0	0
pink					
Alaska	¼ cup	90	0	0	0
fancy	¼ cup	160	0	0	0
regular	¼ cup	90	0	0	0
skinless..boneless	¼ cup	50	0	0	0
red..Alaska sockeye	¼ cup	110	0	0	0
(Chicken of the Sea)					
pink					
chunk-style..skinless..boneless					
in spring water	2 oz	60	0	0	0
traditional	2 oz	90	0	0	0
red					
chunk-style..skinless..boneless	2 oz	60	0	0	0
traditional	2 oz	110	0	0	0
(Deming's) Alaska					
keta	¼ cup	70	0	0	0
pink	¼ cup	90	0	0	0
red sockeye	¼ cup	110	0	0	0
(Ducktrap River)					
Atlantic					
Kendall Brook	2 oz	130	0	0	0
Spruce Point	2 oz	110	0	0	0
pastrami-style..Spruce Point	2 oz	130	0	0	0
roasted	2 oz	100	0	0	0
(Geisha)					
pink..all styles	2 oz	90	0	0	0
red..fresh..Alaska	2 oz	110	0	0	0

Food and Description	Amount	Total Calories	Total Carbs	Fiber	Sugars
(Lasco)					
sliced..smoked	2 oz	60	3	0	<1
tulip pink	¼ cup	90	0	0	<1
fresh					
Atlantic..cooked—dry heat	3 oz	175	0	0	0
chinook..smoked..cooked—dry heat	3 oz	195	0	0	0
chum..keta..cooked—dry heat	3 oz	130	0	0	0
coho..cooked—dry heat	3 oz	150	0	0	0
pink..cooked—dry heat	3 oz	130	0	0	0
red/sockeye..cooked—dry heat	3 oz	150	0	0	0
smoked					
chinook..lox	3 oz	100	0	0	0
(Duck Trap River) pâté	¼ cup	150	1	0	<1
SALMON CAVIAR (See also CAVIAR)					
(Crown Prince) Alaskan coho salmon	1 Tbs	30	1	0	0
SALMON SPREAD (Vita) smoked	¼ cup	180	29	0	na
SALSA (See MEXICAN FOOD; SAUCE)					
SALSIFY..fresh..sliced					
cooked-drained	½ cup	46	10	2	0
raw	½ cup	55	12	2	0
SALT (See also SEASONINGS)					
(Durkee) seasoned or unseasoned	½ tsp	0	0	0	0
(Hain) sea salt..all styles	1 tsp	0	0	0	0
(McCormick/Schilling) Salt 'n' Spice	¼ tsp	0	0	0	0
SALT PORK (See PORK)					
SALT SUBSTITUTE (See also SEASONINGS)					
(Durkee) seasoned or unseasoned	½ tsp	0	0	0	0
(Estee) Salt It	⅛ tsp	0	0	0	0
(Health Valley) Instead of Salt	1 tsp	0	0	0	0
(McCormick/Schilling) Salt-Less..all styles	¼ tsp	0	0	0	0
SANDWICH SPREAD (See also LUNCHEON MEAT SPREAD)					
(Hellman's)					
original	1 Tbs	60	5	3	0
reduced-fat	1 Tbs	35	4	0	3
(Kraft)					
original	1 Tbs	45	3	0	2
reduced-fat	1 Tbs	32	4	0	3
Super Easy Squeeze	1 Tbs	35	2	0	2
(Loma Linda)	¼ cup	80	7	3	–
SAPODILLO..Tropical American	1 medium	140	34	9	0
SAPOTE..fresh	1 medium	300	76	6	0
SARDINE					
(Chicken of the Sea)					
Fancy Brisling					
in chili sauce	2 oz	90	1	1	1
in hot sauce	2 oz	70	1	1	1
in mustard sauce	2 oz	80	1	1	1
in olive oil	2 oz	210	2	0	0
in water	⅓ cup	80	1	0	0
tall sardines in water	2 oz	80	1	0	0

Food and Description	Amount	Total Calories	Total Carbs	Fiber	Sugars
(Crown Prince)					
1-layer brisling					
in mustard..3.79 oz	1 can	210	<1	<1	0
in olive oil..3.5 oz	1 can	230	<1	<1	<1
in water..2.9 oz	1 can	210	0	1	0
2-layer brisling..in olive oil..2.9 oz	1 can	210	0	1	0
skinless..boneless..in water..3.2 oz	1 can	140	1	<1	<1
(Goya)					
in lemon sauce	¼ cup	120	0	0	0
in tomato sauce	¼ cup	130	1	0	0
spiced	¼ cup	120	0	0	0
(King Oscar)					
in pure spring water	3.75 oz	173	0	0	0
(Underwood)					
in mustard sauce	3.73 oz	180	2	1	0
in soybean oil	2.96 oz	220	1	0	0
(Viking's Delight) brisling..in olive oil					
drained	3.75 oz	260	1	0	0
undrained	3.75 oz	460	1	0	0
SAUCE (*See also* ASIAN FOOD, Sauces & Seasonings entry; BARBECUE SAUCE; GRAVY; MARINADE; MEXICAN FOOD; PASTA ENTRÉE/DINNER; SEASONINGS; TOMATO SAUCE)					
MIX					
(Adolph's) Meal Makers..mix only					
beef stew	1 Tbs	10	3	0	0
chili	1 Tbs	30	5	<1	<1
meat loaf	1 Tbs	25	5	0	<1
(Durkee) prepared according to pkg directions					
à la king	1 cup	60	8	0	2
cheese					
nacho	2 Tbs	25	4	0	0
original	¼ cup	25	4	0	0
hollandaise	2 Tbs	10	2	0	0
white	¼ cup	20	20	5	0
(Knorr) as packaged					
Classic Sauce					
béarnaise	1⁄10 pkg	10	2	0	0
hollandaise	1⁄10 pkg	10	2	0	0
hot	1⁄10 pkg	10	2	0	0
meat	1⁄9 pkg	30	7	0	5
Newburg	⅕ pkg	35	5	0	2
peppercorn	⅕ pkg	25	3	0	0
Knorr sauce..made from vegetables & spices	2 Tbs	25	6	0	4
Mexican cooking sauces					
adobo	½ cup	50	7	0	1.5
chipotle	½ cup	60	7	0	3
guajillo	½ cup	50	8	0	2
mole	½ cup	130	20	0	10
pasilla	½ cup	40	6	0	1
pipian	½ cup	120	15	0	4

Food and Description	Amount	Total Calories	Total Carbs	Fiber	Sugars
seasoned tomato	½ cup	45	7	1	1
(Lawry's) mix only					
sauce seasoning mixes					
au jus	1 Tbs	25	4	0	0
beef stew	1 tsp	10	2	0	0
beef Stroganoff	1 tsp	20	5	0	<1
burrito	2 tsp	20	4	<1	0
chicken fajitas	1 tsp	10	2	0	0
chicken taco	2 tsp	20	5	<1	2
chili	1 tsp	10	2	0	0
enchilada	2 tsp	20	4	0	0
hot taco	2 tsp	15	3	<1	0
meat loaf	1 Tbs	30	7	<1	2
Mexican rice	1⅓ Tbs	30	6	0	0
salsa..fresh	½ tsp	5	1	0	0
sloppy joes	2 tsp	20	5	0	3
spaghetti sauce..extra rich & thick	1 Tbs	30	7	<1	2
taco	2 tsp	15	3	<1	0
turkey	1 Tbs	25	4	0	0
(McCormick)					
chicken sauce blends..dry mix only					
Dijon	¼ pkg	40	5	1	1
lemon herb chicken	⅛ pkg	30	5	0	0
teriyaki	¼ pkg	40	5	0	1
McCormick Collection..dry mix only					
béarnaise	1/10 pkg	10	1	0	0
hollandaise	1/10 pkg	15	1	0	0
hunter	¼ pkg	25	4	0	1
pepper medley	¼ cup	30	3	0	0
pesto	¼ pkg	10	1	0	0
pasta sauce blend..dry mix only					
creamy garlic Alfredo	½ pkg	90	4	0	2
pasta rosa	¼ pkg	40	4	0	2
pesto	¼ pkg	10	1	0	0
spaghetti w/mushrooms	⅕ pkg	25	5	0	3
sauces..dry mix only					
beef Stroganoff	⅛ pkg	15	3	0	na
enchilada	⅛ pkg	15	3	0	na
hollandaise	1/10 pkg	15	1	0	0
spaghetti					
thick & zesty	⅕ pkg	25	6	0	3
w/mushroom	⅕ pkg	25	5	0	3
seafood sauce..lemon butter dill	⅛ pkg	120	4	0	0
(Old Bay) mix only					
crab cake classic	1 Tbs	30	2	0	0
salmon classic	5 tsp	40	3	0	0
tuna classic	1 Tbs	30	2	0	0
(A Taste of Thai) mix only					
fish	1 Tbs	15	1	0	0
chicken & rice	¼ pkt	15	3	0	3

Food and Description	Amount	Total Calories	Total Carbs	Fiber	Sugars
garlic chili pepper	1 tsp	10	2	0	2
pad Thai	2 Tbs	90	20	1	16
peanut sauce	¼ pkg	45	7	1	5
satay sauce..peanut	2 Tbs	80	9	1	5
spicy Thai peanut	¼ pkg	45	7	1	5
sweet red chili	1 tsp	10	2	0	2
READY-TO-USE					
(A1) steak sauce					
bold & spicy	1 Tbs	20	5	0	3
Chicago steakhouse	1 Tbs	20	2	0	2
original	1 Tbs	15	3	0	2
steak sauce..regular	1 Tbs	15	3	0	2
(Atkins) Quick Quisine					
regular sauce & marinade	1 Tbs	5	1	0	0
teriyaki sauce & marinade	1 Tbs	10	1	0	0
(Aunt Nellie's) old-style sauce	1 Tbs	70	3	0	3
(Barilla) pasta sauce					
Italian baking sauce	½ cup	210	21	3	11
lasagna	½ cup	210	21	3	11
marinara	½ cup	80	9	3	5
mushroom & garlic	½ cup	80	9	3	5
roasted garlic & onion	½ cup	80	9	3	5
spicy pepper	½ cup	80	9	3	5
sweet peppers & garlic	½ cup	80	9	3	5
tomato & basil	½ cup	80	12	3	7
(Bertolli Lucca) pasta sauces					
creamy Alfredo	¼ cup	110	3	0	1
creamy garlic Alfredo	¼ cup	100	3	0	1
5-cheese..w/Asiago & fontina	½ cup	90	11	3	9
w/Italian sausage, garlic & Romano	½ cup	90	11	3	9
marinara w/burgundy wine	½ cup	80	11	3	9
Mediterranean olive w/sun-dried tomatoes	½ cup	100	13	2	3
mushroom w/white wine	¼ cup	80	3	0	1
olive oil & garlic w/fresh tomatoes	½ cup	90	9	2	8
portobello mushroom w/garlic	½ cup	80	11	3	9
roasted red pepper w/Italian herbs	½ cup	80	13	2	3
summer vegetable w/bell pepper & onion	½ cup	80	11	3	9
tomato & basil w/fresh tomatoes	½ cup	80	10	3	9
traditional basil w/extra-virgin olive oil	½ cup	270	4	0	0
Vidalia onion w/roasted garlic	½ cup	80	10	3	9
(Best Foods)					
dipping sauce..Rockin' Ranch..squeeze	1 Tbs	50	<1	0	0
tartar sauce..original	2 Tbs	80	3	0	2
(Boar's Head)					
cooking sauce					
brown sugar & spice ham glaze	2 Tbs	120	30	0	29
horseradish sauce..pub-style	1 tsp	15	1	0	0
sweet Vidalia onions & sauce	1 Tbs	10	2	0	2

Food and Description	Amount	Total Calories	Total Carbs	Fiber	Sugars
(Buitoni) pasta sauce..refrigerated					
Alfredo					
light	¼ cup	80	5	0	2
regular	¼ cup	140	5	0	2
garden vegetable	½ cup	40	9	2	7
marinara	½ cup	80	11	2	7
roasted garlic	½ cup	60	9	1	6
pesto w/basil					
reduced-fat	¼ cup	230	9	2	5
regular	¼ cup	300	9	2	4
w/sun-dried tomatoes	¼ cup	210	9	2	4
portobello mushroom marinara	½ cup	80	11	2	7
tomato herb	½ cup	120	9	2	7
(Carb Fit) pasta sauce					
portobello mushroom	½ cup	60	7	2	2
puttanesca	½ cup	60	7	1	1
tomato basil	½ cup	60	7	2	2
vodka	½ cup	100	7	2	2
(Carb Options)					
Alfredo sauce	¼ cup	110	2	0	0
double cheddar sauce	¼ cup	90	2	0	0
Italian garlic marinade	1 Tbs	0	0	0	0
steak sauce	1 Tbs	5	1	0	0
(Chef Paul's)					
Magic Sauce & Marinades					
pepper sauce	1 tsp	0	0	0	0
sauce & marinades					
California sun-dried tomato	1 Tbs	17	6	0	4
Louisiana red pepper	1 Tbs	16	5	0	3
Southwest chipotle	1 Tbs	16	2	0	1
(China Bowl)					
chili paste w/garlic	2 Tbs	15	3	<1	<1
hoisin	1 tsp	10	3	0	2
oyster	½ tsp	5	1	0	2
(Classico) pasta sauces					
Alfredo					
regular	¼ cup	100	3	0	1
roasted garlic	¼ cup	100	3	0	1
sun-dried tomato	¼ cup	120	4	2	4
cabernet marinara..w/herbs	½ cup	60	10	2	6
Florentine spinach & cheese	½ cup	80	6	2	5
4-cheese	½ cup	90	10	1	5
garden vegetable primavera	½ cup	60	13	2	8
Italian sausage w/peppers & onions	½ cup	90	13	2	8
mushrooms & ripe olives	½ cup	60	11	2	6
pesto					
basil	¼ cup	230	6	1	2
sun-dried tomato	¼ cup	90	8	1	5
roasted chicken w/Parmesan & garlic	½ cup	90	13	2	8
spicy red pepper & pesto	½ cup	90	7	2	5

Food and Description	Amount	Total Calories	Total Carbs	Fiber	Sugars
sweet basil marinara	½ cup	70	13	1	9
tomato & basil	½ cup	60	11	2	6
triple mushroom	½ cup	80	12	3	5
(Contadina)					
pizza sauce					
flavored w/pepperoni	¼ cup	35	5	<1	3
4-cheese	¼ cup	30	6	2	2
original	¼ cup	30	6	1	2
squeeze bottle	¼ cup	30	6	1	1
sweet & sour sauce w/pineapple	1 Tbs	40	8	0	6
(Crosse & Blackwell) sauce					
brandied hard	2 Tbs	180	26	0	25
mint	1 Tbs	5	1	0	1
seafood cocktail	¼ cup	110	25	0	13
shrimp..zesty	¼ cup	110	25	0	13
steak	1 Tbs	30	7	0	6
Worcestershire	1 Tbs	5	1	0	1
(Crystal)					
cayenne sauce..all styles	1 tsp	0	0	0	0
chicken wing sauce..hot	1 oz	25	6	0	3
habañero sauce	1 tsp	0	0	0	0
hot sauce..all styles	1 tsp	0	0	0	0
soy sauce..original	1 Tbs	20	4	0	1
steak sauce					
bold	1 tsp	5	1	0	1
original	1 Tbs	15	4	0	2
sweet & sour sauce	2 Tbs	60	16	0	14
wing sauce					
barbecue	2 Tbs	45	12	0	6
extra-hot	2 Tbs	25	6	0	3
original	2 Tbs	25	6	0	3
(Del Monte)					
chili sauce	1 Tbs	20	5	0	4
seafood cocktail sauce	¼ cup	100	24	0	22
sloppy joe sauce					
hickory flavor	¼ cup	60	14	0	11
original recipe	¼ cup	60	11	0	9
spaghetti sauce					
4-cheese	½ cup	70	15	3	10
garlic & herb/chunky	½ cup	60	11	<1	9
w/garlic & onion	½ cup	80	16	2	10
w/green peppers & mushrooms	½ cup	80	16	3	10
Italian herb/chunky	½ cup	60	12	<1	8
w/meat	½ cup	60	14	3	9
w/mushrooms	½ cup	60	14	2	9
tomato & basil	½ cup	70	16	3	11
traditional	½ cup	60	14	3	9
(Di Giorno) pasta sauce..refrigerated					
Alfredo	¼ cup	180	3	0	2
basil pesto	¼ cup	310	2	<1	<1

Food and Description	Amount	Total Calories	Total Carbs	Fiber	Sugars
4-cheese	¼ cup	160	3	0	2
marinara	½ cup	70	12	2	10
mushroom marinara	½ cup	60	11	2	8
(Eden)					
pasta sauce..all styles	½ cup	125	12	3	6
soy sauce..shoyu					
imported..all styles	1 Tbs	15	2	0	0
reduced-sodium	1 Tbs	10	2	0	0
tamari					
domestic	1 Tbs	15	2	0	0
imported	1 Tbs	10	2	0	0
(Emeril's) pasta Sauces					
Kicked-Up Tomato	½ cup	70	9	2	4
puttanesca	½ cup	80	9	2	0
roasted garlic	½ cup	70	10	2	3
roasted red pepper	½ cup	60	7	2	3
vodka	½ cup	130	13	2	2
(Five Brothers) pasta sauce					
Alfredo					
creamy	¼ cup	110	3	0	1
creamy garlic	¼ cup	100	3	0	1
mushroom	¼ cup	80	3	0	1
tomato basil	¼ cup	80	10	3	9
basil...traditional w/extra-virgin olive oil	½ cup	270	4	0	0
4-cheese/quattro formaggio	¼ cup	90	11	3	9
5-cheese	½ cup	90	11	3	9
grilled summer vegetable	½ cup	80	11	3	9
marinara w/burgundy wine	½ cup	80	11	3	9
Mediterranean tomato & olive	½ cup	100	13	2	3
mushroom & garlic	½ cup	80	11	3	9
portobello mushroom w/white wine	½ cup	80	3	0	1
roasted red pepper..w/Italian herbs	½ cup	80	13	2	3
Vidalia onion w/roasted garlic	½ cup	80	10	3	9
(Full Circle) organic pasta sauces					
Parmesan cheese	½ cup	50	8	3	4
portobello mushroom	½ cup	50	8	2	5
roasted garlic	½ cup	50	9	2	4
tomato basil	½ cup	60	9	3	4
(Golden Dipt)					
cocktail sauce..all styles	¼ cup	100	18	<1	14
lemon butter dill	2 Tbs	35	7	0	5
tartar sauce					
fat-free	2 Tbs	35	6	0	na
regular	2 Tbs	160	3	0	3
(Healthy Choice) pasta sauce					
creamy Alfredo	¼ cup	45	3	0	0
garlic & herbs	½ cup	60	13	3	6
garlic lovers	½ cup	45	10	3	7

Food and Description	Amount	Total Calories	Total Carbs	Fiber	Sugars
mushroom & sweet peppers..chunky	½ cup	45	16	3	7
super chunky vegetables	½ cup	50	13	3	9
super tomato, mushroom & garlic	½ cup	45	16	3	7
traditional	½ cup	60	13	3	9
(Heinz)					
chili sauce	1 Tbs	15	4	0	4
Heinz 57 steak sauce..all styles	1 Tbs	20	4	0	4
horseradish	1 Tbs	60	3	0	na
sloppy joe sauce	½ cup	70	14	2	3
Worcestershire	1 tsp	0	0	0	0
(Hellmann's)					
Dippin' Sauce					
Honey Mustard Madness..squeeze	1 Tbs	40	4	0	3
Rockin' Ranch..squeeze	1 Tbs	50	<1	0	0
tartar sauce					
low-fat	2 Tbs	40	7	0	0
original	2 Tbs	80	7	3	0
(Hoffman House)					
chili sauce	1 Tbs	10	5	0	4
shrimp & seafood	1 Tbs	110	16	0	13
tartar	2 Tbs	90	4	0	3
(Hormel) Not-So-Sloppy Joe Sauce	¼ cup	60	13	1	8
(House of Tsang)(*See* ASIAN FOOD)					
(Hunt's)					
Family Favorites sauce mixes					
chili sauce	2 oz	25	5	1	3
lasagna	2 oz	30	6	1	5
meat loaf	2 oz	30	7	2	4
pizza sauce	2 oz	25	5	1	3
Manwich					
BBQ	¼ cup	50	12	1	10
bold	¼ cup	60	13	1	11
original	¼ cup	30	7	0	4
spaghetti sauce					
cheese & garlic	½ cup	50	9	2	7
chunky vegetable	½ cup	50	11	3	8
4-cheese	½ cup	50	10	3	7
garlic & herb	½ cup	50	10	3	7
Italian sausage	½ cup	60	10	3	7
light	½ cup	45	9	3	6
meat	½ cup	60	11	3	7
mushroom	½ cup	50	10	3	7
no salt added	½ cup	45	9	3	6
roasted garlic & onion	½ cup	50	10	3	7
traditional	½ cup	50	10	3	7
(Jack Daniel's) grilling sauce					
honey	2 Tbs	50	12	0	11
original	2 Tbs	50	12	0	8
spicy	2 Tbs	50	12	0	8

Food and Description	Amount	Total Calories	Total Carbs	Fiber	Sugars
Tennessee hickory (Kaukauna) cheese sauce	2 Tbs	50	12	0	8
Micro Melts..squeeze..real cheddar	1 oz	90	4	0	3
Micro Melts..real cheddar & jalapeño	1 oz	90	4	0	3
Squeeze..nacho cheese	1 oz	80	4	0	3
(Kikkoman)					
chili sauce..Thai-style	2 Tbs	70	15	1	15
dipping sauce					
plum sauce	1 oz	80	18	0	17
sweet & sour	1 Tbs	35	9	0	7
hoisin sauce	2 Tbs	80	17	0	16
marinade & sauce					
roasted garlic teriyaki	1 Tbs	25	5	0	3
teriyaki	1 Tbs	15	2	0	2
teriyaki light	1 Tbs	15	3	0	3
soy sauce & dressing..ponzu citrus	1 tbs	10	2	0	2
light	1 Tbs	10	1	0	0
regular	1 Tbs	10	0	0	0
sushi & sashimi	1 Tbs	15	2	0	2
steak sauce	1 Tbs	20	5	0	4
stir-fry..regular	1 Tbs	20	4	0	3
sukiyaki	1 Tbs	20	4	0	4
sweet & sour	1 Tbs	35	9	0	7
teriyaki	1 Tbs	15	2	0	2
roasted garlic	1 Tbs	25	5	0	3
teriyaki baste & glaze					
regular	2 Tbs	50	11	0	9
w/honey & pineapple	2 Tbs	80	18	0	14
tonkatsu sauce	1 Tbs	20	5	0	4
(Kiss the Cook) pasta sauce					
Bolognese	½ cup	130	11	4	7
mushroom & wine	½ cup	90	9	3	5
puttanesca	½ cup	100	11	4	7
(Kitchen Bouquet) seasoning sauce	1 tsp	15	3	0	0
(Knorr)					
grilling & broiling sauce..spicy plum	⅛ bottle	60	11	0	na
(Kraft)					
Kraft sandwich spread & burger sauce					
reduced-fat	1 Tbs	35	3	0	3
regular	1 Tbs	50	3	0	2
Sauceworks					
cocktail					
hot & spicy	¼ cup	60	11	1	9
regular	¼ cup	60	13	1	9
horseradish	1 tsp	20	1	0	1
tartar sauce					
fat-free	2 Tbs	25	5	0	4
hot & spicy	2 Tbs	70	4	0	3
lemon & herb	2 Tbs	150	1	0	1
natural lemon & herb flavor	2 Tbs	150	1	0	1

Food and Description	Amount	Total Calories	Total Carbs	Fiber	Sugars
original	2 Tbs	70	4	0	3
(La Choy)					
mandarin orange	1 Tbs	24	6	0	na
plum	1 Tbs	25	6	0	na
soy sauce	1 Tbs	10	1	0	1
stir-fry					
mandarin soy sauce	¼ cup	35	8	1	na
sweet & sour	¼ cup	70	18	1	na
Szechuan	¼ cup	42	9	0	na
sweet & sour..all styles	2 Tbs	60	14	0	0
teriyaki..original	1 Tbs	17	3	1	2
(Lea & Perrins)					
steak					
garlic peppercorn	1 Tbs	25	5	0	3
private label	1 Tbs	25	5	0	3
sweet & spicy	1 Tbs	25	6	0	6
Worcestershire					
for chicken	1 tsp	5	1	0	1
hot pepper..sweet 'n' spicy kick	1 Tbs	25	6	0	6
original	1 tsp	5	1	0	1
pure blend	1 Tbs	25	6	0	5
thick & tangy	1 Tbs	18	4	0	4
white wine	1 tsp	0	0	0	0
(Luna Rossa) premium pasta sauce					
fire-roasted garlic	½ cup	80	8	1	2
Chianti mushroom	½ cup	70	6	1	2
Italian garden vegetable	½ cup	120	19	4	19
Romano pomodoro	½ cup	90	8	1	2
(Luzianne) TryMe Sauces					
Bullfighter steak & burger sauce	1 Tbs	15	4	0	3
Cajun Sunshine hot pepper	1 tsp	0	0	0	0
Caribbean Clipper oyster & shrimp	1 tsp	10	2	0	2
Dragon sauce	1 tsp	5	1	0	0
liquid smoke	1 tsp	0	0	0	0
Tennessee Sunshine..hot pepper	1 tsp	0	0	0	0
Tiger sauce	1 tsp	10	2	0	2
wine & pepper Worcestershire	1 tsp	0	0	0	0
Yucatan Sunshine habañero pepper	1 tsp	0	0	0	0
(Maple Grove Farms) marinade & basting sauces					
Dijon..low-carb..sugar-free	1 Tbs	50	<1	0	0
hickory..low-carb..sugar-free	1 Tbs	20	<1	0	0
lemon rosemary..low-carb..sugar-free	1 Tbs	35	<1	0	0
sweet & sour..low-carb..sugar-free	1 Tbs	40	<1	0	0
teriyaki..low-carb..sugar-free	1 Tbs	<1	<1	0	0
(Manwich) (See (Hunt's) in this section)					
(McCormick) grilling sauces					
hickory BBQ	2 Tbs	80	17	0	16
honey mustard	2 Tbs	70	15	0	13
mesquite	2 Tbs	60	12	0	10
roasted garlic & herb	2 Tbs	35	7	0	5

Food and Description	Amount	Total Calories	Total Carbs	Fiber	Sugars
teriyaki	2 Tbs	60	12	0	11
(Monterey Pasta Co.) pasta sauce					
Carb-Smart sauce..4-cheese	½ cup	190	6	0	4
pesto sauce w/basil, pine nuts & cheese	1 Tbs	280	4	1	1
(Muir Glen) organic..low-fat pasta sauce					
balsamic roasted onion	½ cup	50	12	0	5
cabernet marinara	½ cup	50	11	0	4
chunky tomato–style	½ cup	50	12	0	5
garden vegetable	½ cup	50	10	0	4
garlic & onion	½ cup	55	12	0	5
garlic roasted garlic	½ cup	55	12	0	5
Italian herb	½ cup	55	12	0	5
mushroom marinara	½ cup	45	10	0	4
portobello mushroom	½ cup	50	11	0	4
sun-dried tomato	½ cup	55	10	0	4
tomato basil	½ cup	50	12	0	4
(Nestlé) (See (Contadina) in this section)					
(Newman's Own)					
pasta sauce					
Bombolina tomato & fresh basil	½ cup	100	15	5	9
5-cheese	½ cup	90	14	3	8
Fra Diavolo..hot & spicy	½ cup	70	10	3	4
marinara	¼ cup	60	9	3	7
mushroom marinara	½ cup	60	9	3	7
roasted garlic & peppers	½ cup	70	11	4	6
Socarooni	½ cup	60	9	3	7
tomato & roasted garlic	½ cup	70	11	<1	9
vodka sauce	½ cup	110	11	0	9
steak sauce	1 Tbs	20	4	0	1
(Old Bay)					
cocktail	¼ cup	110	18	1	17
tartar sauce	2 Tbs	130	3	0	3
(Patak's) original cooking sauces					
rich creamy coconut..mild	½ can	210	11	2	4
tangy lemon & cilantro	¼ jar	120	8	1	6
(Prego) sauce					
Pasta Bake Sauce					
hearty meat	⅛ jar	50	12	2	11
Italian sausage	⅛ jar	100	11	2	9
tomato, garlic & basil	⅛ jar	80	11	2	10
Pasta Sauce					
beef & mushroom..hearty meat	½ cup	130	14	2	10
diced onion & garlic	½ cup	120	18	3	12
flavored w/meat	½ cup	140	21	3	13
fresh mushroom..jar	½ cup	120	21	3	13
fresh mushroom..plastic container	½ cup	140	24	3	14
garden combination	½ cup	90	16	3	11
garlic supreme	½ cup	120	17	3	11

Food and Description	Amount	Total Calories	Total Carbs	Fiber	Sugars
Italian sausage & garlic	½ cup	120	16	3	10
Italian sausage..hearty meat	½ cup	150	16	2	12
marinara	½ cup	90	10	3	7
meatball Parmesan..hearty meat	½ cup	160	16	2	10
mini meatball	½ cup	150	20	3	12
mushroom & garlic	½ cup	110	29	2	13
mushroom & green pepper..chunky	½ cup	100	16	3	10
mushroom Parmesan	½ cup	130	22	3	13
mushroom supreme	½ cup	130	19	3	12
mushroom supreme..chunky garden	½ cup	130	19	3	12
Parmesan	½ cup	110	20	3	13
ricotta Parmesan	½ cup	120	20	3	12
roasted garlic & herb	½ cup	110	17	2	11
roasted red pepper & garlic.. chunky	½ cup	120	19	3	12
3-cheese	½ cup	90	16	3	10
tomato, basil & garlic	½ cup	90	17	3	11
tomato, onion & garlic..chunky garden	½ cup	110	18	3	12
traditional..jar	½ cup	110	19	3	13
traditional..plastic container	½ cup	120	18	3	13
zesty mushroom	½ cup	110	18	3	12
(Premier Japan) sauce..wheat-free					
ginger tamari	1 Tbs	5	1	0	1
hoisin	1 Tbs	15	3	0	2
sesame garlic	1 Tbs	10	1	0	1
teriyaki sauce	1 Tbs	15	3	0	2
wabasi tamari	1 Tbs	5	1	0	1
(Progresso) pasta sauce					
creamy clam	½ cup	110	8	0	0
lobster	½ cup	100	6	2	3
red clam	½ cup	60	8	1	4
white clam	½ cup	140	5	0	1
(Ragú)					
Carb Options					
Alfredo	¼ cup	110	2	0	0
double cheddar	½ cup	90	2	0	0
garden-style	½ cup	80	7	2	4
Cheese Creations					
Alfredo					
classic	¼ cup	110	3	0	1
light	¼ cup	80	3	0	1
double cheddar	¼ cup	110	2	0	1
4-cheese	¼ cup	120	2	0	1
roasted garlic Parmesan	¼ cup	120	3	0	1
spicy cheddar & tomato	¼ cup	50	7	1	5
pasta sauce					
Chunky Garden-style					
garden combo..sweet bell pepper	½ cup	110	18	3	12

Food and Description	Amount	Total Calories	Total Carbs	Fiber	Sugars
mushroom					
super	½ cup	80	10	3	7
super chunky	½ cup	80	10	3	7
mushroom & green pepper	½ cup	110	18	3	12
mushroom & onion	½ cup	120	19	3	13
roasted red pepper & onion	½ cup	120	18	2	13
super garlic	½ cup	90	16	2	11
tomato					
garlic & onion	½ cup	120	19	3	13
spinach & cheese	½ cup	120	18	3	13
vegetable primavera	½ cup	110	17	4	10
light					
tomato & basil					
no sugar added	½ cup	60	9	3	5
regular	½ cup	50	11	2	8
Old World–style spaghetti sauce					
beef	½ cup	80	9	3	7
marinara	½ cup	80	9	3	7
mushroom	½ cup	70	10	3	7
traditional	½ cup	70	8	2	7
Robusto!					
beef w/mushroom	½ cup	70	8	2	7
classic Italian meat	½ cup	90	12	2	8
Parmesan & Romano	½ cup	120	18	3	13
red wine & herbs	½ cup	100	16	3	12
roasted garlic	½ cup	120	21	3	15
sautéed beef, onion & garlic	½ cup	120	18	3	13
sautéed onion & garlic	½ cup	90	11	2	9
sautéed onion & mushroom	½ cup	110	17	3	12
spicy red pepper	½ cup	110	21	3	14
7-herb tomato	½ cup	80	11	2	9
6-cheese	½ cup	80	9	2	8
sweet Italian sausage & cheese	½ cup	90	9	2	8
Pizza Quick..sauce					
cheesy mushroom	¼ cup	40	6	1	4
garlic & basil	¼ cup	40	5	1	4
pepperoni snack	¼ cup	50	6	1	3
traditional	¼ cup	45	3	1	3
(S&W)					
Cocktail sauce..seafood	1 Tbs	20	5	0	4
Cooking sauce & marinade					
mesquite steakhouse	1 Tbs	10	3	0	3
Oriental stir-fry	1 Tbs	25	5	0	4
Southwestern fajitas	1 Tbs	10	2	0	3
(Sagawa's) sauce					
Polynesian BBQ	1 Tbs	60	13	1	11
stir-fry	1 Tbs	25	5	0	4
sweet & sassy	1 Tbs	60	14	0	12
sweet & sour	1 Tbs	50	11	0	10
teriyaki	1 Tbs	30	7	0	6

Food and Description	Amount	Total Calories	Total Carbs	Fiber	Sugars
(Sauceworks) (*See* (Kraft) in this section)					
(Snow's)					
Welsh rarebit cheese	½ cup	170	10	0	na
Newburg w/sherry	⅓ cup	120	10	0	na
(Steel's Gourmet)					
gourmet..Rocky Mountain hoisin					
sauce	2 Tbs	15	2	1	1
mango					
curry sauce	1 Tbs	13	2.8	<1	0
ginger chutney sauce	5 Tbs	25	6	5	1
raspberry jalapeño sauce	1 Tbs	9	2	1	<1
sweet & spicy peanut sauce	1 Tbs	34	2	4.5	0
(Tabasco) Sauce					
chipotle pepper	1 tsp	5	1	0	0
garlic pepper	1 tsp	0	0	0	0
green pepper..milder jalapeño	1 tsp	0	0	0	0
habanero	1 tsp	5	1	0	1
pepper	1 tsp	0	0	0	0
(A Taste of Thai)					
chili sauce					
green	1 tsp	10	2	0	2
red	1 tsp	10	2	0	2
garlic chili pepper	1 tsp	10	2	0	2
peanut (satay)	2 Tbs	80	9	1	5
seasoning fish	1 Tbs	15	1	0	0
(Troy's) organic..wheat-free sauce					
ginger	1 Tbs	10	1	0	1
peanut	1 Tbs	25	2	0	1
(Walden Farms)					
cocktail sauce	1 Tbs	0	0	0	0
pasta sauce..scampi	⅓ cup	0	0	0	0
(Walnut Acres) organic sauce					
garlic-garlic	½ cup	50	10	1	6
marinara					
& herbs	½ cup	50	9	1	6
& zinfandel	½ cup	50	9	1	6
roasted garlic	½ cup	60	11	1	7
sweet pepper & onion	½ cup	50	9	1	6
tomato & mushroom	½ cup	50	9	1	6
tomato basil..original	½ cup	50	9	1	7
zesty basil	½ cup	50	9	1	7
(The Wizard's)					
hot stuff sauce	1 tsp	0	<1	0	0
Worcestershire sauce					
vegetarian	1 tsp	5	1	0	<1
wheat-free vegetarian	1 tsp	5	1	0	<1
SAUERKRAUT					
CANNED, JARRED, or BAGGED					
(Bush's Best)					
Bavarian kraut	1 oz	15	3	1	2

Food and Description	Amount	Total Calories	Total Carbs	Fiber	Sugars
shredded	1 oz	5	1	0	0
(Del Monte)					
Bavarian-style	2 Tbs	15	4	3	1
original	2 Tbs	<1	<1	<1	0
(Eden)	½ cup	25	4	3	1
(Hebrew National!)	2 Tbs	50	1	1	0
(Krrrrisp Kraut)					
barrel-cured	1 oz	5	2	1	0
Bavarian-style..barrel-cured	1 oz	10	2	1	1
(Libby's)					
Bavarian-style w/caraway seeds	2 Tbs	10	3	1	2
crispy	2 Tbs	5	1	1	1
(S&W) red cabbage	2 Tbs	5	3	0	2
	½ cup	25	1	0	0
(Silver Floss)					
BAGGED					
barrel-cured	1 oz	5	4	4	5
Bavarian-style barrel-cured	1 oz	10	8	0	4
CANNED					
barrel-cured	4 oz	20	4	4	5
Bavarian-style barrel-cured	4 oz	40	1	1	1
(Stokely's)					
Bavarian..traditional w/caraway seeds	½ cup	35	7	3	1
traditional shredded & chopped	¼ cup	5	1	1	0
SAUERKRAUT JUICE / *CANNED*					
(Biotta)	6 fl oz	20	4	1	0
(Bush's Best)	1 cup	15	1	0	0
SAUSAGE (*See also* FRANKFURTER; LUNCHEON MEAT; SAUSAGE DISH; SAUSAGE STICK)					
■ (Aidell's)					
sausage links					
(NOTE: All link portions are 3.5 oz unless stated otherwise.)					
beef					
chorizo..raw	1 link	400	3	0	0
chicken					
& apple..fresh	1 link	100	1	0	0
& apple..smoked	1 link	210	1	0	0
cocktail..2 oz	6 links	100	1	0	0
lemon..smoked	1 link	210	1	0	0
teriyaki..raw	1 link	210	6	0	0
& turkey..artichoke..smoked	1 link	180	2	0	0
& turkey..curry-smoked Burmese	1 link	220	3	0	0
& turkey..habañero..3.2 oz	1 link	160	2	0	0
& turkey..New Mexico..smoked	1 link	210	2	0	0
& turkey..pesto..smoked	1 link	220	1	0	0
& turkey/Thai..fresh..raw	1 link	200	1	0	0
& turkey w/sun-dried tomatoes & basil..raw	1 link	200	1	0	0
duck & turkey..smoked	1 link	220	1	0	0

Food and Description	Amount	Total Calories	Total Carbs	Fiber	Sugars
lamb & beef w/rosemary..fresh	1 link	220	2	<1	9
pork					
andouille..Cajun..smoked	1 link	240	0	0	0
& veal..bier..smoked	1 link	220	1	<1	0
whiskey fennel	1 link	220	1	<1	0
turkey..cranberry					
smoked	1 link	210	1	<1	0
w/scallions & herbs..fresh	1 link	200	1	<1	0
■ (Amour) Vienna sausage					
CANNED					
BBQ	2 oz	150	3	0	3
chicken	2 oz	110	1	0	0
hot & spicy	2 oz	150	2	0	0
jalapeño	2 oz	170	1	0	0
light..50% less fat	2 oz	90	1	0	1
in sauce	2 oz	150	0	0	0
■ (Beer Baron) smoked sausage	5 oz	420	7	0	1
■ (Big Mama) pickled sausage					
1.4 oz from 57-oz jar	1 sausage	110	1	1	0
2.4 oz from 16-count jar	1 sausage	180	4	0	0
■ (Bilinski's) sausage links					
(NOTE: All link portions are 3.5 oz unless stated otherwise.)					
chicken					
andouille..Cajun-style..2 oz	1 link	80	1	0	1
apple & chardonnay	1 link	70	2.5	0	0
cilantro	1 link	70	1	1	0
jalapeño	1 link	70	0	0	0
pesto	1 link	90	0	0	0
spinach	1 link	70	1	1	0
sun-dried tomato	1 link	70	2	0	0
■ (Bob Evans) express sausage links					
light	2 links	80	0	0	0
maple	2 links	120	2	0	1
original	2 links	160	0	0	0
roll sausage..chub					
Italian	2 oz	210	0	0	0
original recipe	2 oz	210	0	0	0
special seasonings	2 oz	230	0	0	0
sausage..other					
chub..maple log cabin	2 oz	200	2	0	2
links					
Italian-style..5-count pkg	1 link	270	1	0	1
maple..14-count pkg	3 links	170	3	0	2
patties..original..9-count pkg	2 patties	210	1	0	1
■ (Bryan)					
cocktail smokies	6 pieces	180	3	0	2
Polish	1 link	290	2	0	2
cocktail smokies					
Polish					

Food and Description	Amount	Total Calories	Total Carbs	Fiber	Sugars
smoked	2 oz link	160	3	0	2
links..skinless	4 oz link	380	2	0	0
links..w/turkey	1 link	150	3	0	2
rope..skinless	2 oz	180	0	0	0
■ (Butterball)					
Italian..all styles	1 link	170	0	0	0
Polish	1 link	170	0	0	0
turkey					
lean..extra-tender..smoked..2-count	1 link	100	4	0	1
lean..hot fresh Italian links..1-count	1 link	170	0	0	0
lean..sweet fresh Italian links..1-count	1 link	170	0	0	0
original breakfast links	3 links	120	2	0	1
■ (Eckrich)					
country..chub	2.6 oz	230	0	0	0
smoked					
2-count pkg	2.6 oz	170	3	0	1
beef..2-count pkg	2 oz	180	3	0	1
grillers..8-count pkg	2 oz	180	3	0	1
■ (Fire Cracker) sausage..The Original					
pickled sausage..red hot..15-count pkg	1 link	100	2	1	0
The original Giant..15-count pkg	1 link	140	3	1	0
■ (Galileo)					
cappacola..hot	2 oz	140	1	0	1
mortadella	2 oz	160	2	0	2
salami					
cotto..jumbo	2 oz	170	1	0	1
Genoa	2 oz	170	0	0	0
hard	1 oz	120	0	0	0
Italian dry..thin-sliced	5 slices	120	1	0	0
■ (Healthy Choice)					
frozen					
breakfast sausage links..8-count pkg	3 links	70	3	0	1
low-fat..smoked..links..2-count pkg	2 oz	80	6	0	2
patties	3 patties	70	3	0	1
refrigerated..breakfast					
links	3 links	70	3	0	1
patties	3 patties	70	3	0	1
Polska kielbasa	2 oz	80	6	0	2
smoked sausage..beef	2 oz	80	6	0	2
■ (Hebrew National)					
knockwurst..beef..4-count pkg	3 oz	260	1	0	0
pastrami	4 slices	90	1	0	0
salami..beef	3 slices	150	0	0	0
■ (Hillshire Farm)					
sausage..natural casing..Italian..sweet..	1 link	250	2	0	2
smoked					
beef	1 link	190	1	0	1
& cheddar	1 link	270	2	0	2
cheddarwurst..5-count pkg	1 link	270	2	0	2
hot links..5-count pkg	1 link	270	3	0	3

Food and Description	Amount	Total Calories	Total Carbs	Fiber	Sugars
summer..Yard-O-Beef stick	2 oz	190	1	0	0
■ (Hormel)					
breakfast..Little Sizzlers..cooked brown 'n' serve links					
hot & spicy..flavored w/Tabasco	3 links	230	0	0	0
maple-flavored	3 links	220	2	0	2
original	3 links	210	0	0	0
pepperoni..Rosa Grande	1 oz	140	0	0	0
sausage..smoked turkey..packed in vinegar	2 oz	140	1	0	1
smokies	1 link	80	0	0	0
smokies..cocktail..beef	6 links	180	2	0	8
summer sausage..cervelat	2 oz	120	2	0	2
summer sausage..Old Smokehouse	2 oz	200	2	0	2
■ (Jenny-O/The Turkey Store)					
turkey sausage					
breakfast links					
maple	2 oz	140	1	0	0
original	2 oz	140	1	0	0
breakfast lover's..skinless	2 oz	130	0	0	0
breakfast patties..original	2 patties	150	1	0	0
smoked..lean..95% fat-free	2 oz	70	0	0	0
■ (Jimmy Dean)					
breakfast sausage patties..cooked					
formed patty					
1.5 oz	1 patty	130	0	0	0
2 oz	1 patty	230	1	0	0
2.2 oz	2 patties	260	0	0	0
mild	2 oz	170	1	0	1
Patty Master..1.5 oz	1 patty	300	0	0	0
sage..1.5 oz	1 patty	130	0	0	0
turkey	1 patty	140	0	0	0
stuffed & sliced..patty					
1.5 oz	1 patty	150	0	0	0
2.5 oz	2 patties	310	0	0	0
3 oz	2 patties	230	0	0	0
extra sage..1.5 oz	1 patty	170	0	0	0
stuffed & sliced..thick patty					
1.6 oz	2 patties	240	5	0	1
2.5 oz	2 patties	190	0	0	0
breakfast sausage links..cooked					
mild	2 oz	170	1	0	0
mild maple	1.6 oz	140	1	0	1
skinless..2 oz	2 links	270	0	0	0
Trim Breakfast links	1.6 oz	180	0	0	0
turkey..1.35 oz	2 links	110	0	0	0
breakfast sausage–flavored					
pork crumbles	2 oz	180	1	0	0
■ (Johnsonville)					
(NOTE: All portions are cooked unless stated otherwise.)					
bratwurst..fresh varieties					
beef					

Food and Description	Amount	Total Calories	Total Carbs	Fiber	Sugars
beer 'n' bratwurst	1 link	300	2	0	0
bratwurst patty..pan-fried..3.3 oz	1 patty	240	1	0	0
cheddar	1 link	300	2	0	0
German brand	1 link	300	2	0	0
grilling chorizo	1 link	370	2	0	0
honey & garlic	1 link	290	6	0	3
hot 'n' spicy	1 link	300	2	0	0
Irish O' garlic	1 link	300	2	0	0
kielbasa	1 link	300	2	0	0
onion	1 link	300	2	0	0
original	1 link	300	2	0	0
Polish sausage	1 ling	300	2	0	0
roasted garlic	1 link	300	2	0	0
breakfast sausage					
brown sugar & honey..pan-fried	3 links	190	5	0	0
hickory-smoked breakfast	3 links	200	2	0	0
maple breakfast patties..9-oz pkg	2 patties	210	1	0	0
original breakfast patties..9-oz pkg	2 patties	210	1	0	0
Vermont maple syrup..pan-fried					
link	3 links	190	2	0	0
patty	2 patties	180	1	0	0
cocktail links..fully cooked					
beef links	6 links	180	1	0	0
brat bites	6 links	200	1	0	0
little smokies	6 links	180	2	0	0
Heat & Serve products					
bratwurst	1 link	260	3	0	0
Italian sausage	1 link	260	3	0	0
maple breakfast	3 links	230	3	0	2
original breakfast	3 links	230	2	0	0
hot links..all styles	1 link	230	2	0	0
Italian					
hot	1 link	300	2	0	0
Italian..ground..raw	2.5 oz	210	1	0	0
Italian patty..raw	1 patty	340	1	0	0
mild	1 link	300	2	0	0
Italian..ground..raw	2.5 oz	210	1	0	0
patty..pan-fried	3.3 oz	240	1	0	0
perri..raw					
hot	1 link	340	1	0	0
sweet	1 link	230	1	0	0
sweet Italian patty..raw	1 patty	340	1	0	0
simply Italian					
hot..raw	1 link	270	1	0	0
mild..raw	1 link	270	1	0	0
sweet rope..1 portion	2.5 oz	210	0	0	0
sweet sausage..raw	1 link	270	0	0	0
sausages..cooked..all styles	1 link	240	2	0	0
semi-dry sausage..summer sausage					
beef	2 oz	180	1	0	0
beef summer sticks	1 stick	120	0	0	0

Food and Description	Amount	Total Calories	Total Carbs	Fiber	Sugars
garlic	2 oz	180	1	0	0
Old World	2 oz	190	1	0	0
original	2 oz	180	1	0	0
spicy summer sticks	1 stick	120	0	0	0
smoked..cooked sausages					
Beddar w/cheddar	1 link	240	2	0	0
beef brat	1 link	240	2	0	0
bratwurst	1 link	240	2	0	0
hot links	1 link	230	2	0	0
New Orleans brand	1 link	230	2	0	0
Swisswurst	1 link	240	2	0	0
Polish	1 link	240	2	0	0
■ (Jones Dairy Farm) all-natural flavored sausages					
link..maple..skinless	2 links	90	1	<1	0
patty					
hot & zesty	2 patties	170	1	<1	0
maple	2 patties	170	1	<1	0
golden brown pork sausage					
link..casing					
0.8 oz	3 links	80	<1	<2	0
1.6 oz	1 link	160	<1	<2	0
links..skinless					
0.95 oz	2 links	120	<1	<2	0
1.63 oz	2 links	210	<1	<2	0
patty					
0.95 oz	2 patties	120	<1	<2	0
1.43 oz	2 patties	170	<1	<2	0
1.94 oz	1 patty	220	<1	<2	0
2.9 oz	1 patty	330	1	<2	0
Italian					
link..skinless..2.15 oz	1 link	160	1	<1	0
patty..2.68 oz	1 patty	210	1	<1	0
light sausage					
& rice link	1 link	50	1	<2	0
& rice patty	1 patty	100	1	<2	0
poultry sausage..turkey					
link	2 links	30	<1	<2	0
patty	1 patty	60	<1	<2	0
■ (Libby's) Vienna sausage					
in chicken broth	2 oz	100	0	0	0
w/chicken & pork					
in BBQ sauce	2 oz	110	2	0	2
in chicken broth	2 oz	150	1	0	0
■ (Louis Rich)					
turkey kielbasa	2 oz	90	2	0	1
turkey sausage..original	2 oz	120	1	0	0
■ (Old Wisconsin)					
beef sausage					
snack stick	½ oz	60	1	0	0

Food and Description	Amount	Total Calories	Total Carbs	Fiber	Sugars
summer sausage..snack slices	2 oz	210	1	0	0
bratwurst					
light..6-count pkg	1 link	110	1	0	0
premium festival..6-count pkg	1 link	250	1	0	0
Italian..festival..6-count pkg	1 link	210	2	0	2
Polish sausage					
premium smoked	4.66 oz	240	1	0	1
6-count pkg	1 link	260	0	0	0
smoked sausage..premium real					
Wisconsin cheddar links	2.66 oz	250	2	0	2
summer sausage..party..chub	2 oz	220	1	0	0
summer sausage..premier					
beef..chub	2 oz	210	1	0	0
beef stick..chub	2 oz	220	1	0	0
■ (Oscar Mayer)					
Little Smokies					
cheese	2 oz	180	2	0	1
regular	2 oz	170	1	0	1
■ (Owens)					
bratwurst..cooked..beer	1 link	270	1	0	1
fresh pork sausage..chubs					
country-style					
extra-mild	2 oz	180	1	0	1
hot picante..36-count pkg	2 oz	210	1	0	1
maple	2 oz	180	1	0	1
mild	2 oz	210	1	0	1
Italian	2 oz	180	1	0	1
regular..8-count pkg	2 oz	240	1	0	1
special seasoning	2 oz	180	1	0	1
pan-fried links					
hot	2 oz	210	2	0	1
maple	3 links	170	1	0	1
regular	3 links	160	1	0	0
Patties					
hot picante..36-count	2 oz	210	1	0	1
regular..8-count	2 patties	240	1	0	1
■ (Perdue) turkey sausage					
breakfast links..2.3 oz..fully cooked	3 links	170	2	0	0
hot Italian links..2.8 oz..fully cooked	1 link	150	1	0	0
Polish sausages..fully cooked	3.3 oz link	190	3	0	3
sausage links..mild					
2 oz..fully cooked	1 link	120	0	0	0
2 oz..ready-to-cook	2 links	140	0	0	0
sausage patties..mild					
fully cooked	2 oz	110	1	0	0
ready-to-cook	3 oz	210	1	0	0
sweet Italian links..all styles	1 link	150	1	0	0
■ (Purnell's Old Folks)					
bratwurst					
fresh	2 oz	230	0	0	0

Food and Description	Amount	Total Calories	Total Carbs	Fiber	Sugars
old-fashioned..cooked	3.2 oz	270	2	0	0
country..flame-broiled					
links..medium..skinless	2 oz	210	0	0	0
patties..24-count pkg	2 patties	220	19	0	0
Italian sausage..6-count pkg	1 link	210	3	0	0
pork links..fresh..12-count pkg	2 links	150	2	0	0
turkey sausage..patties..16-count pkg	2 oz	180	0	0	0
whole beef sausage	2.67 oz	194	2	1	0
whole hog sausage					
chorizo	2 oz	190	2	0	0
country					
medium	2 oz	220	0	0	0
spicy..medium	2 oz	220	0	0	0
Italian	3.2 oz	210	0	0	0
patties..country..all styles	2 patties	220	0	0	0
■ (Reser's)					
chub					
Hunters..mild	2 oz	140	2	0	2
whole hog..mild	2 oz	210	2	0	1
summer					
Gold Rush	2 oz	210	2	0	1
regular	2 oz	150	2	0	1
■ (Shelton's) turkey sausage					
breakfast links	1 link	140	0	0	0
Italian links	1 link	160	0	0	0
■ (Tennessee Pride)					
sausage					
balls home-style	2.66 oz	280	9	0	1
chub..country..all styles	2 oz	200	0	0	0
links					
country..hot	1 link	190	1	0	0
maple..14-count pkg	2 links	150	3	0	2
original..12-count pkg	3 links	170	0	0	0
original..fully cooked..16-count pkg	2 links	160	0	0	0
patties					
mild..8-count pkg	2 patties	230	0	0	0
original..fully cooked..12-count pkg	2 patties	210	0	0	0
original..real country..6-count pkg	2 patties	190	1	0	0
swirls..home-style	3 oz	310	22	0	2
wraps..home-style	2½ wraps	310	23	0	2
■ (THE TURKEY STORE) (*See* (Jennie-O/The Turkey Store) in this section)					
SAUSAGE DISH (*See also* BREAKFAST SANDWICH; FROZEN ENTRÉE/DINNER; SAUSAGE)					
(Mary Kitchen) sausage hash	1 cup	410	23	2	1
SAUSAGE STICK (*See* MEAT SNACKS)					
SAUSAGE SUBSTITUTE (*See* VEGETARIAN FOODS)					
SCALLION/GREEN ONION/SPRING ONION (*See also* ONION)					
FRESH					
chopped	½ cup	15	4	1.5	0
(Dole)	1 Tbs	2	0	0	0
w/tops	1 large	10	2	1	0

Food and Description	Amount	Total Calories	Total Carbs	Fiber	Sugars
SCALLOP (See also SEAFOOD ENTRÉE/DINNER)					
fresh..breaded & fried..½ oz each	2 scallops	67	3	na	na
imitation					
(Louis Kemp) Scallop Delights..					
bay-style	13 pieces	80	12	0	3
smoked (Ducktrap River)	¼ cup	60	1	0	0
SCONE (See also ROLL)					
(Krusteaz) mix..prepared					
scone					
blueberry	1 scone	280	38	2	12
cranberry orange	1 scone	280	39	2	13
scone & shortcake	1 scone	180	21	1	5
(Otis Spunkmeyer)					
cinnamon chip	3.75 oz	380	59	5	22
maple pecan	3.75 oz	370	60	6	29
wild blueberry	3.5 oz	330	50	7	15
(Wolferman's)					
apple cranberry	1 scone	330	46	2	15
chocolate chunk	1 scone	360	46	2	17
cinnamon chip	1 scone	370	46	1	1
classic currant	1 scone	320	47	2	8
cranberry orange	1 scone	330	46	2	15
wild blueberry	1 scone	330	46	2	16
SCOTCH (See LIQUOR, DISTILLED)					
SCOTCH BROTH (See SOUP)					
SCRAPPLE					
(Jones Dairy Farm) country-style	2 oz	120	7	0	0
SCUP..raw..meat only	3 oz	90	0	0	0
SEA BASS (See also SEAFOOD ENTRÉE/DINNER)					
fresh..cooked—dry heat	3 oz	105	0	0	0
SEA SALT	1 tsp	0	0	0	0
SEA TROUT..raw..meat only	3 oz	88	0	0	0
SEA VEGETABLE (See SEAWEED)					
SEAFOOD CHOWDER (See SOUP)					
SEAFOOD ENTRÉE/DINNER (See also FROZEN ENTRÉE/DINNER; PASTA ENTRÉE/ DINNER; individual listings)					
CANNED					
(Bumble Bee) seafood salad					
ready-to-eat..w/crab & crackers	3.3 oz	200	10	0	4
(Chicken of the Sea)					
fish steaks..in hot sauce	2 oz	70	1	1	1
oysters					
smoked	3 oz	190	8	0	0
whole	4 oz	70	3	1	0
(Crown Prince)					
clams..baby..boiled	2 oz	40	2	0	0
kipper snacks	3.2 oz	190	0	0	0
oysters..smoked	3 oz	290	11	<1	0
(Geisha) snow crab	3 oz	35	1	0	0

Food and Description	Amount	Total Calories	Total Carbs	Fiber	Sugars
FROZEN					
(Avalon Bay)					
fillets					
cod	4 oz	90	0	0	0
gourmet breaded	½ fillet	210	23	0	2
emperor snapper	4 oz	110	4	0	0
grouper	4 oz	100	0	0	0
halibut steaks	3 oz	93	0	0	0
scallops					
gourmet breaded	11 scallops	110	25	0	<1
medallions	2 oz	40	0	0	0
shrimp..stuffed	3 shrimp	330	28	<1	5
(Captain's Cove)					
fish					
chum salmon fillets	4 oz	135	0	0	0
cod fillets	4 oz	90	0	0	0
flounder fillets	4 oz	100	0	0	0
halibut steaks	4 oz	130	0	0	0
orange roughy fillets	4 oz	140	0	0	0
perch fillets	4 oz	110	0	0	0
swordfish steaks	4 oz	150	0	0	0
yellowfin tuna steaks	4 oz	140	4	0	0
scallops					
jumbo	3.2 oz	70	1	0	0
breaded	3.2 oz	120	16	1	1
medium..bacon-wrapped	3.2 oz	220	0	0	0
shrimp					
cooked..tail on..low-fat	4 oz	60	0	0	0
large..cooked ring & sauce	4 oz	80	6	0	3
popcorn	2.85 oz	210	18	1	1
raw..shell on..low-fat	4 oz	70	1	0	0
(Contessa) shrimp..cooked					
shell on	3 oz	60	0	0	0
shelled	3 oz	40	0	0	0
(Dining In)					
crab cakes..Maryland-style	3 oz	150	7	0	0
crab rangoon..handmade	2 oz	160	18	0	2
(Fisher Boy)					
crab cakes..premium.. lightly breaded..6-count pkg	2 oz	110	11	0	3
fish					
fillets..crispy battered	3 oz	130	11	0	1
portions..crispy battered..8-count	⅛ pkg	170	15	0	1
portions..crunchy	1 piece	200	19	2	1
shapes..crunchy..90-count pkg	3 oz	210	22	1	1
sticks..crunchy..128-count pkg	3 oz	190	15	1	0
tenders..crunchy	2.62 oz	220	20	2	1
Qwikstix..crunchy..minced	3 oz	170	27	1	2
School o' Fish Crunch..minced	3 oz	190	19	1	1

Food and Description	Amount	Total Calories	Total Carbs	Fiber	Sugars
(Gorton's)					
clams	½ pkg	240	20	0	2
fish fillets					
beer batter..crispy..10-count pkg	2 pieces	250	19	0	3
crispy battered	2 pieces	270	16	0	4
crunchy golden	2 pieces	270	24	0	3
garlic & herb..crunchy..breaded	2 pieces	270	22	0	4
grilled					
Caesar Parmesan..2-count pkg	1 piece	100	1	0	0
Cajun...blackened..2-count pkg	1 piece	100	1	0	0
classic..char-grilled..2-count pkg	1 piece	100	1	0	0
garlic butter..2-count pkg	1 piece	100	1	0	0
Italian herb..2-count pkg	1 piece	100	1	0	0
lemon butter..2-count pkg	1 piece	100	1	0	0
lemon herb..extra-large	¼ box	180	2	0	0
lemon pepper..2-count pkg	1 piece	100	1	0	0
salmon..lemon..2-count pkg	1 piece	100	1	0	1
lemon herb..crunchy breaded.. 10-count pkg	2 pieces	240	21	0	4
lemon pepper..battered.. 6-count pkg	2 pieces	290	17	0	3
Parmesan..crunchy..breaded.. 6-count pkg	2 pieces	250	19	0	5
premium cod..crunchy..breaded.. extra-large	½ box	220	20	0	4
ranch..crunchy breaded..6-count pkg	2 pieces	240	22	0	3
Southern fried..county-style.. 6-count pkg	2 pieces	230	19	0	3
tenders..extra-crunchy	4.24 oz	260	29	0	5
tenders..original batter	4.24 oz	270	25	0	2
fish portions..batter-dipped.. 10-count pkg	1 piece	170	14	0	2
fish sticks					
crunchy golden	6 sticks	250	20	0	2
garlic & herb..18-count pkg	6 sticks	260	26	0	5
Grilled Fish Fillet Meals					
Alfredo w/broccoli	1 meal	160	14	5	7
lemon & herb butter w/rice & vegetables	1 meal	240	34	3	5
popcorn fish..crispy..golden-battered	4 oz	320	24	0	11
popcorn shrimp					
beer batter..7.2-oz box	½ box	270	24	0	2
garlic & herb..7.2-oz box	½ box	250	28	0	3
original..8-oz box	3.2 oz	240	26	0	2
Shrimp Bowls					
Alfredo-fried rice	1 bowl	270	41	1	4
Alfredo shrimp	1 bowl	270	41	1	4
butter shrimp	1 bowl	260	38	2	6
fried rice shrimp	1 bowl	350	68	1	9
garlic shrimp	1 bowl	320	57	2	4

Food and Description	Amount	Total Calories	Total Carbs	Fiber	Sugars
primavera shrimp	1 bowl	270	41	1	4
teriyaki shrimp	1 bowl	320	57	2	14
Skillet Fillets..all varieties	1 piece	220	13	0	2
(High Liner)					
salmon fillets					
in creamy dill sauce	4 oz	110	1	0	0
stuffed mango & macadamia..					
4-count pkg	¼ pkg	370	21	1	1
scallops..roasted garlic & herb	⅙ pkg	100	5	0	1
sea scallops..breaded..10- to					
30-count pkg	⅙ pkg	220	22	0	0
(Mrs. Paul's)					
cod fillets..breaded..2-count pkg	4 oz	240	19	0	2
crab cakes					
deviled	3 oz	190	23	0	4
fish fillets					
crispy battered					
hearty-size..6-count pkg	⅙ pkg	210	17	0	3
value pack..10-count pkg	⅒ pkg	150	12	0	2
crispy original..breaded..97% fat-free	¼ pkg	130	19	0	3
crunchy..breaded..6-count pkg	⅓ pkg	260	22	0	2
fish sticks..crunchy..18-count pkg	⅓ pkg	230	21	1	2
fish strips..crunchy	4 oz	270	24	0	2
fish tenders..crispy	4 oz	260	22	0	2
flounder fillet..breaded..3-count pkg	⅓ pkg	170	13	0	1
fried clams..breaded	3 oz	250	26	1	1
haddock fillet..breaded..2-count pkg	½ pkg	230	19	0	3
scallops..fried..breaded	3.5 oz	220	27	1	3
shrimp					
Alfredo	11 oz	300	39	2	3
fried rice	11 oz	290	54	2	17
garlic butter	11 oz	290	48	4	7
marinated					
Cajun	5.5 oz	70	2	0	2
scampi	5.5 oz	100	2	0	2
popcorn	4 oz	290	31	1	1
stir-fry	11 oz	330	67	2	25
sweet & sour shrimp	11 oz	310	65	1	16
Thai-style peanut	11 oz	330	51	4	7
tortellini	11 oz	340	58	5	20
(Nancy's) seafood crab cakes	1 pkg	350	28	2	10
(Phillip's)					
bisque..chowder..soup					
crab soup..Maryland-style	7.5 oz	70	13	2	3
crab & corn chowder	7.5 oz	290	17	1	7
crab & shrimp chowder	7.5 oz	150	9	2	5
cream of crab	7.5 oz	340	12	0	6
lobster bisque	7.5 oz	370	22	1	1
New England clam chowder	7.5 oz	260	18	1	3
shrimp bisque	7.5 oz	310	19	1	1
crab					
cocktail crab claws..restaurant-style	2 oz	45	0	0	0

Food and Description	Amount	Total Calories	Total Carbs	Fiber	Sugars
crab balls..Maryland-style	⅛ pkg	250	12	1	4
crab cake..minis..20-count pkg	3 cakes	160	5	1	1
crab cakes..boardwalk..Maryland-style 6-count	⅛ pkg	250	8	1	1
crab meat..pasteurized.. all styles..hand-picked	2 oz	45	0	0	0
crab slammers..jalapeño..20-count pkg	2 oz	160	14	1	2
crab-stuffed shrimp..10-count pkg	⅓ pkg	190	1	0	1
crab & spinach dip	1 oz	60	1	0	0
mahimahi fillets					
Caribbean-style w/pepper jelly	3 oz	220	23	1	8
coconut..w/restaurant-style sauce.. 14-count pkg	¼ pkg	170	18	1	4
shrimp..coconut	5 shrimp	290	23	1	8
tuna..yellowfin steak..w/Oriental peanut sauce..6-count pkg	⅙ pkg	120	0	0	0
(Schwan's)					
breaded seafood					
blue hake	3 oz	190	16	9	1
clam strips	½ cup	270	30	1	1
cod					
battercrisp	2 pieces	280	20	0	0
nuggets	6 nuggets	200	18	1	1
fantail shrimp	4 oz	230	35	1	1
haddock					
squares	4 oz	190	18	2	1
sticks	3 sticks	140	13	1	1
oven-ready shrimp	3 oz	240	24	1	1
unbreaded seafood					
blue hake loins	4 oz	70	0	0	0
buttercrisp cod	2 pieces	280	20	0	0
Caesar Parmesan shrimp	3.3 oz	110	2	0	1
cod fish nuggets	6 nuggets	200	18	1	1
English-style Fish-N-Chips	¼ bag	500	40	1	5
(Sea Pak)					
bay scallops..imported..oven-crunchy	5.5 oz box	420	42	1	2
clam strips..oven..crunchy	3 oz	250	24	0	0
crab cakes					
Boardwalk Maryland–style.. 6-count pkg	1 cake	250	8	1	1
Maryland-style	1 cake	220	14	3	2
6-count pkg	1 cake	170	6	0	0
minis	4 cakes	160	5	1	1
oven-crunchy	1 cake	250	22	1	1
shrimp					
butterfly					
breaded	4 oz	150	22	1	1
jumbo..oven-crunchy	3 oz	200	20	1	1
Oriental breaded	4 oz	150	22	1	1
oven-crunchy	4.5 oz	200	20	1	1

Food and Description	Amount	Total Calories	Total Carbs	Fiber	Sugars
coconut..oven-crunchy	3 oz	250	21	1	3
éntrees					
Alfredo w/broccoli	1 entrée	300	40	4	6
garlic herb	1 entrée	270	35	4	4
teriyaki w/rice	1 entrée	350	54	3	18
marinated					
Caesar Parmesan	3.33 oz	110	3	0	1
garlic herb	3.33 oz	90	2	1	0
spicy Szechuan	3.33 oz	110	3	0	1
popcorn					
Buffalo-style..oven-crunchy	3 oz	230	23	0	1
jumbo..oven-crunchy	3 oz	240	25	1	1
poppers..oven-crunchy	3 oz	220	18	2	0
scampi					
in Baja lime sauce	4 oz	350	4	0	1
in Italian Parmesan sauce	4 oz	350	2	0	0
in traditional garlic sauce	4 oz	350	4	0	0
(Van de Kamp's)					
battered items					
fillets					
fish	1 fillet	170	13	0	3
haddock	2 fillets	220	17	0	4
halibut	3 fillets	220	19	0	4
ocean perch	2 fillets	240	18	0	4
fish					
portions	1 portion	160	13	0	3
tenders	4 pieces	290	24	0	2
breaded items					
fillets					
fish	2 fillets	260	17	0	2
fish sticks					
mini	13 sticks	250	19	0	2
regular	6 sticks	290	22	0	3
fish strips	4 pieces	270	25	0	2
Hearty-Size fish fillets	1 fillet	150	10	0	<1
portions	3 portions	360	23	0	2
Crisp & Healthy..breaded & baked					
fillets					
garlic & herb	2 fillets	170	25	0	3
lemon pepper	2 fillets	170	24	0	5
regular..plain	2 fillets	170	25	0	4
fish sticks	6 sticks	170	24	0	4
grilled Items..3.75-oz fillets..all varieties	1 fillet	120	0	0	0
specialty items					
cheese & crab poppers	4 poppers	320	27	<1	2
clams/fried	18 pieces	250	26	1	1
crab cakes	1 cake	190	20	0	2
mini	4 cakes	260	31	1	3
shrimp					
buffalo	20 shrimp	320	35	0	1

Food and Description	Amount	Total Calories	Total Carbs	Fiber	Sugars
butterfly	7 shrimp	300	30	3	2
linguine	1½ cups	180	30	4	2
popcorn	20 shrimp	270	30	2	2
stir-fry	1⅔ cups	260	54	3	16
stuffed	3 shrimp	290	32	<1	2
MIX (NOTE: The amount of fat and calories in dishes prepared from boxed mixes may vary slightly depending on the fat and calorie content of the seafood used in preparation.)					
(Betty Crocker) Tuna Helper (prepared data are for regular recipe only)					
au gratin	1 cup	310	38	1	5
cheesy broccoli	1 cup	300	38	1	7
cheesy pasta	1 cup	270	31	1	5
creamy broccoli	1 cup	300	33	1	4
creamy pasta	1 cup	290	32	2	5
fettuccine Alfredo	1 cup	300	32	1	5
garden cheddar	1 cup	290	36	1	6
tetrazzini	1 cup	300	31	1	3
tuna casserole	1 cup	280	47	1	4
tuna melt	1 cup	280	34	0	5
(Zatarain's)					
New Orleans–style crab cake..mix only	⅕ box	100	24	0	0
SEASONINGS (*See also* ASIAN FOOD, Sauces & Seasonings entry; BAKE & FRY MIX; GRAVY; MARINADE; MEXICAN FOOD; SAUCE; individual listings)					
(NOTE: Unless stated otherwise, data are for seasoning or seasoning mix only.)					
(Accent)					
flavor enhancer	⅛ tsp	0	0	0	0
Sa-son..all styles	¼ tsp	0	0	0	0
(Adolph's)					
Meal Makers					
beef stew	1 Tbs	10	3	<1	0
chili mix	1 Tbs	30	5	<1	<1
meat loaf	1 Tbs	25	5	0	<1
meat tenderizer					
seasoned	¼ tsp	0	0	0	0
unseasoned	¼ tsp	0	0	0	0
tenderizers..all styles	¼ tsp	0	0	0	0
(Amazing Taste) all styles	½ tsp	<5	1	0	<1
(Chef Paul) Magic Seasoning Blends.. all styles & flavors	¼ tsp	0	0	0	0
(Chi-Chi's) seasoning mix					
fajita seasoning mix	1 tsp	35	7	0	1
fiesta burrito	⅕ pkg	40	6	1	2
fiesta restaurante	1 tsp	10	2	0	0
fiesta taco	⅕ pkg	10	1	0	0
(Duck's Unlimited) seasoning blends					
chili	1⅓ Tbs	30	5	0	<1
lemon lime pepper seasoning & rub	¼ tsp	0	0	0	0
poultry & game seasoning & rub	¼ tsp	0	0	0	0
steak & chop seasoning & rub	¼ tsp	0	0	0	0
taco	2 tsp	15	3	0	1

Food and Description	Amount	Total Calories	Total Carbs	Fiber	Sugars
(French's) seasonings					
meatballs	¼ pkg	35	7	0	0
meat loaf	⅛ pkg	20	5	0	0
(Lawry's) seasoning packets & blends					
beef stew	1 tsp	10	2	0	0
beef Stroganoff	1 Tbs	20	5	0	<1
burrito	2 tsp	20	4	<1	0
chicken taco	2 tsp	20	5	0	1
chili	1 tsp	10	2	0	1
enchilada sauce	2 tsp	20	4	0	0
fajitas	1 tsp	15	3	0	0
garlic pepper	¼ tsp	0	0	0	0
garlic powder w/parsley	¼ tsp	0	0	0	0
garlic salt	1 tsp	4	<1	0	0
guacamole	½ tsp	5	1	0	0
lemon pepper	¼ tsp	0	0	0	0
meat loaf	1 Tbs	30	7	<1	2
Mexican rice	1½ tsp	40	9	<1	0
minced onion w/green onion	¼ tsp	0	0	0	0
pinch of herbs	¼ tsp	0	0	0	0
salt..seasoned					
light	¼ tsp	0	0	0	0
regular	1 tsp	4	1	0	0
salt-free	¼ tsp	0	0	0	0
salt-free 17	¼ tsp	0	0	0	0
sloppy joes	2 tsp	20	5	0	3
spaghetti					
extra rich & thick	1 Tbs	35	6	<1	na
spatini	2 tsp	20	3	0	na
traditional	1½ tsp	30	6	<1	na
taco salad	1 tsp	15	3	0	0
vegetable & herb blends	¼ tsp	0	0	0	0
(McCormick)					
Bag 'N Season					
beef stew	1 tsp	15	1	0	0
buffalo wings	⅙ pkg	30	5	0	3
chicken					
country-style	1 Tbs	25	3	0	1
Italian herb	1 Tbs	15	2	0	1
mesquite	¼ tsp	<5	0	0	<1
Oriental	⅙ pkg	15	4	0	2
original	1 Tbs	20	3	0	<1
Southwest	2 tsp	25	3	1	1
meat loaf	2 tsp	15	2	<1	<1
pork chops	⅙ pkg	15	4	0	2
pork tenderloin	2 tsp	15	2	0	<1
pot roast	1 Tbs	10	1	0	<1
Swiss steak	⅛ pkg	15	2	0	1
turkey w/gravy	1 tsp	15	<1	0	<1
Fry Easy					

Food and Description	Amount	Total Calories	Total Carbs	Fiber	Sugars
all-purpose batter	1/10 pkg	100	20	0	1
all-purpose breading	1/9 pkg	120	20	0	3
beer batter	1/10 pkg	100	19	0	1
Cajun-style	1/30 pkg	35	6	0	0
chicken					
extra-crispy	1/8 pkg	60	9	0	0
herbs & spices	1/16 pkg	70	13	0	1
home-style..original	1/16 pkg	50	9	0	0
hot 'n' spicy	1/16 pkg	50	9	0	0
cracker meal	1/9 pkg	130	23	0	3
fish fry..lightly seasoned	1/13 pkg	35	0	0	0
fish 'n' chips..English-style	1/10 pkg	100	20	0	1
funnel cake batter mix	1/9 pkg	120	23	0	6
hush puppy cornmeal	1/8 pkg	130	25	0	3
onion ring	1/10 pkg	100	20	0	1
seafood-seasoned	1/20 pkg	50	9	0	1
tempura..Japanese-style	1/8 pkg	100	20	0	1
Grill Mates..grilling sauce					
hickory BBQ	1/11 pkg	80	17	0	16
honey mustard	1/11 pkg	70	15	0	13
Montreal chicken & roasted garlic	1 Tbs	15	2	0	1
roasted garlic & herb	1/12 pkg	35	7	0	5
teriyaki	1/11 pkg	60	12	0	11
International Blends..all styles & flavors	1/2 tsp	0	0	0	0
Old Bay (*See* (Old Bay) in this category.)					
Oven Easy					
Cajun-style..for baked seafood	1/6 pkg	90	11	1	3
garlic & herb..for baked seafood	1/6 pkg	100	13	1	2
lemon & pepper..for baked seafood	1/6 pkg	90	12	1	2
shrimp & seafood..for baked seafood	1/6 pkg	70	8	0	1
salt-free blends..all styles & flavors	1/4 tsp	0	0	0	0
seasoning blends					
barbecue	1/4 tsp	<5	0	0	<1
broiled-steak seasoning	1/4 tsp	<5	0	0	<1
Cajun	1/2 tsp	0	0	0	0
Cajun quick..spicy chicken	1/4 tsp	<5	0	0	<1
Caribbean jerk	1/4 tsp	0	0	0	0
celery salt	1/4 tsp	0	0	0	0
chicken..lemon herb	1 Tbs	30	5	0	<1
chili					
hot	1/4 pkg	40	4	2	>1
mild	1/4 pkg	30	5	1	2
Tex-Mex	1/4 pkg	35	4	2	2
white chicken	1/4 pkg	30	5	0	1
chili powder	1/4 tsp	0	0	0	0
citrus pepper	1/4 tsp	0	0	0	0
Creole	1/4 tsp	<5	0	0	<1
fajitas	2 tsp	15	2	0	<1
fried-chicken seasoning	1/4 tsp	<5	0	0	<1
garlic..crushed..California-style	1/4 tsp	10	<1	0	<1

Food and Description	Amount	Total Calories	Total Carbs	Fiber	Sugars
garlic..minced-wet..California-style	1 tsp	15	1	0	0
garlic pepper..California-style	¼ tsp	<5	0	0	<1
garlic salt..all styles	¼ tsp	0	0	0	0
garlic season all	¼ tsp	<5	0	0	<1
garlic spread..all styles	½ Tbs	45	1	0	0
herb & garlic mix	1 Tbs	20	2	0	<1
herb chicken	¼ tsp	0	0	0	0
herb classic chicken	¼ tsp	<5	0	0	<1
imitation butter–flavored salt	¼ tsp	0	0	0	0
lemon herb	¼ tsp	0	0	0	0
lemon pepper..California-style	½ tsp	<5	0	0	<1
meat tenderizer..nonseasoned	¼ tsp	<5	0	0	<1
Mexican seasoning	¼ tsp	<5	0	0	<1
Monterey spice blend	¼ tsp	0	0	0	0
onion salt..California-style	¼ tsp	0	0	0	0
pesto mix	2 tsp	10	<1	0	<1
pizza seasoning..spicy Italian	1 tsp	10	0	0	<1
pork seasoning	½ tsp	<5	0	0	<1
salad supreme seasoning	¼ tsp	0	0	0	0
Santa Fe spice blend	¼ tsp	0	0	0	0
sloppy joe	1 tsp	20	3	0	2
spice blends..all styles & flavors	½ tsp	0	0	0	0
spicy season all	¼ tsp	0	0	0	0
Stroganoff	2 tsp	15	3	0	<1
Swedish meatballs	2 tsp	45	4	0	1
(Molly McButter)					
cheese-flavor sprinkles	½ tsp	5	1	0	0
sour cream–flavor sprinkles	½ tsp	5	1	0	0
(Mrs. Dash) all styles & flavors	¼ tsp	3	<1	0	<1
(Nile Spice) all styles & flavors	⅛ tsp	0	0	0	0
(Old Bay) seasoning					
blackened	⅛ tsp	0	0	0	0
crab cake classic..original Maryland	⅙ pkg	30	2	0	0
for seafood & poultry salt	⅛ tsp	0	0	0	0
salmon classic..original	⅕ pkg	40	3	0	0
seafood..one-step crab boil..spicy	any	0	0	0	0
tuna classic	⅕ pkg	30	2	0	0
(Oven Fry) seasoned Coating					
extra-crispy					
for chicken	⅛ pkg	60	10	0	2
for pork	⅛ pkg	60	11	0	1
fish fry for fish	⅛ pkg	45	9	0	0
home-style flour..for chicken	⅛ pkg	40	7	0	0
(Produce Partners)					
stir-fry	2 tsp	20	4	0	2
super slaw	1 tsp	10	2	0	2
vegetable batter mix	¼ cup	120	16	<1	<1
vegetable seasonings					
onion ring mix	¼ cup	110	18	<1	<1

Food and Description	Amount	Total Calories	Total Carbs	Fiber	Sugars
oven potato fries	1 Tbs	30	3	<1	2
(Shake & Bake)					
French fries					
French fries for fresh potatoes	⅙ pkt	15	3	0	0
Perfect Potatoes seasoning mix					
herb & garlic	⅙ pkt	20	5	0	1
zesty cheddar	⅙ pkt	25	3	0	1
seasoned coating mixture					
Buffalo wings	⅒ pkt	40	8	0	3
for chicken					
crispy chicken nuggets	1/12 pouch	50	9	0	1
original recipe	⅛ pouch	40	7	0	1
for chicken or pork					
classic Italian	⅛ pkt	40	7	0	1
hot & spicy	⅛ pkt	40	7	0	1
original	⅛ pkt	45	8	0	1
for pork..original recipe	⅛ pouch	45	8	0	1
garlic & herb	⅛ pkt	35	7	0	1
hot & spicy	⅛ pkt	40	7	0	1
tangy honey	⅛ pkt	45	9	0	6
seasoning & coating mixture glaze					
barbecue chicken or pork	⅛ pouch	45	9	0	5
honey mustard chicken or pork	⅛ pouch	45	9	0	6
tangy honey chicken or pork	⅛ pouch	45	9	0	6
(A Taste of Thai)					
chicken & rice dinner seasoning	¼ pkg	15	3	0	3
fish seasoning sauce	1 Tbs	15	1	0	0
SEAWEED					
agar					
dried					
(Eden)					
bars	1 Tbs	10	2	2	0
flakes	1 Tbs	10	2	2	0
raw	2 Tbs	3	<1	<1	0
arame (Eden)	½ cup	30	7	7	0
hiziki (Eden)	½ cup	30	6	6	0
kelp..raw	1 oz	12	3	0.5	0
kombu (Eden) 7" sheet	½" sheet	10	10	2	0
laver/Nori..dried					
(Eden) sushi nori sea vegetable	1 sheet	10	1	1	0
spirulina					
dried	3 oz	245	20	na	0
raw	3 oz	24	2	na	0
wakame					
(Eden)	½ cup	25	4	4	0
flakes..instant	1 tsp	3	0	0	0
SEITAN					
(Lightlife) organic					
BBQ	3 oz	120	9	0	2
soy	3 oz	110	6	1	4

Food and Description	Amount	Total Calories	Total Carbs	Fiber	Sugars
(White Wave)					
BOX					
chicken-style..meat of wheat	3 oz	130	12	10	2
traditional	3 oz	140	3	1	0
vegetarian stir-fry strips	3 oz	100	2	0	0
PACK					
chicken-style..water-packed	4.5 oz	130	9	3	0
SELTZER WATER (*See* SOFT DRINK; WATER)					
SEMOLINA (*See also* FLOUR)					
enriched or unenriched	½ cup	310	61	3.5	0
whole-grain	1 cup	600	120	6.5	0
SESAME BUTTER/TAHINI					
(Arrowhead Mills) organic tahini	2 Tbs	190	5	3	0
(Erewhon)					
butter	2 Tbs	190	5	3	0
tahini	2 Tbs	200	3	0	0
(Casbah) sauce mix	¼ pkg	200	10	0.5	0
(Kettle) roaster-fresh sesame butter	2 Tbs	168	6	0	0
(Peloponnese) organic tahini w/ground					
sesame seeds	1 Tbs	100	2	1	0
SESAME FLOUR (*See* FLOUR)					
SESAME SEED					
kernels (Arrowhead Mills)	¼ cup	210	5	5	0
whole					
(Arrowhead Mills) brown	¼ cup	200	8	5	0
generic					
dried	1 Tbs	48	1	<1	0
roasted & toasted	1 oz	160	7	4	0
SHAD, AMERICAN					
cooked-dry heat	3 oz	215	0	0	0
SHALLOT					
freeze-dried	1 Tbs	3	1	0	0
	¼ cup	13	3	0	0
	1 oz	100	4.5	<1	0
fresh..raw..chopped	1 Tbs	7	2	<1	0
SHARK..batter-dipped & fried	3 oz	194	5	0	na
SHEEPSHEAD..cooked—dry heat	3 oz	107	0	0	0
SHELLIE BEAN					
CANNED					
(Allens)	½ cup	35	6	0	0
(Stokely's)	½ cup	45	8	3	1
SPROUTED (La Choy)	1 cup	10	2	1	1
SHERBET (*See also* FRUIT ICES, BARS & POPS)					
(Baskin-Robbins)					
red raspberry	reg scoop	160	36	0	35
all other flavors	reg scoop	160	34	0	34
(Blue Bunny)					
Disney Cool Tubes..all flavors	1 tube	80	18	0	15
Disney Pixar Galactic Buzz Lightyear sherbet	½ cup	80	18	0	15

Food and Description	Amount	Total Calories	Total Carbs	Fiber	Sugars
cups..all flavors	2.28 oz	90	20	0	16
fat-free..all flavors	½ cup	110	25	0	20
regular..all flavors	½ cup	110	25	0	20
(Breyers) natural					
chocolate rainbow	½ cup	140	16	0	14
orange	½ cup	130	28	0	20
rainbow	½ cup	130	27	0	20
raspberry	½ cup	130	28	0	20
Take Two! vanilla ice cream w/orange sherbet	½ cup	140	21	0	17
(Deluxe)					
orange cream bars	1 bar	110	19	0	19
raspberry, orange & lime	½ cup	90	21	0	20
(Dreyer's)					
berry rainbow	½ cup	130	29	0	23
lime	½ cup	130	28	0	23
orange cream	½ cup	120	23	0	19
raspberry	½ cup	130	28	0	22
Swiss orange	½ cup	150	30	0	25
tropical rainbow	½ cup	130	29	0	24
(Edy's)					
berry rainbow	½ cup	130	29	0	23
lime	½ cup	130	28	0	23
orange cream	½ cup	120	23	0	19
raspberry	½ cup	130	28	0	22
Swiss orange	½ cup	150	30	0	25
tropical rainbow	½ cup	130	29	0	24
(Friendly's)					
ice cream & sherbet roll	½ cup	200	31	0	29
Sherbet Sensations					
orange, lemon & raspberry	½ cup	130	28	0	21
watermelon, lemon & chocolate	½ cup	170	35	0	27
(Hiland) raspberry	½ cup	110	25	0	20
(Hiland-Roberts)					
Old Recipe..orange	½ cup	110	24	0	19
orange	½ cup	110	25	0	20
(Hood) Fruit Scoops lime, orange & lemon	½ cup	120	26	0	26
(Kemp's) orange..fat-free	½ cup	120	28	0	21
(Pet)	½ cup	130	30	0	24
lime, orange, or rainbow	½ cup	130	30	0	24
Tom Toms..orange push-up	1 push-up	80	16	0	13
vanilla ice cream w/orange sherbet	½ cup	90	15	0	15

SHORTENING, VEGETABLE (*See also* FAT; LARD; OIL; SHORTENING SUBSTITUTE)

(NOTE: All brands of vegetable shortening contain the same amount of calories and fat, just as all types of vegetable oil do. Because of the flexibility manufacturers are given in rounding off nutritional data, it may appear that one product has slightly fewer calories or less fat than another, but don't be fooled: they all get 100% of their calories from fat.)

(Crisco) regular or butter flavor	1 Tbs	110	0	0	0
	1 cup	1,845	0	0	0

Food and Description	Amount	Total Calories	Total Carbs	Fiber	Sugars
(Snowdrift)	1 Tbs	110	0	0	0
(Wesson)	1 Tbs	100	0	0	0
SHORTENING SUBSTITUTE					
(Smucker's) replacement for baking					
Baking Healthy oil & shortening	1 Tbs	30	7	0	4
SHOYU/SOY SAUCE (*See* ASIAN FOOD, Sauces & Seasonings entry; SAUCE)					
SHRIMP (*See also* ASIAN FOOD; FROZEN ENTRÉE/DINNER; SEAFOOD ENTRÉE/DINNER; SHRIMP, IMITATION; SHRIMP PASTE)					
CANNED					
(3 Diamonds)					
small	3.5 oz	50	1	0	0
tiny..whole	2 oz	90	1	0	0
(Bumble Bee)					
all styles	2 oz	40	0	0	1
Orleans					
all styles	2 oz	40	0	0	1
(Chicken of the Sea)					
deveined					
medium	2 oz	45	1	0	1
small	2 oz	45	1	0	1
medium	2 oz	45	1	0	1
premium shrimp pouch	2.5 oz	55	1	0	1
small	2 oz	45	1	0	1
tiny	2 oz	45	1	0	1
(Crown Prince) tiny..peeled	½ can	60	<1	0	0
(Ducktrap River) smoked	¼ cup	60	0	0	0
fresh					
cooked—moist heat	4 large	112	0	0	0
	3 oz	80	0	0	<1
raw	3 oz	90	<1	0	0
SHRIMP, IMITATION (*See* SEAFOOD ENTRÉE/DINNER)					
SHRIMP PASTE..canned	1 tsp	15	<1	0	0
SMELT (*See also* SEAFOOD ENTRÉE/DINNER)					
rainbow..cooked—dry heat	3 oz	106	0	0	0
SMOKED SALMON (*See* SALMON; SALMON SPREAD; SEAFOOD ENTRÉE/DINNER)					
SNACK BAR (*See* CANDY; GRANOLA/GRANOLA-TYPE BAR)					
SNACK CAKE (*See* CAKE, SNACK; PASTRY; POPCORN & CAKES; RICE CAKES)					
SNACK MIX (*See* SNACKS)					
SNACKS (*See also* FRUIT SNACK; MEXICAN FOOD; NUTS, MIXED; POPCORN; POPCORN CAKES; POTATO CHIPS & SNACKS; PRETZEL; RICE CAKES; TORTILLA CHIPS/CORN CHIPS)					
(AlpineAire) Wild Rice Crunch					
apple cinnamon	½ pkg	143	27	2	na
crunch					
lime	½ pkg	121	28	2	na
orange	½ pkg	117	27	2	na
fruit nuggets..all flavors	½ pkg	91	23	0	na
(Andy Capp) Fries					
BBQ	1 oz	140	19	0	1
cheddar	1 oz	150	17	1	1
hot	1 oz	150	17	2	1

Food and Description	Amount	Total Calories	Total Carbs	Fiber	Sugars
hot chili cheese steak	1.75 oz	130	29	0	1
salsa	1 oz	130	18	0	1
white cheddar	1 oz	260	30	0	1
(Ann's House of Nuts) snack nut mixes					
Cajun	⅓ cup	170	16	2	1
California	¼ cup	130	21	2	16
cranberry fruit..nut	3 Tbs	110	15	2	12
honey nut crunch	3 Tbs	150	14	2	13
nut 'n' fruit mix	3 Tbs	120	16	2	13
nut 'n' raisin mix	3 Tbs	120	14	3	11
Swiss mix	3 Tbs	130	17	1	14
trail mix..raw	3 Tbs	130	12	3	9
(Atkins) Crunchers snack chips					
barbecue	1 oz	100	8	4	0
nacho cheese	1 oz	100	8	4	0
original	1 oz	90	8	4	0
sour cream & onion	1 oz	100	8	3	0
(Baken-ets) fried pork skins & cracklins					
BBQ pork skins	1 oz	70	<1	<1	<1
hot 'n' spicy pork skins	1 oz	80	<1	<1	<1
hot 'n' spicy cracklins	1 oz	80	<1	<1	<1
regular					
cracklins	1 oz	80	<1	<1	<1
pork skins	1 oz	80	<1	<1	<1
sweet 'n' tangy BBQ	1 oz	80	<1	<1	<1
(Barbara's Bakery) natural snacks					
cheese puff bakes..all flavors	1 oz	160	13	0	1
cheese puffs..all flavors	1 oz	150	16	0	0
potato chip snacks..all flavors	1 oz	150	15	1	0
(Betty Crocker)					
Bugles					
chili cheese	1⅓ cups	160	18	0	2
nacho cheese	1⅓ cups	160	18	0	2
original	1⅓ cups	160	18	0	2
smokin' BBQ	1⅓ cups	160	18	0	2
Chex Mix					
bold party blend	½ cup	140	20	2	2
cheddar cheese	⅔ cup	130	22	<1	3
honey nut	½ cup	130	23	1	6
hot 'n' spicy	⅔ cup	130	22	1	2
peanut lovers	½ cup	140	19	1	2
traditional	⅔ cup	130	22	1	2
trail mix	½ cup	140	22	1	7
Fruit by the Foot..all flavors	1 roll	80	17	0	10
Fruit Gushers..all flavors	1 pouch	90	20	0	13
Fruit Roll-Ups..all flavors	1 roll	50	12	0	7
Fruit Snacks..all flavors	1 pouch	80	21	0	14
(Cheetos)					
Asteroids					
hot	1 oz	150	16	<1	<1

Food and Description	Amount	Total Calories	Total Carbs	Fiber	Sugars
regular	1 oz	150	15	<1	1
crunchy	1 oz	160	15	<1	1
curls	1 oz	150	15	<1	1
hot puff rods	1 oz	160	15	<1	<1
jumbo puffs	1 oz	160	13	0	<1
natural white cheddar puffs	1 oz	170	16	0	0
puffs	1 oz	160	15	<1	<1
Wirlz	1 oz	160	14	<1	1
X's & O's	1 oz	160	15	<1	1
(Cheezbits) Cheese snacks..					
white original	1 oz	70	2	0	2
(Chex Mix) (See (Betty Crocker) in this section.)					
(Cornnuts)					
BBQ..crunchy	1.7 oz	220	34	4	3
chile picante..crunchy	1 oz	130	19	2	0
	1.7 oz	210	33	4	0
nacho cheese	1 oz	130	19	2	0
original..crunchy	1.7 oz	210	34	4	0
ranch..crunchy	1 oz	130	19	2	0
	1.7 oz	220	33	4	1
salsa jalisco	1.7 oz	220	34	4	1
(Cracker Jack) (See POPCORN)					
(Crunch & Munch) (See POPCORN)					
(David)					
pumpkin seeds					
all natural	¼ cup	160	3	1	0
2-oz bag	1 bag	250	5	2	<1
2.25-oz bag	1 bag	280	6	2	1
sunflower kernels					
original	¼ cup	200	5	2	1
1-oz bag	1 bag	310	9	4	2
1.75-oz bag	1 bag	330	9	4	1
ranch..1.75 oz bag	1 bag	310	9	4	2
sizzlin' BBQ	¼ cup	190	6	2	1
1.75-oz bag	1 bag	310	9	4	2
sunflower seeds					
BBQ	¼ cup	190	5	2	1
1.75-oz bag	1 bag	160	4	2	1
2.5-oz bag	1 bag	190	5	2	1
jalapeño hot salsa	¼ cup	190	5	2	1
1.75-oz bag	1 bag	160	5	2	1
2.5-oz bag	1 bag	220	6	3	1
nacho cheese	¼ cup	180	6	2	1
0.8-oz bag	1 bag	70	2	<1	0
1.75-oz bag	1 bag	150	5	2	0
original	¼ cup	190	5	2	1
1.75-oz bag	1 bag	160	4	2	1
2.5-oz bag	1 bag	190	5	2	1
ranch	¼ cup	190	6	2	1
1.75-oz bag	1 bag	160	4	2	1

Food and Description	Amount	Total Calories	Total Carbs	Fiber	Sugars
2.5-oz bag	1 bag	220	6	3	1
reduced-sodium	¼ cup	190	5	2	1
toasted corn snacks					
BBQ	⅓ cup	140	29	1	1
1.7-oz bag	1 bag	230	34	2	1
traditional	⅓ cup	140	18	1	0
1.7-oz bag	1 bag	230	31	2	0
(Edward & Sons) brown rice snaps					
buckwheat tamari	8 pieces	60	13	2	0
cheddar	8 pieces	60	12	0	<1
onion garlic	8 pieces	60	13	2	0
plain	8 pieces	50	13	2	0
tamari seaweed	8 pieces	60	13	2	0
tamari sesame	8 pieces	60	13	2	0
toasted onion	8 pieces	60	13	0	<1
unsalted sesame	8 pieces	60	13	2	0
vegetable	8 pieces	60	11	<1	<1
(Fisher) snack mixes					
Nuts & Crunchies					
Bayou blend..spicy sweet	1 oz	150	13	2	4
fiesta	1 oz	140	16	1	2
golden crisp	1 oz	140	15	1	3
honey crunch	1 oz	140	17	1	4
Nuts & Fruits					
California-style	1 oz	140	15	2	8
honey crunch	1 oz	140	17	1	5
pineapple banana	1 oz	140	15	2	10
raisin cranberry	1 oz	150	13	2	9
trail-style	1 oz	150	11	2	8
Snack 'n' Serve Bowl..fiesta mix	1 oz	140	16	1	2
(Flavor Tree)					
party mix..sesame snack blend	1 oz	180	11	2	3
sesame sticks					
garlic	1 oz	170	16	2	0
plain	1 oz	170	13	3	2
(Frito-Lay)					
Doritos..3Ds..corn snacks					
jalapeño cheddar	1 oz	130	20	1	1
KC Masterpiece	1 oz	140	23	<1	3
Nacho Cheesier					
mini	2 oz	270	39	2	7
regular	1 oz	130	19	1	2
zesty sour cream & cheddar..mini	2 oz	270	38	2	3
Funyuns onion-flavored rings	1 oz	140	18	<1	<1
Munchos	1 oz	160	16	1	0
Rold Gold snack mixes					
Colossal Cheddar	¾ cup	160	19	1	2
Munchies	¾ cup	140	18	1	1
original	¾ cup	160	18	1	2

Food and Description	Amount	Total Calories	Total Carbs	Fiber	Sugars
sunflower seeds					
kernels..original	1 oz	180	5	2	<1
seeds					
BBQ	1 oz	200	6	2	3
Flamin' Hot	1 oz	180	5	2	<1
original	1 oz	180	5	2	<1
(Funyuns) (*See* (Frito-Lay) in this section.)					
(Gardetto's)					
deli-style mustard..pretzel mix	½ cup	130	24	1	<1
Italian cheese blend	½ cup	140	20	<1	2
original recipe	½ cup	160	20	1	1
reduced-fat	½ cup	130	20	1	1
sour cream & onion	½ cup	130	21	2	2
special Italian recipe	½ cup	150	20	1	1
(GeniSoy)					
snack bar					
New York–style cheesecake	2.2 oz	220	34	1	28
Xtreme Carrot Cake Quake	1.6 oz	190	24	1	18
soy crisps					
apple cinnamon crunch	1 oz	110	17	2	4
creamy ranch..salted	1 oz	110	15	2	1
deep sea salt	1 oz	100	14	2	1
nacho cheese	1 oz	110	5	2	1
rich cheddar	1 oz	100	14	2	1
roasted garlic	1 oz	100	14	2	1
tangy salt 'n' vinegar	1 oz	100	14	2	1
zesty barbecue	1 oz	110	17	2	2
trail mix					
soy nut Happy Trails	1.23 oz	130	17	2	6
soy nut Mountain Medley	1.23 oz	130	16	2	4
soy nut Tropical Paradise	1.23 oz	119	18	2	11
(Hain) PureSnax					
crudités					
original	1 oz	120	22	1	<1
sour cream & onion	1 oz	120	21	1	<1
kettle corn..original	½ cup	120	24	3	15
Soy Munchies					
caramel	7 pieces	40	8	<1	4
ranch	9 pieces	60	8	1	1
white cheddar	9 pieces	60	6	1	1
Zoinks..corn snacks					
butter	3½ cups	140	23	<1	1
white cheddar	3½ cups	140	22	1	1
(Keebler) Sunshine..Cheez It					
party mix..all styles	½ cup	130	19	1	1
snack mix					
Big Crunch	¾ cup	110	20	<1	1
double cheese	¾ cup	140	19	<1	1
Get Nutty	½ cup	150	17	1	2
original	½ cup	130	21	2	2

Food and Description	Amount	Total Calories	Total Carbs	Fiber	Sugars
(Lance)					
cheese balls	1 oz	150	13	0	1
cheese puffs	1 oz	170	13	0	1
peanut bar	2.2 oz	340	29	3	19
pork skins					
BBQ	1 oz	140	2	0	0
hot & spicy..made w/Texas Pete	1 oz	170	0	0	0
plain	1 oz	150	2	0	0
(Lundberg Family Farms)					
bean & rice chips					
BBQ	1 oz	140	18	1	1
pico de gallo	1 oz	140	18	1	0
sea salt	1 oz	140	18	1	0
sesame & seaweed	1 oz	140	19	1	1
(Michael Season's)					
soy protein chips					
original	1 cup	110	9	4	0
smoky BBQ	1 cup	110	8	4	9
spicy ranch	1 cup	110	9	<1	1
sweet organic..cinnamon twists	1 cup	130	21	0	7
ultimate cheese puffs..all flavors	1 oz	180	13	2	3
(Mike Sell's)					
cheese curls..cheddar..oven-baked	1 oz	160	17	0	1
puffcorn delite..oven-baked	1 oz	180	17	0	0
(Munchos) (See (Frito-Lay) in this section)					
(Nabisco) (See also COOKIES; CRACKERS)					
Nabisco Fruit Snacks					
Blue's Clues	1 pkg	60	14	0	10
Checkers	1 pkg	80	19	0	14
cherry	1 pkg	80	19	0	14
Dora the Explorer	1 pkg	60	14	0	10
Gamesters	1 pkg	80	19	0	14
Jimmy Neutron	1 pkg	80	19	0	14
Wacky Faces	1 pkg	80	19	0	14
Nabisco Teddy Grahams					
graham snacks					
chocolate	1.25 oz	150	26	1	10
chocolate chip	1 oz	130	22	<1	8
mini	1 oz	140	22	1	8
cinnamon	1.25 oz	160	27	1	9
(New York Style)					
bagel chip snack mix..fat-free	1 oz	100	21	1	1
bagel chips..toasted garlic	1 oz	130	20	0	1
(Nutcracker) trail mix..					
The Ultimate Tropical	1 oz	160	20	2	16
(Old Dutch)					
cheese curls					
baked	1 oz	180	15	1	1
Cheez	1 oz	170	15	0	1
crunchy	1 oz	170	13	0	1
snack mix..classical mixers	1 oz	140	20	1	1

Food and Description	Amount	Total Calories	Total Carbs	Fiber	Sugars
(Old London)					
bagel snacks					
cinnamon raisin	5 pieces	60	9	2	0
garlic	5 pieces	60	9	2	0
original	5 pieces	60	9	2	0
poppyseed	5 pieces	60	12	1	0
party snacks					
honey mustard	⅓ cup	70	9	1	0
zesty	⅓ cup	70	8	1	0
waffle snacks..cheddar or Swiss	3 pieces	70	9	0	0
(Planters)					
Cheez Mania Balls	1 oz	160	15	1	1
Cheez Mania Curls	1 oz	150	15	1	1
trail mix					
fruit & nut mix	1 oz	130	14	1	10
honey nut & caramel	1 oz	160	17	1	10
nuts, cheese nips & mini Ritz	1 oz	160	9	2	1
nut & chocolate	1 oz	170	16	2	11
nuts, seeds & raisins	1 oz	160	11	3	5
spicy nuts & Cajun sticks	1 oz	150	13	2	1
(Ralston) snack mix					
cheddar	1 oz	130	22	<1	2
traditional	1 oz	130	22	1	18
(Snyder's of Hanover)					
Eat Smart					
corn & rice puffs..cheddars	1 oz	130	20	1	0
	0.75 oz	100	15	1	0
veggie crisps					
cheddar & jalapeño	1 oz	130	18	2	0
regular	1 oz	140	18	2	0
	1.5 oz	190	26	2	0
sun-dried tomato & pesto	1 oz	140	19	3	0
Nibblers					
cheddar PB-Zels	1 oz	130	14	2	2
garlic bread	1 oz	130	24	<1	<1
honey-roasted PB-Zels	1 oz	140	18	1	1
no salt..fat-free	1 oz	120	25	1	1
sourdough..fat-free	1 oz	120	25	1	1
(SunChips)					
French onion	1 oz	140	18	2	3
harvest cheddar	1 oz	140	19	2	2
original	1 oz	140	19	2	2
(Sunshine) (See (Keebler) this section)					
(Terra Harvest)					
Mr. Krispies..gourmet rice chips					
cheddar salsa	1 oz	120	22	0	0
classic BBQ	1 oz	120	23	0	0
sea salt & cracked pepper	1 oz	110	24	0	0
sticks					
honey-roasted soy	1 oz	150	4	1	3

Food and Description	Amount	Total Calories	Total Carbs	Fiber	Sugars
nacho corn	1 oz	140	6	2	1
poppy & onion	1 oz	150	4	<1	0
salsa corn	1 oz	130	7	2	1
sesame..all styles	1 oz	160	4	<1	0
sesame oat bran	1 oz	160	4	1	0
soy	1 oz	140	4	2	1
unsalted	1 oz	160	4	<1	0
(Utz)					
BBQ pork rinds	½ oz	80	0	0	<1
plain pork rinds	½ oz	80	0	0	<1
pork cracklins	½ oz	90	0	0	<1
(Wise)					
Cheez Doodles					
crunchy	1 oz	150	16	0	1
puffed	1 oz	150	17	0	2
white cheddar	1 oz	150	14	0	1
Cheez Waffies	1 oz	140	15	0	4
Dipsy Doodles	1 oz	160	16	1	0
onion-flavored rings	1 oz	140	20	0	0
pork rinds					
hot & spicy	½ oz	70	1	0	0
original	½ oz	80	1	0	0
sweet & mild BBQ	½ oz	90	1	0	1
SNAIL/ESCARGOT..fresh					
cooked—moist heat	3 oz	235	13	0	0
raw..meat only	3 oz	115	7	0	0
SNAP BEAN (See GREEN BEAN)					
SNAPPER..cooked—dry heat	3 oz	110	0	0	0
SNOW PEA (Frieda's) snow peas & sauce	½ cup	40	8	2	6
SOCKEYE (See SALMON)					
SODA (See COCKTAIL MIXER; SOFT DRINK)					
SOFT DRINK (See also FRUIT PUNCH; SOFT DRINK MIX; TEA; individual juice drink listings)					
(A&W)					
cream soda					
diet	12 fl oz	0	0	0	0
regular	12 fl oz	180	48	0	46
root beer					
diet	12 fl oz	0	0	0	0
regular	12 fl oz	170	46	0	46
(Barq's) root beer					
diet	8 fl oz	0	0	0	0
regular	12 fl oz	160	45	0	45
(Big Red) red soda	8 fl oz	100	25	0	25
	12 fl oz	170	47	0	47
(Blue Sky)					
natural					
black cherry	12 fl oz	150	37	0	37
cherry vanilla cream	12 fl oz	180	46	0	46
cola	12 fl oz	170	42	0	42

Food and Description	Amount	Total Calories	Total Carbs	Fiber	Sugars
Dr. Becker	12 fl oz	150	38	0	38
grape	12 fl oz	140	36	0	36
grapefruit	12 fl oz	150	38	0	38
Jamaican ginger ale	12 fl oz	150	37	0	37
lemon lime	12 fl oz	140	35	0	35
raspberry	12 fl oz	180	45	0	45
root beer	12 fl oz	170	43	0	43
truly orange	12 fl oz	150	38	0	38
organic..natural					
Black Cherry Cherish	12 fl oz	150	37	0	37
Ginger Gale	12 fl oz	160	39	0	39
New Century Cola	12 fl oz	160	40	0	40
Orange Divine	12 fl oz	180	44	0	44
Prime Lime Cream	12 fl oz	160	40	0	40
Root Beer Encore	12 fl oz	170	43	0	43
True Seltzer sparkling waters..all flavors	12 fl oz	0	0	0	0
(Canada Dry)					
birch beer..all styles	8 fl oz	110	27	0	27
bitter lemon	8 fl oz	100	21	0	21
Black Cherry Wish	8 fl oz	120	32	0	32
Cactus Cooler soda	8 fl oz	110	27	0	27
California strawberry soda	8 fl oz	100	27	0	27
club soda..all styles	12 fl oz	0	0	0	0
collins mixer	12 fl oz	130	30	0	30
ginger ale	12 fl oz	120	33	0	33
cranberry					
diet	12 fl oz	5	<1	0	<1
regular	12 fl oz	140	37	0	37
seltzer	12 fl oz	0	0	0	0
tonic water	12 fl oz	130	36	0	36
diet	12 fl oz	0	0	0	0
(Coca-Cola)					
Coca-Cola					
cherry					
diet	8 fl oz	1	0	0	0
regular	8 fl oz	100	27	0	27
classic					
caffeine-free	12 fl oz	100	27	0	27
regular	12 fl oz	100	27	0	27
Diet Coke					
caffeine-free	8 fl oz	1	0	0	0
regular	8 fl oz	1	0	0	0
Vanilla Coke	12 fl oz	100	28	0	28
Fanta..strawberry	12 fl oz	140	38	0	38
Fresca	8 fl oz	0	0	0	0
Mello Yello					
diet	8 fl oz	3	<1	0	<1
regular	8 fl oz	120	32	0	32
Minute Maid					
blueberry	8 fl oz	110	30	0	30

Food and Description	Amount	Total Calories	Total Carbs	Fiber	Sugars
fruit punch..carbonated	8 fl oz	115	32	0	32
grape soda	8 fl oz	120	32	0	32
grapefruit soda	8 fl oz	108	29	0	29
orange soda					
diet	8 fl oz	2	0	0	0
regular	8 fl oz	118	32	0	32
peach soda	8 fl oz	110	29	0	29
pineapple soda	8 fl oz	109	30	0	30
strawberry soda	8 fl oz	120	33	0	33
Mr. Pibb					
diet	8 fl oz	1	0	0	0
regular	8 fl oz	97	26	0	26
Tab	8 fl oz	1	0	0	0
(Crush)					
cherry	8 fl oz	120	34	0	34
orange..regular	12 fl oz	180	50	0	50
(Diet Rite)	12 fl oz	0	0	0	0
(Dr Pepper)					
diet..caffeine-free or regular	12 fl oz	0	0	0	0
Red Fusion..caffeine-free or regular	12 fl oz	150	40	0	40
(Faygo)					
cream cola..vanilla	8 fl oz	110	28	0	27
Frosh					
grape	12 fl oz	200	33	0	32
Moon mist	8 fl oz	120	31	0	30
orange					
diet	8 fl oz	0	0	0	0
regular	8 fl oz	130	33	0	32
(Hansen's) natural					
cherry	12 fl oz	120	32	0	32
ginger beer	8 fl oz	100	28	0	28
orange cream	8 fl oz	110	31	0	31
sarsparilla	8 fl oz	110	30	0	30
(Health Valley)					
ginger ale	12 fl oz	160	40	0	40
root beer..old-fashioned	12 fl oz	160	40	0	40
sarsaparilla root beer	12 fl oz	160	40	0	40
(Hires) root beer					
diet	8 fl oz	5	<1	0	0
regular	8 fl oz	170	45	0	45
(Jones) soda					
naturals					
Bada Bing!	12 fl oz	90	24	0	22
Banana Berry	12 fl oz	90	25	0	25
Berry White	12 fl oz	110	28	0	28
Betty	12 fl oz	90	24	0	24
Bohemian Raspberry	12 fl oz	40	11	0	10
Dave	12 fl oz	80	21	0	2
D'Peach Mode	12 fl oz	90	24	0	23
Fu Cran Fu	12 fl oz	100	27	0	27

Food and Description	Amount	Total Calories	Total Carbs	Fiber	Sugars
Strawbery Manilow	12 fl oz	80	22	9	22
regular					
berry lemonade	12 fl oz	190	48	0	47
blue bubblegum	12 fl oz	190	48	0	48
chocolate fudge	12 fl oz	180	44	0	44
cream soda	12 fl oz	190	48	0	48
fufu berry	12 fl oz	190	46	0	46
green apple	12 fl oz	170	46	0	46
lemon drop	12 fl oz	190	48	0	47
orange & cream	12 fl oz	190	48	0	47
root beer	12 fl oz	180	44	0	44
strawberry lime	12 fl oz	190	48	0	48
vanilla cola	12 fl oz	170	43	0	42
sugar-free..all flavors	12 fl oz	0	0	0	0
(Mountain Dew)					
diet..caffeine-free	8 fl oz	0	0	0	0
regular	8 fl oz	110	32	0	32
(Mug)					
cream soda					
diet	8 fl oz	0	0	0	0
regular	8 fl oz	120	32	0	32
root beer					
diet	8 fl oz	0	0	0	0
regular	8 fl oz	110	0	–	31
(Pepsi)					
diet..caffeine-free or regular	8 fl oz	0	0	0	0
Pepsi 1	8 fl oz	1	0	0	0
Pepsi Blue	8 fl oz	100	27	0	26
Pepsi Twist					
diet	8 fl oz	0	0	0	0
regular	12 fl oz	100	27	0	25
Pepsi Vanilla					
diet	8 fl oz	0	0	0	0
regular	8 fl oz	110	28	0	28
regular or caffeine-free	8 fl oz	100	27	0	27
wild cherry					
diet	8 fl oz	0	0	0	0
regular	8 fl oz	110	29	0	29
(RC)					
cherry cola	12 fl oz	160	44	0	44
cola					
diet	12 fl oz	0	0	0	0
regular or caffeine-free	12 fl oz	160	43	0	43
(R. W. Knudsen) spritzers					
black cherry	12 fl oz	170	42	0	34
boysenberry	12 fl oz	160	40	0	38
cherry cola	12 fl oz	170	42	0	34
cranberry	12 fl oz	190	45	0	45
grape	12 fl oz	170	42	0	37
Jamaican lemonade	12 fl oz	170	41	0	38

Food and Description	Amount	Total Calories	Total Carbs	Fiber	Sugars
kiwi lime	12 fl oz	130	32	0	28
lemon lime	12 fl oz	170	42	0	41
Mandarin lime	12 fl oz	170	42	0	41
Mango Fandango	12 fl oz	190	45	0	45
orange passionfruit	12 fl oz	160	40	0	38
peach	12 fl oz	160	37	0	26
red raspberry	12 fl oz	170	38	0	32
strawberry	12 fl oz	170	42	0	38
tangerine	12 fl oz	170	40	0	35
vanilla cream	12 fl oz	160	35	0	34
(Santa Cruz) organic spritzers					
cherry	12 fl oz	140	34	0	33
ginger ale	12 fl oz	150	37	0	35
lemon lime	12 fl oz	130	33	0	31
lemonade	12 fl oz	100	26	0	23
orange mango	12 fl oz	130	33	0	32
raspberry lemonade	12 fl oz	120	29	0	28
vanilla cream	12 fl oz	160	40	0	39
(Schweppes)					
club soda	10 fl oz	0	0	0	0
collins mixer	10 fl oz	130	30	0	30
ginger ale..plain					
diet	10 fl oz	0	0	0	0
regular	10 fl oz	120	33	0	33
(Seagrams)					
club soda	8 fl oz	0	0	0	0
ginger ale					
diet	8 fl oz	2	0	0	0
raspberry	8 fl oz	90	24	0	24
diet	8 fl oz	2	0	0	0
naturals..seltzer					
black cherry	8 fl oz	2	0	0	0
lemon lime	8 fl oz	1	0	0	0
orange	8 fl oz	1	0	0	0
original	8 fl oz	0	0	0	0
raspberry	8 fl oz	1	0	0	0
tonic water					
diet	8 fl oz	3	0	0	0
regular	8 fl oz	83	22	0	22
w/twist of lime	8 fl oz	93	24	0	24
(7-Up)					
cherry					
diet	12 fl oz	0	0	0	0
regular	12 fl oz	150	39	0	39
regular					
diet	12 fl oz	0	0	0	0
regular	12 fl oz	140	40	0	40
(Slice)					
orange					
diet	8 fl oz	0	0	0	0

Food and Description	Amount	Total Calories	Total Carbs	Fiber	Sugars
w/caffeine	8 fl oz	130	34	0	33
(Squirt)					
original					
diet	12 fl oz	0	0	0	0
regular	12 fl oz	150	40	0	40
ruby red					
diet	12 fl oz	0	0	0	0
regular	12 fl oz	170	46	0	46
(Sunkist) orange	12 fl oz	190	52	0	52
(Vernor's) ginger soda					
diet	8 fl oz	0	0	0	0
regular	12 fl oz	150	39	0	39
(Yoo-Hoo)					
chocolate	8 fl oz	130	29	0	20
double fudge	8 fl oz	140	33	0	27
light	8 fl oz	70	15	0	15
strawberry	8 fl oz	130	29	0	26
SOFT DRINK MIX (See also FRUIT PUNCH; SOFT DRINK; individual fruit drink listings)					
(Crystal Light)					
all flavors..prepared w/water	8 fl oz	5	0	0	0
(Kool-Aid)					
sugar-free..low-calorie					
all flavors..prepared w/water	8 fl oz	0	0	0	0
sugar-sweetened..prepared w/water					
Mad Scientwists	8 fl oz	60	16	0	16
Mega Mountain Twists	8 fl oz	70	17	0	17
unsweetened..all flavors					
prepared w/o sugar	8 fl oz	0	0	0	0
SOLE (See also FROZEN ENTRÉE/DINNER; SEAFOOD ENTRÉE/DINNER)					
cooked—dry heat	3 oz	100	0	0	0
SORBET (See FRUIT ICES, BARS & POPS; SHERBET)					
SORGHUM..whole grain	1 cup	650	143	na	na
SORGHUM SYRUP (See also MOLASSES; SYRUP)					
(Arrowhead Mills)	1 Tbs	60	16	0	16
SORREL (See DOCK)					
SOUP					
(NOTE: Unless stated otherwise, condensed soups were prepared as directed with water. If prepared with milk, whole milk was used unless noted otherwise. Ready-to-serve soups were heated as directed with no added liquid.)					
CANNED					
(Amy's) organic..ready-to-serve					
alphabet..fat-free	1 cup	80	16	2	4
black bean vegetable	1 cup	130	25	5	6
butternut squash..low-fat	1 cup	100	20	2	4
chunky tomato bisque	1 cup	120	21	2	14
cream of mushroom..semi-condensed	1 cup	140	13	2	3
cream of tomato..low-fat	1 cup	100	17	3	11
lentil	1 cup	150	19	9	3
lentil vegetable	1 cup	150	23	6	5
no chicken noodle..low-fat	1 cup	90	12	2	4

Food and Description	Amount	Total Calories	Total Carbs	Fiber	Sugars
pasta & 3-bean	1 cup	130	19	4	6
split pea..low-fat	1 cup	100	19	4	4
vegetable barley..low-fat	1 cup	70	13	3	5
(Baxters) ready-to-serve					
cream of asparagus	1 cup	130	13	6	2
lobster bisque	1 cup	120	11	0	2
(Campbell's)					
condensed/unprepared					
Healthy Request					
chicken noodle	½ cup	60	8	1	2
chicken rice	½ cup	80	13	1	1
cream of celery	½ cup	70	11	0	3
cream of mushroom	½ cup	70	10	1	2
hearty chicken w/white & wild rice	½ cup	110	17	2	2
minestrone	½ cup	80	15	3	4
tomato	½ cup	90	18	1	10
vegetable	½ cup	100	20	3	5
vegetable beef	½ cup	90	20	3	5
Original soups					
98% Fat-Free..prepared					
broccoli cheese	½ cup	70	12	1	2
cream of					
broccoli	½ cup	60	12	1	2
celery	½ cup	60	8	1	1
chicken	½ cup	70	10	<1	1
mushroom	½ cup	70	9	1	1
New England clam chowder	½ cup	80	13	1	1
bean w/bacon	½ cup	170	25	8	4
beef broth..double strength	½ cup	15	1	0	1
beef consommé	½ cup	20	1	0	1
beef noodle	½ cup	70	9	<1	1
beef soup w/vegetables & barley	½ cup	90	15	3	2
beefy mushroom	½ cup	50	6	0	1
black bean	½ cup	110	19	5	4
broccoli cheese	½ cup	100	12	0	2
California-style vegetable	½ cup	70	13	2	3
cheddar cheese	½ cup	100	12	1	2
chicken alphabet	½ cup	80	12	1	1
Chicken consommé	½ cup	25	0	0	0
chicken & dumplings	½ cup	80	10	1	1
chicken & stars	½ cup	80	12	1	1
chicken broth soup	½ cup	20	1	0	1
chicken noodle	½ cup	60	8	<1	1
chicken noodle o's	½ cup	80	12	1	2
chicken w/rice	½ cup	80	14	1	1
chicken w/white & wild rice	½ cup	70	12	1	1
chicken wonton	½ cup	45	6	0	1
cream of asparagus	½ cup	100	10	1	2
cream of broccoli	½ cup	90	12	1	3
cream of celery	½ cup	100	10	1	1

Food and Description	Amount	Total Calories	Total Carbs	Fiber	Sugars
cream of chicken	½ cup	120	11	1	1
cream of chicken mushroom	½ cup	120	9	1	1
cream of chicken w/herbs	½ cup	90	10	1	2
cream of mushroom	½ cup	110	9	1	1
cream of onion	½ cup	100	12	1	5
cream of potato	½ cup	100	15	1	2
cream of shrimp	½ cup	90	8	1	1
creamy chicken noodle	½ cup	120	13	0	2
creamy mushroom & roasted garlic	½ cup	70	11	1	2
curly chicken noodle	½ cup	80	11	1	1
double noodle	½ cup	90	17	2	1
fiesta chili beef w/beans	½ cup	170	25	8	5
fiesta nacho cheese	½ cup	120	10	1	2
French onion	½ cup	45	6	1	4
fun shapes	½ cup	80	12	2	2
golden mushroom	½ cup	80	10	1	1
green pea	½ cup	180	28	4	6
hearty vegetable w/pasta	½ cup	90	19	2	8
home-style chicken noodle	½ cup	70	8	2	1
Manhattan-style clam chowder	½ cup	70	12	2	2
mega noodle in chicken broth	½ cup	80	13	9	1
minestrone	½ cup	90	17	3	3
New England clam chowder	½ cup	90	13	1	1
oyster stew	½ cup	80	5	0	0
pepper pot	½ cup	90	9	1	1
Scotch broth soup	½ cup	70	9	2	1
Southwest-style chicken vegetable	½ cup	110	21	4	3
split pea w/ham	½ cup	180	27	5	4
tomato bisque	½ cup	130	23	1	15
turkey noodle	½ cup	70	9	1	1
vegetable beef	½ cup	80	15	3	2
vegetarian vegetable	½ cup	90	18	2	6
ready-to-serve					
32-oz can					
creamy tomato	1 cup	130	26	2	18
tomato	1 cup	100	21	2	13
tomato w/roasted garlic	1 cup	120	28	2	19
Chunky					
baked potato w/bacon bits & chives	1 cup	160	21	1	4
baked potato w/cheddar & bacon bits	1 cup	180	23	2	3
baked potato w/steak & cheese	1 cup	210	21	3	3
beef w/country vegetables	1 cup	160	22	4	5
beef w/white & wild rice	1 cup	150	24	2	5
cheese tortellini w/chicken & vegetables	1 cup	110	18	2	4
chicken & dumplings	1 cup	190	17	2	3
chicken broccoli	1 cup	190	14	1	2
chicken corn chowder	1 cup	230	19	2	3
chicken mushroom chowder	1 cup	230	12	2	2
classic chicken noodle	1 cup	100	16	2	3

Food and Description	Amount	Total Calories	Total Carbs	Fiber	Sugars
grilled chicken & sausage gumbo	1 cup	140	21	3	5
grilled sirloin steak w/hearty vegetables	1 cup	130	19	4	5
hearty bean 'n' ham	1 cup	180	30	8	5
hearty chicken w/vegetables	1 cup	100	14	2	3
hearty vegetables w/pasta	1 cup	130	23	3	9
herb-roasted chicken w/potatoes	1 cup	110	16	3	4
honey-roasted ham w/potatoes	1 cup	130	20	3	7
Manhattan-style clam chowder	1 cup	130	19	2	4
New England clam chowder	1 cup	240	21	2	1
old-fashioned potato ham chowder	1 cup	190	17	2	1
old-fashioned vegetable beef	1 cup	130	18	6	2
pepper steak	1 cup	120	18	3	4
Salisbury steak, mushrooms & onion	1 cup	150	18	3	7
savory chicken w/white & wild rice	1 cup	120	19	2	2
seasoned rib roast w/potatoes	1 cup	110	17	3	5
sirloin burger w/country vegetables	1 cup	180	17	3	4
slow-roasted beef w/mushrooms	1 cup	120	18	3	5
split pea 'n' ham	1 cup	170	27	4	5
steak & potato	1 cup	130	18	2	2
tomato cheese ravioli w/vegetables	1 cup	150	27	4	12
vegetable	1 cup	130	22	4	5
Chunky..microwaveable bowls					
beef w/country vegetables	1 cup	170	18	3	7
chicken & dumplings	1 cup	190	18	3	4
classic chicken noodle	1 cup	110	15	1	4
grilled chicken w/vegetables & pasta	1 cup	100	13	2	2
grilled sirloin steak w/hearty vegetables	1 cup	130	18	3	6
sirloin burger w/country vegetables	1 cup	160	18	3	5
Healthy Request					
chicken noodle	½ cup	60	8	1	2
chicken rice	½ cup	80	13	1	1
cream					
of celery	½ cup	70	11	0	3
of chicken	½ cup	70	12	1	2
of mushroom	½ cup	70	10	1	2
Hearty					
chicken w/white & wild rice	1 cup	110	17	2	2
minestrone	1 cup	80	15	3	4
tomato ravioli	1 cup	90	18	1	10
vegetable	1 cup	100	20	3	5
vegetable beef	1 cup	90	15	3	2
Kitchen Classics					
bean w/bacon	1 cup	180	28	8	4
chicken noodle	1 cup	90	13	1	1
chicken w/white & wild rice	1 cup	100	18	2	1
cream of potato	1 cup	160	20	2	4
creamy tomato	1 cup	140	24	2	15
lentil	1 cup	120	23	5	1
minestrone	1 cup	110	22	3	3

Food and Description	Amount	Total Calories	Total Carbs	Fiber	Sugars
New England clam chowder	1 cup	240	20	3	1
tomato	1 cup	100	24	1	4
vegetable	1 cup	100	22	3	9
Select soups					
98% fat-free					
New England clam chowder	1 cup	110	19	2	2
bean & ham	1 cup	170	30	7	4
beef w/portobello mushrooms & rice	1 cup	110	15	1	1
beef w/roasted barley	1 cup	150	24	3	3
chicken & pasta w/roasted garlic	1 cup	110	16	2	4
chicken & rice	1 cup	100	17	2	2
chicken vegetable	1 cup	100	18	2	4
chicken w/egg noodles	1 cup	100	14	1	1
creamy chicken Alfredo	1 cup	220	16	2	2
creamy potato w/roasted garlic	1 cup	170	20	2	4
fiesta vegetable	1 cup	120	24	4	6
grilled chicken w/sun-dried tomatoes	1 cup	110	17	2	6
herbed chicken w/roasted vegetables	1 cup	90	14	1	2
honey-roasted chicken	1 cup	100	16	1	7
Italian-style wedding soup	1 cup	120	16	2	3
minestrone	1 cup	100	20	4	3
New England clam chowder	1 cup	200	19	2	1
w/long grain & wild rice	1 cup	100	17	2	2
w/rotini & penne pasta	1 cup	100	16	2	4
rosemary chicken w/roasted potatoes	1 cup	100	18	2	2
savory lentil	1 cup	140	27	6	5
split pea w/ham	1 cup	160	29	5	6
tomato garden	1 cup	100	21	3	12
vegetable	1 cup	100	21	3	6
vegetable beef	1 cup	110	16	3	2
Select..microwaveable bowls					
98% fat-free New England					
clam chowder	1 cup	110	15	3	2
beef w/portobello mushrooms & rice	1 cup	100	13	1	1
chicken w/egg noodles	1 cup	90	11	1	3
Italian-style wedding soup	1 cup	115	15	2	3
Soup At Hand					
blended vegetable medley	1 pkg	110	21	3	9
chicken w/mini noodles	1 pkg	80	12	2	2
classic tomato	1 pkg	120	27	2	16
cream of broccoli	1 pkg	160	16	3	3
Mexican-style fiesta	1 pkg	190	22	3	11
New England clam chowder	1 pkg	130	15	3	1
pizza soup	1 pkg	130	27	2	18
velvety potato	1 pkg	150	21	4	5
(Full Circle) organic..ready-to-serve					
lentil	1 cup	100	21	8	5
mushroom barley	1 cup	70	17	3	4
potato leek	1 cup	70	15	3	5
vegetable	1 cup	80	18	4	5
(Gold's) ready-to-serve					

Food and Description	Amount	Total Calories	Total Carbs	Fiber	Sugars
borscht					
low-cal	1 cup	20	5	0	0
original	1 cup	100	21	0	0
schav	1 cup	25	4	0	0
(Gorton's) ready-to-eat					
corn clam chowder..New England	1 cup	140	17	0	6
cream of crab	½ cup	70	9	0	1
(Health Valley) ready-to-serve					
broths					
fat-free					
beef	1 cup	10	2	0	1
beef-flavored	1 cup	10	0	0	0
chicken	1 cup	30	2	0	1
mushroom	1 cup	10	2	0	1
vegetable	1 cup	15	3	0	0
organic					
beef-flavored	1 cup	15	2	0	1
chicken	1 cup	25	2	0	1
soups					
fat-free					
black bean & vegetable	1 cup	110	24	9	8
corn & vegetable	1 cup	70	17	7	8
5-bean vegetable	1 cup	140	32	10	9
Italian minestrone	1 cup	90	21	8	6
lentil & carrots	1 cup	100	25	7	7
pasta					
cacciatore	1 cup	100	20	4	6
fagioli	1 cup	120	25	4	5
Romano	1 cup	100	20	4	6
rotini & vegetable	1 cup	70	20	4	4
split pea & carrots	1 cup	110	22	2	2
super broccoli carotene	1 cup	70	16	7	12
tomato vegetable	1 cup	80	17	5	9
vegetable barley	1 cup	90	19	4	4
organic					
black bean	1 cup	130	25	5	7
lentil	1 cup	100	21	8	5
minestrone	1 cup	110	17	3	5
mushroom barley	1 cup	70	17	3	4
potato leek	1 cup	70	15	3	5
split pea	1 cup	110	23	8	5
tomato	1 cup	80	18	1	14
vegetable	1 cup	80	18	0	5
organic..no salt added					
black bean	1 cup	130	25	5	7
lentil	1 cup	100	21	8	5
minestrone	1 cup	70	17	3	5

Food and Description	Amount	Total Calories	Total Carbs	Fiber	Sugars
mushroom barley	1 cup	70	17	3	4
potato leek	1 cup	70	15	3	5
split pea	1 cup	110	23	8	5
tomato	1 cup	80	18	1	14
vegetable	1 cup	80	18	4	5
(Healthy Choice) ready-to-serve					
beans & ham	1 cup	170	29	6	4
beef & potato	1 cup	110	19	2	3
chicken..hearty	1 cup	120	29	3	2
chicken					
corn chowder	1 cup	140	26	3	5
fiesta	1 cup	100	17	3	0
roasted Italian-style	1 cup	120	18	4	4
& dumplings	1 cup	130	22	7	0
& pasta	1 cup	110	18	2	3
& rice	1 cup	100	12	2	<1
& roasted garlic	1 cup	120	19	2	4
chili beef	1 cup	170	31	8	5
clam chowder	1 cup	110	21	3	2
country vegetable	1 cup	100	22	4	5
creamy tomato	1 cup	100	22	2	13
fiesta chicken	1 cup	90	17	3	0
garden vegetable	1 cup	120	25	4	6
hearty chicken	1 cup	120	20	3	2
Italian bean & pasta	1 cup	100	18	3	2
old-fashioned chicken noodle	1 cup	110	16	3	<1
split pea & ham	1 cup	170	30	4	4
turkey w/wild rice	1 cup	90	16	3	2
vegetable					
beef	1 cup	130	24	4	5
clam chowder	1 cup	80	16	3	3
country	1 cup	100	22	4	5
garden	1 cup	120	25	4	6
zesty gumbo	1 cup	100	16	3	2
(Imagine) organic					
broths					
free-range chicken	1 cup	20	2	<1	1
no-chicken	1 cup	20	4	<1	2
vegetable	1 cup	30	5	1	3
soups					
broccoli	1 cup	70	10	2	4
butternut squash	1 cup	120	23	2	14
portobello mushroom	1 cup	80	10	2	1
potato leek	1 cup	90	14	2	<1
sweet corn	1 cup	100	15	1	6
tomato	1 cup	90	17	2	10
(Manischewitz) borscht..ready-to-serve					
clear	1 cup	80	21	2	<1
low-calorie	1 cup	20	5	0	<1

Food and Description	Amount	Total Calories	Total Carbs	Fiber	Sugars
original w/beets	1 cup	90	21	3	<1
(Mother's) matzo balls..ready-to-eat					
matzo balls in broth	1 cup	170	23	6	3
(Phillips) seafood soup					
crab..Maryland-style..tub	1 cup	70	13	2	3
cream of crab..restaurant recipe	1 cup	340	12	0	6
(Pritikin) condensed..prepared					
chicken & rice	1 cup	80	13	2	1
chicken broth	1 cup	10	<1	<1	0
chicken pasta	1 cup	80	15	2	0
lentil	1 cup	130	24	6	2
minestrone	1 cup	90	18	4	3
split pea	1 cup	180	32	7	3
vegetable..vegetarian	1 cup	100	21	3	3
(Progresso) ready-to-serve					
99% Fat-Free Soups					
beef barley	1 cup	130	20	4	3
chicken noodle	1 cup	90	13	1	2
minestrone	1 cup	110	19	4	4
New England clam chowder	1 cup	110	18	2	2
roasted chicken w/wild rice	1 cup	90	12	1	1
white cheddar potato	1 cup	100	20	2	2
Other Soups					
cheese & herb tortellini tomato	1 cup	140	23	2	9
chickarina	1 cup	130	12	1	1
clam chowder					
Manhattan	1 cup	110	17	2	3
New England	1 cup	230	23	1	3
creamy cheddar chowder	1 cup	210	25	2	4
creamy mushroom	1 cup	180	12	1	4
escarole in chicken broth	1 cup	25	3	1	1
French onion	1 cup	50	9	1	3
herb & rotini vegetable	1 cup	100	19	5	4
herb & shell minestrone	1 cup	120	22	4	4
lentil	1 cup	140	22	7	2
macaroni & bean	1 cup	160	23	6	1
penne in chicken broth	1 cup	80	14	1	1
potato broccoli & broccoli chowder	1 cup	160	21	1	4
potato ham & cheese chowder	1 cup	170	21	1	3
potato roasted garlic chowder	1 cup	180	23	2	3
Southwestern-style corn chowder	1 cup	200	29	3	9
spicy chicken & penne	1 cup	110	–	–	
split pea w/ham	1 cup	150	20	5	3
vegetable	1 cup	90	17	2	4
vegetable Italiano	1 cup	90	15	4	8
vegetarian vegetable w/barley	1 cup	100	20	4	5
Steak Soup					
beef					
& baked potato	1 cup	100	15	1	2
& mushroom	1 cup	100	14	1	3

Food and Description	Amount	Total Calories	Total Carbs	Fiber	Sugars
& vegetables	1 cup	130	16	2	4
beef barley	1 cup	140	16	3	3
grilled steak	1 cup	120	13	1	4
Tomato Soup					
creamy tomato	1 cup	190	30	1	20
hearty tomato	1 cup	110	23	12	–
tomato					
basil	1 cup	160	29	2	15
rotini	1 cup	140	30	2	12
White Meat Soup					
chicken					
garden herb	1 cup	70	9	1	2
grilled chicken Italiano	1 cup	110	14	1	4
hearty chicken & rotini	1 cup	80	11	<1	1
home-style	1 cup	90	11	1	1
rice w/vegetables	1 cup	90	13	1	1
roasted Italiano	1 cup	80	14	1	4
& wild rice	1 cup	100	15	1	1
turkey					
noodle	1 cup	70	9	1	2
rice w/vegetables	1 cup	110	18	1	2
(Rokeach)					
borscht..ready-to-serve..original	1 cup	100	23	0	na
split pea w/egg barley..condensed..					
prepared	1 cup	130	24	0	na
(ShariAnn's) organic ready-to-serve					
cream of tomato	1 cup	80	17	0	12
French green lentil	1 cup	130	22	1	0
French onion..vegetarian	1 cup	60	9	0	1
Great Plains split pea	1 cup	150	26	2	4
Indian black bean	1 cup	150	30	4	0
Italian white bean	1 cup	170	32	<1	0
minestrone	1 cup	120	20	3	5
potato & cheddar	1 cup	100	15	1	2
spicy Mexican bean	1 cup	210	38	8	9
tomato w/red bell pepper	1 cup	100	19	3	2
tomato w/roasted garlic	1 cup	50	12	0	9
vegetable barley	1 cup	100	18	4	3
(Shelton's) ready-to-serve					
black bean & chicken	1 cup	170	22	7	4
chicken noodle	1 cup	80	9	1	2
vegetable	1 cup	150	28	2	3
(Snow's) New England chowders					
clam chowder..ready-to-serve	1 cup	170	14	1	3
condensed..prepared w/whole milk					
corn	7.5 oz	150	18	0	na
fish	7.5 oz	130	11	0	na
seafood	7.5 oz	140	14	0	na
(Swanson) ready-to-serve broths					
beef					

Food and Description	Amount	Total Calories	Total Carbs	Fiber	Sugars
clear	1 cup	15	0	0	0
reduced-sodium	1 cup	15	1	0	1
w/onions	1 cup	20	2	0	2
chicken					
clear	1 cup	15	1	0	1
Natural Goodness	1 cup	15	1	0	1
w/Italian herbs	1 cup	20	3	0	1
w/roasted garlic	1 cup	10	2	0	2
vegetable	1 cup	15	3	0	2
(Walnut Acres) ready-to-serve					
Autumn harvest	1 cup	100	19	2	5
classic minestrone	1 cup	100	22	3	10
country corn chowder	1 cup	150	28	2	8
Cuban black bean	1 cup	150	30	8	9
4-bean chili	1 cup	140	28	4	12
ginger carrot	1 cup	100	22	3	8
Mediterranean lentil	1 cup	130	26	8	8
savory tomato	1 cup	120	23	2	13
(Westbrae) soups of the World ready-to-serve					
Alabama black bean	1 cup	140	26	6	6
Great Plains savory bean	1 cup	120	23	7	5
Hearty Milano minestrone	1 cup	120	24	6	4
Louisiana bean stew	1 cup	130	25	7	5
Mediterranean lentil	1 cup	140	24	10	5
Old World split pea	1 cup	150	28	6	5
Santa Fe vegetable	1 cup	160	31	8	5
spicy Southwest vegetable	1 cup	130	25	6	5
semi-condensed					
California un-chicken	¾ cup	15	2	0	1
Monte Carlo creamy mushroom	¾ cup	70	10	0	0
Tuscany tomato	¾ cup	70	16	0	12
(Wolfgang Puck's) ready-to-serve					
barley..thick	1 cup	180	25	7	na
chicken w/pasta	1 cup	140	17	2	na
egg	1 cup	150	16	1	na
French onion	1 cup	140	16	1	na
tomato vegetable	1 cup	150	18	2	na
(World Classics) ready-to-serve					
clam chowder					
Manhattan	1 cup	110	17	1	3
New England	1 cup	170	20	1	5
corn chowder..New England..sweet	1 cup	150	21	1	4
lobster bisque..New England	1 cup	120	15	0	3
shrimp bisque..New England	1 cup	130	13	1	3
(Wye River) condensed..prepared w/water					
cream of crab	1 cup	60	8	0	1
red crab	1 cup	40	6	1	2

Food and Description	Amount	Total Calories	Total Carbs	Fiber	Sugars
DEHYDRATED/(MIX OR CUBE) & MICROWAVEABLE					
(Aunt Patsy's Pantry) mix only					
Better Barley	2 Tbs	90	17	4	1
black bean	3 Tbs	130	21	10	1
chicken thyme	2 Tbs	100	22	<1	1
Many Bean	3 Tbs	110	25	8	2
Plentiful Pea	3 Tbs	160	28	3	1
red lentil	2 Tbs	90	16	<1	<1
(Bean Cuisine) soup mix..prepared					
Island Black Bean	1 cup	210	17	7	1
Lots of Lentil	1 cup	230	17	5	1
Santa Fe corn chowder	1 cup	160	18	6	2
13-bean bouillabaisse	1 cup	220	17	5	1
white bean Provençal	1 cup	250	32	11	<1
(Bear Creek) soup mix..prepared					
cheddar broccoli	1 cup	170	26	1	7
cheddar cheese	1 cup	190	29	1	4
chicken noodle	1 cup	120	22	1	3
clam chowder	1 cup	140	25	1	2
hot & sour	1 cup	90	17	1	6
minestrone	1 cup	110	22	2	2
navy bean	1 cup	130	25	4	3
potato..creamy	1 cup	160	28	1	4
Santa Fe chipotle	1 cup	110	22	1	2
split pea	1 cup	110	20	0	2
tortilla	1 cup	110	22	3	4
vegetable beef	1 cup	100	20	2	4
wild rice..creamy	1 cup	140	24	1	2
(Campbell's) Soup At Hand..microwaveable					
blended vegetable medley	1 pkg	110	21	3	9
chicken & stars	1 pkg	60	11	1	0
chicken w/mini noodles	1 pkg	80	12	2	2
classic tomato	1 pkg	120	27	2	16
cream of broccoli	1 pkg	160	16	3	3
creamy chicken	1 pkg	150	15	2	1
Mexican-style fiesta	1 pkg	190	22	3	11
New England clam chowder	1 pkg	130	15	3	1
pizza soup	1 pkg	130	27	2	18
velvety potato	1 pkg	150	21	4	5
(Edward & Sons)					
bouillon cubes					
herb medley	½ cube	10	<1	0	0
vegetable	½ cube	10	1	0	0
miso-cups..prepared					
delicious golden vegetable	1 cup	30	3	<1	1
reduced-sodium	1 cup	25	3	<1	1
savory seaweed	1 cup	30	3	<1	0
traditional w/tofu..organic	1 cup	35	4	<1	<1
(Fantastic Foods) dry mix only					

Food and Description	Amount	Total Calories	Total Carbs	Fiber	Sugars
Carb'tastic Soups					
Asian ginger broccoli	1 pkg	80	11	9	3
broccoli cheddar	1 pkg	110	13	7	5
hot & sour	1 pkg	70	7	1	1
shiitake mushroom	1 pkg	80	9	7	1
sun-dried tomato basil	1 pkg	70	10	7	2
vegetarian					
beef w/barley	1 pkg	70	10	4	2
chicken gumbo	1 pkg	90	9	4	4
mandarin chicken	1 pkg	90	13	10	2
Big Soup Noodle Bowls					
hot & sour	½ pkg	130	22	1	1
Italian tomato noodle	½ pkg	130	26	2	5
mandarin broccoli	½ pkg	110	20	2	1
miso w/tofu	½ pkg	100	19	<1	2
sesame miso	½ pkg	90	17	<1	1
spicy Thai	½ pkg	110	22	1	3
spring vegetable	½ pkg	90	18	<1	1
vegetarian					
beef noodle	½ pkg	100	21	2	1
chicken noodle	½ pkg	90	19	1	0
creamy soups					
broccoli cheddar	½ pkg	130	21	2	11
corn & potato chowder	½ pkg	130	16	2	11
(Goodman's) prepared					
matzo ball & soup					
50% less sodium	1 cup	50	10	1	2
regular	1 cup	40	9	1	2
noodleman					
low-sodium	1 cup	50	9	1	2
regular	1 cup	45	9	0	4
onion					
low-sodium	1 cup	30	6	1	3
regular	1 cup	30	5	1	2
(Health Valley) cups..prepared					
fat-free					
chicken-flavored noodles	½ cup	110	24	3	1
corn chowder	½ cup	100	21	3	1
creamy potato w/broccoli	⅓ cup	80	17	3	2
garden split w/carrots	⅓ cup	110	22	2	2
lentil w/couscous	⅓ cup	130	28	5	1
pasta Italiano	½ cup	140	31	3	1
spicy black bean w/couscous	⅓ cup	130	29	5	3
zesty black bean w/rice	⅓ cup	100	22	4	2
organic					
black bean	1 cup	130	25	5	7
lentil	1 cup	100	21	8	5
minestrone	1 cup	110	17	3	5
mushroom barley	1 cup	70	17	3	4

Food and Description	Amount	Total Calories	Total Carbs	Fiber	Sugars
potato leek	1 cup	70	15	3	5
split pea	1 cup	110	23	8	5
tomato	1 cup	80	18	1	14
vegetable	1 cup	80	18	1	5
(Herb-Ox)					
bouillon cube..all flavors	1 cube	5	0	0	0
instant bouillon..all flavors	1 tsp	5	0	0	0
instant broth/seasoning pkt					
beef					
low-sodium	1 pkg	10	2	0	1
regular	1 pkg	5	0	0	0
chicken					
low-sodium	1 pkg	10	2	0	1
regular	1 pkg	5	0	0	0
(Just Delicious) Gourmet Foods soup mixes..prepared					
black bean chili	1 cup	60	31	20	1
black beans & rice	1 cup	123	22	17	1
champagne					
bean	1 cup	100	19	2	0
split pea	1 cup	150	21	14	5
chicken, rice & curry spice	1 cup	60	10	5	1
chicken vegetable	1 cup	120	21	12	3
corn chowder..golden	1 cup	45	10	0	0
gourmet minestrone	1 cup	30	11	2	1
lentil chili	1 cup	110	18	10	2
potato cheese	1 cup	25	0	0	0
seafood chowder	1 cup	40	8	2	0
sour cream, onion & potato	1 cup	25	4	0	0
spicy chicken vegetable	1 cup	120	21	12	–
tortilla	1 cup	60	21	19	0
(Knorr)					
bouillon cube..½ cube..prepared					
beef	1 cup	20	1	0	0
chicken	1 cup	20	1	0	0
chicken w/tomato	1 cup	15	1	0	0
pumpkin	1 cup	5	0	0	0
pumpkin & ham	1 cup	5	0	0	0
shrimp	1 cup	20	0	0	0
vegetarian vegetable	1 cup	15	1	0	1
concentrated broth					
beef	1/12 container	15	1	0	1
chicken	1/12 container	5	1	0	0
Recipe Classics Mix for soup & dip recipes roasted garlic herb	⅓ box	80	13	0	2
Savory Soups..mix only/ chicken noodle	3 Tbs	70	11	1	2
Soup, Dip, and Recipe mix..mix only					
chicken rice..hearty	⅛ pkg	80	16	0	1
noodle w/beef broth	⅛ pkg	45	8	0	0

Food and Description	Amount	Total Calories	Total Carbs	Fiber	Sugars
noodle w/chicken flavor	⅓ pkg	50	8	0	0
pasta w/chicken	¼ pkg	80	15	0	1
spaghetti-style pasta	¼ pkg	80	17	0	1
Tasty Breaks soup cups..prepared					
beef vegetable	1 cup	150	27	1	5
chicken					
noodle	1 cup	100	17	0	2
low-fat	1 cup	120	20	1	2
w/rice	1 cup	180	36	1	8
corn chowder	1 cup	140	26	2	6
hearty lentil	1 cup	220	39	8	7
navy bean..low-fat	1 cup	130	25	7	4
potato leek					
cup	1 cup	150	27	1	5
packet	1 cup	170	26	1	3
split pea	1 cup	160	30	3	2
(Lipton)					
Cup-A-Soup..mix only					
chicken..cream of	1 pkg	70	12	0	3
chicken noodle w/white meat	1 pkg	50	8	0	0
green pea	1 pkg	80	12	3	1
vegetable..spring	1 pkg	45	19	<1	1
Recipe Secrets..mix only					
herb..fiesta w/red pepper	1 Tbs	30	6	0	1
onion					
beefy	1 Tbs	25	5	0	0
mushroom	2 Tbs	30	5	0	0
regular	1 Tbs	20	4	0	0
ranch	⅙ box	30	6	0	0
vegetable	2 Tbs	30	6	1	2
Soup Secrets..mix only					
chicken noodle w/diced					
white chicken	3 Tbs	80	11	0	1
chicken w/pasta & beans	3 Tbs	110	19	3	1
extra noodle w/real chicken broth	3 Tbs	90	15	1	1
giggle noodle w/real chicken broth	2 Tbs	70	11	0	1
home-style lentil w/bow-tie pasta	3 Tbs	130	22	5	1
noodle w/real chicken broth	2 Tbs	60	9	0	1
ring-o-noodle w/real chicken					
sauce	3 Tbs	90	10	0	1
(Maggi) noodle soup mix..mix only					
beef flavor	¼ pkg	50	9	0	0
chicken noodle	¼ pkg	50	9	0	0
(Manischewitz)					
Mrs. Manischewitz's Soup Cup					
hearty lentil	1 cup	140	26	2	na
minestrone	1 cup	210	39	6	na
regular..mix only					
matzo ball	1 Tbs	40	9	1	na
minestrone	¼ pkg	150	33	7	na

Food and Description	Amount	Total Calories	Total Carbs	Fiber	Sugars
split pea	⅓ pkg	110	21	3	na
(Marachun) cup..prepared					
Instant Lunch					
beef	1 container	290	38	2	1
cheddar cheese	1 container	340	38	2	0
chicken	1 container	280	37	2	2
picante chicken	1 container	280	27	1	0
roasted chicken	1 container	290	38	2	1
shrimp	1 container	290	38	2	1
Ramen Oriental Noodle Soup					
beef	½ pkg	190	26	1	1
chicken	½ pkg	190	26	1	1
pork	½ pkg	190	26	1	1
shrimp	½ pkg	190	26	1	1
tomato	½ pkg	200	28	1	2
(Mrs. Grass) mix only					
chicken w/rice	¼ pkg	80	15	0	na
chicken noodle..home-style	¼ pkg	70	10	1	na
onion					
mushroom	¼ pkg	60	10	0	na
reduced-sodium	¼ pkg	30	10	0	na
regular soup & dip	¼ pkg	50	10	0	na
vegetable soup & dip..home-style	¼ pkg	35	7	1	na
(Nile Spice) home-style cup mix..prepared					
black bean	1 container	170	35	11	4
chicken vegetable	1 container	110	21	2	4
lentil	1 container	170	34	11	3
red beans & rice	1 container	190	40	10	3
split pea	1 container	200	35	8	5
sweet corn chowder	1 container	110	22	3	7
(Produce Partners) mix only					
broccoli, cream of	1⅓ Tbs	35	4	0	1
cheddar cheese broccoli	2 Tbs	70	5	0	3
potato, cream of	1 Tbs	25	3	0	1
(Spice Hunter) bowls..mix					
mix only					
chicken vegetable w/rice	1 bowl	160	29	2	2
chipotle black bean	1 bowl	250	47	19	3
prepared					
creamy Thai noodle	1 bowl	180	29	2	1
spicy Thai noodle	1 bowl	160	33	2	1
split pea	1 bowl	240	43	10	2
Szechuan	1 bowl	160	33	2	2
(A Taste of Thai) mix only					
tangy coconut ginger	2 tsp	15	2	0	2
(Uncle Ben's) Hearty Soup..prepared					
black beans & rice	1.5 oz	150	28	7	2
broccoli, cheese & rice	1 oz	110	19	1	2
(Union Foods)					
noodles..block					

Food and Description	Amount	Total Calories	Total Carbs	Fiber	Sugars
3-oz pkg..all flavors	½ pkg	190	26	1	1
2.25-oz pkg..chicken	1 pkg	190	27	1	1
2.25-oz pkg—all other flavors	1 pkg	320	35	1	1
(Weight Watchers) broth..all flavors	1 pkt	10	2	0	2
(Wyler's)					
bouillon cube					
beef	1 cube	5	1	0	<1
chicken	1 cube	5	1	0	<1
Soup Starter..mix only					
beef vegetable	½ pkg	100	21	2	4
chicken noodle	⅛ pkg	80	15	1	3
Stew Starter..beef..mix only	½ pkg	70	16	2	4
(Zatarain's) Gumbo base..mix only	1 Tbs	45	9	0	0
FROZEN or REFRIGERATED					
(Birds Eye) Hearty Spoonfuls					
cheesy cream of broccoli	11.5 oz	230	25	6	17
chicken rice & vegetables	11.5 oz	160	26	2	3
home-style chicken noodle	11.5 oz	140	19	2	3
Italian minestrone	11.5 oz	240	37	7	10
(Schwan's) soup bowls					
cheesy broccoli	1 bowl	360	18	5	7
chicken wild rice	1 bowl	310	25	4	6
clam chowder	1 bowl	280	25	6	5
SOUR CREAM (*See also* CREAM; DIP; SAUCE; SEASONINGS; SOUR CREAM SUBSTITUTE)					
(Blue Bunny)					
flavored or unflavored					
light	2 Tbs	35	2	0	2
regular	2 Tbs	60	2	0	2
(Breakstone)					
fat-free	2 Tbs	35	6	0	2
original	2 Tbs	60	1	0	1
reduced-fat	2 Tbs	45	2	0	2
(Dairygold)					
fat-free	2 Tbs	25	4	0	3
light	2 Tbs	40	3	0	2
regular	2 Tbs	60	2	0	1
(Daisy) pure & natural					
fat-free	2 Tbs	20	1	0	1
regular	2 Tbs	60	1	0	1
(Hood)					
all-natural	2 Tbs	60	2	0	2
fat-free	2 Tbs	25	4	0	2
low-fat	2 Tbs	35	3	0	2
(Knudsen)					
fat-free	2 Tbs	35	5	0	2
Hampshire	2 Tbs	60	1	0	1
light	2 Tbs	40	2	0	2
(Land O' Lakes)					
fat-free	2 Tbs	30	5	0	2
light	2 Tbs	35	4	0	2

Food and Description	Amount	Total Calories	Total Carbs	Fiber	Sugars
regular	2 Tbs	60	2	0	1
SOUR CREAM SUBSTITUTE (*See also* SEASONINGS)					
(IMO) original	1 Tbs	30	0	0	0
(Pet)	1 Tbs	25	1	0	0
(Tofutti) Sour Supreme/Better Than Sour Cream					
guacamole	2 Tbs	50	1	0	0
plain	2 Tbs	85	9	0	2
SOURSOP..fresh..whole	1 medium	415	105	7	na
SOY CHEESE (*See* CHEESE ALTERNATIVE/IMITATION)					
SOY MILK					
dry..mix only					
(MLO/GeniSoy)					
milk & egg protein drink..chocolate	1.2 oz	105	2	0	2
soy protein drinks					
chocolate	1.2 oz	120	17	2	15
natural	1.1 oz	100	0	0	0
strawberry banana	1.2 oz	120	16	1	14
vanilla	1.2 oz	130	18	0	13
liquid					
(8th Continent)					
chocolate	8 fl oz	140	23	1	21
original	8 fl oz	90	8	0	6
vanilla	8 fl oz	90	11	0	10
(Blue Diamond) almond Breeze					
nondairy soy..soft drinks					
chocolate	8 fl oz	110	22	1	20
original	8 fl oz	60	8	1	7
vanilla	8 fl oz	90	16	1	15
(Eden) organic					
EdenBlend..original	8 fl oz	120	18	<1	8
Edensoy					
carob	8 fl oz	170	28	<1	13
chocolate	8 fl oz	175	28	<1	14
original					
extra	8 fl oz	130	13	3	7
light	8 fl oz	100	14	0	5
regular	8 fl oz	145	14	2	7
unsweetened	8 fl oz	120	5	2	2
vanilla					
extra	8 fl oz	150	23	<1	15
light	8 fl oz	120	20	0	10
regular	8 fl oz	150	24	<1	15
(Full Circle) lactose-free					
chocolate..enriched	8 fl oz	100	11	2	7
vanilla	8 fl oz	110	14	2	9
(Imagine) Power Dream					
natural energy soy drinks					
Java	11 fl oz	240	42	2	24
Vanilla Blast	11 fl oz	240	39	2	24
X-Treme chocolate	11 fl oz	260	48	2	29

Food and Description	Amount	Total Calories	Total Carbs	Fiber	Sugars
(Kikkoman Pearl) organic					
creamy vanilla	8 fl oz	110	11	0	10
green tea	8 fl oz	110	13	1	10
original	8 fl oz	110	12	1	9
tropical delight	8 fl oz	110	14	0	13
(Vitasoy)					
chocolate					
rich	8 fl oz	160	23	2	19
rich..light	8 fl oz	100	17	0	14
original					
classic	8 fl oz	120	11	1	5
creamy smooth	8 fl oz	100	9	2	5
unsweetened	8 fl oz	80	5	0	1
vanilla					
Delight	8 fl oz	120	13	1	8
smooth	8 fl oz	110	11	2	7
(Westsoy)					
Organic					
Chai	8 fl oz	130	25	<1	22
light					
plain	8 fl oz	90	15	2	11
vanilla	8 fl oz	110	19	2	15
nonfat					
plain	8 fl oz	70	10	<1	9
vanilla	8 fl oz	80	12	<1	10
original	8 fl oz	130	18	3	12
unsweetened					
chocolate	8 fl oz	100	6	5	0
plain	8 fl oz	90	5	4	0
vanilla	8 fl oz	100	5	4	0
Smart Plus					
plain	8 fl oz	180	22	5	14
vanilla	8 fl oz	190	25	5	16
Westsoy Plus					
plain	8 fl oz	130	17	3	12
vanilla	8 fl oz	130	19	3	14
(White Wave)					
silk..cultured soy milk..single-serve					
apricot mango	1 serving	160	30	1	20
banana strawberry	1 serving	160	29	1	18
black cherry	1 serving	160	29	1	20
blueberry	1 serving	160	29	1	21
key lime	1 serving	160	30	1	21
lemon	1 serving	160	31	1	22
peach	1 serving	160	32	1	25
plain	1 serving	160	22	1	12
raspberry	1 serving	160	30	1	22
strawberry	1 serving	160	31	1	22
vanilla	1 serving	160	23	1	16
Silk..soy milk creamer					

Food and Description	Amount	Total Calories	Total Carbs	Fiber	Sugars
French vanilla cream	1 Tbs	20	3	0	3
hazelnut	1 Tbs	20	3	0	3
nonflavored	1 Tbs	15	1	0	0
Soylatte coffee..single-serve					
coffee	11 oz	220	38	0	31
spice	11 oz	200	27	0	25
Starbucks..formula	1 cup	120	16	1	13
SOY NUT (See SOYBEAN)					
SOY PROTEIN..concentrate	1 oz	92	9	2	0
SOY SAUCE (See ASIAN FOOD, Sauces & Seasonings entry; SAUCE)					
SOYBEAN					
CANNED					
(Eden) black soybeans	½ cup	120	8	7	1
(Westbrae) organic soy beans	½ cup	150	11	3	3
DRIED (Arrowhead Mills)	¼ cup	170	14	10	0
FROZEN (C&W)					
soybeans/edamame..in the pod	½ cup	60	8	5	1
sweet soybeans	½ cup	100	16	10	2
(MLO/GeniSoy)					
deep sea–salted	1 oz	120	9	5	3
old hickory–smoked	1 oz	120	9	5	5
SPROUTED..raw	10 sprouts	15	1	0	0
	½ cup	45	3	0	0
SOYBEAN CURD (See TOFU; TOFU FROZEN DESSERT; VEGETARIAN FOODS)					
SOYBEAN OIL (See OIL)					
SOYBEAN PASTE (See MISO)					
SPAETZLE (See DUMPLING)					
SPAGHETTI (See PASTA)					
SPAGHETTI SAUCE (See SAUCE)					
SPANISH FOOD (See FROZEN ENTRÉE/DINNER; MEXICAN FOOD; RICE; RICE DISH; VEGETARIAN FOODS)					
SPICES (See SEASONINGS; individual listings)					
SPINACH					
CANNED					
(Bush's Best) chopped	½ cup	30	4	2	0
(Del Monte) all styles	½ cup	30	4	2	0
(S&W) leaf..young & tender	½ cup	30	4	2	1
FRESH..raw (Dole) organic baby..chopped	3½ cups	35	9	4	0
FROZEN					
(Birds Eye) all cuts & styles	3.3 oz	20	3	1	0
(C&W) all cuts & styles	⅓ cup	20	2	2	1
(Green Giant) cut leaf..cooked	⅓ cup	15	2	2	1
SPINACH DISH (See also FROZEN ENTRÉE/DINNER; VEGETABLES, MIXED; VEGETARIAN FOODS)					
FROZEN					
(Birds Eye) creamed in sauce	½ cup	100	7	1	3
(Green Giant)					
creamed	½ cup	80	9	1	5
cut leaf in butter sauce	½ cup	35	4	2	2
SPIRULINA (See SEAWEED)					

Food and Description	Amount	Total Calories	Total Carbs	Fiber	Sugars
SPLIT PEA (*See* PEA)					
SPOONBREAD (*See* BREAD)					
SPOT FISH fresh..cooked—dry heat	3 oz	135	0	0	0
SPRING ONION (*See* SCALLION)					
SQUAB/PIGEON					
RAW					
breast meat only	3 oz	115	0	0	0
meat & skin	3 oz	255	0	0	0
meat only	3 oz	125	0	0	0
SQUASH					
acorn..fresh..boiled..mashed	½ cup	58	30	9	0
banana..fresh..baked	2 oz	35	8	0	0
butternut..fresh..baked..mashed	½ cup	45	11	0	0
crookneck..frozen..cooked	4 oz	45	11	0	0
hubbard..fresh..boiled..mashed	½ cup	35	7.5	3.5	0
scallop..fresh..boiled..mashed	½ cup	20	4	2.5	0
spaghetti..fresh..boiled or baked	1 cup	45	10	2	0
summer..all varieties..fresh..boiled..sliced	1 cup	35	8	3	0
winter..all varieties..baked..cubed	½ cup	40	9	3	0
yellow..frozen..sliced	⅔ cup	23	11	2	0
zucchini					
CANNED					
(Del Monte) w/Italian-style tomato sauce	½ cup	30	7	1	1
FRESH..boiled..drained..mashed	½ cup	20	5	2	0
FROZEN (C&W) yellow & green..sliced	⅔ cup	15	2	1	1
SQUASH SEED..dried..hulled	1 oz	155	5	1	9
	1 cup	747	25	5	0
SQUID					
FRESH					
breaded & fried	3 oz	149	7	0	na
raw	3 oz	78	3	0	0
SQUIRREL..roasted	3 oz	150	0	0	0
STAR FRUIT/CARAMBOLA					
FRESH					
cubed	½ cup	25	5.5	2	na
whole	1 medium	30	7	2	na
STRAWBERRY					
DRIED (Frieda's)	½ cup	150	34	3	29
FRESH (Dole)	8 medium	45	12	4	8
FROZEN					
(Birds Eye)					
deluxe..halves..in light syrup	5 oz	120	31	1	28
halves..in regular syrup	½ cup	120	31	1	28
whole	½ cup	100	25	1	23
(C&W) whole	⅔ cup	50	12	2	8
(Haggen) slices..w/sugar	⅔ cup	150	38	2	35

Food and Description	Amount	Total Calories	Total Carbs	Fiber	Sugars

STRAWBERRY DRINK (*See* FRUIT PUNCH; LEMONADE/LEMONADE-FLAVORED DRINK; SOFT DRINK; SOFT DRINK MIX; STRAWBERRY JUICE/JUICE BLEND/JUICE DRINK; individual juice blend listings)

STRAWBERRY GLAZE

(T. Marzettis)					
regular	1.5 oz	60	14	0	11
sugar-free	1.5 oz	10	3	0	0

STRAWBERRY JUICE/JUICE BLEND/JUICE DRINK (*See also* FRUIT PUNCH; SOFT DRINK MIX)

BOTTLED, BOXED, or CANNED

(Kern's)					
strawberry..aguas frescas	8 fl oz	120	29	0	26
strawberry banana nectar	8 fl oz	150	36	0	33
	12 fl oz	220	52	0	46
(Knudsen) Celebratory					
sparkling..100%	8 fl oz	110	28	0	25
(Minute Maid)					
strawberry passion..juice	12 fl oz	170	46	0	44
strawberry raspberry..juice	8 fl oz	130	34	0	32
(Odwalla) strawberry banana..juice	8 fl oz	120	28	2	24
(Snapple) Whipper Snapple..					
juice drink	10 fl oz	160	40	0	38
(Tropicana)					
strawberry banana..smoothie	11 fl oz	250	59	5	46
strawberry orange..juice	8 fl oz	140	34	0	32
strawberry, orange & banana..juice	8 fl oz	120	28	0	23
(V8 Splash)					
juice drink					
strawberry banana	8 fl oz	110	27	0	27
strawberry kiwi	8 fl oz	110	27	0	27
strawberry kiwi..diet	8 fl oz	10	3	0	2
smoothie..strawberry banana	8 fl oz	130	30	0	29

STUFFING/DRESSING

(Arnold) dry mix..all styles	¾ cup	140	28	1	2
(Brownberry) dry					
home-style for chicken	1 oz	130	16	1	2
home-style for turkey	1 oz	120	18	1	2
traditional sage & onion	¾ cup	140	28	2	2
(Butterball) seasoned..one-step..					
prepared	½ cup	160	28	3	2
(Chatham Village)					
cranberry & herb	1 cup	130	28	2	5
traditional herb	1 cup	150	32	2	4
(Kellogg's) Croutettes stuffing mix	1 cup	120	25	0	0
(Pepperidge Farms) dry mix only..					
seasoned w/herbs	½ cup	170	33	3	2
(Springfield) cornbread..mix only	⅙ pkg	110	20	1	3
(Stove Top) New Meals					

Food and Description	Amount	Total Calories	Total Carbs	Fiber	Sugars
chicken					
lower-sodium	⅙ pkg	110	21	1	3
regular	⅙ cup	110	20	1	3
corn bread					
box	⅙ pkg	110	21	1	3
can	1 oz	120	19	1	3
home-style herb	⅛ pkg	110	19	1	3
pork	1 oz	110	20	1	3
turkey	⅙ pkg	110	20	1	3
STURGEON					
cooked—dry heat	3 oz	115	0	0	0
smoked	3 oz	147	0	0	0
SUCCOTASH (*See also* VEGETABLES, MIXED)					
CANNED					
(Blue Boy) whole kernel	½ cup	90	19	3	4
(Libby) w/whole kernel corn	½ cup	90	19	3	4
FROZEN (HANOVER)	½ cup	80	17	5	3
SUCKER, WHITE cooked—dry heat	3 oz	101	0	0	0
SUGAR					
brown					
(C&H) dark or golden brown	1 tsp	15	4	0	4
(Domino)					
brownulated-style	1 tsp	10	3	0	3
regular brown sugars	1 tsp	15	4	0	4
(Hain)	1 tsp	15	4	0	4
maple	2 Tbs	100	26	0	26
turbinado					
(Hain)	1 tsp	15	4	0	4
(Sugar Foods) Sugar in the Raw	1 pkt	20	5	0	5
white					
(C&H) granulated	1 cube	15	4	0	4
	1 tsp	15	4	0	4
	1 pkt	15	4	0	4
powdered 10-X confectioners					
(C&H) all styles	1 oz	120	30	0	29
(Domino) all styles	¼ cup	120	30	0	29
(Hain)	¼ cup	140	37	0	34
SUGAR APPLE/SWEETSOP fresh..whole	1 medium	145	37	7	na
SUGAR SUBSTITUTE					
(Equal)	1 pkt	<5	1	0	<1
(NutraSweet)	1 tsp	12	3	0	0
	1 pkt	4	1	0	0
(Splenda)					
canister	1 tsp	<5	<1	0	<1
individual packets	1 pkt	<5	<1	0	<1
(Sugar Twin)					
brown sugar	1 tsp	0	0	0	0
regular	1 tsp	0	0	0	0
(Superose) liquid	10 drops	0	0	0	0
(Sweet*10)	⅛ tsp	0	0	0	0

Food and Description	Amount	Total Calories	Total Carbs	Fiber	Sugars
(Sweet 'N Low)					
granulated					
brown..w/measuring spoon	¼ tsp	0	<0.5	0	<0.5
white..w/measuring spoon	¼ tsp	0	<1	0	<1
white..packet	1 pkt	0	<1	0	<1
SUMMER SAUSAGE (*See* SAUSAGE)					
SUN-DRIED TOMATO (*See* TOMATO)					
SUNFISH/PUMPKINSEED					
fresh..cooked—dry heat	3 oz	97	0	0	0
SUNFLOWER SEED BUTTER					
(Kettle) roaster fresh	2 Tbs	160	5	0	0
SUNFLOWER SEED FLOUR (*See* FLOUR)					
SUNFLOWER SEED/NUT					
(Arrowhead Mills) hulled	¼ cup	180	6	4	0
(David)					
kernels..1.75-oz bag					
original	1 bag	330	9	4	1
ranch	1 bag	310	9	4	1
sizzlin' BBQ	1 bag	310	9	4	2
seeds 1.75-oz bag					
BBQ	1 bag	160	4	2	1
jalapeño hot salsa	1 bag	160	5	2	1
nacho cheese	1 bag	150	5	2	0
original	1 bag	160	9	4	1
ranch	1 bag	160	4	2	1
(Fisher)					
dry-roasted	1 oz	170	7	2	1
oil-roasted	1 oz	170	7	2	1
salted in shell..shelled kernels	1 oz	160	6	2	1
(Frito-Lay)					
kernels..original	1 oz	180	5	2	<1
seeds					
BBQ	1 oz	200	6	2	3
Flamin' Hot	1 oz	180	5	2	<1
original	1 oz	180	5	2	<1
(Planters)					
dry-roasted & salted..shelled kernels	¼ cup	190	5	2	1
oil-roasted..shelled kernels	1 oz	170	5	0	0
roasted & salted	1-oz pkg	180	5	2	0
	3-oz pkg	210	8	4	0
SURIMI (*See* CRAB, IMITATION; SEAFOOD ENTRÉE/DINNER; SHRIMP, IMITATION)					
SUSHI (*See* ASIAN FOOD)					
SWEET & SOUR SAUCE (*See* ASIAN FOOD/SAUCES & SEASONINGS; SAUCE)					
SWEET POTATO (*See also* SWEET POTATO LEAVES; YAM)					
CANNED					
(Bruce's) cut					
in heavy syrup	⅔ cup	190	45	3	21
in syrup	⅔ cup	150	36	3	23
(McCain) roasters..oven-roasted	½ cup	120	20	3	8
(Princella) candied..in light syrup	⅔ cup	160	40	3	20

Food and Description	Amount	Total Calories	Total Carbs	Fiber	Sugars
(Royal Prince)					
candied	½ cup	210	50	2	35
in heavy syrup	6.3 oz	200	49	4	17
orange pineapple	½ cup	210	50	3	36
(Trappey's)					
golden sweet..whole in heavy syrup	6.3 oz	200	49	4	16
sugary sam					
golden cut in syrup	⅔ cup	160	39	3	20
golden mashed	⅔ cup	120	28	3	15
FRESH					
baked in skin	1 large	185	44	5	na
boiled-mashed w/o skin	½ cup	175	40	3	na
raw..pieces..cubes	½ cup	70	16	4	na
SWEET POTATO DISH					
FROZEN					
(Mrs. Paul's)					
candied sweet potatoes	5 oz	300	73	3	47
candied sweets 'n' apples	1¼ cups	270	66	3	47
SWEET POTATO LEAVES/fresh..chopped	½ cup	12	2	1	0
SWEET ROLL (*See* PASTRY)					
SWEETBREADS (*See* individual meat listings)					
SWEETENER, ARTIFICIAL (*See* SUGAR SUBSTITUTE)					
SWISS CHARD (*See* CHARD)					
SWORDFISH					
Fresh..cooked—dry heat	3 oz	132	0	0	0
frozen..steaks..boneless..raw	3.5 oz	120	0	0	0
SYRUP (*See also* CORN SYRUP; ICE CREAM TOPPING; MAPLE SYRUP; PANCAKE & WAFFLE SYRUP; RICE SYRUP; SORGHUM SYRUP)					
SYRUP FLAVORING					
(Atkins) sugar-free..all flavors	1 Tbs	0	0	0	0
(Da Vinci) gourmet..sugar-free..all flavors	1 Tbs	0	0	0	0

T

Food and Description	Amount	Total Calories	Total Carbs	Fiber	Sugars
TABASCO SAUCE (*See* SAUCE)					
TABOULI/TABOULE/TABOULY (*See also* VEGETARIAN FOODS)					
(Fantastic Foods) tabouli salad..mix only	2 Tbs	70	15	4	1
(Near East) wheat salad mix..prepared	⅔ cup	110	23	5	1
TACO SAUCE (*See* SAUCE)					

Food and Description	Amount	Total Calories	Total Carbs	Fiber	Sugars
TAHINI (*See* SESAME BUTTER)					
TAMALE (*See* FROZEN ENTRÉE/DINNER; MEXICAN FOOD)					
TAMARIND..fresh	1 medium	5	1	0	na
TANGERINE (*See also* MANDARIN ORANGE)					
fresh (Dole) whole	1 medium	50	15	3	12
TANGERINE JUICE/JUICE DRINK					
BOTTLED					
(R. W. Knudsen) tangerine spritzer	12 fl oz	170	42	0	38
FROZEN CONCENTRATE					
(Minute Maid) prepared	8 fl oz	120	29	0	29
TAPIOCA (*See also* PUDDING & MOUSSE)					
(Minute) quick-cooking	1½ tsp	20	5	0	0
TARO					
chips (*See also* POTATO CHIPS; SNACKS)					
raw..sliced	10 chips	115	16	4	na
TARTAR SAUCE (*See* SAUCE)					
TEA					
BAGS					
(Bigelow) all styles & flavors	1 bag	0	<1	0	0
(Celestial Seasonings) all styles & flavors	1 bag	0	<1	0	0
(Lipton) all styles & flavors	1 bag	0	<1	0	0
(Luzianne) all styles & flavors	1 bag	0	<1	0	0
(Tetley) all styles & flavors	1 bag	0	<1	0	0
BOTTLED, BOXED, OR CANNED					
(AriZona) canned					
black w/ginseng	8 fl oz	60	15	0	14
botanicals..caffeine-free					
black	8 fl oz	70	18	0	17
red	8 fl oz	60	16	0	15
green					
Asia plum	8 fl oz	70	18	0	17
green	8 fl oz	70	18	0	17
mandarin orange	8 fl oz	70	19	0	18
herbal					
RX Memory..caffeine-free	8 fl oz	80	30	0	19
RX Stress..caffeine-free	8 fl oz	60	16	0	16
no-carb					
green decaf	8 fl oz	5	0	0	0
peach green	8 fl oz	5	0	0	0
Palmer's half & half	8 fl oz	50	14	0	13
regular black					
lemon	8 fl oz	90	25	0	24
peach	8 fl oz	70	18	0	17
raspberry	8 fl oz	90	25	0	24
(Lipton) ready-to-drink					
lemon..diet	8 fl oz	0	0	0	0
peach	8 fl oz	110	26	0	26
raspberry..Brisk	11 fl oz	130	35	0	35

Food and Description	Amount	Total Calories	Total Carbs	Fiber	Sugars
regular					
sweetened..Brisk	8 fl oz	80	20	0	20
unsweetened	8 fl oz	0	0	0	0
Southern-style	8 fl oz	100	25	0	25
sweet tea					
extra-sweet	8 fl oz	120	29	0	29
w/lemon	8 fl oz	90	26	0	26
w/o lemon	8 fl oz	100	24	0	24
(Nestea)					
lemon					
diet	8 fl oz	2	<1	0	<1
honey green	8 fl oz	80	22	0	22
sweet	8 fl oz	75	21	0	21
raspberry	8 fl oz	80	21	0	21
sweetened					
decaffeinated	8 fl oz	65	17	0	17
regular	8 fl oz	65	17	0	17
unsweetened	8 fl oz	2	<1	0	<1
(Snapple)					
kiwi strawberry..diet	8 fl oz	20	5	0	4
lemon..decaffeinated	8 fl oz	100	25	0	23
peach					
diet	8 fl oz	<5	1	0	<1
regular	8 fl oz	100	26	0	24
raspberry					
diet	8 fl oz	<5	1	0	<1
regular	8 fl oz	100	26	9	25
sweetened	8 fl oz	100	25	0	23
(SoBe) black..all natural w/ginseng	8 fl oz	100	28	0	27
(Tradewinds) ready-to-drink					
extra-sweet	8 fl oz	120	30	0	30
green	8 fl oz	80	20	0	20
diet	8 fl oz	0	0	0	0
w/honey	8 fl oz	80	20	0	20
honey	8 fl oz	80	20	0	20
lemon	8 fl oz	90	25	0	25
lemon lime	8 fl oz	90	25	0	25
peach	8 fl oz	95	25	0	25
raspberry					
diet	8 fl oz	0	0	0	0
regular	8 fl oz	90	25	0	25
sweet	8 fl oz	80	20	0	20
mix...instant					
(Crystal Light) iced tea..mix only					
all styles & flavors	⅛ tub	5	<1	0	<1
(Lipton) iced tea mix					
lemon					
diet	8 fl oz	5	0	0	0
regular..sugar-sweetened	8 fl oz	70	18	0	18
peach					

Food and Description	Amount	Total Calories	Total Carbs	Fiber	Sugars
diet	8 fl oz	5	1	0	0
regular..sugar-sweetened	8 fl oz	80	19	0	19
raspberry..sugar-sweetened	8 fl oz	80	19	0	19
(Nescafe) liquid concentrate					
100% tea..decaf					
sweetened	1 tsp	60	17	0	16
unsweetened	1 oz	0	1	0	0
green..w/honey	1 oz	80	18	0	17
lemon	1 oz	80	19	0	18
raspberry	1 oz	90	20	0	19
(Oregon Chai)..Chai Tea..mix concentrate					
caffeine-free..4-count pkg	1 pkg	150	26	9	25
decaf original..8-count pkg	1 pkg	100	20	0	16
original..8-count pkg	1 pkg	130	27	0	25
spiced..original	⅛ pkg	100	20	0	16
vanilla..8-count pkg	⅛ pkg	120	25	0	21
(Tetley) cannister..sugar & natural lemon	1 Tbs	80	20	0	20
TEMPEH					
(White Wave)					
5-grain	⅓ block	180	17	8	0
original soy	⅓ block	180	12	8	0
sea veggie	⅓ block	180	14	12	0
soy rice	⅓ block	180	17	5	0
TEMPURA BATTER (See BAKE & FRY MIX)					
TEQUILA (See LIQUOR, DISTILLED)					
TERIYAKI SAUCE (See SAUCE)					
THURINGER SAUSAGE (See SAUSAGE)					
THYME ground	1 tsp	4	0	0	0
TILEFISH..cooked—dry heat	3 oz	125	0	0	0
TOASTER PASTRY (See PASTRY, TOASTER)					
TOFU (See also VEGETARIAN FOODS)					
(Azumaya)					
extra-firm					
light	2.8 oz	60	3	1	0
regular	2.8 oz	70	2	1	0
firm..silken	2.8 oz	90	3	1	<1
light	3.2 oz	40	3	0	0
regular	3.2 oz	40	1	<1	0
seasoned..all flavors	3 oz	90	3	1	<1
(Mori-Nu)					
extra-firm					
light	1" slice	35	1	0	<1
regular	1" slice	45	2	0	<1
firm					
light	1" slice	30	1	0	<1
regular	1" slice	45	2	0	>1
silken	1" slice	50	2	0	>1
(Nasoya)					
extra-firm	⅕ pkg	80	2	1	0

Food and Description	Amount	Total Calories	Total Carbs	Fiber	Sugars
firm	⅕ pkg	70	2	<1	0
light	⅕ pkg	40	0	<1	0
garlic onion	¼ pkg	90	3	1	<1
marinated cubes					
ginger sesame	5.5 oz	210	27	2	20
sweet & sour	5.5 oz	190	26	1	20
teriyaki	5.5 oz	240	25	1	17
Thai peanut	5.5 oz	240	24	2	18
silken	⅕ pkg	45	2	0	<1
light	⅕ pkg	30	0	<1	0
soft	⅕ pkg	60	1	<1	0
(White Wave)					
extra firm	¼ pkg	110	4	2	0
organic					
extra firm	¼ pkg	110	4	2	0
firm					
box	⅕ box	90	1	1	0
box..transitional	⅕ box	90	1	1	0
water-packed	⅕ pkg	110	4	2	0
soft	⅕ pkg	110	4	2	0
TOFU DAIRY YOGURT					
(White Wave) silk..cultured soy					
apricot mango	1 container	160	29	1	18
banana strawberry	1 container	160	29	1	18
key lime	1 container	160	30	1	21
lemon	1 container	160	31	1	22
peach	1 container	160	32	1	25
plain	1 container	120	22	1	12
raspberry	1 container	160	30	1	22
strawberry	1 container	160	31	1	22
vanilla	1 container	120	23	1	16
TOFU DISH (See VEGETARIAN FOODS)					
TOFU FROZEN DESSERT					
(Tofutti)					
CHEESECAKE SUPREME					
cheesecake..all styles & flavors	½ cup	200	20	0	15
LOW-FAT SUPREME					
chocolate fudge coffee	½ cup	145	25	0	18
marshmallow swirl	½ cup	120	24	0	14
vanilla fudge	½ cup	130	24	0	16
NO SUGAR ADDED					
chocolate	½ cup	115	12	0	0
strawberry	½ cup	110	12	0	0
NOVELTY BARS					
Hooray Hooray	1 bar	150	10	0	0
Marry Me	1 bar	168	22	0	18
Monkey..peanut butter	1 bar	220	22	0	18

Food and Description	Amount	Total Calories	Total Carbs	Fiber	Sugars
PREMIUM					
butter pecan	½ cup	210	22	0	17
chocolate cookie crunch	½ cup	210	26	0	13
chocolate supreme	½ cup	180	18	0	8
mint chocolate chip	½ cup	210	21	0	16
vanilla almond bark	½ cup	210	21	0	16
vanilla fudge	½ cup	190	25	0	18
wild berry supreme	½ cup	190	24	0	19
SANDWICHES..Cuties					
chocolate	1 sdw	130	16	0	9
Chocolate Wave	1 sdw	140	20	0	12
Jazzy	1 sdw	120	17	0	9
mint chocolate chip	1 sdw	120	19	0	11
peanut butter	1 sdw	165	20	0	10
Strawberry Wave	1 sdw	140	20	0	12
wildberry	1 sdw	140	17	0	9
SANDWICHES..Too-Too's..chocolate chip	1 sdw	230	30	0	18
SUPER SOY SUPREME					
Bella Vanilla	½ cup	160	20	0	13
Cool Cappuccino	½ cup	170	21	0	14
Plum Krazy	½ cup	160	26	0	18
NY NY Chocolate	½ cup	170	22	0	15
TOFU PÂTÉ					
(Toby's) all flavors					
light	2 Tbs	70	2	0	0
regular	2 Tbs	30	2	0	0
TOMATO					
CANNED or JARRED					
(Contadina)					
crushed..recipe-ready					
w/Italian herbs	¼ cup	20	3	<1	0
w/roasted garlic	¼ cup	20	3	1	0
diced					
original	½ cup	30	6	1	0
primavera	½ cup	60	13	2	0
w/Italian herbs	½ cup	45	10	1	0
w/roasted garlic	½ cup	45	10	<1	0
w/roasted red pepper	½ cup	60	13	2	0
stewed					
Italian-style	½ cup	35	8	1	7
original w/onions, celery & green pepper	½ cup	35	9	1	0
(Del Monte)					
diced					
original	½ cup	25	6	2	4
w/basil, garlic & oregano	½ cup	50	11	1	8
w/garlic & onion	½ cup	40	8	<1	6
w/green pepper & onion	½ cup	40	9	2	7
w/jalapeños	½ cup	30	6	1	3

Food and Description	Amount	Total Calories	Total Carbs	Fiber	Sugars
zesty chili–style	½ cup	30	8	2	6
stewed					
Cajun recipe	½ cup	35	9	2	7
Italian recipe	½ cup	30	8	2	6
Mexican recipe	½ cup	35	9	2	7
original	½ cup	35	9	2	7
whole..peeled in juice	½ cup	25	4	1	3
(Full Circle)					
Italian..whole..peeled	½ cup	30	5	5	5
organic..crushed	¼ cup	25	5	3	1
(Furmano's)					
crushed					
chunky	¼ cup	18	4	1	3
w/garlic & oregano	¼ cup	15	3	1	2
diced					
Italian-style..w/juice	½ cup	40	8	1	7
petite					
w/cilantro & lime	½ cup	30	6	1	4
w/green chilies	½ cup	25	5	2	3
w/juice	½ cup	25	5	1	3
w/green peppers & onions	½ cup	30	7	2	5
(Hunt's)					
diced					
original	½ cup	20	5	<1	4
w/balsamic vinegar	½ cup	60	8	1	6
w/basil, garlic & oregano	½ cup	25	6	1	5
w/green pepper, celery & onions	½ cup	45	10	1	8
w/roasted garlic	½ cup	30	6	1	5
w/sweet onions	½ cup	45	10	<1	7
diced..petite					
original	½ cup	20	5	1	3
w/mild green chilis	½ cup	30	6	2	5
w/mushrooms	½ cup	40	6	<1	5
pear-shaped	½ cup	20	5	1	3
stewed..original	½ cup	30	7	1	5
whole	2 tomatoes	20	4	1	3
(Muir Glen) organic					
crushed..w/basil	¼ cup	20	5	1	4
diced..all styles & flavors	½ cup	25	4	1	4
fire-roasted					
crushed	¼ cup	20	5	1	4
diced..all styles	½ cup	30	6	1	4
(Progresso) peeled					
Italian-style..peeled	½ cup	30	5	1	5
Recipe ready..crushed	¼ cup	20	3	0	2
(Rosoff's)..pickled..half sour	1 oz	5	1	0	0
(Ro*Tel)					
diced					
chunky..w/green chilis	½ cup	20	4	1	3
extra-hot	½ cup	25	4	1	3

Food and Description	Amount	Total Calories	Total Carbs	Fiber	Sugars
Italian harvest	½ cup	30	6	1	3
Mexican festival	½ cup	30	6	1	3
w/green chilis..chili fixin's	½ cup	30	8	3	5
whole..w/green chilis	½ cup	20	4	1	3
(S&W)					
ready-cut..diced					
Italian recipe	½ cup	25	4	1	4
Mexican recipe	½ cup	35	7	2	5
no salt	½ cup	25	4	1	3
original	½ cup	25	4	1	4
peeled	½ cup	25	4	1	3
roasted garlic	½ cup	30	5	1	3
stewed..all styles & flavors	½ cup	35	7	2	5
(Tuttorosso) peeled					
crushed..in thick purée..all styles	¼ cup	10	4	1	2
plum-shaped in tomato juice	½ cup	30	5	2	5
plum-shaped w/basil	½ cup	30	5	1	3
FRESH					
green	1 medium	30	6	1	0
red					
chopped or diced	1 cup	35	8	2	0
whole	1 medium	25	6	1	0
sun-dried (Sonoma) bits	2–3 tsp	15	3	1	0
TOMATO JUICE/JUICE BLEND					
(Campbell's)					
Healthy Request					
low-sodium	8 fl oz	50	10	1	8
regular	8 fl oz	50	12	1	8
original	8 fl oz	50	10	2	7
(Del Monte)					
from concentrate	8 fl oz	50	10	1	7
Snap-E-Tom..tomato & chili cocktail					
32-oz bottle	8 fl oz	50	11	2	6
individual can	11.5 fl oz	70	15	3	8
(Full Circle) organic tomato juice	8 fl oz	40	10	0	7
(Knudsen) organic	8 fl oz	60	14	0	8
(Sacramento)					
bottle..from concentrate	8 fl oz	45	10	2	7
can..individual	6 fl oz	35	8	1	5
(Springfield)					
100% pure tomato juice	8 fl oz	40	7	0	7
tomato clam juice..32-oz glass bottle	8 fl oz	60	11	1	8
tomato clam..juice cocktail	8 fl oz	40	7	0	7
(V8 Splash) 100% vegetable juice					
calcium-enriched	8 fl oz	50	11	2	8
lightly tangy	8 fl oz	60	11	1	9
low-sodium	8 fl oz	50	11	2	8
picante or spicy hot	8 fl oz	50	10	1	7
TOMATO PASTE..canned					
(Contadina)					

Food and Description	Amount	Total Calories	Total Carbs	Fiber	Sugars
100% tomatoes	2 Tbs	30	6	1	0
Italian					
w/Italian seasonings	2 Tbs	35	7	1	0
w/roasted garlic	2 Tbs	35	6	1	0
w/tomato pesto	2 Tbs	35	5	1	0
(Hunt's) all styles & flavors	2 Tbs	25	6	2	4
(Muir Glen) organic	2 Tbs	30	6	1	3
(Red Gold)	2 Tbs	30	6	1	3
TOMATO PURÉE..canned					
(Contadina)	¼ cup	20	4	<1	0
(Hunt's)	¼ cup	30	7	2	4
(Progresso)	¼ cup	25	5	1	3
(Red Gold)	¼ cup	25	5	1	3
(S&W) w/medium-diced tomatoes	½ cup	30	6	2	3
(Tuttorosso) all styles & flavors	½ cup	25	5	1	3
TOMATO SAUCE (See also MEXICAN FOOD; SAUCE)					
canned					
(Contadina)					
garlic & onion	¼ cup	20	4	<1	1
Italian	¼ cup	15	4	1	1
original	¼ cup	15	3	<1	1
thick & zesty	¼ cup	20	3	1	2
(Del Monte)	¼ cup	20	4	1	2
(Hunt's)					
basil, garlic & oregano	¼ cup	15	3	<1	2
no salt added	¼ cup	30	6	2	4
original	¼ cup	15	3	<1	2
roasted garlic	¼ cup	15	3	<1	2
(Muir Glen) organic..chunky	¼ cup	20	4	1	2
(Red Gold) thick 'n' rich					
hot w/garlic, onion & jalapeño	¼ cup	15	4	0	0
w/garlic, onion & green pepper	¼ cup	20	4	0	1
(S&W) home-style	¼ cup	20	4	1	2
TONIC WATER (See COCKTAIL MIXER)					
TORTELLINI (See PASTA)					
TORTILLA (See MEXICAN FOOD)					
TORTILLA CHIPS/CORN CHIPS					
(Barbara's Bakery) blue corn chips..					
all styles	1 oz	140	16	1	–
(Doritos)					
Cooler Ranch	1 oz	140	18	1	<1
3D's	2 oz	270	39	2	7
jalapeño cheddar–flavored	1 oz	130	20	1	1
K. C. Masterpiece BBQ	1 oz	140	23	<1	3
Nacho Cheesier	1 oz	130	19	1	2
original	1 oz	270	39	2	7
WOW..Nacho Cheesier	1 oz	90	18	1	1
zesty ranch	2 oz	270	38	2	3
EXTREME..bold BBQ	1 oz	140	18	1	2
4-cheese–flavored	1 oz	140	17	1	0

Food and Description	Amount	Total Calories	Total Carbs	Fiber	Sugars
Nacho Cheesier					
baked	1 oz	120	21	2	1
original	1 oz	140	17	1	2
salsa verde	1 oz	140	18	1	1
spicier nacho	1 oz	140	18	1	1
taco	1 oz	140	18	1	1
toasted corn	1 oz	140	18	1	0
WOW..Nacho Cheesier	1 oz	90	18	1	1
(Fritos)					
Bar-B-Q	1 oz	150	16	1	<1
chili cheese	1 oz	160	15	1	1
flamin' hot	1 oz	160	15	1	<1
flavor twists cheddar ranch	1 oz	150	17	1	<1
honey BBQ	1 oz	160	16	1	1
Hoops..honey BBQ..mini	1 oz	160	17	1	1
king-size	1 oz	160	16	1	0
original	1 oz	160	15	1	<1
Sabrositas					
flamin' hot	1 oz	160	15	1	<1
lime 'n' chili	1 oz	150	17	1	0
Scoops!	1 oz	160	16	1	0
(Full Circle)					
cheesy nacho	1 oz	140	19	1	0
sesame stone-ground blue corn	1 oz	150	16	2	0
stone-ground..white or yellow	1 oz	140	20	1	0
(Garden of Eatin')					
blue corn tortilla chips					
Little Soy Blues	1 oz	140	17	2	0
no salt or original	1 oz	140	18	2	0
Red Hot Blues	1 oz	140	18	2	0
Sesame Blues	1 oz	150	17	2	0
Sunny Blues	1 oz	150	17	2	0
red corn tortilla chips					
red chips	1 oz	140	18	1	0
salsa reds	1 oz	140	18	3	0
white corn tortilla chips					
chili lime	1 oz	140	18	2	1
guacamole	1 oz	140	19	2	<1
pico de gallo	1 oz	140	18	3	0
tamari	1 oz	140	18	3	0
white chips	1 oz	140	19	2	0
yellow corn tortilla chips					
black bean	1 oz	140	18	4	0
chili	1 oz	140	17	4	0
garden grains	1 oz	140	18	2	0
nacho cheese	1 oz	140	18	2	<1
yellow chips	1 oz	140	18	2	0
(GeniSoy) low-carb chips					
all styles & flavors	1 oz	140	12	4	0

Food and Description	Amount	Total Calories	Total Carbs	Fiber	Sugars
(Guiltless Gourmet) baked					
chili lime	1 oz	110	22	2	2
Mucho Nacho	1 oz	110	22	2	2
others..all styles & flavors	1 oz	110	22	2	0
(Kettle)					
blue corn	1 oz	140	18	2	0
5-grain yellow	1 oz	140	18	2	0
Little Dippers	1 oz	140	18	2	0
Sesame Blue Moons	1 oz	150	19	2	0
sesame rye w/caraway	1 oz	140	17	2	0
sweet brown rice & black bean	1 oz	120	16	2	0
(Michael Season's)					
sesame blue	1 oz	150	16	2	0
sesame yellow	1 oz	140	20	1	0
yellow corn	1 oz	140	20	1	0
(Mike Sell's)					
baked..low-fat	1 oz	110	24	2	0
miestos					
nacho cheese	1 oz	140	19	1	0
restaurant-style	1 oz	140	18	2	0
tortilla chips..original	1 oz	130	20	0	0
(Mission) authentic Mexican tortilla					
rounds..all styles & flavors	1 oz	140	17	1	0
(Nana's) fried..salted					
cocina triangles	19 chips	150	21	2	0
guacamole green triangles	1 oz	160	17	2	0
white	1 oz	140	18	1	0
(Old Dutch)					
Arriba nacho cheese	1 oz	140	18	2	0
restaurant-style					
bite-size	1 oz	150	18	1	0
original	1 oz	140	20	2	0
(Santitas)					
tortilla chips					
white corn	1 oz	130	19	1	0
yellow corn	1 oz	130	20	1	0
tortilla strips					
yellow corn	1 oz	130	19	1	0
(Snyder's of Hanover)					
EatSmart..organic					
blue corn-tillas	1 oz	140	17	5	0
w/sesame seeds	1 oz	140	17	4	0
tortilla chips					
white corn	1 oz	140	23	2	0
yellow corn	1 oz	140	23	2	0
(Tostitos)					
baked					
bite-size	1 oz	110	24	2	0
white	1 oz	110	24	2	0
yellow	1 oz	140	19	1	0

Food and Description	Amount	Total Calories	Total Carbs	Fiber	Sugars
original					
100% white corn..bite-size	1 oz	140	17	1	0
blue corn..natural..restaurant-style	1 oz	140	19	1	0
restaurant-style	1 oz	140	18	1	0
crispy rounds..white corn.. restaurant-style	1 oz	140	18	1	0
hint of lime	1 oz	140	19	1	<1
white corn	1 oz	140	19	1	0
Santa Fe gold	1 oz	140	20	1	0
spicy quesadilla..bite-size round	1 oz	150	16	1	<1
Scoops!	1 oz	140	18	1	0
WOW! restaurant-style	1 oz	90	20	1	0
(Wise) Bravos..all styles	1 oz	150	18	1	0
TRAIL MIX (*See* CEREAL; FRUIT SNACK; NUTS, MIXED; SNACK MIX)					
TROUT					
mixed species..cooked—dry heat	3 oz	165	0	0	0
rainbow					
farmed..cooked-dry heat	3 oz	145	0	0	0
wild..cooked-dry heat	3 oz	130	0	0	0
sea..mixed species..cooked—dry heat	3 oz	115	0	0	0
TUNA (*See also* SEAFOOD ENTRÉE/DINNER; TUNA DISH; VEGETARIAN FOODS)					
CANNED/DRAINED					
(3 Diamonds)					
chunk light..in water	2 oz	60	0	0	0
chunk white..in water..albacore	2 oz	60	0	0	0
solid white..in water					
fancy albacore	2 oz	90	0	0	0
premium albacore	2 oz	70	0	0	0
(Bumble Bee)					
albacore chunk white..in water	2 oz	60	0	0	0
albacore solid white..in water	2 oz	70	0	0	0
albacore solid white prime fillet					
chunk light..in oil	2 oz	110	0	0	0
chunk light..in water	2 oz	60	0	0	0
in water	2 oz	70	0	0	0
(Chicken of the Sea)					
chunk light..in canola oil	2 oz	110	0	0	0
chunk light..in spring water					
50% less salt	2 oz	60	0	0	0
low-sodium	2 oz	60	0	0	0
premium					
can	2 oz	60	0	0	0
pouch	1 pouch	90	0	0	0
regular	2 oz	60	0	0	0
salad kit..single					
reduced-fat mayo	3.5 oz	180	11	1	2
savory smoked	3.5 oz	280	7	1	2
w/mayo & onion	3.5 oz	300	7	1	2
w/sweet pickle relish	3.5 oz	220	7	1	4
solid light Genova tonno	2 oz	130	0	0	0

Food and Description	Amount	Total Calories	Total Carbs	Fiber	Sugars
yellowfin chunk light..in spring water	2 oz	60	0	0	0
yellowfin solid light..in spring water	2 oz	60	0	0	0
(Crown Prince)					
chunk light tongol					
no salt added	¼ cup	70	0	0	0
regular	¼ cup	60	0	0	0
solid white albacore					
no salt added	¼ cup	60	0	0	0
regular	¼ cup	60	0	0	0
yellowfin..in olive oil	¼ cup	110	0	0	0
(StarKist)					
chunk light					
in oil	2 oz	110	0	0	0
in water..drained	2 oz	60	0	0	0
chunk white..low-salt..low-fat					
in distilled water	2 oz	60	0	0	0
in spring water	2 oz	60	0	0	0
Lunch-To-Go..pouch..chunk light	4.5 oz	210	27	3	8
solid light					
Gourmet's Choice..drained..					
in olive oil	2 oz	90	0	0	0
solid white..in oil	2 oz	90	0	0	0
StarKist Flavor Fresh..pouch					
chunk light..in water	2 oz	90	0	0	0
StarKist Select..yellowfin..chunk light	2 oz	60	0	0	0
Tuna Creations..hickory-smoked	2 oz	60	0	0	0
FRESH					
bluefin..cooked—dry heat	3 oz	157	0	0	0
skipjack..cooked—dry heat	3 oz	112	0	0	0
yellowfin..cooked—dry heat	3 oz	118	0	0	0

TUNA DISH (*See also* FROZEN ENTRÉE/DINNER; SEAFOOD ENTRÉE/DINNER)
MIX
(Betty Crocker)

Food and Description	Amount	Total Calories	Total Carbs	Fiber	Sugars
Tuna Helper (prepared as directed)					
au gratin	1 cup	310	38	1	5
cheesy pasta	1 cup	270	31	1	5
creamy broccoli	1 cup	300	33	1	4
creamy pasta	1 cup	290	32	2	5
fettuccini Alfredo	1 cup	300	32	1	5
garden cheddar	1 cup	290	36	1	6
tetrazzini	1 cup	300	31	1	3
tuna melt	1 cup	280	34	0	5

TURBINADO SUGAR (*See* SUGAR)
TURBOT..cooked—dry heat | 3 oz | 104 | 0 | 0 | 0
TURKEY (*See also* BACON; LUNCHEON MEAT; SAUSAGE; TURKEY ENTRÉE/DINNER; VEGETARIAN FOODS)
■ **TURKEY & TURKEY PARTS..BRAND NAME**
CANNED, FRESH, or FROZEN
(Best Yet) breast

Food and Description	Amount	Total Calories	Total Carbs	Fiber	Sugars
97% fat-free	1.25 oz	30	0	0	0
oven-roasted	1.25 oz	25	1	1	0
smoked	1.25 oz	30	0	0	0
young..lean	4 oz	170	0	0	0
(Briar Street Market)					
chunk..smoked breast w/white meat	2 oz	50	1	0	0
diced..white & dark meat..½" pieces	¼ cup	70	1	0	0
ground	4 oz	210	0	0	0
logs..rolls					
cured dark picnic log	2 oz	60	0	0	0
roasted breast roll	2 oz	45	1	1	0
cooked white roll	2 oz	100	0	0	0
meatballs..Italian..6 pieces	3 oz	210	0	0	0
pulled white..½" pieces	3 oz	120	0	0	0
(Butterball) fresh..premium cuts					
breast					
boneless roast	4 oz	110	1	0	1
fillets	2.85 oz	80	0	0	0
ground..99% fat-free	4 oz	110	0	0	0
London broil	4 oz	110	1	0	0
packaged..sliced					
breast..London broil..fresh prime	4 oz	110	1	0	0
honey-roasted..smoked..hearty.. thick-sliced	1 oz	30	1	0	1
oven-roasted..hearty..thick-sliced	1 oz	30	1	0	0
tenderloin..young..boneless	4 oz	110	1	0	0
ground					
43% less fat	4 oz	220	0	0	0
7% fat	4 oz	160	0	0	0
stuffed	4 oz	130	0	0	0
whole..Great on the Grill.. dark & white	4 oz	140	1	0	0
whole..smoked cured.. dark & white	½ oz	35	0	0	0
(Honeysuckle White) fresh (unless specified otherwise)					
breast					
99% fat-free..for scallopini & Milanese	4 oz	120	0	0	0
boneless roast	4 oz	110	1	0	0
split	4 oz	190	0	0	0
tenderloins					
boneless	4 oz	110	3	0	0
97% fat-free					
lemon garlic	4 oz	130	4	0	1
rotisserie	4 oz	130	5	0	1
other..fresh (unless specified otherwise)					
drumstick	4 oz	180	6	<1	1
drumettes	3 oz	190	0	0	0
ground					
93% lean..chub	4 oz	160	0	0	0

Food and Description	Amount	Total Calories	Total Carbs	Fiber	Sugars
w/natural flavoring..chub	4 oz	240	0	0	0
rotisserie					
Italian herb flavor	4 oz	170	3	0	2
original flavor	4 oz	170	2	0	1
thigh	4 oz	190	0	0	0
whole					
frozen..boneless	2 oz	160	1	0	1
hickory-smoked	3 oz	140	3	0	1
young					
Cajun-style	3 oz	140	3	0	1
fresh	4 oz	170	0	0	0
frozen	4 oz	170	0	0	0
wing	4 oz	220	0	0	0
(Hormel)					
whole..hickory-smoked	2 oz	60	1	0	1
natural shape..boneless	2 oz	50	0	0	0
chunk..canned in water					
mixed	2 oz	60	0	0	0
white premium	2 oz	50	0	0	0
(Jennie-O)					
ground..chub	4 oz	170	0	0	0
whole young..prime	5 oz	180	4	0	1
whole..smoked..premium..young	3 oz	110	1	0	1
(Jennie-O Turkey Store)					
all meat					
burger patties..lean..7% fat	4 oz	160	0	0	0
burger patties..lean..7% fat..					
seasoned	4 oz	180	5	0	0
burgers..original	4 oz	160	0	0	0
burgers..savory-seasoned	4 oz	160	0	0	0
drumsticks	4 oz	190	7	0	3
ground	4 oz	180	0	0	0
thighs	4 oz	190	7	0	3
wings	4 oz	190	7	0	3
young					
premium fresh	4 oz	180	0	0	0
whole premium	4 oz	180	0	0	0
breast					
hickory-smoked..half..97% fat free	2 oz	60	0	0	0
honey-cured..half..97% fat-free	2 oz	60	0	0	0
oven-roasted..w/broth	2 oz	50	0	0	0
slices..extra-lean..99% fat-free	4 oz	180	5	0	0
breast..stuffed					
cheddar, cheese & broccoli	2 oz	60	1	0	0
pepper, cheese & rice	2 oz	60	1	0	0
Swiss cheese & rice	2 oz	60	1	0	0
breast tenderloins..marinated					
lemon garlic	4 oz	120	1	0	0
seasoned pepper	4 oz	100	1	0	0
tequila lime	4 oz	190	7	0	0

Food and Description	Amount	Total Calories	Total Carbs	Fiber	Sugars
(Louis Rich)					
turkey breast portions					
hickory-smoked	2 oz	50	1	0	0
honey-roasted	2 oz	60	3	0	2
oven-roasted	2 oz	50	1	0	0
ground..bulk	4 oz	190	0	0	0
(Perdue) fresh..cooked					
carving breast					
Cajun-style	2 oz	50	1	0	0
honey-smoked	2 oz	50	2	0	2
mesquite-smoked	2 oz	50	0	0	0
Carving Classics..breast..pan-roasted					
braised home-style	2 oz	70	1	0	0
cracked pepper	2 oz	50	2	0	0
hickory-smoked	2 oz	70	1	0	1
deli breast..oven-roasted	2 oz	50	0	0	0
Fit'N Easy..fresh lean ground					
cooked	3 oz	160	0	0	0
raw	4 oz	170	0	0	0
fresh..cooked					
burgers..lean	4 oz	170	0	0	0
ground..lean turkey breast					
cooked	3 oz	110	0	0	0
raw	4 oz	120	0	0	0
whole hen					
dark	3 oz	180	0	0	0
white	3 oz	150	0	0	0
whole tom					
dark	3 oz	160	0	0	0
white	3 oz	140	0	0	0
wing					
drumettes	3 oz	180	0	0	0
portions	3 oz	160	0	0	0
wing portions	3 oz	160	0	0	0
wings	3 oz	160	0	0	0
frozen..cooked					
whole hen					
dark	3 oz	180	0	0	0
white	3 oz	150	0	0	0
whole tom					
dark	3 oz	160	0	0	0
white	3 oz	140	0	0	0
(Plantation) whole breast					
fiesta-oven-roasted	2 oz	50	1	0	0
hickory-smoked	2 oz	50	2	0	1
honey mesquite–smoked	2 oz	50	2	0	1
mesquite-smoked	2 oz	50	1	0	0
oven-roasted	2 oz	45	1	0	0
peppered..hickory-smoked	2 oz	50	1	0	0
(Shady Brook) fresh..raw					

Food and Description	Amount	Total Calories	Total Carbs	Fiber	Sugars
breast					
99% fat-free..boneless					
for London broil	4 oz	130	0	0	0
for scallopini	4 oz	110	0	0	0
chops..boneless	4 oz	110	0	0	0
cutlets..boneless	4 oz	110	0	0	0
split..natural	4 oz	190	0	0	0
tenderloin..97% fat-free	4 oz	130	0	0	0
lemon garlic	4 oz	130	4	0	1
rotisserie-flavor	4 oz	130	5	0	1
young					
fresh	4 oz	190	0	0	0
hotel-style	4 oz	180	0	0	0
burgers..93% lean patties	4 oz	170	0	0	0
ground					
85% fat-free	4 oz	240	0	0	0
93% lean	4 oz	160	0	0	0
meatballs..Italian-style	3 oz	190	6	1	1
meatballs..w/sweet & sour sauce	3 oz	190	6	1	1
turkey ham..chub..hickory-smoked	2 oz	60	2	0	0
whole..young	4 oz	180	0	0	0
(Shelton's) free-range..cooked..frozen					
ground..chub	4 oz	170	0	0	0
meatballs	6 pieces	180	6	<1	0
(Wampler-Longacre)					
burgers					
100% pure turkey	4 oz	210	0	0	0
BBQ	4 oz	220	3	0	3
specially seasoned	4 oz	180	1	0	0
The Diamond Line					
5 Diamond breast					
oil-browned..w/skin	2 oz	70	0	0	0
oil-browned..w/o skin	2 oz	45	0	0	0
w/ skin	2 oz	70	0	0	0
w/o skin	2 oz	50	0	0	0
smoked..w/skin	2 oz	70	0	0	0
4 Diamond breast					
honey-cured..smoked	2 oz	70	4	0	3
no salt..w/o skin	2 oz	60	0	0	0
oil-browned	2 oz	60	1	0	0
petite..honey-cured..smoked	2 oz	50	4	0	0
smoked	2 oz	60	2	0	1
2 Diamond breast..smoked	2 oz	60	2	0	1
1 Diamond breast					
oven-roasted	2 oz	50	1	0	1
smoked	2 oz	50	1	9	1
ground	4 oz	210	0	0	0

TURKEY ALTERNATIVE (*See* VEGETARIAN FOODS)
TURKEY BACON (*See* BACON)
TURKEY ENTRÉE/DINNER (*See also* FROZEN ENTRÉE/DINNER; PASTA ENTRÉE/DINNER)

Food and Description	Amount	Total Calories	Total Carbs	Fiber	Sugars
CANNED OR MICROWAVEABLE					
(Dinty Moore) American Classics					
turkey & dressing w/gravy	1 bowl	290	33	3	4
turkey stew..microwaveable	1 cup	140	19	2	3
READY-TO-SERVE					
(Hormel) fully cooked..refrigerated					
sliced turkey breast & gravy	5.6 oz	130	4	0	2
teriyaki turkey tenderloin	4 oz	130	6	0	4
(Jennie-O Turkey Store)					
stuffed turkey breast..pepper cheese	2 oz	60	1	0	0
turkey roast w/white meat w/gravy in roasting pan	4 oz	150	3	0	2
(Schwan's)					
boneless breast of turkey w/gravy	4 oz	140	3	0	1
pot pie	1 pie	690	57	3	6
mignon	1 filet	220	3	0	1
(Shady Brook)					
meatballs..fully cooked					
Italian-style	3 oz	190	6	1	1
w/sweet & sour sauce	3 oz	190	6	1	1
meat balls	6 pieces	180	6	1	0
TURKEY HAM (*See* HAM; LUNCHEON MEAT; TURKEY..BRAND NAME..CANNED..FRESH)					
TURKEY SAUSAGE (*See* SAUSAGE)					
TURKEY SUBSTITUTES (*See* VEGETARIAN FOODS)					
TURMERIC..ground	1 tsp	8	2	0	0
TURNIP *FRESH*					
boiled..mashed	½ cup	25	5.5	2.5	0
raw..cubed	½ cup	18	4	1	0
TURNIP GREENS					
CANNED					
(Bush's Best)					
chopped	½ cup	25	3	2	1
w/diced turnips	½ cup	30	5	2	0
(The Allens)					
seasoned Southern-style	½ cup	35	5	2	1
w/diced turnips	½ cup	35	5	2	1
w/ mustard greens	½ cup	45	6	1	2
verduras de nabo..chopped	½ cup	25	3	2	1
verduras de nabo picadas w/diced turnips	½ cup	30	5	3	1
(The Allens Sunshine)					
seasoned Southern-style	½ cup	35	5	2	1
fat-free	½ cup	35	5	2	1
w/diced turnips	½ cup	35	5	2	1
FROZEN					
(Bird's Eye)					
chopped	1 cup	30	3	2	0
w/diced turnips	1 cup	25	2	2	1
TURTLE..green					

CANNED	3 oz	91	0	0	0
RAW	3 oz	76	0	0	0

V

Food and Description	Amount	Total Calories	Total Carbs	Fiber	Sugars
VEAL					

(NOTE: All serving sizes are for cooked portions, unless otherwise stated. "Lean" means veal trimmed of separable fat before cooking. "Lean & fat" means untrimmed and cooked or eaten as purchased. In most cases, 4 ounces of raw veal yields approximately 3 ounces cooked.)

Food and Description	Amount	Total Calories	Total Carbs	Fiber	Sugars
ground/broiled	4 oz	195	0	0	0
loin					
lean					
braised or broiled	3 oz	195	0	0	0
roasted	3 oz	150	0	0	0
lean & fat					
braised or broiled	3 oz	240	0	0	0
roasted	3 oz	180	0	0	0
organs					
brain					
braised	3 oz	115	0	0	0
fried	3 oz	180	0	0	0
heart..braised	3 oz	160	0	0	0
kidney..braised	3 oz	140	0	0	0
liver					
braised	3 oz	140	0	0	0
fried	3 oz	210	0	0	0
spleen..braised	3 oz	110	0	0	0
tongue..braised	3 oz	170	0	0	0
rib roast					
lean					
braised or broiled	3 oz	185	0	0	0
roasted	3 oz	150	0	0	0
lean & fat					
braised or broiled	3 oz	215	0	0	0
roasted	3 oz	195	0	0	0
round w/rump					
roasts & leg cutlets..lean..broiled	3 oz	160	0	0	0
sirloin					

Food and Description	Amount	Total Calories	Total Carbs	Fiber	Sugars
lean					
braised or broiled	3 oz	175	0	0	0
roasted	3 oz	145	0	0	0
lean & fat					
braised or broiled	3 oz	215	0	0	0
roasted	3 oz	175	0	0	0
top round					
lean					
roasted	3 oz	130	0	0	0
lean & fat					
roasted	3 oz	135	0	0	0
VEAL DISH (*See also* FROZEN ENTRÉE/DINNER)					
frozen (Redi-Serve Tray) veal patties					
breaded & cooked	1 patty	320	25	4	2
VEGETABLE DISH (*See* FROZEN ENTRÉE/DINNER; VEGETARIAN FOODS; individual vegetable listings)					
VEGETABLE JUICE/JUICE COCKTAIL/JUICE DRINK					
BOTTLED, BOXED, OR CANNED					
(Campbell's)					
Invigor8					
Energy Boost	8 fl oz	110	27	1	22
Nutrition Boost	8 fl oz	110	27	1	20
V8 Splash vegetable juice..100% juice					
100% A-C-E vitamin rich	8 fl oz	50	11	2	8
calcium-enriched V8	8 fl oz	50	11	2	8
lemon twist V8	8 fl oz	50	10	2	7
lightly tangy V8	8 fl oz	60	11	1	9
low-sodium V8	8 fl oz	50	11	2	8
picante V8	8 fl oz	50	10	1	7
spicy hot V8	8 fl oz	50	10	1	7
V8 100% vegetable juice	8 fl oz	50	10	2	7
(DelMonte) vegetable blended cocktail					
Snap-E-Tom..tomato & chili	8 fl oz	50	11	2	6
cocktail	11.5 oz	70	15	3	8
(Knudsen) Very Veggie..100% juice					
low-sodium	8 fl oz	50	11	0	6
organic	8 fl oz	50	11	2	7
original	8 fl oz	50	11	2	7
spicy	8 fl oz	50	11	2	7
Vita Juice	8 fl oz	120	29	0	25
(Muir Glen) organic..100% vegetable					
juice	8 fl oz	70	15	3	11
(RedGold) vegetable juice	8 fl oz	50	11	2	6
VEGETABLE OIL (*See* COOKING SPRAY; OIL)					
VEGETABLE SOUP (*See* SOUP)					
VEGETABLES, MIXED (*See also* ASIAN FOOD; FROZEN ENTRÉE/DINNER; SUCCOTASH)					
CANNED OR JARRED					
(Allens)					
okra & tomatoes	½ cup	30	5	3	1

Food and Description	Amount	Total Calories	Total Carbs	Fiber	Sugars
okra, tomatoes & corn	½ cup	30	6	4	1
(Del Monte)					
regular	½ cup	40	8	2	3
w/potatoes	½ cup	45	10	2	3
(Freshlike)					
sweet corn & diced peppers					
Freshlike Selects	½ cup	80	16	1	4
sweet peas & carrots	½ cup	60	12	4	4
(Green Giant)					
garden medley	½ cup	40	9	1	4
Mexicorn	⅓ cup	60	14	1	4
mixed vegetables	½ cup	60	20	4	10
3-bean salad	½ cup	90	20	4	10
(LeSueur) early peas w/mushrooms					
& pearl onions	½ cup	60	12	3	4
(S&W)					
peas & carrots	⅔ cup	50	11	2	4
peas & onions	⅔ cup	40	11	3	1
(Stokely's)	⅔ cup	35	7	2	3
(Trappey's)					
okra & tomatoes	½ cup	30	5	3	1
okra, tomatoes & corn	½ cup	30	6	4	1
(Veg-All)					
Cajun	½ cup	50	10	3	2
chicharos y zanahorias	½ cup	60	11	4	5
chunky vegetables mixtos en tracitos	½ cup	45	9	2	2
home-style..large cut	½ cup	40	8	2	2
hot 'n' spicy	½ cup	40	8	2	2
original	½ cup	40	8	2	2
sweet peas & carrots	½ cup	60	12	4	4
FROZEN					
(Birds Eye)					
Baby Vegetable Blends					
baby bean & carrot	1 cup	30	5	2	3
baby broccoli	1 cup	70	8	3	3
baby corn blend	⅔ cup	60	12	2	2
baby corn & bean	¾ cup	60	12	2	4
baby pea blend	¾ cup	40	7	2	3
baby sweet peas & pearl onions	⅔ cup	60	12	4	6
Farm Fresh Mixtures					
broccoli, cauliflower & red peppers	1 cup	20	4	2	2
broccoli, corn & red peppers	1 cup	60	4	2	2
broccoli, green beans, pearl onions					
& red peppers	1 cup	25	5	2	3
brussel sprouts, cauliflower & carrots	1 cup	35	6	3	3
cauliflower, carrots & snow pea pods	1 cup	30	5	2	3
Simply Grillin' Vegetables					
garden herb	¼ box	140	19	4	6
potatoes & onions	¼ box	180	25	3	1
roasted corn & potatoes	⅕ box	140	19	3	6

Food and Description	Amount	Total Calories	Total Carbs	Fiber	Sugars
roasted garlic	⅕ box	120	17	3	5
Southern vegetables					
gumbo blend	¾ cup	40	10	2	3
seasoning blend	¾ cup	20	5	1	4
vegetables for stew	¾ cup	40	9	1	2
Traditional..vegetables for soup..bag	⅔ cup	45	10	2	3
Vegetable blends					
Asian blend in sesame sauce	½ box	60	12	2	8
Szechuan vegetables in sesame sauce	½ box	60	9	2	6
Tuscan vegetables in herbed tomato sauce	½ box	50	7	2	3
Vegetable Mix..classic..16-oz bag	⅕ bag	60	11	2	4
(C&W)					
organic					
fancy mixed vegetables	¾ cup	60	11	2	4
plain					
baby pea pods w/water chestnuts	⅔ cup	40	6	2	3
Vegetable Stand combinations					
Early Harvest corn, broccoli florets & julienne red peppers	⅔ cup	60	14	1	4
Healthy Garden vegetables					
Farmer's Harvest	1 cup	25	4	2	2
Ultimate					
petite mixed vegetables	¾ cup	60	11	2	4
Southwest blend	⅔ cup	90	15	6	2
stir-fry	¾ cup	30	6	1	2
(Cascadian Farm) as packaged					
California blend	⅔ cup	20	4	0	4
gardener's blend	¾ cup	57	12	4	7
peas & carrots	⅔ cup	50	10	3	4
peas & pearl onions	¾ cup	60	11	4	5
Santa Fe blend	¾ cup	60	12	3	6
stir-fry blends					
Chinese	1 cup	25	6	2	3
Thai	¾ cup	25	6	2	2
vegetable medley..w/cheese sauce	½ cup	60	7	3	3
(Green Giant) as packaged..boil-in-bag					
Italian-style vegetables	1 cup	90	6	2	2
roasted potatoes					
w/broccoli & cheese	¾ cup	120	19	2	4
Szechuan vegetables	¾ cup	50	9	2	5
teriyaki vegetables	1¼ cups	80	6	2	3
(McKenzie's)					
soup mix w/tomatoes	3 oz	40	9	2	2
vegetable gumbo mixture	2.66 oz	35	8	2	3
(Schwan's)					
California blend	1 cup	25	4	2	2
fire-roasted vegetable blend	1 cup	60	9	2	1

Food and Description	Amount	Total Calories	Total Carbs	Fiber	Sugars
herb garlic–roasted Yukon Gold potato & vegetable blend	1 cup	90	15	2	2
stir-fry vegetables	1 cup	40	8	2	2

VEGETARIAN FOODS

(NOTE: Some of the foods listed in this category were designed to be substitutes for meat and foods traditionally made with meat, and their names may therefore reflect the items they are intended to replace. However, all products listed here are meatless.)

■ **(Amy's) organic**

Food and Description	Amount	Total Calories	Total Carbs	Fiber	Sugars
frozen					
bowls					
brown rice & vegetable	1 bowl	240	36	5	8
country cheddar	1 bowl	400	41	4	3
pesto tortellini	1 bowl	470	58	3	4
Santa Fe enchilada	1 bowl	340	47	10	5
stuffed pasta shells	1 bowl	300	30	5	7
teriyaki	1 bowl	300	59	3	12
dessert..apple pie	4 oz	240	37	2	15
entrées					
black bean vegetable enchilada	4.75 oz	170	26	3	2
cheese enchilada	4.75 oz	220	18	2	2
cheese lasagna	10.25 oz	330	38	5	6
garden vegetable lasagna	10.25 oz	290	41	5	7
macaroni & cheese	9 oz	410	37	3	7
macaroni & soy cheese	9 oz	370	42	4	2
pasta primavera	9.5 oz	300	37	3	7
ravioli w/sauce	8 oz	340	43	3	3
rice mac & cheese	9 oz	410	47	3	6
tofu vegetable lasagna	9.5 oz	300	41	6	6
vegetable lasagna	9.5 oz	300	35	5	5
pizzas					
cheese	⅓ pizza	300	38	2	4
mushroom & olive	⅓ pizza	250	33	2	3
pesto w/tomato & broccoli	⅓ pizza	310	39	2	3
rice crust cheese	⅓ pizza	300	31	2	5
roasted vegetable	⅓ pizza	260	42	2	5
soy cheese	⅓ pizza	290	37	2	3
spinach	⅓ pizza	300	38	2	4
veggie combo	⅓ pizza	290	36	1	4
pocket sandwiches					
broccoli & cheese	4.5 oz	270	37	3	4
Mediterranean vegetable	4.5 oz	220	39	4	4
spinach feta	4.66 oz	300	34	3	4
tofu scramble	4 oz	180	23	<1	2
vegetable pie	5 oz	300	45	3	5
vegetarian pizza	4.5 oz	250	39	4	4
pot pies					
broccoli	1 pie	430	49	4	3
country vegetable	1 pie	370	48	4	5
Mexican tamale	1 pie	150	28	1	2
shepherd's	1 pie	160	28	5	5

Food and Description	Amount	Total Calories	Total Carbs	Fiber	Sugars
vegetable..nondairy	1 pie	360	50	4	3
snacks					
cheese pizza	5–6 pieces	190	22	2	3
nacho	5–6 pieces	210	26	<1	1
spinach feta	5–6 pieces	170	24	2	3
toaster pops					
apple	1 piece	140	26	<1	8
cheese pizza	1 piece	150	23	<1	2
strawberry & cream cheese	1 piece	160	24	<1	8
whole meals..burgers..sandwiches					
All American veggie burger	1.5 oz	120	15	3	2
bean & cheese burrito	6 oz	280	43	6	1
bean & rice burrito	6 oz	280	48	5	2
bean, rice & cheese burrito	6 oz	280	48	5	2
black bean burrito	6 oz	320	44	4	4
black bean enchilada	10 oz	320	55	9	4
burrito especial	6 oz	260	45	3	4
California veggie burger	2.5 oz	130	19	5	2
cheese enchilada	9 oz	330	38	6	6
Chicago veggie burger	2.5 oz	160	20	3	2
chili & corn bread	10.5 oz	340	59	10	14
Indian Mattar Paneer	10 oz	320	54	6	8
macaroni & soy cheese	1 serving	360	42	4	2
stir-fry					
Asian noodle	10 oz	240	41	6	6
Thai	9.5 oz	310	45	5	2
Texas veggie burger	2.5 oz	120	14	3	2
tofu vegetable lasagna	9.5 oz	300	41	6	6
vegetable lasagna w/cheese	9.5 oz	300	35	5	5
veggie loaf dinner	10 oz	280	47	7	6
■ (BOCA Burgers) (*See* Oscar Mayer in this section)					
■ (Cascadian Farm) frozen					
Meals For A Small Planet					
Aztec	3½ cups	290	54	10	1
Indian	3½ cups	340	61	6	5
Moroccan	3½ cups	310	59	11	12
organic meals					
fettuccine alfredo w/mushrooms	1 meal	360	42	1	6
fiesta vegetarian enchiladas	1 meal	370	54	9	10
spaghetti marinara w/vegetables	1 meal	230	38	4	9
spinach lasagna	1 meal	330	42	4	9
3-cheese pasta w/red peppers	1 meal	340	42	1	7
vegetable blends					
California	⅔ cup	20	4	0	4
Chinese stir-fry	1 cup	25	6	2	3
Gardener's	¾ cup	57	12	4	7
Santa Fe	¾ cup	60	12	3	6
Thai stir-fry	¾ cup	25	6	2	2
veggie & chicken bowls					
Caribbean veggies & rice	1 bowl	280	52	7	10

Food and Description	Amount	Total Calories	Total Carbs	Fiber	Sugars
cascade veggies au gratin	1 bowl	170	24	4	7
fiesta casserole	1 bowl	340	52	7	10
Japanese noodles & vegetables	1 bowl	180	29	4	7
pasta marinara	1 bowl	180	37	2	7
pasta primavera	1 bowl	270	37	2	7
Szechuan rice	1 bowl	210	45	3	11
teriyaki rice	1 bowl	270	42	3	7
■ (CedarLane) Natural Cuisine..organic appetizers, sides & snacks					
3-cheese quesadilla	1 quesadilla	250	27	0	4
five-layer Mexican dip	2 Tbs	60	4	1	2
mini bistro pizza	3 pizzas	280	27	2	3
pesto, mozzarella, tomato bruschetta	1 piece	100	10	0.5	2
burritos & wraps..low-fat					
beans, rice & cheese–style burrito	1 burrito	260	48	7	2
couscous & vegetable veggie wrap	1 wrap	220	36	3	2
roasted vegetable & cheese burrito	1 burrito	330	48	3	8
vegetable & rice teriyaki veggie wrap	1 wrap	320	56	2	5
vegetarian pizza veggie wrap	1 wrap	220	32	2	3
veggie ham & cheese veggie wrap	1 wrap	350	36	1	1
carb-buster entrées					
chili relleno pie	1 pkg	520	9	1	6
eggplant Parmesan	1 pkg	220	15	4	8
quiche					
broccoli cheddar	1 pkg	320	7	2	3
4-cheese	1 pkg	500	5	<1	3
spinach artichoke	1 pkg	330	7	2	2
spinach and feta enchiladas	1 pkg	490	11	4	2
vegetable lasagna	1 pkg	504	19	9	3
focaccia..stuffed					
Mediterranean-stuffed	⅓ focaccia	296	37	1	4
Roma tomato & basil	⅓ focaccia	275	33	2	5
veggie pepperoni	⅓ focaccia	250	34	1	3
specialty dinner entrées					
cheese enchiladas	1 enchilada	270	19	2	3
garden vegetable enchilada..low-fat	1 enchilada	140	20	3	4
garden vegetable lasagna..low-fat	1 pkg	180	20	2	2
lasagna w/meatless ground round	1 pkg	380	45	3	3
3-layer enchilada pie	½ pie	215	27	3	0
■ (Forkless Gourmet)					
filled-bun meals					
beef & broccoli	1 bun	300	43	2	14
beef asada	1 bun	280	41	2	14
black bean adobo	1 bun	270	45	4	10
chicken sesame teriyaki	1 bun	320	47	2	15
chipotle chicken	1 bun	280	42	3	15
kung pao shrimp	1 bun	320	47	2	12
margarita chicken	1 bun	260	41	2	14
pork & vegetables w/fortune cookies & BBQ sauce	1 bun	310	48	2	13

Food and Description	Amount	Total Calories	Total Carbs	Fiber	Sugars
pork w/ancho..honey BBQ sauce	1 bun	270	44	2	11
Thai-style chicken	1 bun	310	43	2	16
vegetarian feast w/tofu & edamame	1 bun	320	49	5	15
■ **(Gardenburger)**					
frozen burgers					
fire-roasted vegetable	1 burger	120	18	4	1
flame-grilled hamburger-style	1 burger	120	7	4	0
garden vegan	1 burger	90	12	2	0
original whole-grain veggie	1 burger	110	16	3	1
Santa Fe	1 burger	130	20	4	2
savory portobello	1 burger	120	18	4	1
veggie medley	1 burger	90	18	3	2
meatless, other					
BBQ chick'n	1 patty	250	30	5	20
buffalo chick'n wings	3 pieces	170	8	5	0
chick'n flamed grill	1 patty	100	5	3	0
country-fried chick'n w/gravy	1 patty	190	16	2	2
herb-crusted cutlet	1 cutlet	170	12	2	0
meatballs	6 pieces	110	8	4	0
meat loaf w/gravy	1 slice	130	12	4	1
riblets w/sauce	1 riblet	210	10	4	7
soy BBQ ribs in smoky BBQ sauce	5 oz	210	10	4	7
soy breakfast patties	1 patty	50	2	2	0
sweet 'n' sour pork	½ pouch	170	30	2	19
veggie nuggets..crispy 'n' crunchy					
pizza-spiced	2.66 oz	180	22	3	2
■ **(Lightlife)**					
frozen					
hot dogs					
Deli Jumbos..Smart	1 link	80	3	1	2
Tofu Pups	1 link	60	2	0	2
links					
country breakfast–style	2 links	80	7	3	1
grill-ready brats	1 link	120	5	1	0
grill-ready..2 oz	1 link	110	5	0	2
Old World Italian–style	1 link	90	8	2	1
meatless..slices					
3 peppercorn–style pastrami	2 oz	60	1	0	0
ham..country-style	2 oz	90	5	1	0
Italian-style..Smart Links	2 oz	120	7	3	2
pepperoni-style	1 oz	45	3	1	1
roast-style turkey	2 oz	80	4	1	0
seitan..organic					
BBQ	3 oz	130	8	0	2
teriyaki	3 oz	120	9	0	2
Smart ground burgers & sausage					
Gimme Lean	2 oz	50	4	2	1
ground beef–style	2 oz	50	4	2	1

Food and Description	Amount	Total Calories	Total Carbs	Fiber	Sugars
ground					
original..meatless	2 oz	80	7	3	1
taco & burrito..meatless	2 oz	70	5	4	1
meatballs	5 pieces	160	6	2	1
Smart Menu					
burger	1 burger	100	9	4	0
chick'n nuggets	4 nuggets	220	16	2	1
crumbles	⅓ cup	80	7	3	1
cutlets					
Salisbury steak w/mushroom					
gravy	4.5 oz	130	13	6	1
seasoned chicken	4.0 oz	180	11	4	3
veggie burger	1 burger	80	14	2	1
tempeh..organic					
Fakin' Bacon strips	3 slices	80	6	1	1
garden veggie	4 oz	240	21	8	0
soy	4 oz	210	14	10	0
3-Grain	4 oz	240	21	8	0
wild rice	4 oz	280	14	10	0
■ (Linda McCartney)					
FROZEN MEALS					
butternut squash ravioli	1 meal	450	49	3	11
Caribbean-style ragout	1 meal	310	29	7	10
cheese enchiladas w/Mexican-style					
corn risotto	1 meal	250	23	2	2
fettuccini Alfredo	1 meal	360	35	4	3
fire-grilled vegetarian chicken & veg	1 meal	340	35	4	10
macaroni & cheese	1 meal	420	32	3	3
portobello mushroom barley pilaf	1 meal	250	33	8	3
spicy peanut pasta w/vegetarian					
chicken	1 meal	340	44	4	16
vegetarian chicken fajita	1 meal	320	31	4	7
vegetarian chicken Parmesan	1 meal	510	40	4	9
■ (Loma Linda)					
CANNED or DRY-PACKED					
Big Franks					
low-fat	1 link	80	3	2	0
original	1 link	110	2	2	0
dinner cuts	2 slices	90	3	2	0
fried chik'n w/gravy	2 pieces	150	5	2	0
Gravy Quik..dry mix only					
brown	1 Tbs	20	4	0	0
chicken-style	1 Tbs	20	3	0	0
country-style	1 Tbs	20	4	0	0
mushroom	1 Tbs	15	3	0	0
onion	1 Tbs	15	3	0	0
Linketts	1 link	70	1	1	0
Little Links	2 links	90	2	2	0

Food and Description	Amount	Total Calories	Total Carbs	Fiber	Sugars
Nuteena luncheon loaf	⅜" slice	160	6	2	<1
Redi-Burger	⅝" slice	120	4	0	1
sandwich spread	¼ cup	80	7	3	<1
Swiss Stake	1 piece	120	8	4	<1
Tender Bits	6 pieces	110	7	3	0
Tender Rounds	8 pieces	120	6	1	1
Vege-Burger	¼ cup	70	2	2	0
Vitaburger..dry mix only..granules	3 Tbs	70	6	3	1
FROZEN					
Chik Nuggets	5 pieces	240	13	4	<1
corn dog	1 piece	150	22	3	4
mix..Soyagen..mix only					
all-purpose	¼ cup	130	12	3	7
carob	¼ cup	130	13	2	7
■ **(Morningstar Farms)**					
FROZEN or REFRIGERATED					
America's original veggie dog	1 link	80	6	1	2
Better 'n Burgers	1 patty	100	6	3	<1
Better 'n Eggs	¼ cup	20	9	0	1
breakfast sausage links	2 links	80	3	2	0
breakfast sausage patties	1 patty	80	3	2	1
breakfast sandwiches					
English muffin Scramblers..patty	1 sdw	240	32	5	3
w/cheese	1 sdw	280	35	5	5
breakfast strips..bacon	2 strips	60	2	1	0
Chik patties					
Parmesan ranch	1 patty	170	17	2	1
regular	1 patty	150	16	2	1
Chik'n					
nuggets	4 nuggets	190	18	2	1
pot pies	1 pie	350	45	9	6
chili & corn bread pot pies..home-style	1 pie	330	49	7	11
corn dogs					
mini	4 pieces	170	21	1	6
regular	1	150	22	3	4
fajita burgers	1 burger	130	7	3	1
Grillers					
burger-style recipe crumbles	⅔ cup	80	4	2	<1
Prime	1 patty	170	5	2	0
ground meatless crumbles	½ cup	60	4	2	0
Harvest burgers..patties..original	1 patty	140	8	5	<1
oven-roasted veggie burgers	1 patty	120	9	3	1
pizza..supreme	½ pizza	360	49	3	6
portobello mushrooms & oven-roasted					
peppers veggie burgers	1 burger	120	9	3	1
sausage-style recipe crumbles	⅔ cup	90	5	2	<1
Scramblers..egg substitute	¼ cup	35	2	0	2
spicy black bean burgers	1 patty	150	16	5	2
tomato & basil pizza burgers	1 patty	130	7	3	2

Food and Description	Amount	Total Calories	Total Carbs	Fiber	Sugars
■ (Natural Touch)					
CANNED					
vegetarian chili	1 cup	170	21	11	2
FROZEN or REFRIGERATED					
breakfast patty made w/organic soy	1 patty	80	4	1	<1
classic burger	1 burger	150	10	3	2
corn dog..veggie	1	170	22	3	5
herb chik'n made w/organic soy	1 patty	110	9	2	1
lentil rice loaf	1" slice	160	13	5	<1
9-bean loaf	1" slice	160	13	5	<1
okra patty	1 patty	120	6	3	<1
Tex Mex burger made w/organic soy	1 patty	120	17	2	4
Thai burger	1 burger	100	7	3	1
vegan burger made w/organic soy	1 patty	100	8	5	2
veggie medley made w/organic soy	1 patty	120	11	1	1
zesty tomato basil burger	1 burger	130	7	4	3
MIX					
Kaffree Roma	1 rounded tsp	10	2	0	0
■ (Near East)					
falafel vegetable patty mix..prepared	2½ patties	230	18	5	3
tabouli salad mix..prepared	~⅔ cup	110	23	5	2
■ (Oscar Mayer) BOCA..soy					
breakfast					
links					
regular	2 links	100	6	4	2
70% less fat	2 links	90	8	2	3
patties..6-count pkg					
regular	⅙ pkg	80	5	3	1
70% less fat	⅙ pkg	80	6	2	2
burgers					
All American Classic..70% less fat	¼ pkg	110	6	4	0
cheese	¼ pkg	130	6	4	1
garden vegetable..70% less fat	¼ pkg	120	9	4	2
grilled vegetable	¼ pkg	90	6	4	0
roasted garlic..70% less fat	¼ pkg	100	7	5	1
roasted onion..90% less fat	¼ pkg	90	8	5	1
vegan original	¼ pkg	90	6	4	0
ground					
burger..meatless..original	2 oz	70	7	3	0
sausage..Italian	2 oz	60	6	4	0
nuggets..original..chik'n..65% less fat	2.85 oz	190	16	2	2
patties					
original chik'n..50% less fat	¼ pkg	150	12	2	1
spicy chik'n	¼ pkg	150	12	2	1
pizza..meatless					
pepperoni					
regular	4 oz	240	27	2	3
tomato & herb	4 oz	240	36	2	4
supreme w/pepperoni & sausage	4 oz	250	36	2	5

Food and Description	Amount	Total Calories	Total Carbs	Fiber	Sugars
sausages					
bratwurst					
natural ingredients	¼ pkg	120	6	2	2
60% less fat	¼ pkg	130	6	1	2
Italian..65% less fat	¼ pkg	120	6	5	3
smoked..65% less fat	¼ pkg	130	7	2	2
■ (Quorn)					
cutlets					
garlic & herb..chicken-style	1 cutlet	200	20	4	2
naked	1 cutlet	80	5	2	0
links..meat-free	2 links	70	2	1	0
pasta meals					
fettuccini Alfredo	1 pkg	360	40	4	5
lasagna..meat-free	1 pkg	360	43	4	13
nuggets..chicken-style	3–4 nuggets	180	18	3	2
patties..chicken-style	1 patty	160	12	3	2
roast..turkey-style	⅓ pkg	90	8	6	0
tenders..chicken-style recipe	1 cup	90	8	3	1
■ (Turtle Island Foods)					
Tofurky					
deli slices					
cranberry & stuffing	3 slices	98	8	3	2
hickory-smoked	3 slices	103	6	3	1
Italian	3 slices	103	7	4	2
original	3 slices	103	6	3	1
peppered	3 slices	103	6	3	1
Philly-style	3 slices	110	7	3	0
gourmet sausages					
beerbrats	3.5 oz	250	8	2	1
kielbasa	3.5 oz	240	8	2	2
sweet Italian	¾ oz	260	12	8	3
Holiday Products..Tofurky					
w/cranberry apple potato dumplings	2 pieces	210	45	6	7
w/wild rice & mushroom stuffing	½ cup	115	21	1	2
Jurky..all flavors	4 pieces	110	9	1	3
Super Burgers					
original	1 burger	120	15	2	0
smoked	1 burger	120	16	2	0
Tex Mex	1 burger	120	14	3	0
■ (White Wave)					
Tofu Tenders					
Havana black bean	½ pkg	200	15	2	10
Mediterranean tahini	½ pkg	240	11	2	6
sesame ginger teriyaki	½ pkg	220	18	3	12
tamari	⅓ pkg	150	5	2	3
■ (Worthington)					
CANNED or DRY-PACKED					
Chik					
diced..drained	¼ cup	50	2	1	0

Food and Description	Amount	Total Calories	Total Carbs	Fiber	Sugars
sliced..drained	3 slices	80	3	2	0
chili					
low-fat	1 cup	170	21	11	2
original	1 cup	290	21	9	2
choplets	2 slices	90	3	2	0
corned beef	4 slices	140	5	0	1
country stew	1 cup	210	20	5	3
cutlets..multigrain	2 slices	100	5	4	0
FriChik					
low-fat	2 pieces	80	4	1	0
original	2 pieces	140	3	1	0
meatless					
chicken roll	⅜" slice	90	2	<1	0
chicken slices	3 slices	90	2	<1	0
corned beef..roll	⅜" slice	140	5	0	1
salami	3 slices	120	3	2	0
smoked beef	3 slices	130	7	<1	2
smoked turkey..vegetable protein	3 slices	140	5	0	2
smoked turkey..vegetable protein roll	⅜" slice	140	5	0	2
multigrain cutlets	2 slices	100	5	4	0
Numete	⅜" slice	130	5	3	1
Prime Stakes	1 piece	120	6	1	0
Prosage					
patties	1 patty	80	3	2	0
vegetable & grain protein roll	⅝" slice	140	5	3	<1
Protose	⅜" slice	130	5	3	<1
Saucettes	1 link	90	1	1	0
savory slices	3 slices	150	7	0	<1
sliced Chik	3 slices	80	3	2	0
sloppy joe	½ cup	140	21	3	11
Stakelets patties	1 patty	150	7	2	0
Stripples	2 strips	40	2	1	0
Stroganoff	½ cup	110	10	2	2
Super Links	1 link	110	2	1	0
turkee slices	3 slices	180	5	0	1
vegetable skallops	½ cup	90	3	3	0
vegetarian burger	¼ cup	60	2	1	0
vegetarian cutlets	1 slice	70	3	2	0
Veja-Links					
low-fat	1 link	40	1	0	0
original	1 link	50	1	0	0
Wham					
vegetable protein roll	⅜" slice	110	3	0	2
vegetable protein slices	3 slices	110	3	0	2
FROZEN					
BBQ FriChik w/BBQ sauce	2 pieces	240	27	3	13
Bolono	3 slices	80	3	2	1
Chic-ketts roll	2⅜" slice	120	2	2	0
Chik Stiks	1 piece	100	4	2	0

Food and Description	Amount	Total Calories	Total Carbs	Fiber	Sugars
Crispy Chik	1 patty	150	16	2	2
dinner roast	¾" slice	180	5	3	1
fillet	2 fillets	180	8	4	<1
Fripats	1 patty	130	4	3	0
golden croquettes	4 pieces	210	14	2	3
Leanies..vegetable & grain protein links	1 link	100	2	1	<1
Tuno..tuna substitute	½ cup	80	2	1	0
■ (Yves) veggie dogs					
hot 'n' spicy chili	1.85 oz	74	2.7	0	0
original..jumbo	1.7 oz	104	6.8	0	0
tofu dogs	1.35 oz	47	2.2	0	0
veggie	1.6 oz	56	1.4	0	0
VENISON..boneless					
raw					
caribou	3 oz	105	0	0	0
ground..antelope	3.5 oz	110	0	0	0
roasted..deer	3 oz	135	0	0	0
VICHYSSOISE (See SOUP)					
VINEGAR					
(Bertolli)					
balsamic of Modena	1 Tbs	15	3	0	0
red wine	1 Tbs	3	0	0	0
white wine	1 Tbs	3	0	0	0
(China Bowl) white rice	1 Tbs	0	0	0	0
(Consorzio) balsamic..organic	1 Tbs	6	2	0	2
(Eden) all styles except plum	1 Tbs	0	0	0	0
plum..Ume	1 Tbs	2	0	0	0
(Filippo Berio) all styles	1 Tbs	0	0	0	0
(Four Monks) all styles	1 Tbs	0	0	0	0
(Hain) balsamic..from Italy	1 Tbs	10	2	0	2
(Nakano) rice vinegar					
balsamic blend	1 Tbs	15	4	0	4
basil & oregano	1 Tbs	20	5	0	5
roasted garlic..original seasoned	1 Tbs	20	5	0	5
roasted garlic..pesto	1 Tbs	20	5	0	5
seasoned red pepper	1 Tbs	20	5	0	5
(Progresso) balsamic	1 Tbs	10	2	0	2
(Regina) balsamic	1 Tbs	5	2	0	2
(S&W) all styles & flavors	1 Tbs	0	0	0	0
VODKA (See LIQUOR, DISTILLED)					

W

Food and Description	Amount	Total Calories	Total Carbs	Fiber	Sugars
WAFFLE (*See also* PANCAKE & WAFFLE MIX)					
(Aunt Jemima) frozen					
blueberry	2 waffles	190	32	1	5
buttermilk	2 waffles	200	33	1	3
home-style..10-count pkg	2 waffles	190	32	1	3
low-fat	2 waffles	160	30	1	2
(Belgian Chef) frozen Belgian	2 waffles	180	34	0	6
(Haggen) frozen..10-count pkg					
blueberry	2 waffles	230	33	1	8
buttermilk	2 waffles	210	29	1	5
cinnamon toast	2 waffles	240	37	1	11
home-style	2 waffles	210	29	1	5
strawberry	2 waffles	220	31	1	8
(Kashi) GoLean..all styles	2 waffles	170	33	6	4
(Kellogg's) frozen					
Eggo Waf-Fulls..all flavors	1 piece	150	25	<1	8
Eggo Waffles					
apple cinnamon	2 waffles	200	30	2	5
banana bread	2 waffles	190	30	2	5
blueberry	2 waffles	200	30	1	5
buttermilk	2 waffles	190	30	1	5
chocolate chip	2 waffles	200	32	1	9
cinnamon toast	2 waffles	290	46	1	17
Froot Loops	2 waffles	200	30	1	5
home-style					
mini..3 sets of	4 waffles	290	46	1	17
regular-size	2 waffles	190	29	2	2
Minis..chocolate chip cookie dough	8 waffles	180	31	1	7
Nutri-Grain					
whole wheat	2 waffles	170	28	3	3
low-fat	2 waffles	140	28	3	3
Special K	2 waffles	120	26	1	3
SpongeBob SquarePants	2 waffles	190	28	1	5
strawberry	2 waffles	200	30	2	4
(Krusteaz) mix..prepared..					
Belgian/ 7" round	1 waffle	440	56	2	11
(Nature's Path)					
natural					
buckwheat wild berry	2 waffles	230	44	1	6
8-grain	2 waffles	240	35	3	6
flax plus	2 waffles	240	34	4	5

Food and Description	Amount	Total Calories	Total Carbs	Fiber	Sugars
hemp plus	2 waffles	240	35	3	6
mesa sunrise	2 waffles	240	40	1	4
soy plus	2 waffles	230	35	2	6
organic					
Envirokidz Gorilla..banana	2 waffles	220	35	2	5
Envirokidz Koala Choco	2 waffles	240	38	2	4
Optimum Power	2 waffles	190	33	4	3
(Pillsbury)					
apple cinnamon	2 waffles	210	34	<1	7
blueberry	2 waffles	220	34	<1	7
buttermilk	2 waffles	190	30	<1	4
home-style	2 waffles	190	30	<1	4
home-style..rounds	2 waffles	170	27	<1	3
(Thomas') fresh					
blueberry	2 waffles	230	34	1	15
buttermilk	2 waffles	220	32	1	12
carb counting..home-style	1 waffle	110	17	6	2
home-style	1 waffle	110	16	1	5
(Van's) frozen..eggless..dairy-free					
Belgian					
blueberry	2 waffles	184	33	2	4
original	2 waffles	172	30	6	4
7-grain	2 waffles	180	42	7	5
Carb Manager..all styles	2 waffles	200	21	6	0
gourmet					
97% fat-free	2 waffles	180	30	5	4
blueberry	2 waffles	157	24	2	4
buckwheat	2 waffles	260	34	6	5
flax	2 waffles	230	37	4	6
multigrain	2 waffles	190	30	5	4
original	2 waffles	145	24	2	3.5
mini..2 sets of 4 = serving size					
blueberry	1 serving	119	21	2	4
chocolate chip	1 serving	119	18	2	5
home-style	1 serving	107	18	2	4
wheat-free	1 serving	160	30	<1	1
organic					
blueberry	2 waffles	202	33	6	6
original	2 waffles	190	30	6	4
soy..flax	2 waffles	190	28	6	4
wheat-free					
apple cinnamon	2 waffles	220	30	5	5
blueberry	2 waffles	232	35	5	7
flax	2 waffles	230	42	5	3
mini..2 sets of	4 waffles	160	30	1	<1
original	2 waffles	220	32	5	5
WAFFLE SYRUP (*See* MAPLE SYRUP; PANCAKE & WAFFLE SYRUP)					
WAKAME (*See* SEAWEED)					
WALNUT					
(Alma) chopped	½ cup	90	4	<1	<1

Food and Description	Amount	Total Calories	Total Carbs	Fiber	Sugars
(Arroyo Seco) gourmet-quality..all sizes	1 oz	190	4	1	1
(Azar) English..pieces	1 oz	190	4	1	1
(Best Yet) shelled..all sizes	1 oz	190	5	1	1
(Diamond) English					
pieces	¼ cup	190	15	2	0
shelled	¼ cup	190	15	2	0
(Fisher Chef's Naturals)					
chopped	1 oz	200	3	3	0
ground..fine	1 oz	200	3	3	0
halves & pieces	1 oz	200	3	3	0
in the shell..shelled	1 oz	200	3	3	0
(Hammons) black..recipe-ready	1 oz	190	4	2	<1
(Planters)					
black	2 oz	340	8	3	2
English or Persian..all sizes	1.17 oz	210	6	2	1
WATER (*See also* COCKTAIL MIXER; SOFT DRINK)					
BOTTLED					
(Arrowhead) all styles	1 liter	0	0	0	0
(Canada Dry)					
seltzer/sparkling water..all flavors	8 fl oz	0	0	0	0
(Cascadia) sparkling water w/juice					
all flavors	6 fl oz	2	0	0	0
(Coor's) Rocky Mountain sparkling					
water..all flavors	8 fl oz	0	0	0	0
(Evian) spring water	8 fl oz	0	0	0	0
(Perrier) mineral water with-a-twist	12 fl oz	0	0	0	0
(Propel) fitness water..all flavors	8 fl oz	10	3	0	2
(Quest) Sparkling water..all flavors	8 fl oz	0	0	0	0
(Schweppes) Seltzer/Sparkling water	8 fl oz	0	0	0	0
(Water Joe) caffeine-enhanced					
natural artesian water	8 fl oz	0	0	0	0
WATER CHESTNUT (*See also* ASIAN FOOD)					
CANNED					
(3 Diamonds) all styles	½ cup	40	6	6	4
(Geisha)					
sliced	4.6 oz	50	12	4	3
whole..peeled	4.6 oz	45	11	3	0
(La Choy) sliced	1.33 oz	10	3	1	0
WATERCRESS..fresh..raw..chopped	½ cup	2	0	0	0
WATERCRESS SOUP (*See* SOUP)					
WATERMELON (*See also* WATERMELON RIND)					
FRESH					
wedges..10" dia	1/16 wedge	152	35	2	na
cubed	1 cup	50	11	1	na
WATERMELON RIND (Reese)	2 cubes	70	17	0	0
WATERMELON SEEDS/KERNELS					
dried kernels	1 oz	158	4	na	0
WAX BEAN					
CANNED					
(Best Yet) cut wax..all styles	½ cup	20	4	2	2

Food and Description	Amount	Total Calories	Total Carbs	Fiber	Sugars
(Blue Boy) cut wax	½ cup	25	4	2	2
(Del Monte) cut golden	½ cup	20	4	2	1
(S&W)					
premium golden—cut	½ cup	20	4	1	2
young & tender w/green beans	½ cup	20	3	2	2
WAX GOURD..fresh					
boiled	1 cup	23	5	2	0
raw	1 cup	17	4	4	0
WELSH RAREBIT (See FROZEN ENTRÉE/DINNER; SAUCE)					
WHEAT (See also BULGUR; CEREAL; FLOUR; WHEAT GERM)					
(Arrowhead Mills) whole grain					
hard red	2 oz	190	41	8	0
soft red	2 oz	190	41	8	0
(Grain Gourmet) cracked-wheat mix					
Side Dish Solutions..dry mix only	⅒ box	150	32	6	0
(Hodgson Mill) vital wheat gluten					
w/vitamin C	4 tsp	40	3	1	0
(White Wave) seitan					
traditional	3 oz	140	3	1	0
vegetarian stir-fry strips	3 oz	100	2	0	0
WHEAT GERM (See also CEREAL)					
(Arrowhead Mills) raw	2 oz	210	26	7	0
(Hodgson Mill) untoasted	2 Tbs	55	7	4	0
(Kretschmer)					
honey crunch	1⅔ Tbs	50	8	1	na
plain	2 Tbs	50	6	2	0
(Mother's) toasted	2 Tbs	50	6	2	0
WHELK (See SNAIL)					
WHEY					
dried					
acid	1 cup	193	42	0	0
sweet	1 cup	512	108	0	0
fluid					
acid	1 cup	60	13	0	0
sweet	1 cup	65	13	0	0
WHIPPED TOPPING (See also CREAM)					
(NOTE: Unless specified otherwise, 1 serving of mix = the amount in 2 Tbs prepared.)					
(Cool Whip)					
extra-creamy	2 Tbs	25	2	0	2
free	2 Tbs	15	3	0	1
light	2 Tbs	20	2	0	1
original	2 Tbs	25	2	0	1
(Dream Whip) dry mix only	2 Tbs	20	2	0	2
(Haggen)					
light whipped cream..aerosol	1 Tbs	20	1	0	1
whipping cream					
grade A	1 Tbs	45	1	0	1
heavy	1 Tbs	55	0	0	0
(Hood)					
whipped cream					

Food and Description	Amount	Total Calories	Total Carbs	Fiber	Sugars
aerosol..instant					
light	2 Tbs	15	1	0	<1
regular	2 Tbs	20	<1	0	<1
whipping cream	1 Tbs	45	<1	0	1
(Keller's) real whipped..aerosol..light..					
sweetened..ultra-pasteurized	2 Tbs	20	1	0	1
(Kraft)					
free..fat-free	2 Tbs	15	2	0	2
light cream..whipped	2 Tbs	10	<1	0	<1
(Reddi-wip)					
chocolate	2 Tbs	20	2	0	<1
deluxe extra-creamy	2 Tbs	15	<1	0	<1
fat-free	2 Tbs	5	1	0	<1
original	2 Tbs	15	<1	0	<1
real whipped					
heavy cream	2 Tbs	30	<1	0	0
light cream	2 Tbs	20	<1	0	<1
(Rich's)					
nondairy					
aerosol	2 Tbs	25	1	0	0
bowl	2 Tbs	25	1	0	0
Richwhip					
liquid	2 Tbs	25	1	0	0
whipped	2 Tbs	25	1	0	0
WHISKEY (*See* LIQUOR, DISTILLED)					
WHITE BEAN					
CANNED					
(Goya) Spanish-style	7.5 oz	130	30	12	<1
(S&W) lightly seasoned..low-fat	½ cup	80	19	6	1
(Trappey's)..white lima beans					
flavored w/slab bacon	½ cup	130	21	6	2
DRIED					
(Best Yet) small white	1.33 oz	70	22	14	1
WHITE SAUCE (*See* SAUCE)					
WHITEFISH..mixed species (*See also* GEFILTE FISH)					
FRESH					
cooked—dry heat	3 oz	145	0	0	0
JARRED					
(Mother's) 12-oz jar					
jellied	1 ball	45	3	0	0
regular..in liquid	1 ball	55	5	0	0
SMOKED	3 oz	95	0	0	0
(Ducktrap River)	2 oz	70	0	0	0
	4 oz	122	0	0	0
WHITEFISH & PIKE					
JARRED					
(Mother's)					
jellied in broth					
24-oz jar	1 ball	60	4	0	0
Old World	1 ball	60	5	0	0

Food and Description	Amount	Total Calories	Total Carbs	Fiber	Sugars
regular..in liquid	1 ball	70	7	0	0
(Rokeach) jellied in broth	1 ball	45	3	0	0
WHITING (*See also* SEAFOOD ENTRÉE/DINNER)					
cooked—dry heat	3 oz	100	0	0	0
WIENER (*See* FRANKFURTER; FRANKFURTER, VEGETARIAN; SAUSAGE; VEGETARIAN FOODS)					
WILD CELERY (*See* CELERIAC)					
WINE (NOTE: For the calories in a 4-oz glass of wine, simply multiply calorie figures by 4.)					
(Carlo Rossi)					
blush	1 fl oz	21	1	0	0
burgundy	1 fl oz	22	<1	0	0
chablis	1 fl oz	21	<1	0	0
paisano	1 fl oz	23	<1	0	0
red sangria	1 fl oz	24	2	0	<1
Rhine	1 fl oz	21	1	0	0
vin rosé	1 fl oz	21	1	0	0
white grenache	1 fl oz	20	1	0	<1
white zinfandel..new vintage	1 fl oz	18	<1	0	<1
(Four Monks) cooking sherry	1 fl oz	40	2	0	1
(Gallo)					
Ernest & Julio Gallo Vineyards label					
burgundy	1 fl oz	22	<1	0	<1
cabernet sauvignon	1 fl oz	23	1	0	<1
café zinfandel	1 fl oz	21	2	0	1.5
chardonnay	1 fl oz	24	1	0	1
hearty burgundy	1 fl oz	24	2	0	1
Malvasia chardonnay	1 fl oz	24	1	0	<1
merlot	1 fl oz	24	1	0	<1
pink chablis	1 fl oz	20	1	0	<1
red rose	1 fl oz	23	1	0	0
sauvignon blanc	1 fl oz	22	<1	0	<1
shiraz	1 fl oz	23	1	0	<1
white zinfandel	1 fl oz	20	1.6	0	3.5
Gallo of Sonoma					
cabernet sauvignon	1 fl oz	24	1	0	0
chardonnay	1 fl oz	25	<1	0	<1
merlot	1 fl oz	25	<1	0	0
pinot noir/Russian River Valley	1 fl oz	25	1	0	0
sangiovese/Alexander Valley	1 fl oz	25	1	0	0
zinfandel	1 fl oz	25	1	0	<1
(Holland House) cooking wine					
Marsala	1 fl oz	45	4	0	4
red	1 fl oz	20	0	0	0
sherry	1 fl oz	45	2	0	2
vermouth	1 fl oz	35	2	0	2
white	1 fl oz	20	0	0	0
white w/lemon flavor	1 fl oz	20	0	0	0
(Regina) cooking wine					
burgundy	2 Tbs	20	3	0	0

Food and Description	Amount	Total Calories	Total Carbs	Fiber	Sugars
sauterne..white	2 Tbs	20	3	0	0
sherry	2 Tbs	35	5	0	0
WINE COOLER					
(Bartles & Jaymes)					
malt-based					
blackberry	12 fl oz	228	39	0	36
black cherry	12 fl oz	200	32	0	29
classic original	12 fl oz	190	29	0	25
exotic berry	12 fl oz	210	33	0	31
fuzzy navel	12 fl oz	230	39	0	38
hard lemonade	12 fl oz	230	39	0	36
juicy peach	12 fl oz	210	33	0	31
kiwi strawberry	12 fl oz	214	39	0	32
margarita	12 fl oz	260	46	0	42
pina colada	12 fl oz	270	48	0	45
raspberry daiquiri	12 fl oz	216	36	0	33
raspberry hard lemonade	12 fl oz	226	39	0	36
strawberry cosmopolitan	12 fl oz	219	37	0	34
strawberry daiquiri	12 fl oz	220	36	0	34
tropical burst	12 fl oz	230	37	0	35
wine-based coolers					
blackberry	12 fl oz	240	40	0	36
classic original	12 fl oz	200	29	0	26
exotic berry	12 fl oz	220	34	0	30
fuzzy navel	12 fl oz	250	43	0	38
hard lemonade	12 fl oz	240	38	0	34
kiwi strawberry	12 fl oz	230	37	0	32
raspberry hard lemonade	12 fl oz	230	37	0	33
strawberry daiquiri	12 fl oz	230	38	0	33
tropical burst	12 fl oz	240	39	0	35
WINGED BEAN					
mature seeds..cooked	½ cup	126	23	9	0
mature seeds..raw	½ cup	375	38	na	0
WOLFFISH					
Atlantic..fresh..cooked—dry heat	3 oz	105	0	0	0
WON TON (See ASIAN FOOD)					
WON TON SOUP (See SOUP)					
WON TON WRAPPER (See ASIAN FOOD)					
WORCESTERSHIRE SAUCE (See SAUCE)					

Y

Food and Description	Amount	Total Calories	Total Carbs	Fiber	Sugars
YAM (*See also* SWEET POTATO)					
CANNED					
(Bruce's) cut					
in syrup	⅔ cup	150	36	3	23
in heavy syrup	⅔ cup	190	45	3	21
(McCain) roasters..oven-roasted	½ cup	120	20	3	8
(Princella) candied..in light syrup	⅔ cup	160	40	3	20
(Royal Prince)					
candied	½ cup	210	50	2	35
in heavy syrup	6.3 oz	200	49	4	17
orange pineapple	½ cup	210	50	3	36
(Trappey's)					
golden sweet..whole..in heavy syrup	6.3 oz	200	49	4	16
sugary sam					
cut golden in syrup	⅔ cup	160	39	3	20
mashed	⅔ cup	120	28	3	15
FRESH					
baked in skin	1 large	185	44	5	na
boiled-mashed w/o skin	½ cup	175	40	3	na
Hawaiian Mountain					
cooked..cubed	½ cup	59	15	na	<1
raw..pieces..cubes	½ cup	70	16	4	na
YAM BEAN-TUBER (*See* JICAMA)					
YARDLONG BEAN					
FRESH					
boiled..drained..sliced	½ cup	25	5	na	0
raw..sliced	½ cup	22	4	na	0
mature seeds					
boiled	½ cup	100	18	3	0
raw	½ cup	290	50	9	0
YEAST					
baker's					
(Fleischmann's)					
active dry & rapid rise..pocket					
or jar	¼ oz	20	3	0	0
fresh active	⅓ pkt	0	0	0	0
household	0.5 oz	15	2	0	0
(Red Star)					
active dry	¼ oz	15	2	0	0
flakes	3 Tbs	45	5	4	1

Food and Description	Amount	Total Calories	Total Carbs	Fiber	Sugars
brewer's..tormula	1 oz	80	10	<1	0
YELLOWTAIL					
mixed species..fresh..cooked—dry heat	3 oz	160	0	0	0
YOGURT, DAIRY					
(Altadena)					
fat-free					
black cherry	1 cup	190	38	0	34
lemon	1 cup	190	38	0	36
peach	1 cup	190	38	0	35
raspberry	1 cup	190	38	0	33
strawberry	1 cup	180	36	0	32
vanilla	1 cup	180	30	0	3
wild berries	1 cup	180	37	0	32
low-fat					
black cherry	1 cup	220	41	0	36
peach	1 cup	220	41	0	36
raspberry	1 cup	220	40	0	34
strawberry	1 cup	210	39	0	34
strawberry banana	1 cup	210	39	0	35
(Blue Bunny)					
Carb Freedom..all Flavors	6 oz	90	5	0	5
Disney					
Swirl 'n' Magic..all flavors	1 cup	80	12	0	9
Yo-pals..all flavors	1 cup	120	19	0	18
Lite 85					
bananas Foster	6 oz	80	14	0	9
black cherry	6 oz	80	14	0	9
black forest	6 oz	80	14	0	9
blackberry crème	6 oz	80	13	0	9
coconut cream pie	6 oz	80	13	0	8
lemon chiffon	6 oz	80	14	0	8
peach	6 oz	80	14	0	9
piña colada	6 oz	80	13	0	8
raspberry	6 oz	80	13	0	8
strawberry	6 oz	80	13	0	8
strawberry banana	6 oz	80	14	0	9
vanilla cream	6 oz	80	13	0	8
vanilla pear	6 oz	80	13	0	8
(Breyers)					
Creme Savers..low-fat					
4-oz cups..all flavors	4 oz	120	22	0	18
8-oz cups					
blueberries & cream or					
peaches & cream	8 oz	240	45	0	35
other flavors..all	8 oz	240	45	0	36
Fruit on the Bottom					
low-fat					
black cherry	8 oz	240	46	0	44
blueberry	8 oz	230	44	0	42
peach	8 oz	230	45	0	43

Food and Description	Amount	Total Calories	Total Carbs	Fiber	Sugars
raspberry	8 oz	240	46	0	44
strawberry	8 oz	240	46	0	44
light					
Nonfat					
4-oz cups..all flavors	4 oz	60	11	0	8
8-oz cups					
apple cinnamon	8 oz	120	22	0	17
black cherry jubilee	8 oz	120	21	0	16
blueberries 'n' cream	8 oz	120	21	0	15
raspberries 'n' cream	8 oz	120	22	0	15
strawberry cheesecake	8 oz	120	22	0	16
Smooth & Creamy					
4-oz cups					
black cherry parfait	4 oz	110	23	0	18
raspberries 'n' cream	4 oz	120	24	0	19
8-oz cups					
apple cobbler	8 oz	230	46	0	37
black cherry parfait	8 oz	230	46	0	36
raspberries 'n' cream	8 oz	240	48	0	37
strawberry cheesecake	8 oz	230	47	0	37
(Colombo)					
classic..low-fat..99% fat-free					
banana strawberry	8 oz	230	47	0	42
black cherry parfait	8 oz	220	47	0	42
vanilla	8 oz	180	32	0	26
all other flavors	8 oz	220	42	0	35
fat-free..all flavors	8 oz	120	21	0	15
light					
blended..6-count multipack..					
all flavors	4 oz	110	22	0	19
low-fat..32-oz container					
French vanilla	1 cup	180	32	0	26
plain	1 cup	130	16	0	20
strawberry	1 cup	190	31	0	27
(Dannon)					
Carb Control..Light 'n' Fit					
peaches 'n' cream	4 oz	160	3	0	3
raspberries 'n' cream	4 oz	160	3	0	3
strawberries 'n' cream	4 oz	160	3	0	3
vanilla cream	4 oz	60	3	0	2
Danimals..super creamy..all					
flavors	4 oz	130	20	0	18
Fruit Blends..4-oz mini packs..					
all flavors	4 oz	110	21	0	19
Fruit Blends..6-oz cups					
blueberry	6 oz	170	34	0	31
peach	6 oz	170	34	0	31
strawberry	6 oz	170	32	0	29
Fruit on the Bottom..low-fat					
apple cinnamon	6 oz	160	31	<1	26

Food and Description	Amount	Total Calories	Total Carbs	Fiber	Sugars
blueberry	6 oz	150	29	0	26
boysenberry	6 oz	150	28	0	26
cherry	6 oz	150	29	<1	27
mixed berry	6 oz	150	29	0	27
peach	6 oz	160	30	0	28
raspberry	6 oz	150	29	0	27
strawberry	6 oz	160	30	0	28
La Creme					
banana	4 oz	150	21	0	19
other flavors...all	4 oz	140	20	0	18
La Creme Mousse..all flavors	2.6 oz	120	15	0	14
Light 'n' Fit					
creamy..all flavors	6 oz	100	16	0	10
multipack..all flavors	4 oz	60	11	0	6
natural flavors..low-fat					
coffee	6 oz	150	26	0	25
lemon	6 oz	150	26	0	25
vanilla	6 oz	150	39	0	38
nonfat yogurt					
blackberry pie	6 oz	90	16	0	12
lemon chiffon	6 oz	90	16	0	12
orange mango	6 oz	90	16	0	11
strawberry kiwi	6 oz	90	17	0	12
white chocolate raspberry	6 oz	90	16	0	12
(Go-Gurt) all flavors	1 tube	80	13	0	11
(Horizon) organic					
baby yogurt..all flavors	½ cup	120	18	0	17
blended..low fat..all flavors	6 oz cups	160	30	1	28
fat-free..all flavors	6 oz cups	130	26	<1	25
fat-free..32-oz carton					
plain or vanilla	1 cup	170	33	0	32
tubes..low-fat..all flavors	1 tube	70	12	0	11
(Kemp's)					
classic..low-fat..all flavors	6 oz	160	30	0	28
fat-free..all flavors	6 oz	90	15	0	12
JR'S..4-oz cups..all flavors	1 cup	130	24	0	23
100 calorie..all flavors	5 oz	100	22	0	18
(La Yogurt)					
blended..low-fat..light..6-oz cups					
banana cream	6 oz	90	15	0	11
blueberry	6 oz	90	16	0	13
cherry cheesecake	6 oz	160	32	0	28
cherry vanilla	6 oz	170	33	0	29
cinnamon bun	6 oz	160	31	0	26
piña colada	6 oz	150	30	0	26
strawberry	6 oz	90	15	0	12
strawberry banana	6 oz	90	16	0	12
strawberry fruit cup	6 oz	150	30	0	26
vanilla	6 oz	90	15	0	11

Food and Description	Amount	Total Calories	Total Carbs	Fiber	Sugars
blended..low-fat..8-oz cups					
blueberries 'n' cream	8 oz	200	39	0	36
peaches 'n' cream	8 oz	200	39	0	37
raspberries 'n' cream	8 oz	190	39	0	36
strawberries 'n' cream	8 oz	200	38	0	36
vanilla 'n' cream	8 oz	200	39	0	37
Sabor Latino..blended					
guava	6 oz	170	34	0	33
mango	6 oz	170	33	0	33
papaya	6 oz	170	33	0	32
pear	6 oz	170	333	0	25
(Mountain High)					
classic..low-fat..all flavors	6 oz	140	29	0	21
European Delight..all flavors	4 oz	110	20	0	17
fat-free					
plain	6 oz	110	19	0	15
raspberry	6 oz	110	29	0	28
strawberry garden	6 oz	110	29	0	28
low-fat					
plain	1 cup	150	22	0	15
vanilla	1 cup	200	34	0	33
Naturally Nutritious..all flavors	4 oz	100	18	2	16
original					
plain	1 cup	190	18	0	15
vanilla	1 cup	240	36	0	27
(Nancy's) organic cultured soy					
blackberry	6 oz	140	24	4	13
blueberry	6 oz	140	24	3	13
kiwi lime	6 oz	160	31	4	21
mango	6 oz	170	33	3	23
plain	6 oz	150	25	2	15
raspberry	6 oz	140	24	4	13
(Stonyfield Farm) organic					
99% fat-free					
caramel	6 oz	130	38	2	35
Just Peachy	6 oz	130	25	2	23
Luscious Lemon	6 oz	140	25	3	23
maple vanilla	6 oz	130	23	2	20
mocha latte	6 oz	140	25	2	23
plain	6 oz	90	13	2	11
all natural..fat-free					
apricot mango	6 oz	130	26	2	23
Berry Bash	6 oz	130	25	2	23
blackberry	6 oz	140	29	2	26
Chocolate Underground	6 oz	180	39	2	36
key lime	6 oz	140	29	2	26
Lotsa Lemon	6 oz	140	28	2	25
strawberry cheesecake	6 oz	140	29	2	26
fat-free..32-oz cups					

Food and Description	Amount	Total Calories	Total Carbs	Fiber	Sugars
French vanilla	1 cup	180	36	3	33
plain	1 cup	110	18	3	15
strawberry	1 cup	180	36	3	32
Moo-La-La					
double chocolate	4 oz	150	25	2	22
lemon chiffon	4 oz	140	22	2	19
strawberry cheesecake	4 oz	140	20	2	17
white chocolate raspberry	4 oz	140	20	2	17
O'Soy..6-pack..6-oz cups					
blueberry	6 oz	170	33	4	27
lemon	6 oz	170	33	4	28
peach	6 oz	170	32	4	27
raspberry	6 oz	170	32	4	27
strawberry	6 oz	170	32	4	27
vanilla	6 oz	150	26	4	21
whole milk..6-oz cups					
French vanilla	6 oz	170	27	3	24
strawberries & cream	6 oz	170	24	2	22
vanilla truffle	6 oz	220	41	3	37
(Trix) all flavors	4 oz	120	23	0	19
(White Wave) cultured soy					
apricot mango	6 oz	160	30	1	20
banana strawberry	6 oz	160	29	1	18
black cherry	6 oz	150	29	1	20
blueberry	6 oz	160	29	1	21
key lime	6 oz	160	30	1	21
lemon	6 oz	160	31	1	22
peach	6 oz	160	32	1	25
raspberry	6 oz	160	30	1	22
vanilla	6 oz	120	23	1	16
(Yoplait)					
custard-style..all flavors	6 oz	190	32	0	28
light..fat-free					
apple turnover	6 oz	100	19	0	14
apricot mango	6 oz	100	19	0	14
banana cream pie	6 oz	100	19	0	14
blackberry	6 oz	100	19	0	14
Boston cream pie	6 oz	110	20	0	15
lemon cream pie	6 oz	100	20	0	15
orange cream	6 oz	100	19	0	14
raspberry peach melba	6 oz	100	19	0	14
strawberry orange sunrise	6 oz	100	19	0	14
white chocolate strawberry	6 oz	100	19	0	14
original..99% fat-free*					
(*except for coconut cream pie)					
banana cream	6 oz	170	33	0	27
blackberry harvest	6 oz	170	33	0	27
boysenberry	6 oz	170	33	0	27
coconut cream pie	6 oz	190	34	0	27

Food and Description	Amount	Total Calories	Total Carbs	Fiber	Sugars
harvest peach	6 oz	170	33	0	27
lemon	6 oz	180	36	0	31
Mandarin orange	6 oz	170	33	0	27
orange cream	6 oz	170	33	0	27
piña colada	6 oz	170	33	0	26
red raspberry	6 oz	170	33	0	27
strawberry cheesecake	6 oz	170	33	0	27
strawberry mango	6 oz	170	33	0	27
tropical peach	6 oz	170	33	0	27
white chocolate raspberry	6 oz	170	33	0	27
Ultra..Low-carb..all flavors	6 oz	90	8	0	5
Whips..all flavors	4 oz	140	25	0	21
Yumsters..all flavors	4 oz	120	21	0	18
YOGURT, FROZEN					
(Baskin-Robbins)					
low-fat					
Maui Brownie Madness	½ cup	210	39	1	34
Perils of Praline	½ cup	190	37	1	34
Raspberry Cheese Louise	½ cup	190	36	1	32
nonfat..soft-serve					
chocolate	½ cup	120	25	1	22
peppermint	½ cup	110	24	0	23
red raspberry	½ cup	110	25	0	24
vanilla	½ cup	110	23	0	22
nonfat..soft-serve..no sugar added					
Truly Free					
butter pecan	½ cup	90	17	1	6
café mocha	½ cup	90	18	1	74
chocolate	½ cup	80	14	0	6
strawberry patch	½ cup	90	17	1	6
vanilla	½ cup	90	17	1	6
(Ben & Jerry's)					
Cherry Garcia	½ cup	170	32	0	27
Chocolate Fudge Brownie	½ cup	190	36	1	31
Half Baked	½ cup	210	39	<1	29
Phish Food	½ cup	230	42	1	30
(Blue Bunny)					
Brownie Fudge Fantasy	½ cup	110	24	0	16
cookies 'n' cream	½ cup	100	21	0	16
homemade chocolate	½ cup	100	19	0	16
homemade vanilla	½ cup	100	19	0	17
strawberry cheesecake	½ cup	100	21	0	18
(Breyers)					
All Natural					
chocolate	½ cup	130	23	1	18
vanilla					
natural	½ cup	120	22	0	17
no sugar added	½ cup	150	17	0	17
vanilla, chocolate & strawberry	½ cup	120	22	0	17

Food and Description	Amount	Total Calories	Total Carbs	Fiber	Sugars
Carb Smart					
chocolate	½ cup	90	15	5	4
vanilla	½ cup	90	14	4	4
(Dreyer's)					
fat-free					
black cherry vanilla swirl	½ cup	90	20	0	14
caramel praline crunch	½ cup	100	23	0	17
vanilla	½ cup	90	19	0	13
vanilla chocolate swirl	½ cup	90	19	0	13
regular					
cookies 'n' cream	½ cup	120	19	0	14
Heath Toffee Crunch	½ cup	120	18	0	15
raspberry vanilla	½ cup	100	17	0	13
(Edy's)					
fat-free					
black cherry vanilla swirl	½ cup	90	20	0	14
caramel praline crunch	½ cup	100	23	0	17
vanilla	½ cup	90	19	0	13
vanilla chocolate swirl	½ cup	90	19	0	13
regular					
cookies 'n' cream	½ cup	120	19	0	14
Heath Toffee Crunch	½ cup	120	18	0	15
raspberry vanilla	½ cup	100	17	0	13
(Häagen-Dazs) pints					
chocolate fudge brownie	½ cup	290	28	1	24
coffee	½ cup	200	31	0	20
dulce de leche	½ cup	190	35	0	25
strawberry	½ cup	140	31	0	20
vanilla	½ cup	200	31	0	21
vanilla raspberry swirl	½ cup	170	31	1	24
(Hood)					
nonfat					
caramel & brownie sundae	½ cup	120	28	0	26
double raspberry	½ cup	110	27	0	25
mocha fudge	½ cup	110	27	0	25
old-fashioned vanilla	½ cup	110	24	0	23
strawberry	½ cup	100	23	0	22
regular..low-fat					
chocolate almond praline	½ cup	140	24	0	23
classic trio	½ cup	120	22	0	21
coffee toffee chunk sundae	½ cup	150	27	0	26
cookies & cream	½ cup	140	26	0	22
vanilla Swiss almond sundae	½ cup	150	25	0	24
(Kemp's)					
fat-free					
caramel praline crunch	½ cup	110	25	0	20
chocolate	½ cup	90	19	0	15
cookies 'n' cream	½ cup	110	23	0	14
peach	½ cup	90	19	0	14

Food and Description	Amount	Total Calories	Total Carbs	Fiber	Sugars
strawberry	½ cup	80	16	0	13
vanilla	½ cup	90	18	0	14
fat-free..no sugar added					
strawberry	½ cup	70	17	0	5
vanilla	½ cup	70	18	0	5
low-fat					
caramel brownie	½ cup	140	25	0	18
chocolate almond	½ cup	140	20	1	16
chocolate chip	½ cup	140	23	0	18
Moose Lake fudge	½ cup	170	24	0	19
peach	½ cup	110	20	0	16
raspberry	½ cup	110	21	0	16
strawberry	½ cup	110	20	0	16
(Schwan's) premium low-fat					
black cherry	½ cup	120	23	0	16
chocolate	½ cup	120	20	0	13
chocolate fudge brownie	½ cup	130	24	0	16
orange pineapple	½ cup	110	22	0	14
(Stonyfield Farm) organic					
chocolate mint chip	½ cup	130	22	<1	20
crème caramel	½ cup	120	23	0	23
decaf coffee	½ cup	90	19	0	18
mocha almond fudge	½ cup	130	23	1	21
raspberry	½ cup	100	21	0	19
vanilla fudge swirl	½ cup	110	23	0	21
(TCBY) soft-serve yogurt & fruit sorbet					
96% fat-free	½ cup	140	23	0	20
nonfat	½ cup	110	23	0	20
no sugar added	½ cup	90	20	0	7
w/nondairy sorbet	½ cup	100	24	0	19
YOGURT DRINK					
(Breyer's) Creme Savers..smoothies					
all flavors	10 fl oz	190	32	0	29
(Dannon)					
Actimel..cultured dairy drink					
orange	3.3 fl oz	100	18	0	17
original	3.3 fl oz	90	16	0	15
vanilla	3.3 fl oz	100	18	0	17
DanActive..cultured dairy drink					
orange	3.3 fl oz	100	18	0	17
original	3.3 fl oz	90	16	0	15
strawberry	3.3 fl oz	100	18	0	17
vanilla	3.3 fl oz	100	18	0	17
Danimals drinkable					
fruit punch	3.1 fl oz	90	16	0	16
Rockin' Raspberry	3.1 fl oz	90	16	0	15
Strawberry Explosion	3.1 fl oz	90	16	0	15
strawberry kiwi	3.1 fl oz	90	16	0	13
Swingin' Banana	3.1 fl oz	90	16	0	13

Food and Description	Amount	Total Calories	Total Carbs	Fiber	Sugars
Danimals XL drinkable..all flavors	5.75 oz	170	29	0	28
Frusion smoothies..blends					
banana berry	10 fl oz	270	52	0	49
cherry berry	10 fl oz	280	53	<1	51
peach passion fruit	10 fl oz	270	51	0	49
strawberry kiwi	10 fl oz	270	52	0	50
tropical fruit	10 fl oz	270	52	0	50
(Stonyfield Farm) organic					
peach	1 bottle	250	49	4	44
raspberry	1 bottle	240	45	4	41
strawberry	1 bottle	250	46	4	41
tropical banana	1 bottle	250	46	4	41
vanilla	1 bottle	250	46	4	41
wild berry	1 bottle	250	46	4	41
(TCBY) Fruithead Smoothies					
20-oz w/yogurt					
A Lotta Colada	1 smoothie	550	99	3	94
Berry Slim	1 smoothie	410	95	2	91
Healthy Balance	1 smoothie	410	95	2	91
Holy-Cal	1 smoothie	470	114	3	107
Peachy Lean	1 smoothie	470	116	<1	113
Raspberry DeLITE	1 smoothie	360	85	4	81
Raspberry Revitalizer	1 smoothie	370	84	3	77
Tropical Replenisher	1 smoothie	370	87	1	85
Workout Whey	1 smoothie	460	112	1	108
32-oz w/yogurt					
A Lotta Colada	1 smoothie	710	142	4	130
Berry Slim	1 smoothie	600	143	4	135
Healthy Balance	1 smoothie	590	138	4	131
Holy-Cal	1 smoothie	610	149	4	139
Peachy Lean	1 smoothie	620	151	1	147
Raspberry DeLITE	1 smoothie	510	116	7	112
Raspberry Revitalizer	1 smoothie	530	124	4	113
Tropical Replenisher	1 smoothie	520	121	2	115
Workout Whey	1 smoothie	600	145	2	139
(Tropicana) smoothies					
cherry vanilla	11 fl oz	250	59	5	46
peach	11 fl oz	250	59	5	46
piña colada	11 fl oz	250	50	5	46
raspberry chocolate dip	11 fl oz	250	59	5	46
strawberry	11 fl oz	250	59	5	46
tropical orange	11 fl oz	250	59	5	36
(Yami)					
low-fat..strawberry	8 oz	240	44	0	42
Yami-Free					
blueberry	8 oz	100	17	0	14
strawberry	8 oz	100	16	0	13
strawberry banana	8 oz	100	17	0	14
(Yoplait) Nouriche smoothies					
low-fat..all flavors	11 fl oz	170	33	6	18
regular..all flavors	11 fl oz	290	60	6	46

Z

Food and Description	Amount	Total Calories	Total Carbs	Fiber	Sugars

ZUCCHINI (*See* SQUASH)

ZWIEBACK (*See* COOKIE)

FAST FOOD

Food and Description	Amount	Total Calories	Total Carbs	Fiber	Sugars
A&W					
■ **BEVERAGES**					
shakes					
chocolate	1 shake	700	92	0	61
strawberry	1 shake	670	90	0	52
vanilla	1 shake	720	100	2	6
■ **BURGERS & HOT DOGS**					
burgers					
deluxe					
¼ lb					
bacon cheeseburger	1 burger	600	44	4	9
cheeseburger	1 burger	500	43	4	8
hamburger	1 burger	500	40	4	8
bacon double cheeseburger	1 burger	830	49	4	9
double cheeseburger	1 burger	750	48	4	9
jr.					
cheeseburger	1 burger	470	41	3	8
hamburger	1 burger	430	38	3	8
hot dogs					
cheese	1 hot dog	500	25	1	4
Coney..chili	1 hot dog	310	24	2	5
Coney..chili..cheese	1 hot dog	350	27	2	5
plain	1 hot dog	280	22	7	4
■ **CHICKEN**					
sandwiches					
crispy	1 sdw	580	57	5	5
grilled	1 sdw	430	37	4	10
strips & fries	3 strips	500	32	2	2
■ **SIDE ORDERS**					
fries					
cheese	1 order	350	47	4	0
chili	1 order	370	49	5	2
chili cheese	1 order	400	51	5	2
regular					
kid's..small	1 order	310	45	4	0
large	1 order	430	61	6	1
onion rings	1 order	350	45	2	3
■ **SWEETS & TREATS**					
ice cream					
cones..chocolate	1 cone	250	41	1	27

Food and Description	Amount	Total Calories	Total Carbs	Fiber	Sugars
Float..A&W Root Beer	1 float	300	63	0	59
Freeze..A&W Root Beer	1 freeze	480	89	0	42
Polar Swirls					
M&M Polar	1 swirl	720	107	1	92
Oreo Polar	1 swirl	720	107	2	77
Reese's Polar	1 swirl	750	97	2	84
sundaes					
chocolate	1 sundae	320	53	0	15
hot caramel	1 sundae	340	57	0	13
hot fudge	1 sundae	350	54	1	15
strawberry	1 sundae	300	47	0	12
vanilla	1 sundae	310	52	0	18
ARBY'S					
■ BEVERAGES					
shakes					
chocolate	large	660	110	<1	106
jamocha	large	650	107	<1	102
strawberry	large	650	107	<1	101
vanilla	large	650	107	0	106
■ BREAKFAST					
biscuit..plain	1 biscuit	230	26	<1	3
add butter	1 Tbs	100	0	0	0
add scrambled eggs	1 serving	80	2	0	1
add Swiss cheese	1 slice	40	0	0	0
biscuit..other					
bacon	1 biscuit	300	27	<1	3
ham	1 biscuit	270	27	<1	4
sausage	1 biscuit	390	26	<1	3
croissant					
bacon 'n' egg	1 croissant	410	31	<1	4
ham 'n' cheese	1 croissant	410	30	<1	5
sausage 'n' egg	1 croissant	510	31	<1	4
sourdough					
bacon, & egg 'n' Swiss	1 sdw	500	33	1	2
egg 'n' cheese	1 sdw	330	31	1	2
ham, egg 'n' Swiss	1 sdw	450	33	1	3
■ CONDIMENTS					
Arby's sauce	1 pkt	15	4	0	1
BBQ sauce	1 oz	40	10	0	9
Bronco Berry sauce	2 oz	120	30	0	28
Buffalo dipping sauce	2 oz	20	3	0	1
honey mustard dipping sauce	1 oz	130	5	0	5
Horsey sauce	1 pkt	60	3	0	1
Tangy Southwest sauce	2 oz	330	5	0	4
■ DESSERT					
gourmet chocolate cookie	1 cookie	200	26	<1	16
turnovers..apple or cherry	1 turnover	250	35	2	15
turnover icing	1 pkt	130	29	0	26
■ SALADS & SALAD DRESSINGS					
salads					

Food and Description	Amount	Total Calories	Total Carbs	Fiber	Sugars
chicken club	530	32	5	4	
Martha's Vineyard	1 salad	250	23	4	23
Santa Fe	1 salad	520	40	5	6
salad dressings					
buttermilk ranch	2.28 oz	330	4	0	2
light	2 oz	100	12	1	4
raspberry vinaigrette	2.28 oz	170	16	0	14
Santa Fe	2.28 oz	300	10	0.5	0
■ SANDWICHES					
chicken					
bacon 'n' Swiss	1 sdw	550	49	2	10
breast fillet	1 sdw	490	46	2	7
Cordon Bleu	1 sdw	570	46	2	34
grilled chicken deluxe	1 sdw	380	40	2	9
hot ham 'n' cheese	1 sdw	300	35	1	7
hot ham 'n' Swiss melt	1 sdw	270	35	1	7
roast chicken club	1 sdw	470	39	2	7
roast beef					
Arby Q in BBQ sauce	1 sdw	360	51	2	20
beef 'n' cheddar	1 sdw	440	44	2	8
Big Montana	1 sdw	590	41	3	6
French dip 'n' Swiss	1 sdw	320	56	3	2
original					
giant	1 sdw	450	41	2	6
junior	1 sdw	320	34	2	5
regular	1 sdw	320	34	2	5
super	1 sdw	440	48	3	11
Philly beef supreme	1 sdw	450	59	3	6
other sandwiches..market fresh					
chicken salad	1 sdw	860	92	6	33
roast beef & Swiss	1 sdw	780	74	6	15
roast ham & Swiss	1 sdw	700	74	5	18
roast turkey	1 sdw	830	75	5	16
roast turkey & Swiss	1 sdw	720	74	5	16
ultimate BLT	1 sdw	780	75	6	18
other sandwiches.. Market Fresh..low carb..wraps					
chicken Caesar	1 wrap	520	46	30	2
roast turkey & bacon	1 wrap	710	48	30	3
Southwest chicken	1 wrap	550	45	30	1
ultimate BLT	1 wrap	650	47	31	4
■ SIDE ORDERS					
baked potato					
broccoli 'n' cheddar	1 potato	460	56	6	4
deluxe	1 potato	570	50	5	23
plain	1 potato	200	46	4	3
chicken fingers					
4-pack	1 order	640	42	0	0
combo w/curly fries	1 order	1,050	89	5	0
snack w/curly fries	1 order	590	53	3	0
curly fries	medium	410	47	5	na
	large	630	73	7	na

Food and Description	Amount	Total Calories	Total Carbs	Fiber	Sugars
home-style fries	medium	380	55	4	1
	large	570	82	6	1
jalapeño bites					
large	10 bites	610	58	4	5
regular	5 bites	310	29	2	3
mozzarella sticks					
large	8 sticks	850	76	4	9
regular	4 sticks	430	38	2	5
onion petals					
large	1 order	830	88	5	18
regular	1 order	330	35	2	7
potato cakes	2 cakes	220	26	2	na
AU BON PAIN					
■ **BAGELS**					
Asiago cheese	1 bagel	380	59	3	5
cinnamon crisp	1 bagel	430	96	3	25
cinnamon raisin	1 bagel	330	71	3	5
Dutch apple w/walnut strudel	1 bagel	470	98	5	28
everything	1 bagel	330	63	3	5
French toast	1 bagel	420	76	3	15
honey 9-grain	1 bagel	360	75	6	5
jalapeño double cheddar	1 bagel	350	56	2	5
plain	1 bagel	300	61	3	5
sesame	1 bagel	340	62	3	5
■ **BREADS, LOAVES & ROLLS**					
apple spice loaf	1 slice	190	29	0	15
artisan..baguette or ficelle	1 slice	150	30	1	0
Asiago flatbread	1 slice	330	63	3	1
braided roll	1 roll	420	63	3	8
bread bowl	1 bowl	640	127	6	3
chocolate cherry bread	1 slice	170	33	2	8
country white loaf	1 slice	110	23	1	0
focaccia	10.3 oz	740	137	7	4
4-grain	1 slice	310	59	2	2
French sandwich roll	1 roll	290	60	3	0
hearth roll	1 roll	240	44	2	1
lahvash	1 roll	240	55	4	0
multigrain loaf	1 slice	130	24	1	0
Parisienne loaf	1 slice	120	25	1	0
petit pain roll	1 roll	200	40	2	0
rosemary garlic breadstick	1 stick	200	33	2	2
3-seed sandwich roll	1 roll	330	63	5	1
tomato herb loaf	1 slice	140	26	2	0
■ **COOKIES**					
chocolate chip	1 cookie	270	39	1	24
chocolate-dipped cranberry almond	1 cookie	320	42	3	33
double chocolate shortbread	1 cookie	340	42	2	24
English toffee	1 cookie	210	28	1	17
macaroon chocolate-dipped shortbread	1 cookie	300	52	1	17
oatmeal raisin	1 cookie	250	41	2	14

Food and Description	Amount	Total Calories	Total Carbs	Fiber	Sugars
shortbread					
plain	1 cookie	340	35	1	11
white chocolate–dipped chocolate	1 cookie	380	46	2	26
■ CROISSANTS					
apple	1 croissant	230	47	2	1
chocolate	1 croissant	380	61	3	26
cinnamon raisin	1 croissant	340	69	3	15
ham & cheese	1 croissant	340	46	2	6
plain	1 croissant	250	44	2	6
raspberry	1 croissant	340	55	2	20
spinach & cheese	1 croissant	250	32	2	5
sweet cheese	1 croissant	350	52	1	17
■ FICELLES					
goat cheese & field greens	1 ficelle	320	40	3	4
grilled salmon salad	1 ficelle	280	40	1	4
grilled tarragon chicken	1 ficelle	330	35	0	1
roasted vegetable	1 ficelle	270	42	2	4
roma tomato & mozzarella	1 ficelle	470	40	0	4
tuna, carrot & dill salad	1 ficelle	320	40	1	4
turkey tenderloin	1 ficelle	310	40	2	4
■ MUFFINS					
apple spice	1 muffin	420	65	33	2
banana walnut	1 muffin	440	60	3	24
blueberry	1 muffin	510	76	5	33
carrot nut	1 muffin	550	71	4	40
chocolate cake..low-fat	1 muffin	320	74	4	48
chocolate chunk	1 muffin	590	83	5	46
corn	1 muffin	440	64	2	30
cranberry walnut	1 muffin	560	69	5	30
pumpkin	1 muffin	580	84	3	41
raisin bran	1 muffin	530	100	12	42
triple berry..low-fat	1 muffin	290	61	2	31
■ PASTRIES					
cinnamon roll	1 roll	390	67	2	20
crème de fleur	1 piece	550	71	1	32
crumb cake					
apple	1 piece	540	62	1	23
butter	1 piece	790	96	2	48
raspberry	1 piece	770	94	2	47
Danish					
cranberry cheese	1 Danish	460	57	2	23
lemon	1 Danish	430	57	1	22
sweet cheese	1 Danish	470	54	1	22
pecan roll	1 roll	750	112	4	48
strudel					
apple	1 piece	410	56	1	19
cherry	1 piece	390	49	1	5
■ SALAD DRESSINGS & SALADS					
salad dressings					
bleu cheese	2.5 oz	370	3	0	2

Food and Description	Amount	Total Calories	Total Carbs	Fiber	Sugars
Caesar	2.5 oz	390	6	0	5
honey mustard..light	2.5 oz	240	26	0	18
Mediterranean	2.5 oz	200	4	0	3
olive oil vinaigrette..light	2.5 oz	150	7	0	5
Parmesan & peppercorn	2.5 oz	400	5	0	4
ranch..light	2.5 oz	200	5	0	3
raspberry vinaigrette..fat-free	2.5 oz	80	19	0	16
salads					
Caesar	1 serving	320	31	4	4
chef	1 serving	260	9	4	4
chicken					
Caesar	1 serving	400	32	4	4
pesto	1 serving	420	14	5	2
Cobb	1 serving	460	26	8	5
garden	1 small	80	12	3	1
gorgonzola & walnut	1 serving	340	20	5	10
Mediterranean chicken	1 serving	230	13	5	2
pear & gorgonzola	1 serving	340	20	5	10
Thai chicken	1 serving	140	14	6	2
tomato mozzarella w/basil pesto	1 serving	280	11	3	7
tuna garden	1 serving	420	25	6	4
turkey medallion Cobb	1 serving	440	27	6	2
■ SANDWICHES & WRAPS					
sandwiches					
baguette					
Dijon albacore tuna	1 sdw	450	56	3	1
grilled chicken club					
w/chili dressing	1 sdw	670	64	4	4
honey Dijon Cordon Bleu	1 sdw	590	71	3	16
roast beef & Swiss	1 sdw	690	57	2	1
Tuscan	1 sdw	710	60	3	2
breakfast					
egg on a bagel..cholesterol & fat free	1 sdw	400	63	3	5
w/bacon	1 sdw	480	63	3	5
w/bacon & cheese	1 sdw	560	63	3	5
w/cheese	1 sdw	480	63	3	5
Fresh sandwiches					
chicken					
Arizona	1 sdw	580	58	4	3
honey Dijon	1 sdw	630	58	3	16
grilled w/mozzarella focaccia	1 sdw	740	73	6	3
honey Dijon chicken salad	1 sdw	630	78	3	16
tarragon w/field greens	1 sdw	800	71	4	5
Thai	1 sdw	490	71	6	5
mozzarella, tomato & pesto	1 sdw	820	67	4	4
turkey, ham & provolone	1 sdw	1030	140	7	7
wraps					
chicken Caesar	1 wrap	600	63	5	3
Cobb turkey	1 wrap	570	65	6	2
fields & feta	1 wrap	560	90	14	5
Mediterranean	1 wrap	580	80	9	14

Food and Description	Amount	Total Calories	Total Carbs	Fiber	Sugars
Southwestern tuna	1 wrap	650	68	7	5
■ **SOUPS**					
baked stuffed potato	8 oz	240	20	1	1
broccoli cheddar	8 oz	230	13	2	5
chicken Florentine	8 oz	170	17	1	2
chicken noodle..low-fat	8 oz	90	11	0	2
clam chowder	8 oz	220	16	1	1
corn chowder	8 oz	240	25	2	4
curried rice & lentil..low-fat	8 oz	100	18	4	1
French Moroccan tomato lentil	8 oz	110	19	6	3
French onion..low-fat	8 oz	80	11	2	3
garden vegetable..low-fat	8 oz	40	7	2	3
harvest pumpkin	8 oz	140	15	4	2
Italian wedding	8 oz	100	12	2	3
Jamaican black bean..low-fat	8 oz	110	26	14	3
Mediterranean pepper	8 oz	190	30	7	3
old-fashioned tomato	8 oz	130	17	2	10
Southern black-eyed pea	8 oz	190	34	12	2
Southwest tortilla	8 oz	140	17	3	3
Southwestern vegetable	8 oz	150	23	4	3
BLIMPIE					
■ **9 GRAMS OF FAT OR LESS FOODS**					
cookie..oatmeal raisin	1 cookie	190	27	1	16
salads					
chef	regular	212	9	3	5
grilled chicken	regular	139	7	3	3.5
seafood	regular	122	16	3	4.5
sandwiches..subs					
Buffalo chicken	6" regular	320	50	3	6
grilled chicken	6" regular	425	50	3	7
MexiMax	6" regular	425	65	7	9
roast beef	6" regular	388	49	3	7.5
seafood	6" regular	355	58	3.8	9
turkey	6" regular	320	49	3	7.5
VegiMax	6" regular	395	60	8	8
■ **COOKIES**					
chocolate chunk	1 cookie	200	26	1	16
macadamia white chunk	1 cookie	210	26	1	15
oatmeal raisin	1 cookie	190	27	1	16
peanut butter	1 cookie	220	23	1	14
sugar	1 cookie	330	24	0	24
■ **SALADS**					
antipasto	regular	244	10	3	6
chef	regular	212	9	3	5
Chili Ole	regular	480	42	3	2
grilled chicken w/Caesar dressing	regular	347	9	3	5
Roast Beef 'n' Bleu	regular	390	29	0	0
seafood	regular	122	16	3	5
tuna	regular	261	7	3	3
Zesto Pesto Turkey	regular	370	31	0	1

Food and Description	Amount	Total Calories	Total Carbs	Fiber	Sugars
■ SANDWICHES					
café-style					
Cable Car Club					
BCC IT!..(Blimpie Carb Counter)	6" regular	300	16	5	4
regular	6" regular	350	36	2	5
Fisherman's Wharf tuna melt					
BCC IT!	6" regular	300	16	7	3
regular	6" regular	350	35	3	4
Golden Gate Gourmet					
BCC IT!	6" regular	350	20	5	8
regular	6" regular	400	40	2	8
Union Square Ultimate Veggie					
BCC IT!	6" regular	280	19	6	4
regular	6" regular	330	38	2	5
subs					
cold..fresh-sliced					
BLIMPIE Best	6" regular	476	52	3	10
club	6" regular	440	50	3	9
ham & Swiss cheese	6" regular	436	51.5	3	10
roast beef	6" regular	468	49	3.3	7
seafood	6" regular	355	58	4	9
tuna	6" regular	493	50.5	3	7
turkey	6" regular	424	49	3	7
hot					
BLT	6" regular	588	49	3	8
Buffalo chicken melt	6" regular	400	50	3	7
ChikMax	6" regular	511	71	8	10
grilled chicken	6" regular	373	50	3	8
meatball..Italian-style	6" regular	572	55	2	12
MexiMax	6" regular	425	65	7	9
pastrami	6" regular	507	53	3	11
steak & onion melt	6" regular	440	49	3	9
VegiMax	6" regular	395	60	8	8
panini sub..grilled					
beef, turkey & cheddar	6" regular	600	49	3	8.5
Cuban	6" regular	462	50	3	9
Pastrami Special	6" regular	462	52	3	10.5
Reuben	6" regular	630	55	2.5	15
Ultimate Club	6" regular	724	51	3	10
wraps					
beef & cheddar	regular	714	57	3	5
chicken Caesar	regular	649	56	3	5.5
Southwestern	regular	674	54	3	4
steak & onion	regular	716	64	3	7
Ultimate BLT	regular	831	60	3	7
Zesty Italian	regular	638	74	3	13
■ SIDE ORDERS					
coleslaw	5 oz	180	13	1	13
macaroni salad	5 oz	360	25	1	6
mustard potato salad	5 oz	160	21	1	23
potato salad	5 oz	270	19	1	10

Food and Description	Amount	Total Calories	Total Carbs	Fiber	Sugars
■ **SOUPS**					
chicken w/white & wild rice	8 oz	230	21	2	2
cream of broccoli	8 oz	190	15	3	5
cream of potato	8 oz	190	24	3	3
garden vegetable	8 oz	80	13	2	3
grande chili w/beans & beef	8 oz	250	30	18	7
home-style chicken noodle	8 oz	120	18	1	4
tomato basil w/raviolini	8 oz	110	22	<1	5
vegetable beef	8 oz	80	14	3	5
BOSTON MARKET					
■ **BAKED GOODS**					
apple pie	1 slice	550	66	3	36
brownie					
caramel pecan	1 brownie	900	114	6	88
chocolate	1 brownie	580	88	6	65
chocolate					
cake	1 slice	650	86	2	68
mania	1 slice	490	36	1	28
cookies					
chocolate chip	1 cookie	390	51	2	28
oatmeal Scotchie	1 cookie	390	47	2	24
■ **ENTRÉES..**individual meals					
chicken					
crispy-baked country	1 serving	420	31	5	1
mango..grilled	1 serving	390	26	0	23
marinated..grilled	1 serving	230	1	0	0
pot pie	1 pie	750	57	0	3
ham..honey-glazed	1 serving	210	10	0	10
meat loaf..Angus					
w/beef gravy	1 serving	360	19	1	3
w/chunky Creole sauce	1 serving	350	25	2	9
w/double sauce	1 serving	310	16	1	3
rotisserie chicken					
¼ chicken					
dark meat..garlic					
w/skin	1 serving	320	2	0	2
w/o skin	1 serving	190	1	0	1
white meat..garlic				0	
w/skin & wing	1 serving	280	2	0	2
w/o skin & wing	1 serving	170	2	0	1
½ chicken..sweet garlic w/skin	1 serving	590	4	0	4
rotisserie turkey breast w/o skin	1 serving	170	3	0	3
■ **SALADS**					
Caesar					
chicken..marinated..grilled	1 salad	800	18	3	4
entrée	1 salad	470	17	3	3
side	1 salad	300	13	<1	2
Oriental grilled chicken					
w/dressing & noodles	1 salad	570	56	8	13
Southwest grilled chicken					
w/dressing & chips	1 salad	890	46	7	17

Food and Description	Amount	Total Calories	Total Carbs	Fiber	Sugars
■ SANDWICHES					
chicken carver					
marinated..grilled	1 sdw	670	45	2	5
w/cheese & sauce	1 sdw	640	61	4	13
w/o cheese & sauce	1 sdw	400	60	4	12
meat loaf carver w/cheese	1 sdw	730	85	5	18
turkey carver					
w/cheese & sauce	1 sdw	630	64	4	14
w/o cheese & sauce	1 sdw	400	61	4	12
■ SIDE DISHES..hot					
butternut squash	¾ cup	150	25	6	12
creamed spinach	¾ cup	260	11	2	2
garlic new potatoes	¾ cup	130	25	2	2
macaroni & cheese	¾ cup	280	33	1	8
mashed potatoes					
home-style w/gravy	¾ cup	230	32	3	4
plain	⅔ cup	210	30	2	4
rice pilaf	⅔ cup	140	24	1	2
savory stuffing	¾ cup	190	27	2	5
sesame broccoli	½ cup	80	13	2	10
squash casserole	¾ cup	330	20	3	8
sweet corn	¾ cup	180	30	2	13
sweet potato casserole	¾ cup	280	39	2	23
tomato au gratin..roasted	¾ cup	160	14	1	2
BURGER KING					
■ BEVERAGES					
shakes					
chocolate	1 medium	600	97	2	94
	1 large	850	133	2	128
strawberry	1 medium	590	96	0	94
	1 large	840	131	<1	128
vanilla	1 medium	540	76	0	74
	1 large	800	113	<1	110
■ BREAKFAST					
biscuit					
bacon, egg & cheese	1 biscuit	510	30	1	3
sausage	1 biscuit	590	41	1	2
sausage, egg & cheese	1 biscuit	600	25	1	3
Croissan'wich					
w/bacon, egg & cheese	1 sdw	360	25	<1	4
w/egg & cheese	1 sdw	320	24	<1	3
w/ham, egg & cheese	1 sdw	360	25	<1	3
w/sausage & cheese	1 sdw	420	23	<1	4
w/sausage, egg & cheese	1 sdw	520	24	1	4
French toast sticks	5 pieces	390	46	2	11
hash browns	small	230	23	2	0
sourdough breakfast sandwich					
w/bacon, egg & cheese	1 sdw	380	30	2	3
w/ham, egg & cheese	1 sdw	380	30	2	3
w/sausage, egg & cheese	1 sdw	540	30	2	3

Food and Description	Amount	Total Calories	Total Carbs	Fiber	Sugars
■ BURGERS					
fire-grilled					
bacon cheeseburger	1 burger	390	31	1	5
double	1 burger	530	32	2	6
BK veggie	1 burger	380	46	4	6
cheeseburger..regular	1 burger	350	31	1	5
double					
cheeseburger	1 burger	530	32	2	5
hamburger	1 burger	440	30	1	5
hamburger..regular	1 burger	310	30	1	5
Whopper					
double sandwich					
¾ low-carb	1 burger	540	52	4	8
w/mayo	1 burger	970	52	4	8
double w/cheese sandwich					
¾ low-carb	1 burger	630	5	<1	2
w/mayo	1 burger	1,060	53	4	0
original sandwich					
¾ low-carb	1 burger	280	3	<1	2
w/mayo	1 burger	700	52	4	8
original w/cheese sandwich					
¾ low-carb	1 burger	370	5	<1	2
w/mayo	1 burger	800	53	4	9
Whopper Jr. sandwich					
¾ low-carb	1 burger	140	1	0	1
w/mayo	1 burger	390	31	2	5
Whopper Jr. w/cheese sandwich					
¾ low-carb	1 burger	190	2	0	1
w/mayo	1 burger	430	32	2	5
■ CHICKEN & FISH					
chicken					
sandwich					
original w/mayo	1 sdw	560	52	3	5
Santa Fe..baguette	1 sdw	370	57	4	7
savory mustard fire-grilled baguette	1 sdw	380	58	3	9
Tendercrisp w/mayo	1 sdw	810	72	6	9
Whopper	1 sdw	160	3	1	1
low carb..w/mayo	1 sdw	570	48	4	5
tenders	4 pieces	170	19	9	9
	5 pieces	210	13	<1	0
	8 pieces	340	29	<1	9
fish..BK fish fillet sdw w/tartar sauce	1 sdw	520	44	2	4
■ DESSERT					
Dutch apple pie	1 pie	340	52	1	23
Hershey's sundae pie	1 pie	300	31	1	23
Nestle Toll House chocolate chip cookie	2 cookies	440	68	0	32
■ SIDE ORDERS					
chili	1 serving	190	17	5	5
French fries..salted or unsalted	medium	360	46	4	1
	large	500	63	5	1

Food and Description	Amount	Total Calories	Total Carbs	Fiber	Sugars
onion rings	medium	320	40	3	5
	large	480	60	5	7
CHICK-FIL-A					
■ **CHICKEN**					
nuggets	8-pack	260	12	<1	3
sandwiches					
chargrilled	1 sdw	270	1	0	2
club..no sauce	1 sdw	380	33	3	7
chicken salad	1 sdw	350	32	5	6
Chick-Fil-A	1 sdw	410	38	1	5
deluxe	1 sdw	420	39	2	5
wraps..Cool Wrap	1 wrap	390	54	3	7
Caesar	1 wrap	460	52	3	5
spicy	1 wrap	380	52	3	5
■ **DESSERT**					
cheesecake	1 slice	340	30	2	25
w/blueberry topping	1 slice	370	39	2	32
w/strawberry topping	1 slice	360	38	2	31
fudge nut brownie	1 brownie	330	45	2	29
ice cream cup	1 small	230	38	0	38
lemon pie	1 slice	320	51	3	39
■ **DIPPING SAUCES**					
honey mustard	1 pkt	45	10	0	10
honey-roasted BBQ	1 pkt	60	2	0	1
Polynesian	1 pkt	110	13	0	13
■ **SALADS & SOUPS**					
salads					
carrot & raisin	1 salad	170	28	2	18
chargrilled chicken					
garden	1 salad	180	9	3	6
Southwest	1 salad	240	17	5	6
Chick-fil-A Chick-n Strips	1 salad	390	22	4	8
side	1 salad	60	4	2	2
soup..chicken breast	1 cup	140	18	1	2
■ **SIDE ORDERS**					
coleslaw	small	260	17	2	11
fruit cup	medium	60	16	2	13
waffle potato fries	small	280	37	5	0
CHURCH'S CHICKEN					
■ **CHICKEN**					
with batter and skin removed					
breast	2.5 oz	145	1	0	0
leg	2 oz	118	1.25	0	0
thigh	2.25 oz	180	3	0	0
wing	2.25 oz	160	2	0	0
with skin					
breast	2.8 oz	200	4	0	0
leg	2 oz	140	2	0	0
tender crunchers	6–8 pieces	411	32	1	0

Food and Description	Amount	Total Calories	Total Carbs	Fiber	Sugars
tender strip	2 oz	137	11	<1	0
thigh	2.8 oz	230	5	0	0
wing	3.1 oz	250	8	0	0
■ **DESSERT**					
apple pie	1 piece	280	41	1	13
Edward's double lemon pie	1 piece	380	39	0	29
Edward's strawberry cream cheese pie	1 piece	280	32	2	22
■ **SIDE ORDERS**					
biscuit w/honey butter	1 biscuit	250	26	1	3
Cajun rice	1 serving	130	16	<1	0
coleslaw	1 serving	92	8	2	6
collard greens	1 serving	25	5	2	0
corn on the cob	1 piece	139	24	9	2
French fries	1 serving	210	29	2	0
jalapeño cheese bombers	1 serving	240	29	3	5
macaroni & cheese	1 serving	210	23	1	6
okra	1 serving	210	19	4	<1
potatoes..mashed w/gravy	1 serving	90	14	1	2
steak..country-fried w/white gravy	1 serving	470	36	1	4
sweet corn nuggets	regular	250	30	2	6
DAIRY QUEEN					
■ **BEEF, CHICKEN & PORK**					
beef..BBQ beef sandwich	1 sdw	300	37	2	15
chicken					
basket..strip	1 basket	1,000	102	5	3
sandwich..breaded chicken	1 sdw	510	47	4	9
pork..BBQ pork sandwich	1 sdw	280	36	2	8
■ **BEVERAGES**					
malt..chocolate	medium	870	153	2	134
shake..chocolate	small	560	93	1	83
	medium	760	129	2	115
	large	1,140	186	2	165
■ **BURGERS & HOT DOGS**					
hamburger..DQ home-style					
double					
deluxe	1 burger	340	29	2	5
w/bacon & cheese	1 burger	610	31	2	6
w/cheese	1 burger	540	30	2	5
single	1 burger	290	29	2	5
w/cheese	1 burger	340	29	2	5
Ultimate	1 burger	670	29	2	6
hot dog	1 hot dog	240	15	1	4
chili 'n' cheese	1 hot dog	330	22	2	4
Super Dog	1 hot dog	580	39	2	6
chili 'n' cheese	1 hot dog	710	42	3	6
■ **FROZEN DESSERT SPECIALTIES**					
banana split	1 serving	510	96	3	82
Blizzard					
banana split	medium	580	97	1	83

Food and Description	Amount	Total Calories	Total Carbs	Fiber	Sugars
chocolate chip cookie dough	medium	1,030	150	0	112
Oreo cookie	medium	700	103	1	77
cone					
chocolate	regular	340	53	0	34
dipped	medium	490	59	1	43
vanilla	medium	330	53	0	38
Brownie Earthquake	1 serving	740	112	0	86
Dilly Bar..chocolate	1 bar	210	21	0	17
Peanut Buster parfait	1 serving	730	99	2	85
pecan praline parfait	1 serving	720	105	1	81
strawberry shortcake	1 serving	430	70	1	47
sundae					
chocolate	medium	400	71	0	61
strawberry	medium	340	58	<1	51
Triple Chocolate Utopia	1 serving	770	96	5	76
■ SALADS & SALAD DRESSINGS					
salads					
crispy chicken..no dressing	1 salad	350	21	6	5
grilled chicken..no dressing	1 salad	240	12	4	7
side	1 salad	60	6	2	4
salad dressings..DQ					
blue cheese	2 oz	210	4	0	2
honey mustard	2 oz	260	18	0	11
ranch	2 oz	310	3	0	2
■ SIDE ORDERS					
French fries	medium	300	56	4	<1
onion rings	1 serving	470	45	3	7
DAVANNI'S					
■ CALZONES					
chicken tomato	1 calzone	660	66	2	4
pepperoni sausage	1 calzone	730	66	2.5	2
sausage green pepper	1 calzone	696	67	3	4
3-cheese	1 calzone	700	64	2	2
■ GARLIC CHEESE BREAD					
half order..w/sauce	2 pieces	369	24	1	5
whole order..w/sauce	4 pieces	687	42	2	7
■ HOAGIES					
cheese	½ hoagie	401	21	1	4
chicken					
breast	½ hoagie	495	23	1	5
parmigiana	½ hoagie	383	22	1	4
club	½ hoagie	400	22	1	4
ham	½ hoagie	379	22	1	5
Italian sausage	½ hoagie	522	28	2	8
meatball	½ hoagie	465	31	2	7
Mediterranean	½ hoagie	511	22	1	4
pastrami	½ hoagie	459	22	1	5
pizza	½ hoagie	315	23	2	4
roast beef	½ hoagie	385	21	1	4
salami	½ hoagie	484	21	1	4
tuna	½ hoagie	563	24	1	4

Food and Description	Amount	Total Calories	Total Carbs	Fiber	Sugars
turkey	½ hoagie	372	22	1	4
veggie	½ hoagie	445	29	3	9
■ LASAGNA					
half lasagna w/toast	1 serving	547	31	4	11.5
whole lasagna w/toast	1 serving	989	50	6	16
DOMINO'S PIZZA					
■ BUFFALO WINGS, BREADS & DIPPING SAUCES					
bread					
cheesy	1 piece	142	18	<1	<1
Cinna Stix	1 piece	111	15	<1	3
sweet icing	2.5-oz cup	283	60	0	51
sticks	1 piece	116	18	<1	<1
dipping sauces					
blue cheese	1.5 oz	223	2	0	2
hot	1.5 oz	15	4	<1	<1
ranch	1.5 oz	197	2	0	2
wings..Kickers					
BBQ	1 piece	50	2	0	1
hot Buffalo	1 piece	45	1	0	0
■ 12" MEDIUM PIZZA					
America's Favorite Feast					
deep-dish	⅛ pizza	309	29	2	3
hand-tossed	⅛ pizza	257	29	2	2
thin-crust	⅛ pizza	208	15	1	2
Bacon Cheeseburger Feast					
deep-dish	⅛ pizza	325	28	2	3
hand-tossed	⅛ pizza	273	26	2	2
thin-crust	⅛ pizza	224	14	1	2
Barbecue					
deep-dish	⅛ pizza	304	32	2	5
hand-tossed	⅛ pizza	252	31	1	4
thin-crust	⅛ pizza	203	17	1	4
Beef					
deep-dish	⅛ pizza	277	28	2	3
hand-tossed	⅛ pizza	225	28	2	2
thin-crust	⅛ pizza	175	14	1	2
Cheese					
deep-dish	⅛ pizza	238	28	2	3
hand-tossed	⅛ pizza	186	28	1	2
thin-crust	⅛ pizza	137	14	1	2
Deluxe Feast					
deep-dish	⅛ pizza	287	29	2	3
hand-tossed	⅛ pizza	234	29	2	2
thin-crust	⅛ pizza	185	15	1	2
ExtravaganZZa Feast					
deep-dish	⅛ pizza	341	30	2	3
hand-tossed	⅛ pizza	289	30	2	3
thin-crust	⅛ pizza	240	16	1	2
Green Pepper, Onion & Mushroom					
deep-dish	⅛ pizza	244	30	2	3

Food and Description	Amount	Total Calories	Total Carbs	Fiber	Sugars
hand-tossed	⅛ pizza	191	29	2	2
thin-crust	⅛ pizza	142	15	1	2
Ham					
deep-dish	⅛ pizza	250	28	2	3
hand-tossed	⅛ pizza	198	28	1	2
thin-crust	⅛ pizza	148	14	1	2
Ham & Pineapple					
deep-dish	⅛ pizza	252	30	2	4
hand-tossed	⅛ pizza	200	29	2	3
thin-crust	⅛ pizza	150	15	1	3
Hawaiian Feast					
deep-dish	⅛ pizza	275	30	2	4
hand-tossed	⅛ pizza	223	30	2	3
thin-crust	⅛ pizza	174	16	1	3
MeatZZa Feast					
deep-dish	⅛ pizza	333	29	2	3
hand-tossed	⅛ pizza	281	29	2	2
thin-crust	⅛ pizza	232	15	1	2
Pepperoni					
deep-dish	⅛ pizza	275	28	2	3
hand-tossed	⅛ pizza	223	28	2	2
thin-crust	⅛ pizza	174	14	1	2
Pepperoni & Sausage					
deep-dish	⅛ pizza	307	29	2	3
hand-tossed	⅛ pizza	200	29	2	3
thin-crust	⅛ pizza	150	15	1	3
Pepperoni Feast					
deep-dish	⅛ pizza	317	29	2	3
hand-tossed	⅛ pizza	265	28	2	2
thin-crust	⅛ pizza	216	14	1	2
Sausage					
deep-dish	⅛ pizza	283	29	2	3
hand-tossed	⅛ pizza	231	28	2	2
thin-crust	⅛ pizza	181	14	1	2
Vegi Feast					
deep-dish	⅛ pizza	270	30	2	3
hand-tossed	⅛ pizza	218	29	2	2
thin-crust	⅛ pizza	168	15	1	2
■ 14" LARGE PIZZA					
America's Favorite Feast					
deep-dish	⅛ pizza	433	42	3	4
hand-tossed	⅛ pizza	353	39	2	3
thin-crust	⅛ pizza	285	20	2	2
Bacon Cheeseburger Feast					
deep-dish	⅛ pizza	459	41	2	4
hand-tossed	⅛ pizza	379	38	2	3
thin-crust	⅛ pizza	311	19	1	3
Barbecue					
deep-dish	⅛ pizza	424	46	2	7
hand-tossed	⅛ pizza	344	43	2	6
thin-crust	⅛ pizza	276	24	1	5

Food and Description	Amount	Total Calories	Total Carbs	Fiber	Sugars
Beef					
deep-dish	⅛ pizza	392	38	2	3
hand-tossed	⅛ pizza	312	38	2	3
thin-crust	⅛ pizza	243	19	1	2
Cheese					
deep-dish	⅛ pizza	336	41	2	4
hand-tossed	⅛ pizza	256	38	2	3
thin-crust	⅛ pizza	188	19	1	2
Deluxe Feast					
deep-dish	⅛ pizza	397	42	3	4
hand-tossed	⅛ pizza	316	39	2	3
thin-crust	⅛ pizza	247	20	2	3
ExtravaganZZa Feast					
deep-dish	⅛ pizza	468	43	3	5
hand-tossed	⅛ pizza	388	40	3	3
thin-crust	⅛ pizza	320	21	2	3
Green Pepper, Onion & Mushroom					
deep-dish	⅛ pizza	343	42	3	4
hand-tossed	⅛ pizza	263	39	2	3
thin-crust	⅛ pizza	201	21	2	3
Ham					
deep-dish	⅛ pizza	352	41	2	4
hand-tossed	⅛ pizza	272	38	2	3
thin-crust	⅛ pizza	204	19	12	3
Ham & Pineapple					
deep-dish	⅛ pizza	355	42	2	6
hand-tossed	⅛ pizza	275	40	2	5
thin-crust	⅛ pizza	207	21	1	4
Hawaiian Feast					
deep-dish	⅛ pizza	389	43	3	6
hand-tossed	⅛ pizza	309	41	1	5
thin-crust	⅛ pizza	240	21	2	4
MeatZZa Feast					
deep-dish	⅛ pizza	458	42	3	4
hand-tossed	⅛ pizza	378	39	2	3
thin-crust	⅛ pizza	310	20	2	3
Pepperoni					
deep-dish	⅛ pizza	385	41	2	4
hand-tossed	⅛ pizza	305	38	2	2
thin-crust	⅛ pizza	237	19	1	2
Pepperoni & Sausage					
deep-dish	⅛ pizza	430	41	3	4
hand-tossed	⅛ pizza	350	39	2	3
thin-crust	⅛ pizza	282	19	2	2
Pepperoni Feast					
deep-dish	⅛ pizza	443	42	3	4
hand-tossed	⅛ pizza	363	35	2	3
thin-crust	⅛ pizza	295	29	1	3
Sausage					
deep-dish	⅛ pizza	400	42	3	4

Food and Description	Amount	Total Calories	Total Carbs	Fiber	Sugars
hand-tossed	⅛ pizza	320	39	2	3
thin-crust	⅛ pizza	252	20	2	2
Vegi Feast					
deep-dish	⅛ pizza	380	43	3	4
hand-tossed	⅛ pizza	300	40	3	3
thin-crust	⅛ pizza	231	21	2	3

DUNKIN' DONUTS

■ BAGELS

Food and Description	Amount	Total Calories	Total Carbs	Fiber	Sugars
berry berry	1 bagel	340	69	4	12
blueberry	1 bagel	350	69	2	10
cinnamon raisin	1 bagel	330	65	3	12
everything	1 bagel	430	75	3	6
garlic	1 bagel	410	79	3	6
onion	1 bagel	370	71	4	12
plain	1 bagel	360	69	2	6
poppyseed	1 bagel	440	72	3	6
salsa	1 bagel	320	62	3	5
salt	1 bagel	360	69	2	6
sesame	1 bagel	450	71	3	6
sourdough	1 bagel	340	65	2	4
wheat	1 bagel	350	66	4	7

■ BEVERAGES

Food and Description	Amount	Total Calories	Total Carbs	Fiber	Sugars
coffee					
Coolatta					
flavored					
lemonade	16 fl oz	240	59	0	56
orange mango	16 fl oz	270	66	2	58
strawberry	16 fl oz	290	72	1	65
vanilla bean	16 fl oz	440	70	1	69
unflavored					
w/cream	16 fl oz	350	40	0	35
w/skim milk	16 fl oz	170	41	0	40
w/2% milk	16 fl oz	190	41	0	40
w/whole milk	16 fl oz	210	42	0	40
Dunkaccino	10 fl oz	230	35	0	25
hot chocolate	10 fl oz	220	38	2	28
hot espresso drinks					
cappuccino w/sugar	10 fl oz	130	21	0	20
espresso w/sugar	2 fl oz	30	7	0	7
latte..caramel or mocha swirl	10 fl oz	230	37	1	35
iced latte	16 fl oz	120	11	0	10
iced latte..caramel or mocha swirl	16 fl oz	240	37	0	36
w/sugar	16 fl oz	170	23	0	21

■ BREAKFAST SANDWICHES

Food and Description	Amount	Total Calories	Total Carbs	Fiber	Sugars
bagel					
bacon, egg & cheese	1 sdw	500	71	2	7
ham, egg & cheese	1 sdw	500	70	2	7
sausage, egg & cheese	1 sdw	670	71	2	7
biscuit					
egg & cheese	1 sdw	360	31	1	3

Food and Description	Amount	Total Calories	Total Carbs	Fiber	Sugars
sausage, egg & cheese	1 sdw	560	31	1	4
croissant..egg, ham & cheese	1 sdw	470	38	0	3
English muffin					
bacon, egg & cheese	1 sdw	310	35	1	3
egg & cheese	1 sdw	270	35	1	3
ham, egg & cheese	1 sdw	310	35	1	3
New England maple cheddar	1 sdw	700	42	0	6
■ **CROISSANTS**					
plain	1 croissant	330	37	0	3
reduced-carb	1 croissant	370	19	2	1
■ **DONUTS & PASTRIES**					
cruller..French	1 cruller	150	17	1	8
Danish					
apple	1 Danish	250	36	0	15
cheese	1 Danish	270	32	0	11
strawberry cheese	1 Danish	250	33	0	12
donuts					
apple crumb	1 donut	230	34	1	12
apple 'n' spice	1 donut	200	29	1	7
Bavarian cream	1 donut	210	30	1	9
black raspberry	1 donut	210	32	1	10
blueberry					
cake	1 donut	290	35	1	16
crumb	1 donut	240	36	1	15
Boston cream	1 donut	240	36	1	14
chocolate					
coconut cake	1 donut	300	31	1	12
cinnamon cake	1 donut	330	34	1	14
double chocolate cake	1 donut	310	37	2	18
glazed					
cake donut	1 donut	350	41	1	21
donut	1 donut	180	25	1	6
jelly-filled	1 donut	210	32	1	14
Kreme-filled frosted	1 donut	270	35	1	16
cake donut	1 donut	360	40	1	15
donut	1 donut	200	29	1	10
lemon cake					
burst	1 donut	300	35	3	25
frosted	1 donut	240	28	0	17
glazed	1 donut	240	28	0	16
maple-frosted	1 donut	210	30	1	12
marble-frosted	1 donut	200	29	1	11
old-fashioned cake	1 donut	300	28	1	9
powdered cake	1 donut	330	36	1	17
strawberry	1 donut	210	32	1	11
frosted	1 donut	210	30	1	12
sugar-raised	1 donut	170	22	1	4
vanilla cream–filled	1 donut	270	36	1	17
whole wheat glazed cake	1 donut	310	32	2	14

Food and Description	Amount	Total Calories	Total Carbs	Fiber	Sugars
fancies					
apple fritter	1 fritter	300	41	1	12
bow-tie donut	1 donut	300	34	1	10
chocolate-frosted coffee roll	1 roll	290	36	1	12
chocolate-iced Bismark	1 Bismark	340	50	1	31
coffee roll	1 roll	270	36	1	13
éclair	1 éclair	270	39	1	17
glazed fritter	1 fritter	260	31	1	7
maple-frosted coffee roll	1 roll	290	36	1	13
vanilla-frosted coffee roll	1 roll	290	36	1	13
Munchkins					
cinnamon cake	4 pieces	270	31	1	14
glazed					
cake	3 pieces	280	38	1	22
chocolate cake	3 pieces	200	26	1	13
jelly-filled	5 pieces	210	30	1	15
lemon-filled	4 pieces	170	23	0	9
powdered cake	4 pieces	270	31	2	15
sticks					
cinnamon cake	1 stick	450	42	1	17
glazed					
cake	1 stick	490	51	1	26
chocolate cake	1 stick	470	49	2	24
jelly	1 stick	530	61	1	32
powdered cake	1 stick	450	42	1	18
■ MUFFINS					
banana walnut	1 muffin	540	73	3	35
blueberry	1 muffin	490	75	2	39
carrot walnut spice	1 muffin	600	81	3	49
chocolate chip	1 muffin	590	85	3	47
coffee cake w/topping	1 muffin	710	102	2	59
corn	1 muffin	510	81	1	35
cranberry orange	1 muffin	460	71	3	35
honey bran raisin	1 muffin	490	81	5	45
■ OTHER BAKERY ITEMS					
apple pie à la mode	1 serving	810	107	4	54
scones					
maple walnut	1 scone	470	62	1	25
raspberry white chocolate	1 scone	450	59	2	29
EINSTEIN BROTHERS BAGELS					
■ BAGELS					
Asiago cheese	1 bagel	360	71	2	4
chocolate chip	1 bagel	370	76	3	10
chopped garlic	1 bagel	380	79	4	3
chopped onion	1 bagel	330	71	2	4
cinnamon raisin swirl	1 bagel	350	78	2	14
cinnamon sugar	1 bagel	330	74	2	10
Chicago-style	1 bagel	500	72	2	4
cranberry	1 bagel	350	78	3	13
dark pumpernickel	1 bagel	320	68	3	3

Food and Description	Amount	Total Calories	Total Carbs	Fiber	Sugars
egg	1 bagel	340	69	2	5
everything	1 bagel	340	75	2	5
honey whole wheat	1 bagel	320	71	3	11
lower-carb 9-grain	1 bagel	210	28	10	1
marble rye	1 bagel	340	73	3	3
nutty banana	1 bagel	360	74	2	5
poppy dip'd	1 bagel	350	74	2	3
potato	1 bagel	350	69	2	5
power	1 bagel	410	81	4	18
w/peanut butter	1 bagel	750	92	7	22
pumpkin	1 bagel	330	72	3	6
sesame dip'd	1 bagel	380	75	3	3
sun-dried tomato	1 bagel	320	69	3	3
wild blueberry	1 bagel	350	77	3	9
■ BAGELS..TOP-SHELF					
roasted red pepper & pesto	1 bagel	410	73	2	5
6-cheese	1 bagel	390	72	2	4
spicy nacho	1 bagel	450	77	3	5
spinach Florentine	1 bagel	410	72	3	5
■ BEVERAGES					
coffee..specialty	12 fl oz	90	9	0	8
cafe latte	12 fl oz	140	13	0	13
nonfat	12 fl oz	100	14	0	12
cappuccino					
low-fat	12 fl oz	130	19	0	18
nonfat	12 fl oz	60	9	0	8
mocha	12 fl oz	230	34	0	32
low-fat	12 fl oz	190	34	0	31
smoothie..mocha	10 fl oz	470	98	0	61
■ CREAM CHEESE..whipped					
blueberry	2 Tbs	70	6	0	5
cappuccino	2 Tbs	70	5	0	4
garden vegetable	2 Tbs	60	3	0	1
honey almond	2 Tbs	70	6	0	4
jalapeño salsa	2 Tbs	60	3	0	1
maple raisin walnut	2 Tbs	60	4	0	3
onion & chive	2 Tbs	70	3	0	1
plain	2 Tbs	70	1	0	1
reduced-fat	2 Tbs	60	2	0	1
smoked salmon	2 Tbs	60	2	0	1
strawberry	2 Tbs	70	5	0	4
sun-dried tomato & basil	2 Tbs	60	2	0	1
■ SALADS..entrées					
Asiago					
Caesar	1 salad	660	25	3	6
chicken Caesar	1 salad	740	25	3	6
Bros. Bistro	1 salad	810	37	4	23
chicken chipotle	1 salad	630	38	7	19
Jamaican Jerk	1 salad	340	43	4	30

Food and Description	Amount	Total Calories	Total Carbs	Fiber	Sugars
■ SANDWICHES					
bagel dogs..Chicago					
Asiago	1 sdw	740	78	2	6
chili cheese	1 sdw	810	83	4	9
everything	1 sdw	730	80	3	6
onion..w/o cheese	1 sdw	680	78	2	6
frittatas					
Denver omelet breakfast panini	1 sdw	750	70	2	7
egg					
Black Forest ham	1 sdw	660	76	2	9
plain	1 sdw	590	74	2	7
Santa Fe	1 sdw	720	78	2	8
sausage	1 sdw	660	76	2	9
thick-cut bacon	1 sdw	840	75	2	7
lower carb..9-grain bagel					
bagel dog	1 sdw	560	35	10	3
Denver omelet panini	1 sdw	650	35	10	7
frittata..egg	1 sdw	470	31	10	4
egg & bacon	1 sdw	720	32	10	4
egg					
w/Black Forest ham	1 sdw	550	33	10	6
w/turkey sausage	1 sdw	550	31	10	4
Tasty Turkey	1 sdw	490	49	11	4
tuna salad	1 sdw	360	34	12	4
turkey deli	1 sdw	330	32	11	3
panini					
Cali club	1 sdw	990	71	4	3
ham & cheese	1 sdw	640	68	2	6
Italian chicken	1 sdw	690	68	3	4
Signature Sandwiches					
100% albacore tuna w/artisan wheat	1 sdw	400	40	5	6
Black Forest ham on challah	1 sdw	620	65	3	14
Calypso chicken salad	1 sdw	460	72	3	7
Club Mex on challah	1 sdw	920	65	3	10
Cobbie on challah	1 sdw	810	65	5	11
Einstein club on rustic white	1 sdw	840	55	4	4
hummus Mediterranean w/feta					
on ciabatta	1 sdw	450	77	5	8
New York lox & bagel	1 sdw	660	79	3	10
roasted turkey on artisan wheat	1 sdw	610	51	5	7
Tasty Turkey on Asiago bagel	1 sdw	630	83	3	6
Veg Out on sesame seed bagel	1 sdw	500	82	4	10
■ SWEETS					
coffee cake					
apple cinnamon	1 slice	570	87	0	42
blueberry	1 slice	600	94	0	48
chocolate chip	1 slice	660	96	2	50
cookies					
heavenly chocolate chip	1 cookie	565	70	2	42
honey-roasted peanut butter	1 cookie	610	63	3	39

Food and Description	Amount	Total Calories	Total Carbs	Fiber	Sugars
trail-mix	1 cookie	500	74	5	39
pastries..cinnamon					
twists	1 twist	370	41	1	18
walnut strudel	1 slice	550	63	3	25
FAZOLI'S					
■ DESSERT					
cheesecake	1 piece	290	17	0	17
chocolate chip	1 piece	300	22	1	19
turtle	1 piece	420	24	2	21
cookie..milk chocolate chunk	1 cookie	360	54	0	33
Freezi					
strawberry	1	510	115	0	99
strawberry banana	1	530	118	0	101
triple berry	1	520	116	0	100
■ ENTRÉES..Italian Specialties					
baked					
chicken Alfredo	1 serving	790	82	3	3
chicken Parmesan	1 serving	740	99	6	10
pizza baked spaghetti	1 serving	750	78	5	8
spaghetti Parmesan	1 serving	700	76	5	8
ziti					
classic meaty	1 small	430	47	6	11
	1 regular	670	73	9	16
twice-baked..w/meat sauce	1 serving	810	73	9	16
broccoli					
fettucine Alfredo..regular	1 serving	830	125	8	7
lasagna..6-layer	1 serving	690	70	6	12
fettuccine..shrimp & scallop	1 serving	610	80	3	3
lasagna					
broccoli..6-layer	1 serving	690	70	6	12
classic..w/6 layers	1 serving	810	108	6	12
six-layer..w/meat sauce	1 serving	630	63	4	13
twice-baked	1 serving	820	67	4	13
ravioli..cheese					
w/marinara sauce	1 sering	480	65	4	9
w/meat sauce	1 serving	510	65	4	8
ultimate sampler platter	1 serving	1,030	123	8	16
■ ENTRÉES..Pasta					
fettuccine					
Alfredo	1 serving	530	80	3	3
regular	1 serving	800	119	5	5
broccoli	1 serving	560	85	6	5
penne					
chicken..garden-style	1 serving	830	100	7	7
spicy marinara penne..w/chicken	1 serving	990	178	13	36
peppery chicken Alfredo	1 serving	610	80	3	3
spaghetti					
w/marinara	1 serving	420	74	5	8
w/marinara..regular	1 serving	620	111	7	12
w/meatballs	1 serving	720	80	6	9

Food and Description	Amount	Total Calories	Total Carbs	Fiber	Sugars
w/meatballs..regular	1 serving	1,020	119	8	13
w/meat sauce	1 serving	450	74	5	8
w/meat sauce..regular	1 serving	670	111	8	11
■ PIZZA					
cheese	double slice	460	58	2	6
combination	double slice	570	63	3	7
pepperoni	double slice	530	61	2	6
■ SALADS & BREADSTICKS					
breadstick	1 stick	140	18	1	1
dry..no oil or butter	1 stick	90	17	1	1
salad					
chicken & pasta Caesar	1 salad	370	33	3	7
chicken Caesar	1 salad	420	17	4	5
chicken finger					
regular	1 salad	190	8	2	4
w/bacon	1 salad	400	17	2	13
Italian chef	1 salad	260	13	3	3
side pasta	1 salad	240	29	2	4
■ SUBMARINOS & PANINI					
panini					
chicken					
Caesar club	1 sdw	660	61	4	1
pesto	1 sdw	510	51	3	1
4-cheese & tomato	1 sdw	720	55	3	3
ham & Swiss	1 sdw	600	53	2	4
Italian					
club	1 sdw	670	54	3	3
deli	1 sdw	660	61	4	1
smoked turkey	1 sdw	710	57	3	3
subs..Submarino					
club	½ sub	1,100	121	7	8
ham & Swiss	½ sub	1,000	120	7	8
w/meatballs	½ sub	1,260	128	8	10
original	½ sub	1,160	124	8	8
pepperoni pizza	½ sub	1,060	133	6	11
turkey	½ sub	990	121	7	8
GREAT AMERICAN COOKIES					
Big Bites					
chocolate chip	1 cookie	120	17	1	10
double fudge	1 cookie	110	18	2	12
M&M	1 cookie	140	20	2	12
peanut butter supreme	1 cookie	130	14	<1	9
sugar	1 cookie	130	19	2	10
white chunk macadamia	1 cookie	130	15	1	9
Big Bite Doozies					
chocolate chip w/Imperial fudge	1 cookie	340	47	3	31
chocolate chip w/Xtra smooth icing	1 cookie	350	47	3	33
M&M					
w/Imperial fudge	1 cookie	380	52	4	35
w/Xtra smooth icing	1 cookie	390	53	3	38

Food and Description	Amount	Total Calories	Total Carbs	Fiber	Sugars
sugar					
w/Imperial fudge	1 cookie	330	48	3	28
w/Xtra smooth icing	1 cookie	340	49	3	31
brownies					
cheesecake	1 brownie	400	48	0	37
chocolate cheesecake swirl	1 brownie	470	60	3	42
fudge	1 brownie	470	67	3	46
fudge nut	1 brownie	510	63	4	42
Colossal M&M	1 cookie	500	68	2	40
Double Doozies					
chocolate chip	1 cookie	581	79	2	50
M&M	1 cookie	601	79	2	50
sugar	1 cookie	491	67	0	48
regular cookies					
chewy					
chocolate supreme	1 cookie	190	30	1	26
pecan supreme	1 cookie	200	25	1	20
chocolate chip	1 cookie	230	32	1	19
Cookie Monster	1 cookie	180	27	1	20
double fudge	1 cookie	220	34	1	22
Elmo	1 cookie	200	29	1	15
M&M	1 cookie	240	32	1	10
oatmeal raisin	1 cookie	240	34	2	19
peanut butter					
M&M	1 cookie	265	30	<1	18
supreme	1 cookie	250	28	<1	16
pecan supreme	1 cookie	250	30	1	18
snickerdoodle	1 cookie	240	32	0	17
sugar	1 cookie	185	26	0	13
triple chocolate	1 cookie	240	31	<1	21
white chunk macadamia	1 cookie	240	32	<1	16
HARDEE'S					
■ **BEVERAGES**					
shakes & malts					
chocolate	regular	710	137	12	85
strawberry	regular	720	139	10	85
vanilla	regular	580	99	10	89
■ **BREAKFAST**					
Big Country Breakfast Platter					
w/bacon	1 serving	980	90	3	13
w/chicken	1 serving	1,140	105	4	12
w/country ham	1 serving	970	90	3	12
w/country steak	1 serving	1,150	98	4	12
w/sausage	1 serving	1,060	91	4	13
biscuits					
bacon	1 serving	560	37	0	4
bacon, egg & cheese	1 serving	560	37	0	4
biscuit 'n' gravy	1 serving	530	47	0	6
chicken fillet	1 serving	600	50	1	3
country ham	1 serving	440	36	0	3

Food and Description	Amount	Total Calories	Total Carbs	Fiber	Sugars
country steak	1 serving	620	44	0	3
ham, egg & cheese	1 serving	560	37	0	5
loaded omelet	1 serving	500	36	0	4
sausage & egg	1 serving	610	36	0	4
smoked sausage	1 serving	620	37	0	5
Frisco breakfast sandwich/ham	1 serving	360	38	2	4
low-carb breakfast bowl	1 serving	620	6	2	2
pancakes	3 pancakes	300	55	2	12
Made-from-Scratch	1 serving	370	35	0	3
Sunrise Croissant					
w/bacon	1 serving	450	28	0	5
w/ham	1 serving	430	28	0	5
w/sausage patty	1 serving	550	29	0	5
tortilla scrambler	1 serving	310	18	0	2
■ **BREAKFAST SIDES**					
biscuit gravy	5 oz	160	12	0	3
cinnamon roll	1 roll	390	96	2	43
croissant	1 croissant	210	26	0	4
grits	1 serving	110	16	0	0
hash rounds	small	260	25	2	1
	medium	350	34	3	1
sausage					
patty	1 patty	150	1	0	1
smoked	2.78 oz	250	2	0	2
scrambled egg	1 serving	160	1	0	1
■ **BURGERS & SANDWICHES**					
Burgers					
⅓-lb bacon cheese Thickburger	1 burger	910	50	3	10
⅓-lb cheeseburger	1 burger	680	51	3	10
⅓-lb chili cheese..Thickburger	1 burger	870	55	4	11
⅓-lb low-carb Thickburger	1 burger	420	5	2	3
⅓-lb mushroom 'n' Swiss Thickburger	1 burger	720	48	2	7
⅓-lb Thickburger	1 burger	850	54	3	12
½-lb Six-dollar Burger	1 burger	1,120	72	5	25
½-lb grilled sourdough Thickburger	1 burger	1,100	61	5	19
⅔-lb bacon cheese Thickburger	1 burger	1,340	60	5	17
⅔-lb double Thickburger	1 burger	1,230	53	3	12
⅔-lb double bacon cheese Thickburger	1 burger	1,300	51	3	11
sandwiches					
chicken					
big	1 sdw	770	73	4	9
charbroiled chicken					
low-carb	1 sdw	420	11	2	8
regular	1 sdw	590	53	4	11
spicy	1 sdw	430	46	2	6
hot dog w/condiments	1 sdw	420	22	1	4
hot ham 'n' cheese					
big	1 sdw	570	59	3	4
regular	1 sdw	420	39	2	4
roast beef					

Food and Description	Amount	Total Calories	Total Carbs	Fiber	Sugars
big	1 sdw	470	38	2	3
regular	1 sdw	330	29	2	2
Slammers					
w/cheese	1 sdw	280	20	0	2
w/o cheese	1 sdw	240	19	0	2
■ **CHICKEN..fried**					
individual pieces					
breast	1 serving	370	29	0	0
leg	1 serving	170	15	0	0
thigh	1 serving	330	30	0	0
wing	1 serving	200	23	0	0
kid's meal					
chicken strips..no sauce	1 order	500	50	3	1
Slammer	1 order	720	71	4	4
strips					
3-piece	1 order	380	27	1	1
5-piece	1 order	630	45	2	1
■ **SIDE ORDERS**					
chili cheese fries	1 order	700	67	7	2
coleslaw	small	170	20	2	16
crispy curls potatoes	medium	410	52	4	0
	large	480	60	5	0
French fries	kid's	250	32	3	0
	medium	520	67	5	1
	large	610	89	6	1
mashed potatoes	small	90	17	0	1
IN-N-OUT BURGER					
■ **BEVERAGES**					
shakes					
chocolate	15 oz	690	83	0	62
strawberry	15 oz	690	91	0	75
vanilla	15 oz	680	78	0	57
■ **CHEESEBURGERS**					
w/mustard & ketchup..no spread	1 burger	400	41	3	10
w/onions & spread	1 burger	480	39	3	10
protein-style..lettuce leaves w/o bun	1 burger	330	11	3	7
■ **DOUBLE-DOUBLE HAMBURGERS**					
w/mustard & ketchup..no spread	1 burger	590	41	3	10
w/onions & spread	1 burger	670	39	3	10
protein-style..lettuce leaves w/o bun	1 burger	520	11	3	7
■ **FRENCH FRIES**	1 order	400	54	2	0
■ **HAMBURGERS**					
w/mustard & ketchup	1 burger	310	41	3	10
w/onions	1 burger	390	39	3	10
protein-style	1 burger	240	11	3	7
JACK-N-THE-BOX					
■ **BEVERAGES**					
Minute Maid					
lemonade	1 regular	190	65	0	65
orange juice	1 regular	210	56	0	56

Food and Description	Amount	Total Calories	Total Carbs	Fiber	Sugars
strawberry	1 regular	220	59	0	59
shakes w/ice cream					
chocolate	small	660	89	1	79
	medium	850	111	1	98
creamy caramel	small	670	87	0	74
	medium	860	109	0	93
strawberry	small	640	84	0	71
	medium	830	106	0	89
vanilla	small	570	65	0	54
	medium	750	85	0	71
■ **BREAKFAST**					
Breakfast Jack	1 sdw	305	34	0	3
Extreme Sausage Sandwich	1 sdw	690	37	0	5
French toast sticks	1 serving	560	89	2	38
hash browns	1 serving	150	13	2	0
sausage biscuit	1 biscuit	600	41	2	3
sausage croissant	1 croissant	605	42	1	4
sausage, egg & cheese biscuit	1 biscuit	970	50	2	5
Sourdough Breakfast Sandwich	1 sdw	445	37	2	2
Supreme Croissant	1 croissant	475	41	1	4
Ultimate Breakfast Sandwich	1 sdw	605	58	2	8
■ **BURGERS & SANDWICHES**					
burgers					
cheeseburger					
bacon bacon	1 burger	780	50	2	8
Bacon Ultimate	1 burger	1,025	53	2	11
Ultimate	1 burger	945	52	2	10
hamburger					
deluxe	1 burger	370	32	0	6
w/cheese	1 burger	460	34	0	7
regular	1 burger	310	30	0	6
w/cheese	1 burger	355	31	0	6
Jumbo Jack	1 burger	600	52	2	10
Junior bacon	1 burger	525	32	0	6
w/cheese	1 burger	695	55	2	11
Sourdough Jack	1 burger	715	36	2	7
sandwiches					
deli trio pannido	1 sdw	645	53	2	4
ham & turkey pannido	1 sdw	610	54	2	3
Ultimate club sandwich	1 sdw	630	52	2	6
Zesty Turkey pannido	1 sdw	740	51	2	3
■ **CHICKEN..FISH..MEXICAN ITEMS**					
chicken					
breast strips	1 order	630	39	3	1
sandwich					
Jack's spicy	1 sdw	615	62	3	7
w/cheese	1 sdw	655	63	3	7
regular	1 sdw	390	39	1	3
sourdough grilled club	1 sdw	505	35	2	4
w/cheese	1 sdw	430	40	1	3

Food and Description	Amount	Total Calories	Total Carbs	Fiber	Sugars
fish & chips	1 serving	840	69	4	1
Mexican taco					
monster	1 taco	240	18	2	2
regular	1 taco	160	15	2	4
■ DESSERTS					
cheesecake	1 piece	310	34	0	23
double fudge cake	1 slice	310	49	4	37
■ SALADS					
Asian chicken salad	1 salad	595	58	8	29
chicken club	1 salad	825	34	5	11
side salad	1 salad	155	16	0	3
Southwest chicken	1 salad	735	46	4	13
■ SIDE ORDERS					
curly fries	small	270	30	3	1
	medium	400	45	5	1
French fries	small	330	44	3	0
	medium	410	55	4	0
onion rings	1 serving	500	51	3	3
■ SNACKS					
bacon cheddar potato wedges	1 order	620	45	5	2
egg rolls	1 piece	175	26	2	7
	3 pieces	445	55	6	10
stuffed jalapeños	3 pieces	230	22	2	2
KENTUCKY FRIED CHICKEN					
■ CHICKEN					
Extra Crispy					
breast	1 piece	480	19	0	0
drumstick	1 piece	160	5	0	0
thigh	1 piece	370	12	0	0
wing/whole	1 piece	190	10	0	0
Hot & Spicy					
breast	1 piece	460	20	0	0
drumstick	1 piece	150	4	0	0
thigh	1 piece	400	14	0	0
wing/whole	1 piece	180	9	0	0
Original Recipe					
breast w/skin	1 piece	380	11	0	0
breast w/o skin or breading	1 piece	140	0	0	0
drumstick	1 piece	140	4	9	9
thigh	1 piece	360	12	9	9
wing/whole	1 piece	150	5	0	0
popcorn chicken	individual	450	25	9	9
	kid's	270	16	9	9
	large	660	36	9	9
pot pie..chunky chicken	1 pot pie	770	70	5	2
strips..crispy	3 pieces	400	17	0	0
wings					
boneless..honey BBQ	7 pieces	600	49	2	7
honey BBQ	6 pieces	540	36	1	15

Food and Description	Amount	Total Calories	Total Carbs	Fiber	Sugars
hot	8 pieces	450	23	1	1
■ **DESSERTS**					
cheesy cheesecake parfait	1 serving	300	45	2	37
Colonel's Pies					
apple	1 slice	279	45	4	22
lemon meringue	1 slice	310	47	3	36
pecan	1 slice	370	56	2	20
strawberry crème	1 slice	270	37	0	23
double chocolate chip cake	1 slice	400	31	2	27
Little Bucket Parfaits					
chocolate crème	1 serving	270	37	0	23
fudge brownie	1 serving	270	44	1	38
strawberry shortcake	1 serving	200	34	0	34
■ **SANDWICHES..chicken w/sauce**					
honey BBQ–flavored	1 sdw	300	41	4	16
original recipe	1 sdw	450	22	0	0
tender roast	1 sdw	390	24	1	0
triple crunch	1 sdw	670	42	1	3
zinger	1 sdw	650	42	1	3
■ **SIDE ORDERS**					
BBQ baked beans	1 serving	230	46	7	22
buttermilk biscuits	1 biscuit	190	23	0	1
coleslaw	1 serving	232	22	3	13
corn on the cob..5.5"	1 piece	150	26	7	10
macaroni & cheese	1 serving	130	15	1	1
mashed potatoes & gravy	1 serving	110	18	1	<1
potato salad	1 serving	180	22	1	5
potato wedges..small size	1 serving	240	30	3	0
LONG JOHN SILVER'S					
■ **DESSERTS..pie**					
chocolate cream	1 piece	310	24	1	18
pecan	1 piece	370	55	2	20
pineapple cream cheese	1 piece	290	39	1	26
■ **ENTRÉES**					
chicken..batter-dipped plank	1 piece	140	9	0	0
clams..breaded	1 order	240	22	1	5
fish					
baked cod	1 piece	120	1	0	0
batter-dipped	1 piece	230	16	0	0
shrimp					
battered	1 piece	45	3	0	0
crunchy	1 basket	340	32	2	1
giant	1 piece	80	5	0	0
■ **SALAD DRESSINGS & SALADS**					
salad dressings					
garden ranch	1 pouch	230	2	0	2
light Italian	1 pouch	20	3	0	2
Thousand Island	1 pouch	220	7	0	6
salads					
chicken club	1 salad	510	35	5	4

Food and Description	Amount	Total Calories	Total Carbs	Fiber	Sugars
shrimp & seafood	1 salad	280	22	4	6
■ SANDWICHES					
chicken	1 sdw	380	41	3	4
fish					
plain	1 sdw	440	48	3	2
ultimate	1 sdw	500	47	3	4
■ SIDE ORDERS					
cheese sticks	3 sticks	140	12	1	0
clam chowder	1 bowl	220	23	0	8
corn cobbette	1 cobbette	90	14	3	6
crumblies	1 oz	170	14	1	0
fries	regular	230	34	3	0
	large	390	56	5	1
hushpuppy	1 piece	60	9	1	1
lobster-stuffed crab cake	1 piece	170	16	1	0
rice pilaf	1 serving	180	34	3	1
slaw	1 serving	200	15	3	19

McDONALD'S

Food and Description	Amount	Total Calories	Total Carbs	Fiber	Sugars
■ BEVERAGES..shakes..triple-thick					
chocolate	12 fl oz	430	70	1	61
strawberry	12 fl oz	420	67	<1	59
vanilla	12 fl oz	430	67	0	57
■ BREAKFAST					
bagels	1 bagel	260	54	2	7
ham, egg & cheese	1 bagel	550	58	2	10
Spanish omelet	1 bagel	710	59	3	10
steak, egg & cheese	1 bagel	640	57	2	9
Big Breakfast	1 serving	700	45	3	3
biscuits	1 biscuit	240	30	1	1
bacon, egg & cheese	1 biscuit	430	31	1	3
sausage	1 biscuit	410	30	1	2
sausage & egg	1 biscuit	490	31	1	2
cinnamon roll..warm	1 roll	440	60	2	33
deluxe..warm	1 roll	510	81	4	35
Deluxe Breakfast	1 serving	1,190	130	3	40
Egg McMuffin	1 McMuffin	300	28	2	2
English muffin w/spread	1 muffin	150	27	2	2
hash browns	1 serving	140	15	2	0
hotcakes & sausage	1 serving	780	104	0	40
hotcakes w/margarine & syrup	1 serving	600	104	0	40
McGriddles					
bacon, egg & cheese	1 serving	440	43	1	16
sausage	1 serving	420	42	1	15
sausage, egg & cheese	1 serving	550	43	1	16
sausage burrito	1 burrito	290	24	2	2
Sausage McMuffin	1 McMuffin	370	28	2	2
w/egg	1 McMuffin	450	29	2	2
scrambled eggs	2 eggs	160	1	0	1
■ BURGERS					
Big Mac	1 burger	600	50	4	8

Food and Description	Amount	Total Calories	Total Carbs	Fiber	Sugars
Big N' Tasty	1 burger	540	38	3	9
w/cheese	1 burger	590	39	3	9
cheeseburger	1 burger	330	36	2	7
double	1 burger	490	38	2	8
hamburger	1 burger	280	36	2	7
Quarter Pounder	1 burger	430	38	3	9
double w/cheese	1 burger	770	39	3	10
w/cheese	1 burger	540	39	3	9
■ CHICKEN & FISH					
Chicken McNuggets & sauce					
McNuggets	4 pieces	170	10	0	0
	10 pieces	420	26	0	0
	20 pieces	840	51	0	0
sauces					
barbecue	1 pkt	45	10	0	10
honey	1 pkt	45	12	0	11
hot mustard	1 pkt	60	7	<1	6
sweet & sour	1 pkt	50	11	0	10
sandwiches					
chicken					
crispy	1 sdw	510	47	3	7
hot 'n' spicy	1 sdw	450	40	1	5
McChicken	1 sdw	430	41	–	6
McGrilled w/mayonnaise	1 sdw	400	37	3	7
Filet-O-Fish	1 sdw	410	41	1	5
■ DESSERTS					
Apple Dippers w/low-fat caramel dip	1 serving	100	22	0	15
baked apple pies	1 pie	260	34	<1	13
cookies					
chocolate chip	1 cookie	170	37	1	20
McDonaldland					
chocolate chip	1 pkg	280	37	1	20
cookies	1 pkg	230	38	1	12
oatmeal raisin	1 cookie	150	23	1	12
sugar	1 cookie	140	20	0	10
fruit 'n' yogurt parfaits					
w/granola	1 serving	160	30	<1	21
w/o granola	1 serving	130	25	0	19
ice cream					
cones					
kiddie	1 cone	45	7	0	6
vanilla..reduced-fat	1 cone	150	23	0	17
sundaes					
hot caramel	1 serving	360	61	0	47
hot fudge	1 serving	340	52	1	47
strawberry	1 serving	290	50	<1	46
McFlurry					
M&M	1 serving	630	90	1	81
Oreo	1 serving	570	82	<1	69

Food and Description	Amount	Total Calories	Total Carbs	Fiber	Sugars
■ SALADS					
bacon ranch..no chicken	1 salad	130	7	3	3
Caesar salad..no chicken	1 salad	90	7	3	3
California Cobb	1 salad	150	7	3	3
crispy chicken					
bacon ranch	1 salad	350	20	3	4
Caesar	1 salad	310	20	3	4
California Cobb	1 salad	370	20	3	4
Fiesta					
w/salsa	1 salad	390	26	5	2
w/sour cream	1 salad	420	21	4	3
w/sour cream & salsa					
14 oz	1 salad	450	28	5	3
13 oz	1 salad	360	26	5	2
grilled chicken					
bacon ranch	1 salad	250	9	3	3
Caesar	1 salad	200	9	3	3
California Cobb	1 salad	270	9	3	4
■ SIDE ORDER..French fries	small	220	28	3	0
	medium	350	44	4	0
	large	520	66	6	0
MRS. FIELDS COOKIES					
■ BREAKFAST COOKIES					
banana nut	1 cookie	340	34	2	18
blueberry	1 cookie	330	43	2	25
chocolate chip	1 cookie	320	42	2	21
mandarin orange	1 cookie	290	37	<1	19
raspberry	1 cookie	280	38	<1	20
■ BROWNIES					
cheesecake	1 brownie	520	43	<1	35
double fudge	1 brownie	360	49	2	39
frosted fudge	1 brownie	440	62	2	41
German chocolate	1 brownie	570	69	4	57
peanut butter dream bar	1 bar	670	70	3	52
pecan					
fudge	1 brownie	340	40	2	30
pie	1 brownie	140	20	<1	15
Rocky Mountain Mogul	1 brownie	610	76	4	60
walnut fudge	1 brownie	340	40	2	30
■ COOKIE CUPS					
butter toffee	1 cup	420	60	<1	39
chewy fudge	1 cup	410	61	3	46
coconut macadamia	1 cup	440	55	2	37
milk chocolate macadamia	1 cup	450	56	2	41
w/walnuts	1 cup	440	58	2	42
oatmeal raisin	1 cup	410	60	2	42
peanut butter	1 cup	430	54	1	35
pumpkin harvest	1 cup	370	47	1	32

Food and Description	Amount	Total Calories	Total Carbs	Fiber	Sugars
semisweet chocolate	1 cup	420	62	2	45
w/walnuts	1 cup	440	58	2	43
triple chocolate	1 cup	430	60	2	47
white chunk macadamia	1 cup	460	58	1	42
■ JUMBO COOKIES..snickerdoodle	1 cup	640	90	2	49
■ MISCELLANEOUS ITEMS					
carrot cake w/cream cheese icing	1 piece	420	51	1	37
cinnamon roll w/cream cheese icing	1 roll	1,070	147	2	75
cinnamon roll w/sticky bun topping	1 roll	1,100	152	4	79
cookies					
cookie monster	1 cookie	370	52	<1	38
lemon..w/cream cheese icing	1 cookie	300	44	<1	26
■ REGULAR COOKIES					
butter toffee	1 cookie	290	40	<1	24
chewy fudge	1 cookie	300	40	3	27
cinnamon sugar	1 cookie	300	41	<1	23
coconut macadamia	1 cookie	280	39	2	25
Debra's special	1 cookie	280	39	2	25
egg nog	1 cookie	300	41	<1	22
gingersnap	1 cookie	250	46	<1	29
M&M	1 cookie	330	45	<1	27
milk chocolate	1 cookie	280	38	<1	18
w/macadamia nuts	1 cookie	320	36	<1	25
w/walnuts	1 cookie	320	37	1	26
oatmeal chocolate chip	1 cookie	280	40	1	17
peanut butter	1 cookie	310	34	<1	18
w/milk chocolate chips	1 cookie	300	35	<1	16
pumpkin harvest	1 cookie	260	32	<1	18
semisweet chocolate	1 cookie	280	40	1	26
w/pecans	1 cookie	300	37	2	25
w/walnuts	1 cookie	310	38	2	25
white chunk macadamia	1 cookie	310	37	<1	25
■ SMOOTHIES					
Banana Berry Blastoff	20 fl oz	400	113	3	110
Colada Combustion	20 fl oz	420	96	3	93
Latte Cooler	20 fl oz	410	94	3	81
Pina Chill-ada	20 fl oz	420	96	3	93
Raspberry Rush	20 fl oz	400	98	6	92
Strawberry Surge	20 fl oz	400	94	3	91
PANDA EXPRESS					
■ APPETIZERS					
chicken egg roll	1 roll	190	21	3	<1
fried shrimp	6 pieces	260	26	<1	0
veggie spring roll	1 roll	80	14	<1	0
■ BEEF					
w/broccoli	1 order	150	9	1	2
w/string beans	1 order	170	11	2	0
■ CHICKEN					
black pepper	1 order	180	10	2	2
mandarin	1 order	250	8	2	2

Food and Description	Amount	Total Calories	Total Carbs	Fiber	Sugars
orange-flavored	1 order	480	50	2	5
sweet & sour	1 order	310	28	2	0
w/mushrooms	1 order	130	7	2	2
w/peanuts	1 order	200	17	4	2
w/potato	1 order	220	17	1	1
w/string beans	1 order	170	12	3	2
■ PORK					
BBQ	1 order	350	13	<1	5
sweet & sour	1 order	410	17	3	0
■ RICE & NOODLES					
steamed rice	1 order	330	74	2	0
vegetable					
chow mein	1 order	330	74	2	0
fried rice	1 order	390	61	2	0
■ SAUCES					
hot	2 tsp	10	2	0	1
hot mustard	2 tsp	18	1	0	0
mandarin	1.5 oz	70	16	0	14
sweet & sour	1.5 oz	60	15	0	13
■ TOFU..string beans w/fried tofu	1 order	180	11	3	3
PIZZA HUT					
■ APPETIZERS					
breadsticks	1 breadstick	150	20	<1	4
cheese	1 breadstick	200	21	<1	4
breadstick dipping sauce	1 serving	50	11	2	6
Buffalo wings	2 pieces	110	1	0	0
hot	2 pieces	110	<1	0	0
wing dipping sauce					
blue cheese	1.5 oz	230	2	0	2
ranch	1.5 oz	210	4	0	2
■ DESSERT					
apple dessert pizza	1 slice	260	53	1	14
cherry dessert pizza	1 slice	240	46	1	24
cinnamon sticks	2 pieces	170	27	<1	16
white icing dipping cup	2 oz	190	46	0	39
■ P'ZONE					
classic	½ order	610	71	3	9
Meat Lover's	½ order	680	70	3	8
■ PIZZA					
extra-large..16					
cheese	1 slice	420	51	3	11
chicken supreme	1 slice	400	53	4	12
ham..quartered	1 slice	380	50	3	11
Meat Lover's	1 slice	500	51	3	12
pepperoni	1 slice	430	50	3	11
Pepperoni Lover's	1 slice	520	51	3	12
Sausage Lover's	1 slice	510	51	3	11
super supreme	1 slice	490	45	3	19
supreme	1 slice	460	44	3	8

Food and Description	Amount	Total Calories	Total Carbs	Fiber	Sugars
Veggie Lover's	1 slice	390	45	3	19
Fit 'n' Delicious..12" medium					
diced chicken					
w/mushroom & jalapeño	1 slice	170	22	2	5
w/red onion & green pepper	1 slice	170	23	2	6
green pepper, red onion & tomato	1 slice	150	22	2	6
ham					
w/pineapple & diced red tomato	1 slice	160	24	2	7
w/red onion & mushrooms	1 slice	150	22	2	6
tomato, mushroom & jalapeño	1 slice	150	26	2	8
Fit 'n' Delicious..14" large					
diced chicken					
w/mushroom & jalapeño	1 slice	160	22	2	5
w/red onion & green pepper	1 slice	160	22	2	6
green pepper, red onion & jalapeño	1 slice	140	24	2	6
ham					
w/pineapple & diced red tomato	1 slice	150	22	1	7
w/red onion & mushrooms	1 slice	150	21	2	6
tomato, mushroom & jalapeño	1 slice	140	21	2	5
Hand-tossed..12" medium					
cheese	1 slice	240	30	2	5
chicken supreme	1 slice	230	30	2	6
ham..quartered	1 slice	220	29	2	5
Meat Lover's	1 slice	300	29	2	6
pepperoni	1 slice	250	29	2	6
Pepperoni Lover's	1 slice	300	30	2	6
Sausage Lover's	1 slice	280	30	2	6
super supreme	1 slice	300	31	2	6
supreme	1 slice	270	30	2	6
Veggie Lover's	1 slice	220	31	2	6
Hand-tossed..14" large					
cheese	1 slice	220	27	1	5
chicken supreme	1 slice	210	28	2	6
ham..quartered	1 slice	200	27	1	5
Meat Lover's	1 slice	280	27	2	5
pepperoni	1 slice	230	27	2	5
Pepperoni Lover's	1 slice	280	27	2	5
Sausage Lover's	1 slice	260	27	2	4
super supreme	1 slice	270	28	2	6
supreme	1 slice	250	28	2	6
Veggie Lover's	1 slice	200	28	2	8
Pan..12" medium					
cheese	1 slice	280	29	1	6
chicken supreme	1 slice	280	30	2	7
ham..quartered	1 slice	260	29	1	6
Meat Lover's	1 slice	340	29	2	5
pepperoni	1 slice	290	29	2	6
Pepperoni Lover's	1 slice	340	29	2	6
Sausage Lover's	1 slice	330	29	2	6
super supreme	1 slice	340	30	2	7

Food and Description	Amount	Total Calories	Total Carbs	Fiber	Sugars
supreme	1 slice	320	30	2	7
Veggie Lover's	1 slice	260	30	2	7
Pan..14" large					
cheese	1 slice	270	27	1	6
chicken supreme	1 slice	260	26	1	6
ham..quartered	1 slice	250	26	1	6
Meat Lover's	1 slice	320	27	2	6
pepperoni	1 slice	280	26	1	6
Pepperoni Lover's	1 slice	330	27	2	6
Sausage Lover's	1 slice	300	27	2	6
super supreme	1 slice	320	28	2	6
supreme	1 slice	300	27	2	6
Veggie Lover's	1 slice	250	28	2	6
Personal Pan..6"					
cheese	1 pizza	160	18	<1	4
chicken supreme	1 pizza	160	19	<1	4
ham..quartered	1 pizza	150	18	<1	4
Meat Lover's	1 pizza	200	18	1	4
pepperoni	1 pizza	170	18	<1	4
Pepperoni Lover's	1 pizza	200	18	1	4
Sausage Lover's	1 pizza	190	18	1	4
super supreme	1 pizza	200	19	1	4
supreme	1 pizza	190	19	1	4
Veggie Lover's	1 pizza	150	19	1	4
Stuffed Crust..14"					
cheese	1 slice	360	43	2	8
chicken supreme	1 slice	380	44	3	10
ham..quartered	1 slice	340	42	2	8
Meat Lover's	1 slice	450	43	3	9
pepperoni	1 slice	370	42	3	8
Pepperoni Lover's	1 slice	420	43	3	8
Sausage Lover's	1 slice	430	43	3	9
super supreme	1 slice	440	45	3	10
supreme	1 slice	400	44	3	9
Veggie Lover's	1 slice	360	45	3	10
Thin 'n' Crispy..12" medium					
cheese	1 slice	200	21	1	4
chicken supreme	1 slice	200	22	1	6
ham..quartered	1 slice	180	21	1	5
Meat Lover's	1 slice	270	21	2	5
pepperoni	1 slice	210	21	1	5
Pepperoni Lover's	1 slice	260	21	2	5
Sausage Lover's	1 slice	240	21	2	5
super supreme	1 slice	260	23	2	6
supreme	1 slice	240	22	2	5
Veggie Lover's	1 slice	180	23	2	5
PRETZEL TIME					
■ **DELI POCKET** turkey..no cheese or butter	1 pocket	390	59	2	6
■ **PRETZEL BITES**					

Food and Description	Amount	Total Calories	Total Carbs	Fiber	Sugars
plain	medium	280	59	2	6
Whirl & Salt	regular	310	59	2	6
■ PRETZEL DOGS	1 order	490	39	<1	10
■ PRETZELINIS					
Canadian bacon & pineapple	1 pretzelini	460	64	3	9
cheese	1 pretzelini	430	62	3	8
pepperoni	1 pretzelini	480	62	3	8
■ PRETZELS					
caramel crunch	1 pretzel	350	69	2	10
cinnamon & sugar	1 pretzel	330	65	2	9
garlic	1 pretzel	340	57	3	6
Parmesan	1 pretzel	340	66	2	7
plain	1 pretzel	280	57	2	6
regular w/butter & salt	1 pretzel	310	59	2	6
sour cream & onion	1 pretzel	340	66	2	49
■ PRETZEL STIX..regular w/butter & salt	1 order	370	72	2	16
■ TOPPINGS					
caramel	2 oz	100	22	0	22
cheddar cheese	2 oz	80	4	0	1
honey glaze	2 oz	180	45	0	43
honey mustard	2 oz	120	27	0	21
nacho cheese	2 oz	80	4	0	1
pizza sauce	2 oz	135	24	0	33
PRETZELMAKER					
■ PRETZELS					
caramel crunch	1 pretzel	390	74	2	19
cinnamon	1 pretzel	380	74	2	19
garlic	1 pretzel	380	72	2	16
original	1 pretzel	340	70	2	16
Parmesan	1 pretzel	390	72	2	16
poppyseed	1 pretzel	380	71	2	16
sesame	1 pretzel	380	71	2	16
■ SAUCES					
caramel	1.5 oz	100	22	0	22
cheddar cheese	1.5 oz	130	6	0	3
chili spice	1.5 oz	360	72	2	16
cream cheese	1.5 oz	145	3	0	3
nacho cheese	1.5 oz	105	4	0	4
pizza sauce	1.5 oz	135	24	0	33
■ WRAPZEL					
ham & Swiss	1 wrapzel	540	73	2	16
pepperoni	1 wrapzel	570	76	3	17
turkey & Swiss	1 wrapzel	580	71	2	16
SCHLOTZKY'S DELI					
■ DESSERTS					
cake..fudge brownie	1 slice	410	46	3	30
cheesecake					
cookies & cream	1 slice	330	36	1	25
New York cream-style	1 slice	310	31	0	22
strawberry swirl	1 slice	300	30	0	20

Food and Description	Amount	Total Calories	Total Carbs	Fiber	Sugars
cookies					
chocolate chip	1 cookie	160	23	9	14
cookies w/real M&M's	1 cookie	140	20	0	11
fudge chocolate chip	1 cookie	170	22	1	13
oatmeal raisin	1 cookie	150	24	1	15
peanut butter	1 cookie	170	21	1	12
sugar	1 cookie	160	23	0	11
white chocolate macadamia nut	1 cookie	170	22	0	13
cranberry walnut crunch	1 serving	160	23	1	13
golden oatmeal raisin	1 serving	160	23	1	13
triple chocolate chip	1 serving	170	21	1	11
■ DRINKS					
lemonade					
original	12 oz	150	39	0	38
raspberry	12 oz	165	45	0	42
■ PIZZAS..8" sourdough crust					
BBQ chicken	1 pizza	683	93	2	19
double cheese & pepperoni	1 pizza	721	77	4	7
kid's..cheese	1 pizza	460	72	3	5
kid's..pepperoni	1 pizza	507	72	3	5
Kung Pao chicken	1 pizza	718	92	5	16
Thai chicken	1 pizza	663	89	5	16
"The Original" combination	1 pizza	625	79	5	8
3-meat	1 pizza	805	74	3	6
Tuscan herb	1 pizza	541	80	5	9
vegetarian special	1 pizza	551	76	4	7
■ SALADS & SALAD EXTRAS					
deli salads					
albacore tuna	1 salad	218	8	3	2
California pasta	1 serving	58	10	1	8
chicken & pesto	1 salad	454	55	6	6
chicken salad	1 salad	376	13	5	5
coleslaw..home-style	1 serving	188	24	3	19
fruit..fresh	1 salad	123	30	5	23
macaroni..elbow	1 serving	275	23	2	8
potato					
choice	1 serving	288	35	4	10
mustard & egg	1 serving	250	31	4	6
leaf salads w/o salad extras					
Caesar	1 salad	30	3	2	1
chicken Caesar	1 salad	111	4	2	1
garden	1 salad	48	7	3	3
smoked turkey..chef's	1 salad	199	13	3	3
■ SANDWICHES..hot					
albacore tuna	regular	496	77	5	7
chicken breast	regular	499	80	4	8
deluxe original	regular	930	84	4	11
fiesta chicken	regular	839	79	4	10
original..ham & cheese	regular	749	82	4	11
original	regular	738	79	4	8

Food and Description	Amount	Total Calories	Total Carbs	Fiber	Sugars
pastrami & Swiss	regular	882	81	4	11
roast beef & cheese	regular	855	83	4	11
smoked turkey breast	regular	498	75	3	6
turkey & bacon club	regular	834	79	5	8
turkey..original	regular	822	81	4	8
vegetarian	regular	482	79	6	9
SANDWICHES..hot..where available					
albacore tuna melt	regular	740	83	6	8
BLT	regular	578	70	3	5
chicken club	regular	686	75	4	6
corned beef	regular	593	78	4	11
corned beef Reuben	regular	838	82	4	12
Dijon chicken	regular	496	74	6	6
pastrami Reuben	regular	944	83	4	12
pesto chicken	regular	512	73	4	5
Philly	regular	840	86	4	14
roast beef	regular	623	78	3	9
Santa Fe chicken	regular	605	81	5	9
Texas Schlotzky's	regular	776	76	3	9
turkey guacamole	regular	643	84	3	9
turkey Reuben	regular	823	80	4	7
vegetable club	regular	541	76	5	6
Western vegetarian	regular	611	76	4	6
■ **WRAPS**					
asian almond chicken	1 wrap	459	72	4	30
chicken Caesar	1 wrap	511	40	3	1
salsa chicken w/cheddar	1 wrap	460	44	3	5
zesty albacore tuna	1 wrap	311	45	3	4
SONIC					
■ **BREAKFAST**					
Breakfast Burrito	1 burrito	616	45	3	2
Sonic Sunrise	regular	224	60	1	56
	large	368	100	2	94
Sonic Toasters					
bacon, egg & cheese	1 order	500	40	2	3
ham, egg & cheese	1 order	436	41	2	4
sausage, egg & cheese	1 order	570	44	2	3
■ **BURGERS & CONEYS**					
burgers					
bacon cheeseburger	1 burger	727	44	2	7
Jr. burger	1 burger	353	27	1	7
Sonic					
burger					
No. 1	1 burger	577	43	2	7
No. 2	1 burger	481	43	2	7
cheeseburger					
No. 1	1 burger	647	44	2	7
No. 2	1 burger	551	44	2	7
SuperSonic					

Food and Description	Amount	Total Calories	Total Carbs	Fiber	Sugars
No. 1	1 burger	929	45	2	7
No. 2	1 burger	839	46	3	7
coneys					
corn dog	1 corn dog	262	22	1	5
extra-long					
cheese	1 coney	666	47	2	9
plain	1 coney	483	44	1	9
regular..cheese	1 coney	366	24	1	5
■ CHICKEN					
sandwich					
breaded	1 sdw	582	66	2	6
grilled	1 sdw	343	31	2	8
strip					
dinner	1 dinner	749	86	5	5
snack	1 snack	272	22	0	0
■ FROZEN FAVORITES					
banana split	1 banana split	467	75	3	72
floats					
Coca-Cola	regular	379	41	0	37
Dr Pepper	regular	377	41	0	36
root beer	regular	386	44	0	40
shakes					
banana cream pie	regular	775	92	2	82
chocolate	regular	564	58	0	64
chocolate cream pie	regular	795	96	1	86
coconut cream pie	regular	721	79	1	71
strawberry	regular	510	46	1	44
vanilla	regular	454	32	0	31
shakes..Sonic Blasts					
Butterfinger	regular	636	56	1	56
M&M's	regular	641	58	1	54
Oreo	regular	638	57	1	56
Reese's	regular	658	52	1	48
■ SANDWICHES..TOASTER					
bacon cheddar burger	1 sdw	675	60	4	6
BLT	1 sdw	581	42	3	4
chicken club	1 sdw	675	75	3	10
grilled cheese	1 sdw	282	39	2	2
steak..country-fried	1 sdw	708	55	3	4
■ SIDE ORDERS..FAVE..CRAVES					
Ched 'R' Peppers	1 order	256	29	4	5
French fries	regular	195	22	4	1
cheese	regular	265	23	4	1
chili cheese	regular	299	24	4	2
Super Sonic	1 order	358	44	7	2
Fritos chili pie	1 piece	611	36	3	1
mozzarella sticks	1 order	382	35	0	5
onion rings	regular	331	66	7	23
tater tots	regular	259	27	3	1

Food and Description	Amount	Total Calories	Total Carbs	Fiber	Sugars
cheese	regular	329	28	3	1
chili cheese	regular	363	28	3	2
■ WRAPS					
Fritos chili cheese wrap	1 wrap	743	68	5	3
grilled chicken strip w/ranch dressing	1 wrap	574	55	2	2
SOUPLANTATION & SWEET TOMATOES					
■ DESSERTS					
apple cobbler	½ cup	350	64	1	19
apple medley..fat-free	½ cup	70	18	1	12
banana pudding	½ cup	160	27	1	26
Blissful Blueberry Cobbler	½ cup	380	70	3	45
butterscotch					
praline cake	½ cup	220	24	<1	17
pudding..low-fat	½ cup	140	24	0	24
caramel apple cobbler	½ cup	390	65	2	50
cherry cobbler	½ cup	340	61	2	10
chocolate lava cake	1 serving	295	55	0	40
cranberry apple cobbler	½ cup	370	58	3	42
deep chocolate winter mint lava cake	1 serving	295	55	0	39
Pauline's apple walnut cake	1 serving	180	28	1	21
peach cobbler	½ cup	360	65	2	40
raspberry apple cobbler	½ cup	380	67	2	39
rice pudding..low-fat	½ cup	110	20	1	12
■ MUFFINS					
banana nut	1 muffin	150	22	1	9
black forest	1 muffin	230	36	1	19
cappuccino chip	1 muffin	160	28	1	15
Caribbean key lime	1 muffin	170	28	1	15
carrot pineapple..w/oat bran	1 muffin	150	23	2	13
cherry nut	1 muffin	150	22	1	9
chili corn..low-fat	1 muffin	140	27	2	5
chocolate brownie muffin	1 muffin	170	22	1	10
chocolate chip	1 muffin	170	22	1	10
country blackberry	1 muffin	170	27	1	13
cranberry orange bran..99% fat-free	1 muffin	80	17	1	15
French Quarter praline	1 muffin	290	38	2	21
Georgia peach poppyseed	1 muffin	150	20	1	10
lemon	1 muffin	140	24	1	13
macadamia nut spice	1 muffin	220	33	1	18
mango tropics	1 muffin	180	28	1	17
maple walnut	1 muffin	230	33	1	21
nutty peanut butter	1 muffin	170	21	1	9
pumpkin raisin	1 muffin	150	25	1	14
strawberry buttermilk	1 muffin	140	21	1	8
sweet orange & cranberry	1 muffin	200	33	1	20
taffy apple	1 muffin	160	25	1	18
tropical papaya coconut	1 muffin	180	28	1	18
Wildly Blue Blueberry	1 large	310	46	2	20
zucchini nut	1 muffin	150	22	1	9

Food and Description	Amount	Total Calories	Total Carbs	Fiber	Sugars
■ **SOUPS & CHILI**					
chili					
Arizona Red	1 cup	220	25	7	3
Cheatin' Heart	1 cup	300	23	6	6
Deep Kettle House					
More Meat!..33%	1 cup	250	26	7	7
More Meat!..50%	1 cup	290	29	6	5
house/low-fat	1 cup	230	26	7	4
longhorn beef	1 cup	190	25	4	5
Rock n' Mole	1 cup	240	22	5	6
Santa Fe black bean..low-fat	1 cup	190	26	8	2
Texas Red	1 cup	240	30	7	4
3-bean turkey..low-fat high-fiber	1 cup	170	24	7	6
vegetarian	1 cup	150	25	6	6
white bean & chicken	1 cup	220	28	7	5
soups					
albino bean chicken cuisine	1 cup	190	18	4	3
Albondigas Locas..a meat-ball soup	1 cup	210	19	2	4
autumn root vegetable w/wild rice	1 cup	80	18	2	3
baked potato & cheese	1 cup	290	22	2	6
Be Wild w/mushroom	1 cup	220	14	2	5
beef & barley stew	1 cup	240	19	3	5
Better Than Mom's beef stew	1 cup	270	19	2	3
big chunk chicken noodle..low-fat	1 cup	160	17	2	3
black bean sausage fling	1 cup	350	21	5	3
Bombay lentil..low-fat..vegetarian	1 cup	160	25	9	5
border black bean & chorizo	1 cup	230	27	6	6
brocon	1 cup	220	13	2	4
broccoli cheese	1 cup	280	15	2	7
butternut squash..vegetarian	1 cup	140	15	4	4
Canadian cheese w/ham	1 cup	370	20	1	9
cheese-stuffed cappelletti	1 cup	130	20	1	8
Chesapeake corn chowder	1 cup	280	30	2	8
chicken					
fajitas & black beans	1 cup	280	33	7	4
Get Smoked	1 cup	350	28	2	6
pot-pie stew	1 cup	310	21	2	7
tortilla..low-fat	1 cup	100	5	1	2
classical					
French onion	1 cup	130	16	2	12
minestrone..low-fat..vegetarian	1 cup	120	20	3	4
shrimp bisque	1 cup	240	15	1	5
country corn & red potato chowder	1 cup	160	24	4	6
cream of					
broccoli	1 cup	210	14	7	3
chicken	1 cup	250	21	2	3
mushroom	1 cup	290	15	2	3
rosemary potato	1 cup	270	22	2	4
creamy vegetable chowder	1 cup	200	23	3	6
Devotion to the Ocean	1 cup	220	14	2	7
Do the Stew!	1 cup	280	25	2	8
8-vegetable chicken stew	1 cup	190	17	2	5

Food and Description	Amount	Total Calories	Total Carbs	Fiber	Sugars
El Paso lime & chicken	1 cup	160	24	2	5
Field of Creams..cauliflower..w/cheese	1 cup	260	15	1	3
Field of Creams..celery vegetarian	1 cup	210	15	2	2
Field of Creams..spinach vegetarian	1 cup	280	18	2	3
Field of Creams..tomato basil	1 cup	220	20	2	4
Fire-roasted green chile corn chowder	1 cup	230	21	1	7
garden-fresh vegetable..low-fat	1 cup	110	22	4	4
garlic-kickin' roasted chicken	1 cup	140	10	3	4
green chile stew	1 cup	150	14	3	2
herbed turkey w/cranberries	1 cup	290	17	1	5
Hungarian vegetable..low-fat	1 cup	120	20	2	5
Living on the Veg	1 cup	90	15	3	3
Lonely for Minestrone	1 cup	150	18	4	5
Make Room for Mushroom	1 cup	240	15	1	4
Manhattan clam chowder	1 cup	130	16	2	4
Marvelous Minestrone	1 cup	210	31	5	7
minestrone w/Italian sausage	1 cup	210	14	5	3
Mulligatawny	1 cup	210	18	2	5
navy bean w/ham	1 cup	340	30	6	3
Neighbor Joe's Gumbo	1 cup	280	36	3	5
New Mexican corn tortilla w/chicken	1 cup	200	20	2	3
New Orleans–style jambalaya	1 cup	210	18	3	7
Not Skimpy on the Shrimpy	1 cup	290	18	2	5
old-fashioned vegetable..low-fat	1 cup	100	18	5	5
posole	1 cup	150	8	2	1
potato					
chunky potato cheese..w/thyme	1 cup	210	19	2	3
Irish leek	1 cup	250	23	1	7
Sprung a Leek	1 cup	190	22	1	4
ratatouille Provençale..fat-free	1 cup	110	25	2	3
roasted mushroom	1 cup	320	20	1	7
rustic Tuscan stew..low-fat	1 cup	140	25	4	3
savory turkey harvest	1 cup	210	18	2	7
Southwest					
tomato cream	1 cup	120	14	2	5
turkey chowder w/bacon	1 cup	240	21	2	3
spicy 4-bean minestrone..low-fat	1 cup	140	23	6	4
spicy sausage & pasta	1 cup	310	36	5	8
split pea w/ham	1 cup	350	32	6	3
stuffed herbed turkey w/cranberries	1 cup	310	17	1	4
sweet tomato onion..low-fat	1 cup	90	11	2	5
tomato chipotle bisque	1 cup	240	30	7	4
tomato Parmesan vegetable..low-fat	1 cup	120	18	3	3
Toot Your Horn for Crab & Corn	1 cup	290	18	2	8
U.S. Senate bean w/smoked ham	1 cup	150	20	3	4
vegetable beef stew..low-fat	1 cup	250	21	7	4
vegetarian harvest	1 cup	190	23	4	5
vegetarian lentils & brown rice..low-fat	1 cup	130	25	6	2
Veggie Jackson	1 cup	100	18	5	5
Very Nice chicken & rice	1 cup	160	15	2	5

Food and Description	Amount	Total Calories	Total Carbs	Fiber	Sugars
Yankee clipper clam chowder	1 cup	330	21	2	3

STARBUCKS (See also ICE CREAM & FROZEN DESSERTS)

■ **CLASSIC & SEASONAL FAVORITES**

Food and Description	Amount	Total Calories	Total Carbs	Fiber	Sugars
apple cider					
caramel	16 fl oz	300	72	0	64
steamed	16 fl oz	270	57	0	52
eggnog	16 fl oz	410	41	0	38
hot chocolate					
regular	16 fl oz	340	42	2	35
white	16 fl oz	480	63	0	62
milk					
chocolate	16 fl oz	340	42	2	35
steamed	16 fl oz	270	21	0	21
pumpkin spice					
crème	16 fl oz	400	52	0	52
Frappuccino blended coffee					
light	16 fl oz	190	37	3	29
regular	16 fl oz	300	61	0	53
latte	16 fl oz	380	52	0	49

■ **ESPRESSO..HOT**

Food and Description	Amount	Total Calories	Total Carbs	Fiber	Sugars
caffe latte	16 fl oz	260	21	0	19
caffe misto/café au lait	16 fl oz	140	11	0	11
caffe mocha					
w/whipped cream	16 fl oz	400	42	2	33
w/o whipped cream	16 fl oz	300	41	2	31
cappuccino	16 fl oz	150	13	0	11
caramel macchiato	16 fl oz	310	37	0	34
cinnamon spice mocha	16 fl oz	330	45	<1	45
syrup-flavored latte	16 fl oz	320	39	0	36
vanilla latte	16 fl oz	320	39	0	36
white chocolate mocha	16 fl oz	410	56	0	53

■ **ESPRESSO..ICED**

Food and Description	Amount	Total Calories	Total Carbs	Fiber	Sugars
caffe latte	16 fl oz	160	13	0	11
caffe mocha	16 fl oz	220	35	2	25
caramel macchiato	16 fl oz	270	34	0	31
caramel mocha	16 fl oz	290	54	2	42
syrup-flavored latte	16 fl oz	210	31	0	28
vanilla latte	16 fl oz	210	31	0	28
white chocolate mocha	16 fl oz	360	56	0	52

■ **FRAPPUCCINO BLENDED COFFEE**..light & regular blends w/o whipped cream

Food and Description	Amount	Total Calories	Total Carbs	Fiber	Sugars
caffe vanilla					
light	16 fl oz	230	49	4	38
regular..original	16 fl oz	340	72	0	63
caramel					
light	16 fl oz	180	36	3	26
regular	16 fl oz	280	57	0	48
coffee					
light	16 fl oz	150	30	3	20
regular	16 fl oz	260	52	0	44
espresso					

Food and Description	Amount	Total Calories	Total Carbs	Fiber	Sugars
light	16 fl oz	140	27	3	18
regular	16 fl oz	230	46	0	38
java chip					
light	16 fl oz	260	46	5	32
regular	16 fl oz	370	69	2	56
mocha					
light	16 fl oz	180	36	4	25
regular	16 fl oz	290	58	0	48
white chocolate mocha					
light	16 fl oz	200	40	3	30
regular	16 fl oz	320	62	0	54
■ **FRAPPUCCINO BLENDED CRÈME**					
double chocolate chip	16 fl oz	460	79	3	64
strawberries & crème	16 fl oz	450	90	<1	83
Tazo chai crème Frappuccino blended tea	16 fl oz	380	72	0	63
■ **TAZO TEA**					
tazo chai iced tea latte	16 fl oz	270	48	0	45
■ **FRESH FOOD ITEMS**					
almond-filled croissant	1 croissant	330	39	2	16
apple Danish..w/mocha swirls	1 Danish	370	44	2	18
apple harvest torte	1 piece	350	53	4	34
apple walnut coffee cake	1 piece	320	41	1	28
apricot currant scone	1 scone	450	67	3	17
bagel..plain	1 bagel	430	92	3	5
banana pound cake	1 piece	360	47	1	24
banana pullman	1 pullman	400	57	2	31
black & white cookie	1 cookie	430	68	2	53
blueberry muffin	1 muffin	380	49	1	28
blueberry scone	1 scone	460	68	3	24
blueberry walnut coffee cake	1 piece	340	43	1	30
butter croissant w/apricot glaze	1 croissant	320	36	1	13
butterscotch pecan scone	1 scone	520	64	2	22
caramel apple bar	1 bar	310	38	2	21
caramel brownie	1 brownie	580	60	2	44
caramel pecan sticky roll	1 roll	730	75	7	39
carrot cake bar	1 bar	420	46	<1	35
cheese Danish w/mocha swirls	1 Danish	460	44	1	18
chocolate big baby bundt cake	1 piece	330	45	4	29
chocolate cream cheese muffin	1 muffin	450	53	1	31
chocolate-filled croissant	1 croissant	350	43	2	21
chocolate hazelnut biscotti	1 biscuit	110	15	1	8
chocolate pullman	1 pullman	380	54	2	33
cinnamon chip scone w/icing	1 scone	510	71	2	29
cinnamon-flavored twist	1 twist	320	37	1	13
cinnamon raisin bagel	1 bagel	440	96	3	14
cinnamon roll	1 roll	620	80	3	41
cinnamon walnut coffee cake	1 piece	360	46	1	31
classic coffee cake	1 piece	570	75	2	45
cranberry bliss bar	1 bar	320	38	<1	26

Food and Description	Amount	Total Calories	Total Carbs	Fiber	Sugars
cranberry orange muffin	1 muffin	410	53	2	31
cranberry walnut pound cake	1 piece	390	45	1	26
cranberry walnut pullman	1 pullman	360	53	2	28
crisp cinnamon twist	1 twist	60	9	0	4
crumb cake	1 piece	670	89	1	44
crumble berry coffee cake	1 piece	520	69	2	40
dark chocolate graham	1 graham	140	17	<1	12
double chocolate chunk cookie	1 cookie	430	58	3	37
enrobed espresso brownie	1 brownie	430	48	3	32
espresso brownie	1 brownie	370	43	2	30
hazelnut coffee cake	1 piece	630	74	2	43
holiday gingerbread	1 piece	480	81	1	56
home-style oatmeal raisin cookie	1 cookie	390	65	3	34
iced carrot pound cake	1 piece	540	101	3	64
iced lemon pound cake	1 piece	500	69	<1	46
key lime crumb cake	1 piece	550	71	1	44
lemon bar	1 bar	310	44	0	32
lemon glazed pullman	1 pullman	370	55	<1	31
lemon yogurt bundt cake	1 piece	350	56	<1	34
madeleine	1 madeleine	80	11	0	6
maple oat scone w/icing	1 scone	490	69	2	28
marble chocolate chip pullman	1 pullman	440	61	1	37
marble pound cake	1 piece	400	49	<1	29
milk chocolate graham	1 graham	140	17	<1	12
milk chocolate peanut butter brownie	1 brownie	460	45	2	34
morning sunrise muffin	1 muffin	330	54	2	32
oatmeal cranberry mountain	1 serving	430	49	3	22
orange poppy cheese pullman	1 pullman	450	55	1	34
orange poppy pound cake	1 piece	490	55	2	32
Oreo Dream bar	1 bar	420	33	2	22
pecan diamond	1 diamond	490	38	2	24
peppermint brownie	1 brownie	440	48	2	36
pumpkin pound cake	1 piece	310	47	2	27
pumpkin pullman	1 pullman	370	51	2	22
raspberry and cream cheese–filled croissant	1 croissant	260	34	1	11
raspberry Danish w/mocha swirls	1 Danish	370	45	1	17
raspberry sammy	1 sammy	300	41	1	18
raspberry scone	1 scone	440	65	2	20
sesame bagel	1 bagel	440	92	6	5
shortbread	1 piece	100	12	0	4
sour cream coffee cake	1 piece	420	43	1	29
toffee cream cheese chew	1 chew	440	38	2	26
toffee crunch bar	1 bar	430	56	1	37
vanilla almond biscotti	1 biscotti	110	15	1	8
white chocolate macadamia nut cookie	1 cookie	470	54	2	34
zucchini pound cake	1 piece	370	47	2	27

SUBWAY

Food and Description	Amount	Total Calories	Total Carbs	Fiber	Sugars
Atkins Friendly Salads					
classic club w/ranch dressing	1 salad	590	14	5	5
grilled chicken & baby spinach w/Atkins Sweet as Honey Mustard dressing	1 salad	620	11	5	2
Atkins Friendly Wraps					
chicken bacon ranch	1 wrap	440	17	9	1
turkey bacon melt	1 wrap	430	20	9	3
turkey breast & ham	1 wrap	390	19	9	3
■ **BREADS..6" long**					
hearty Italian	2.78 oz	210	41	3	5
herb & cheese	3.4 oz	240	40	3	5
honey oat	3 oz	250	48	4	9
Italian white bread	2.5 oz	200	38	3	5
Monterey cheddar	3 oz	240	39	3	5
Parmesan oregano	2.8 oz	210	40	3	4
■ **COOKIES**					
Atkins Friendly double chocolate	1 cookie	100	37	1	25
chocolate chip	1 cookie	210	30	1	18
chocolate chunk	1 cookie	220	30	1	17
double chocolate chip	1 cookie	210	30	1	20
M&M	1 cookie	210	30	1	17
oatmeal raisin	1 cookie	200	30	2	16
peanut butter	1 cookie	220	26	1	16
sugar	1 cookie	230	28	0	14
white chocolate macadamia nut	1 cookie	220	28	1	17
■ **FRENCH TOAST & OMELETS**					
French toast w/syrup	1 serving	350	57	2	33
omelets					
bacon & egg	1 omelet	240	2	0	0
cheese & egg	1 omelet	240	2	0	0
ham & egg	1 omelet	230	2	0	1
vegetable & egg	1 omelet	210	4	1	1
Western & egg	1 omelet	220	4	1	0
■ **SALAD DRESSINGS & SALADS**					
salad dressings					
Atkins Sweet as Honey Mustard	1 pkt	200	1	0	0
Greek vinaigrette	1 pkt	200	3	0	2
Italian..fat-free	1 pkt	35	7	0	4
ranch	1 pkt	200	2	0.5	0
red wine vinaigrette	1 pkt	80	17	0	7
salads					
classic club	1 salad	390	13	4	5
garden fresh	1 salad	60	14	5	6
grilled chicken & baby spinach	1 salad	420	10	5	2
Mediterranean chicken	1 salad	170	11	5	5
■ **SANDWICHES & SUBS**					
6" 6 grams of fat or less sandwiches					
chicken					
oven-roasted breast	1 sdw	330	47	5	9

Food and Description	Amount	Total Calories	Total Carbs	Fiber	Sugars
teriyaki..sweet onion	1 sdw	370	58	4	18
ham	1 sdw	290	46	4	8
honey mustard ham	1 sdw	310	54	5	14
roast beef	1 sdw	290	45	4	7
turkey breast					
w/ham & roast beef	1 sdw	320	47	4	8
savory	1 sdw	280	46	4	7
savory & ham	1 sdw	290	47	4	8
Veggie Delight	1 sdw	230	44	4	7
6" cold sandwiches					
Classic Italian BMT	1 sdw	450	47	4	8
cold cut combo	1 sdw	410	46	4	7
Seafood Sensation	1 sdw	450	51	5	8
tuna	1 sdw	530	44	4	7
6" double meat (DM) sandwich					
cheese steak	1 sdw	450	50	6	11
chicken	1 sdw	430	50	5	11
chicken..sweet onion teriyaki	1 sdw	450	59	4	18
cold cut combo	1 sdw	550	48	4	8
ham	1 sdw	350	49	4	9
Italian BMT	1 sdw	630	49	4	10
meatball marinara	1 sdw	740	61	5	10
roast beef	1 sdw	360	46	4	9
Seafood Sensation	1 sdw	490	60	5	10
Southwest chipotle cheese steak	1 sdw	530	52	6	11
tuna..classic	1 sdw	610	35	3	3
turkey					
breast	1 sdw	330	48	4	8
breast & ham	1 sdw	360	48	4	9
breast..ham & bacon melt	1 sdw	490	51	4	9
breast..ham & roast beef	1 sdw	410	49	4	10
6" hot sandwiches					
cheese steak	1 sdw	360	47	5	9
chipotle Southwest cheese steak	1 sdw	440	49	5	10
Dijon turkey, ham & bacon melt	1 sdw	470	48	5	8
meatball marinara	1 sdw	500	52	5	9
turkey breast, ham & bacon melt	1 sdw	380	46	4	7
breakfast sandwiches					
6" Italian or wheat bread					
bacon & egg	1 sdw	450	42	3	5
cheese & egg	1 sdw	440	42	3	5
ham & egg	1 sdw	430	42	3	5
steak & egg	1 sdw	460	43	4	6
vegetable & egg	1 sdw	410	44	4	5
Western & egg	1 sdw	430	44	4	6
deli round					
bacon & egg	1 sdw	320	34	3	3
cheese & egg	1 sdw	320	34	3	3
ham & egg	1 sdw	310	34	3	4
steak & egg	1 sdw	330	35	3	4

Food and Description	Amount	Total Calories	Total Carbs	Fiber	Sugars
vegetable & egg	1 sdw	290	36	3	4
Western & egg	1 sdw	300	36	3	4
deli-style sandwiches					
ham	1 sdw	210	36	3	4
roast beef	1 sdw	220	35	3	4
tuna..classic	1 sdw	350	35	3	3
turkey breast..savory	1 sdw	210	36	3	4
■ **SOUPS**					
broccoli					
& cheese..golden	1 cup	180	16	2	3
cream of	1 cup	130	15	2	0
cheese w/ham & bacon	1 cup	240	17	1	5
chicken					
& dumpling	1 cup	130	16	1	2
& rice..Spanish-style	1 cup	90	13	1	1
roasted noodle	1 cup	60	7	1	1
w/brown & wild rice	1 cup	190	17	2	3
chili con carne	1 cup	240	23	8	14
minestrone	1 cup	90	7	1	1
New England clam chowder	1 cup	110	16	1	1
potato..cream of..w/bacon	1 cup	200	21	2	3
tomato garden vegetable w/rotini	1 cup	100	20	2	7
vegetable beef	1 cup	90	15	3	3
■ **WRAPS**					
chicken & bacon ranch	1 wrap	440	17	9	1
Mediterranean chicken	1 wrap	350	17	9	2
turkey					
bacon melt	1 wrap	430	20	9	3
breast & ham	1 wrap	390	19	9	3
TACO BELL					
■ **BREAKFAST**					
burrito	1 burrito	510	48	6	4
gordita	1 gordita	380	28	2	6
quesadilla	1 quesadilla	400	38	3	3
steak					
burrito	1 burrito	500	40	3	4
quesadilla w/green sauce	1 quesadilla	480	39	3	4
■ **BURRITOS**					
7-layer	1 burrito	530	67	10	6
bean	1 burrito	370	55	8	4
Burrito Supreme					
beef	1 burrito	440	51	7	6
chicken	1 burrito	410	50	5	5
steak	1 burrito	420	50	6	5
chili cheese	1 burrito	390	40	3	3
Fiesta Burrito					
beef	1 burrito	390	50	5	4
chicken	1 burrito	370	48	3	4
steak	1 burrito	370	48	4	4
Grilled Stuft					

Food and Description	Amount	Total Calories	Total Carbs	Fiber	Sugars
beef	1 burrito	730	79	10	7
chicken	1 burrito	680	76	8	6
steak	1 burrito	680	76	7	6
■ CHALUPAS					
Baja					
beef	1 chalupa	430	32	3	4
chicken	1 chalupa	400	30	1	4
steak	1 chalupa	400	30	2	4
Nacho Cheese					
beef	1 chalupa	380	33	2	5
chicken	1 chalupa	350	31	1	4
steak	1 chalupa	350	31	2	4
Supreme					
beef	1 chalupa	390	31	3	5
chicken	1 chalupa	370	30	1	4
steak	1 chalupa	370	29	2	4
■ GORDITAS					
Baja					
beef	1 gordita	350	31	4	7
chicken	1 gordita	320	29	2	7
steak	1 gordita	320	29	2	7
Nacho Cheese					
beef	1 gordita	300	32	3	7
chicken	1 gordita	270	30	2	7
steak	1 gordita	270	30	2	7
Supreme					
beef	1 gordita	310	30	3	7
chicken	1 gordita	290	28	2	7
steak	1 gordita	290	28	2	7
■ NACHOS & SIDES					
cinnamon twists	1 twist	160	28	0	13
Mexican rice	1 serving	210	23	3	<1
nachos	1 serving	320	33	2	3
BellGrande	1 serving	780	80	12	6
Supreme	1 serving	450	42	7	4
pintos 'n' cheese	1 serving	180	20	6	1
■ SAUCES & CONDIMENTS					
guacamole	1 oz	50	3	1	<1
nacho cheese sauce	1 oz	50	3	0	1
pepper jack cheese sauce	1 oz	50	2	0	1
3-cheese blend	1 oz	50	1	0	0
zesty dressing	1 oz	50	3	0	<1
■ SPECIALTY ITEMS					
enchirito					
beef	1 enchirito	380	35	6	3
chicken	1 enchirito	350	33	5	3
steak	1 enchirito	360	33	5	3
express taco salad w/chips	1 salad	620	69	13	9
Mexican pizza	1 pizza	550	46	7	3
MexiMelt	1 serving	290	23	3	3

Food and Description	Amount	Total Calories	Total Carbs	Fiber	Sugars
quesadilla					
cheese	1 quesadilla	490	39	3	4
extreme	1 quesadilla	470	41	2	4
chicken	1 quesadilla	540	40	3	4
steak	1 quesadilla	540	40	3	4
Southwest steak bowl	1 bowl	700	73	13	4
taco salad w/salsa	1 salad	790	73	13	10
w/salsa..w/o shell	1 salad	420	33	11	9
tostada	1 tostada	250	29	7	2
Zesty Border Bowl..chicken w/dressing	1 bowl	730	65	12	5
w/o dressing	1 bowl	500	60	12	4
■ TACOS					
Double Decker	1 taco	340	39	6	3
Taco Supreme	1 taco	380	40	6	4
plain..original	1 taco	170	13	3	1
soft					
beef	1 taco	210	21	2	2
chicken	1 taco	190	19	<1	2
grilled steak	1 taco	280	21	1	3
Supreme	1 taco	220	14	3	2
soft					
beef	1 taco	260	22	3	3
chicken	1 taco	230	21	1	3
WENDY'S					
■ BURGERS					
Big Bacon Classic on kaiser roll	1 burger	580	45	3	11
cheeseburger					
bacon..junior	1 burger	380	34	2	6
deluxe..junior	1 burger	350	36	2	6
junior..plain	1 burger	310	34	2	7
kid's meal	1 burger	310	33	1	7
hamburger					
junior	1 burger	270	34	2	7
kid's meal	1 burger	270	33	1	6
single..classic..w/everything	1 burger	410	37	2	8
hamburger..patty only					
junior..2 oz	1 oz patty	100	0	0	0
¼ lb	1 patty	200	0	0	0
■ CHICKEN					
chicken nuggets & sauce					
chicken	5 pieces	220	13	0	0
kid's meal	4 pieces	180	10	0	0
sauce					
barbecue	1 pkt	40	10	0	5
honey mustard	1 pkt	130	6	0	5
sweet & sour	1 pkt	45	12	0	7
chicken strip sauce					
deli honey mustard	1 pkt	170	6	0	4
heartland ranch	1 pkt	200	1	0	1
spicy Southwest chipotle	1 pkt	140	5	0	1

Food and Description	Amount	Total Calories	Total Carbs	Fiber	Sugars
chicken strips..home-style	3 pieces	410	33	0	0
'Chicken Temptations' Sandwiches					
home-style chicken fillet	1 sdw	540	57	2	8
spicy chicken fillet	1 sdw	510	57	2	8
ultimate chicken grill	1 sdw	360	44	2	11
■ CHILI					
small	1 serving	200	21	5	5
large	1 serving	300	31	7	7
■ DESSERT					
Frosty..dairy	6 oz	160	28	0	21
	12 oz	330	56	0	42
	16 oz	430	74	0	55
■ FRENCH FRIES					
Biggie	1 order	440	63	7	0
Great Biggie	1 order	530	75	8	1
kid's meal	1 order	250	36	4	0
medium	1 order	390	56	6	0
■ POTATOES..baked	1 potato	270	61	7	3
w/bacon & cheese	1 potato	560	67	7	6
w/broccoli & cheese	1 potato	440	70	9	6
w/sour cream & chives	1 potato	340	62	7	3
■ SALADS & SALAD DRESSINGS					
fresh salads					
chicken BLT	1 salad	360	10	4	4
home-style chicken strips	1 salad	450	34	5	6
mandarin chicken	1 salad	190	16	3	11
spring mix	1 salad	180	12	5	5
taco supreme	1 salad	360	29	8	8
side salads					
Caesar	1 salad	70	2	1	1
traditional	1 salad	35	7	3	4
salad dressings					
Caesar	1 pkt	150	1	0	0
creamy ranch..reduced-fat	1 pkt	100	6	1	3
French..fat-free	1 pkt	80	19	0	16
honey mustard..low-fat	1 pkt	110	21	0	16
WHATABURGER					
■ BEVERAGES					
shakes					
chocolate	small	616	100	0	na
	medium	904	145	0	na
	large	1,216	196	0	na
strawberry	small	620	191	9	na
	medium	909	146	0	na
	large	1,159	181	0	na
vanilla	small	559	82	0	na
	medium	834	122	0	na
	large	1,118	163	0	na
■ BREAKFAST					
biscuit					

Food and Description	Amount	Total Calories	Total Carbs	Fiber	Sugars
plain..buttermilk	1 biscuit	300	34	0	na
w/bacon	1 biscuit	375	34	0	na
w/bacon, egg & cheese	1 biscuit	475	35	0	na
w/egg & cheese	1 biscuit	445	35	0	na
w/egg, cheese & sausage	1 biscuit	662	35	1	na
w/gravy & sausage	1 biscuit	490	47	0	na
w/sausage	1 biscuit	517	34	1	na
Breakfast Platter					
w/bacon	1 platter	697	52	3	na
w/sausage	1 platter	839	52	4	na
Breakfast-On-A-Bun					
w/bacon	1 serving	398	28	2	na
w/sausage	1 serving	539	28	2	na
Breakfast-On-A-Bun..Ranchero					
w/bacon	1 serving	403	29	3	na
w/sausage	1 serving	545	29	3	na
cinnamon roll	1 roll	860	126	4	na
egg sandwich	1 sdw	322	28	1	na
hash brown sticks	1 order	140	16	3	0
Mexican breakfast					
taquito					
bacon & egg	1 taquito	387	25	1	na
bacon, egg & cheese	1 taquito	432	25	1	na
potato & egg	1 taquito	382	33	4	na
potato, egg & cheese	1 taquito	427	33	4	na
sausage & egg	1 taquito	390	26	1	na
sausage, egg & cheese	1 taquito	434	26	1	na
pancakes	1 order	614	118	3	na
w/bacon	1 serving	689	118	3	na
w/sausage	1 serving	831	118	5	na
Texas toast	1 slice	328	42	2	na
■ **BURGERS**					
Justaburger	1 burger	309	28	1	na
Whataburger					
double meat	1 burger	857	53	3.5	na
junior	1 burger	315	29	2	na
regular	1 burger	607	53	3	na
special request					
no bun	1 burger	270	4	1	na
small bun..no bun oil	1 burger	428	31	2	na
triple meat	1 burger	1,108	53	4	na
w/bacon & cheese	1 burger	810	54	3	na
special request..no bun	1 burger	473	5	1	na
w/cheese special request..no bun	1 burger	360	4	1	na
■ **CHICKEN & FISH**					
chicken strips	2 pieces	382	22	4	na
	3 pieces	574	33	6	na
	4 pieces	765	44	8	na
grilled chicken fajita taco	1 taco	363	35	2.5	na
grilled chicken sandwich..regular	1 sdw	473	49	4	na

Food and Description	Amount	Total Calories	Total Carbs	Fiber	Sugars
Whatacatch sandwich	1 sdw	472	53	3	na
Whatachick'n sandwich	1 sdw	523	63	5	na
■ SALADS & SALAD DRESSINGS					
garden	1 salad	49	10	4	na
w/cheddar cheese	1 salad	218	10	4	na
w/cheddar cheese & bacon	1 salad	293	11	4	na
grilled chicken	1 salad	229	19	5	na
w/cheddar cheese	1 salad	398	19	4	na
w/cheddar cheese & bacon	1 salad	473	19	5	na
salad dressings					
ranch..					
low-fat	1 pkt	66	9	2	na
regular	1 pkt	310	3	0	na
Thousand Island	1 pkt	150	11	0	na
vinaigrette..low-fat	1 pkt	35	6	0	na
■ SIDE ORDERS					
French fries	medium	386	20	4	na
	large	514	66	5	na
onion rings	medium	200	23	1	na
■ SWEETS..cookies					
chocolate chunk	1 cookie	210	33	2	na
oatmeal raisin	1 cookie	185	36	2	na
peanut butter	1 cookie	215	29	1	na
white chocolate macadamia nut	1 cookie	230	30	1	na
WHITE CASTLE					
■ BEVERAGES..shakes					
chocolate	14 oz	220	32	0	28
vanilla	14 oz	230	35	0	28
■ BREAKFAST..breakfast sandwich	1 sdw	340	17	0	2
■ BURGERS					
cheeseburger					
bacon	1 burger	200	12	3	0
double	1 burger	285	16	5	0
single	1 burger	160	11	2	0
hamburger					
double	1 burger	235	16	2	0
single	1 burger	135	11	2	0
■ CHICKEN & FISH					
chicken					
rings	1 order	310	14	0	0
sandwich	1 sdw	190	21	0	1
fish sandwich w/o tartar sauce	1 sdw	160	18	0	1
■ SIDE ORDERS					
cheese sticks	1 order	290	19	0	0
chicken rings	1 order	310	14	0	0
chili	1 bowl	375	45	0	0
French fries	1 order	115	15	2	2
onion rings	1 order	540	69	0	0

Personal Food Diary

Date	Food	Amount	Total Calories	Total Carbs	Fiber	Sugars

Personal Food Diary

Date	Food	Amount	Total Calories	Total Carbs	Fiber	Sugars

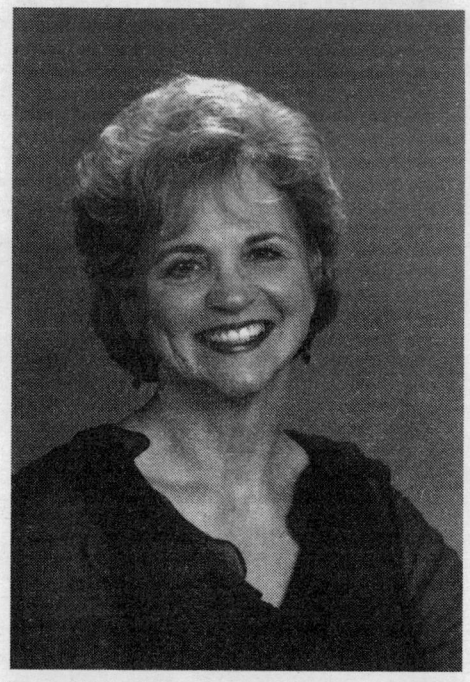

Karen J. Bellerson is the author of *The Shopper's Guide to Fat in Your Food; Low-Fat, No-Fat Cookbook*; and *The Complete & Up-to-Date Fat Book*. She has been a nutritional consultant for more than twenty years and makes her home in the Southwest.